Illustrated
Medical
Biochemistry

Illustrated
Medical
Biochemistry

SM Raju
BSc MBBS MD (Biochemistry)
Professor and Head
Department of Biochemistry
Sri Siddartha Medical College, Tumkur

Bindu Madala
MD
The Hospitalist, Group of El Paso
Texas, USA

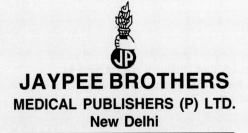

JAYPEE BROTHERS
MEDICAL PUBLISHERS (P) LTD.
New Delhi

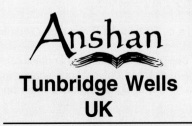

Tunbridge Wells
UK

First published in the UK by

Anshan Ltd
in 2005
6 Newlands Road
Tunbridge Wells
Kent TN4 9AT, UK

Tel/Fax: +44 (0)1892 557767
E-mail: info@anshan.co.uk
www.anshan.co.uk

ISBN 1 904798 322

British Library Cataloguing in Publication Data
A catalogue record for this book is available from the British Library

Printed in India by Brijbasi Art Press Ltd., Okhla Indl. Area, New Delhi

Dedicated to
Dr TN Pattabiraman
Our teacher, philosopher and guide

Preface

This book is intended primarily for medical and dental students. However, it also meets the needs of students of life sciences who study biochemistry as a separate subject, both at undergraduate and postgraduate levels.

In this book an effort has been made to illustrate concepts of biochemistry using multicolored sketch diagrams.

A new chapter has been included on *Molecular Tools in Medicine* to give a glimpse of advances made in biochemistry that have direct application in modern day medicine.

All efforts have been made to make this book as comprehensive as possible. There is always scope for improvement. Constructive suggestions are welcome from all quarters that will enable us to make the book more useful in the subsequent editions.

SM Raju
Bindu Madala

Acknowledgements

At the outset, we must express our sincere thanks to Dr CS Ramadoss for having gone through the manuscript and made valuable suggestions.

We thank Mr Sunil R for the computer diagrams made for this book, and the assistance provided by him in preparing the manuscript in a readable form. He taught us use computers to a nicety.

It is always a pleasant experience to work with Mr Jitendar P Vij, Chairman and Managing Director of M/s Jaypee Brothers Medical Publishers (P) Ltd. Indeed we thank every member of the publishing house, not the least Mr Tarun Duneja, General Manager (Publishing), Mr RN Mandal, Regional Manager and Mr Venu, Assistant Branch Manager for the sustained efforts in publishing this book.

Contents

Unit-I
General Biochemistry

Unit-II
Metabolism and Biochemical Genetics

UNIT-I
General Biochemistry

Cell Structure and Function

1

CELL THEORY

1. All living creatures are made from one or more cells
2. All cells are produced from previously existing cells (no spontaneous generation)
3. All cells appear to be descended from the first cell, which existed about 4 billion years ago
4. For a species to exist its reproductive cells must be potentially immortal (no aging)
5. Our bodies start from a single cell and contain about 100,000,000,000,000 (10^{13}) cells at maturity.

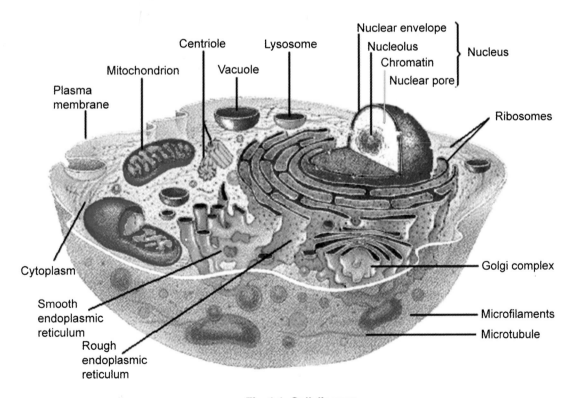

Fig. 1.1: Cell diagram

Cells are of two types: *Prokaryotic* and *Eukaryotic*

Prokaryotic cells are more primitive, small and without organelles. Examples: bacteria, and blue-green algae.

Eukaryotic cells are more advanced, larger, and contain organelles. Examples: cells of all higher species (animals, plants), fungi, and protozoa. Human cells are of the eukaryotic type.

Small Prokaryotic Cells are Simple but Fast Multiplying

Size: mycoplasmas are 0.1 to 1 micron in diameter; other bacteria are 1 to 10 micron in diameter. A few much larger exceptions are known. Small cells such as bacteria divide faster (once in 20 min). Have no nucleus, hence DNA is less protected and mutates faster. Our bodies are not made of prokaryotic cells, but our gut is inhabited by approximately 1.3 kg of bacteria. Bacteria inhabiting our gut are small in size and outnumber our body cells by a factor of 10:1. Intestinal bacteria are believed to be beneficial, because they produce vitamins and stimulate the immune system.

Large Eukaryotic Cells are Slow but Versatile

Size: typically 10 to 100 micron in diameter and are much larger than prokaryotes. Cell division is very slow (once in 20 hours). Have nucleus, hence DNA is better protected and mutation rate is low. Organelles are present, which allow many activities to take place within the same cell but in different compartments. Organelles can be isolated for study by centrifuge techniques.

What are the biological advantages of having cell organelles?

Some of the Organelles Found in Eukaryotic Cells are the Result of Endosymbiosis during Evolution

Cells often ingest other cells and digest them for food. Sometimes the ingested cell is not digested, but the two cells learn to live together for mutual benefit (endosymbiosis). Mitochondria and plant chloroplasts are believed to have originated in this way. These organelles have their own DNA and plasma membrane made of lipid bi-layer.

Cell Organelles are Found within the Cytosol

Cytosol is the liquid matrix of the cell, which is mostly water that contains cell organelles (except nucleus), salts, dissolved molecules, and enzymes. Glycolysis (anaerobic energy metabolism:) takes place in the cytoplasm.

Cell Membrane Separates the Cytoplasm from its Surrounding

Cell membrane is a lipid bi-layer made of phospholipids and proteins. It forms a barrier for the movement of molecules in and out of the cell; hydrophobic molecules pass through it more readily than hydrophilic ones. Specialized transport mechanisms allow selective movement of materials across the membrane.

Cell Shape is Supported and Determined by Cytoskeleton

Tubules are imbedded in the cytosol to form a meshwork of fibers that give shape to the cell. These tubules help the transport of structures within the cell (example: movement of chromosomes during cell division) and are also involved in movement of the whole cell.

There are three basic types of fibers:

Microtubules made of tubulin is 25 nm in diameter

Intermediate filaments made of several proteins, is 8 to 12 nm in diameter)

Microfilaments made of actin, is 7 nm in diameter).

Nucleus Contains the Molecule of Heredity (DNA)

The DNA (genetic information) does not leave the nucleus and functions as an archival copy of the genes. Genes are encoded in the DNA that is organized into chromosomes. There are many proteins associated with DNA, which are involved in DNA repair and turning the genes on and off. Nucleus has one or more nucleoli that make ribosomes. The RNA copy of gene (messenger RNA) is made in nucleus by transcription. Nuclear membrane is a lipid bi-layer with special pores that allow RNA to move out of the nucleus. Most cells contain single nucleus, but a few have more. Examples: some liver cells have multiple nuclei (polyploidy); muscle cells are very long and have hundreds of nuclei. Whereas mature red blood cell has lost its nucleus.

Centrioles Organize the Mitotic Spindle for Cell Division

Centrioles are a pair of small structures found in the centrosome near the nucleus; its structure is similar to that of cilia made of 9 triplet tubules. In animal cells, centrioles divide before cell division and help to organize the mitotic spindle (made of tubulin).

Mitochondria are the Powerhouses of the Cell

Mitochondria are covered by two bi-layer membranes, the inner of the two membranes is thrown into folds to increases the surface area of the site of cell respiration (electron transport and oxidative phosphorylation) where molecular oxygen functions as final acceptor of electrons that are generated during oxidation of energy yielding biomolecules (oxidation of one molecule of glucose yield 36 ATP). Typical cells have about 1000 mitochondria, but active cells like muscles will have more. Mitochondria have small amounts of DNA left over from when they were independent microorganisms. All your mitochondria come from your mother (very few in sperm)!

The diagram below (Fig.1.2) shows the internal structure of a mitochondrion.

Krebs cycle reactions take place in the internal matrix (blue). NADH and FADH2 (produced by glycolysis and the Krebs cycle) deliver their hydrogens and electrons to the electron transport chain

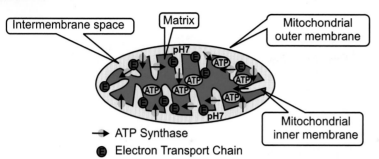

→ ATP Synthase

Ⓔ Electron Transport Chain

Fig. 1.2: Structure of mitochondria

(ETC). The ETC pumps hydrogen ions into the intermembrane space (yellow); this sets up a pH gradient- pH 8 in the matrix and pH 7 in the intermembrane space. Hydrogen ions flow through a channel in the enzyme ATP synthase from the intermembrane space to the matrix (see arrows). This causes a protein shaft in the ATP synthase to rotate and generates ATP in the matrix (Fig. 1.2)

Proteins are Made on the Ribosomes

Ribosomes are made in the nucleolus and are composed of rRNA and protein. Each unit of ribosome has two subunits. Ribosomes synthesize proteins (translation) by decoding the genetic code of mRNA. Some ribosomes are found free in the cytosol, but others are attached to the endoplasmic reticule to form rough endoplasmic reticule (RER). Proteins that are secreted by the cell, or which go to other organelles are made on the RER. Rough ER is prominent in cells that are secreting hormones and enzymes. Example: pancreatic cells.

Smooth Endoplasmic Reticule (SER)

Smooth endoplasmic reticulum is involved in lipid synthesis and detoxification of drugs. SER is made up of lipid membranes, has no ribosomes, makes cell membranes, steroid hormones, etc. Liver smooth SER has enzymes that detoxify drugs (cytochrome P450 system). In muscle, special smooth ER (sarcoplasmic reticulum) accumulates Ca ions (trigger for muscle contraction). Smooth ER can be seen best in cells that make lipid hormones (ovary, testes, adrenal cortex) and in cells that detoxify drugs (liver).

Golgi Apparatus Finishes, Sorts, and Targets Proteins

Golgi apparatus is a set of stacked membrane compartments found near the nucleus. Golgi finishes proteins: adds sugar molecules to side groups that make proteins water soluble, packages proteins into vesicles for secretion or internal use, sorts proteins and routes them to the right destination (some go to mitochondria, others to lysosomes, some to cell membranes, etc.) Golgi is found in all cells but is especially well developed in cells that secrete proteins. Examples: plasma cells (secrete antibodies), and pancreatic acinar cells (secrete digestive enzymes).

Lysosomes Digest Materials within the Cell

Lysosomes are small vesicles surrounded by lipid bi-layer. They contain digestive enzymes (acid hydrolases active at pH 4.5) that breakdown proteins, lipids, and defective cell parts so that they can be recycled. These enzymes also digest food brought into cell by phagocytosis and are involved in apoptosis (programmed cell death).

Peroxisomes Deal with Reactive Oxygen Molecules such as Peroxides

Peroxisomes contain the enzymes catalase, which converts hydrogen peroxide to O_2 and water, and another enzyme oxidase, that plays an important role in fat metabolism.

Cilia and Flagella help Cell Movement

Eukaryotic cilia and flagella are whip like projections from the cell, both have same internal structure: 9 pairs of tubules arranged in circle, surrounding a central pair of tubules (called the 9 + 2 structure). They beat repetitively (a bending motion) and cause cell to move (or move fluids along a surface of cells). Bending caused by a contractile protein, dynein enclosed within the cell membrane is made of at least 200 different proteins (Fig. 1.3).

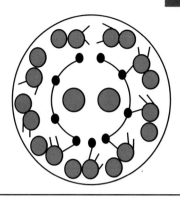

9 pairs of tubules arranged in circle, surrounding the central pari of tubules.

Fig. 1.3: Cross-section of cilia

Differences between Cilia and Flagella

Flagellated cells usually have only 1 or 2 flagella measuring 50 to 200 microns in length. Example: sperms.

Ciliated cells usually have hundreds of cilia that measure 5 to 10 microns in length. Examples are: cells lining respiratory tract that helps expel mucus secretions, cells lining fallopian tube that help to move egg cells, cells lining spinal canal that help move cerebrospinal fluid.

Microvilli Increase the Surface Area of Cells

Projections of cell surface form the brush borders of cells, which are sometimes confused with cilia, but they are much smaller (1 micron length) and with a different structure. Projections are supported by cytoskeletal filaments mostly the protein actin. Such projections increase the cell surface for faster absorption and secretion of materials.

Example of absorptive cells with microvilli is intestinal epithelium cells.

Examples of secretory cells with microvilli are choroid plexus cells of brain that secrete cerebrospinal fluid.

Specialized microvilli called stereocilia (misnamed) are found on the surface of the hair cells of the inner ear. The stereocilia respond to sound vibrations and are involved in hearing

Defective Cell Organelles are Responsible for Some Diseases

a. *Tay-Sachs* is a lysosomal storage disease in which gangliosides accumulate in lysosomes since they lack hydrolases that are responsible for its breaking down. phospholipids

b. *Cilia paralyzed by tobacco smoke* and other pollutants cannot move mucus. Mucus accumulates in the lungs that impair respiration.

c. *Abnormal mitochondria* with defective aerobic metabolism can lead to accumulation of lactic acid that causes lactic acidosis.

There are about 250 Types of Specialized Cells in the Body

Cells specialize by turning their genes on and off, and by structural modifications.

Few examples of specialized cells are:

Red blood cells have lost their nuclei and mitochondria, and are specialized for transport of gases in blood. These cells are loaded with hemoglobin (O_2 carrying protein) specialized for carrying O_2 to the tissues.

Nerve cells have long axons measuring a meter or more in length and are specialized for transmitting electrical impulses, they have specialized Na^+ and K^+ channels for generating electricity. These cells have a single nucleus in the cell body with special axonal transport mechanism to deliver proteins made in the cell body to the ends of the cell.

Muscle cells have special contractile proteins actin and myosin arranged in a sarcomere, which is specialized for producing force by contraction. These are very long cells often attached to two bones. Muscle cells are formed by fusion of many smaller cells, so they have many nuclei.

Insulin-secreting cells (beta cells of pancreas) have large amounts of rough endoplasmic reticulum needed for insulin secretion. Gene for making the insulin hormone is turned on in beta cells of Langerhans'.

CELL DIVISION

Reasons for Cell Division

Cell division is required for: (a) growth, (b) repair and replacement of damaged parts, and (c) reproduction of the species.

In Cell Division Copies of the DNA must be Sent to both New Cells

Since the instructions for making cell parts are encoded in the DNA, each new cell must get a complete set of the DNA molecules. This necessitates the DNA be copied (replicated or duplicated) before cell undergo division.

Genetic Blueprints for Cells are Organized into Chromosomes

The plans for making cells are coded in DNA, which is organized into giant molecules called chromosomes. Each chromosome is a single DNA molecule containing many genes. Each gene gives the directions for making one protein. In humans, each chromosome has approximately 2000 genes.

Chromosomes have Distinct Parts

Centromere is the part that holds duplicated chromosomes together before they are separated during mitosis. Kinetochore proteins bind to centromere and attach chromosome to spindle during mitosis. *Telomeres* are the ends of chromosomes important in cell aging.

DNA in chromosomes is associated with proteins. These proteins strengthen DNA fiber, help package chromosomes when they condense, and control activity of genes.

Human's Cells have 23 Pairs of Chromosomes (Diploid = pair of each chromosome = 46 total)

The members of a chromosome pair are called homologues. One of each pair came from mother, the other from father. Human reproductive cells (sperms and eggs) have 23 single chromosomes (Haploid = single copy of each chromosome = 23 total).

Genetic Instructions are Organized Into Genes

A section of DNA, which codes for a protein, is called a gene ("One gene, one enzyme"). We have approximately 50,000 genes (approx. 2000 per chromosome). Most of DNA in chromosome (about 95%) is "junk" DNA (function not known).

Before a Cell can Divide it Must Duplicate its Chromosomes

To make a new cell the old cell must duplicate all its parts. Duplication takes place in interphase. DNA (chromosomes) duplicated in the S sub-phase. Entire chromosome is duplicated at the same time. The duplicated chromosome remains attached to the original chromosome by its centromere. The original chromosome and its duplicated partner are called sister chromatids (Fig. 1.4).

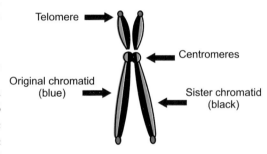

Fig. 1.4: Structure of chromosome

During Duplication the DNA Strands Separate ("unzip")

DNA is a double helix spiral with the two strands held together by hydrogen bonds. During replication the two strands come apart and each acts as a template to form a new strand. The coming apart ("unzipping") is made possible because the strands are held together by hydrogen bonds.

Chromosomes must be Tightly Packaged for Division

DNA must be tightly packaged for division otherwise it would tangle. This is made possible by histones and other proteins on which DNA is wound up to enable strands get 10,000 times shorter and much thicker (called condensation). Condensation occurs during prophase and they become visible under microscope.

Mitosis is Used for Growth and Repair

Object of mitosis is to produce two identical cells with same number of chromosomes. This is required for growth, repair and reproduction (in single-cell organisms). During mitosis cell divides only once after DNA duplicates, giving each cell the original number of chromosomes.

Some cells such as those lining the gut and skin, and white blood cells must be repaired often whose cell lifespan is only a few days.

Others such as nerve and muscle cells do not divide at all after birth.

Red blood cells have an intermediate lifespan of about 120 days.

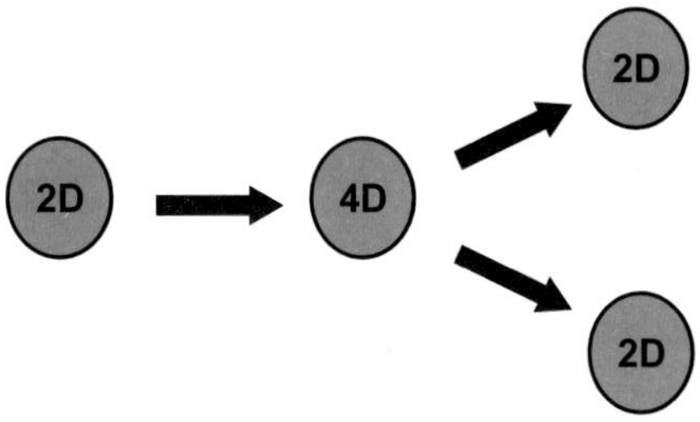

General Scheme of Mitosis

The DNA duplicates to form two sister chromatids, then chromosomes attach to spindle and separate (Fig. 1.5).

2D = DNA content of diploid cell; 4D = amount after duplication.

Fig. 1.5: General scheme of mitosis

Meiosis is Used for Sexual Reproduction

Object of meiosis is to reduce the number of chromosomes to single copy of each (haploid), for making sperm and eggs that are haploid. When a sperm fertilizes an egg to form a zygote the diploid number of chromosomes is restored (23 + 23 = 46). In meiosis, cells divide twice after a single DNA duplication.

General Scheme of Meiosis

DNA duplicates to form 2 sister chromatids, then chromosomes attach to spindle and separate. First division separates homologue chromatids, and the second division separates sister chromatids, which results in 4 haploid cells each with half the original number of chromosomes (Fig. 1.6).

2D = amount of DNA in diploid cell; 4D = amount after duplication; 1D = amount of DNA in haploid cells (sperm and eggs).

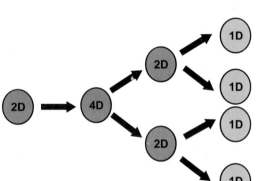

Fig. 1.6: General scheme of meiosis

Spindle Apparatus Separates Chromosomes both in Mitosis and Meiosis

Spindle is formed of microtubule fibers between the two centrosomes, spindles attach to chromosomes at centromere. Separation of chromosomes requires energy (ATP).

Cell Division Cycle has Five Stages

Interphase is the longest phase during which essentially the cell must duplicate all its parts. During this phase DNA replicates, proteins synthesized, centrioles duplicated, and chromosomes replicated (sister chromatids) but sister chromatids remain attached by centromeres until anaphase.

Prophase is the phase during which chromosomes condense and become visible, centrosomes move to opposite ends of cell to form spindle, and nuclear membrane dissolves.

Metaphase: Chromosomes attach to spindle fibers at their centromeres, line up in center of spindle apparatus.

Anaphase: Centromeres split to free the sister chromatids, and chromosomes move toward centrosomes to opposite polls of cell.

Telophase/Cytokinesis: Cell cleaves to form two cells (cytokinesis), and the nuclear membrane reforms. The last four phases are called mitosis (Fig. 1.7).

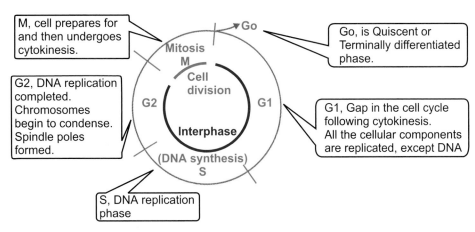

Fig. 1.7: Simple diagram of cell cycle

Mitosis = Prophase + Metaphase + Anaphase + Telophase (PMAT)

Cancer is Uncontrolled Mitosis

Mitosis must be controlled otherwise growth will occur without limit (cancer). Special proteins produced by oncogenes control cell growth. Mutations in control proteins can cause cancer.

MEMBRANE STRUCTURE AND FUNCTION

Cell Membranes are Primarily Phospholipid Bi-layers (2 layers)

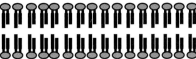

Phospholipid bi-layer forms a barrier to passage of molecules in and out of cell. In addition, presence of cholesterol in the lipid bi-layer stabilizes cell membranes. In the Fig. 1.8, note that the hydrophobic tails of the phospholipids (fatty acids) are together in the center of the bi-layer that keeps them out of the water.

Fig. 1.8: Lipid bi-layer of cell membrame

Membranes also Contain Proteins

Proteins that penetrate the membrane have hydrophobic sections of about 25 amino acids long (Fig. 1.9).
   Membrane proteins have many functions:
1. Receptors for hormones
2. Pumps for transporting materials across the membrane
3. Ion channels
4. Adhesion molecules for holding cells to extracellular matrix, and
5. Cell recognition antigens

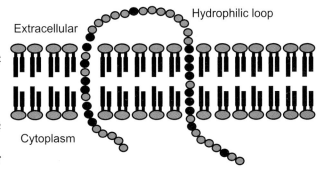

Fig. 1.9: Hydrophobic portion of protein in the membrane

All Molecules move Continuously by Simple Diffusion

Heat energy causes molecules to move randomly. If the concentration of molecules is different in 2 regions diffusion will cause molecules to move from a region of high concentration to one of low concentration. Higher the concentration gradient more rapid is the net diffusion. Diffusion tries to even out the concentrations so they are equal everywhere.

Simple Diffusion Across a Membrane is called Permeability

Diffusion is most efficient over short distances about the diameters of cells (Fig. 1.10). This type of penetration does not require energy from ATP. Hydrophobic substances have a high permeability through lipid bi-layer membranes, since they cross membranes faster than those that like water. Many biological chemicals are deliberately made hydrophobic to increase their rate of penetration into cells. Examples: many drugs, pesticides such as DDT.

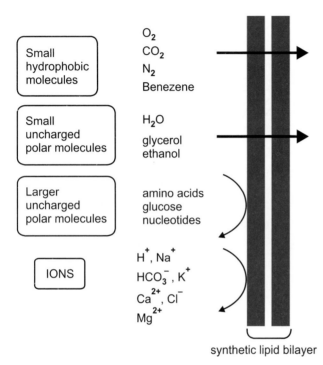

Fig. 1.10: Membrane permeability

Osmosis Moves Water Across Biological Membranes

Osmosis is movement of water from low osmotic pressure (dilute solution) to high osmotic pressure (concentrated solution). Except for blood flow almost all water movement in body is by osmosis. It is useful to think of a dilute solution as having a high water concentration and a concentrated solution as having a lower water concentration. Then the water flow goes from high water to low water concentration. In the figure 1.11, the blue dots represent the solute (the higher the solute concentration the lower the water concentration).

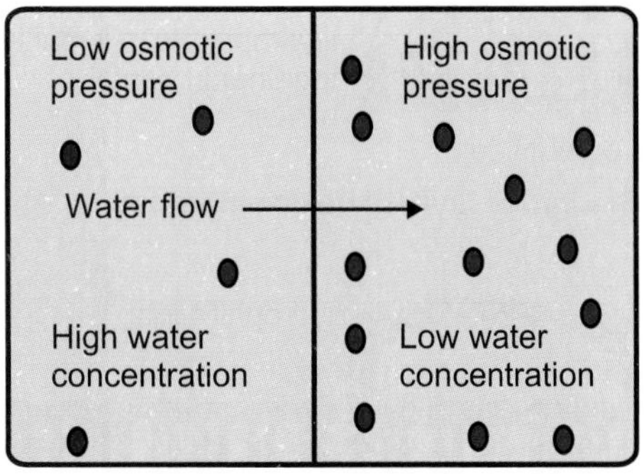

Osmosis is Passive it does not Require ATP Energy

Osmotic flow through most biological membranes is not by simple diffusion, it is by bulk flow and is similar to the flow caused by a pressure gradient. The kidney is an osmotic machine it adjusts body water volume by osmosis. Medical problems involving osmosis are pulmonary edema, childhood diarrhea, cholera, and inflammation of tissues.

Cholera is caused by Osmotic Imbalances, Which can be Treated Using Principle of Osmosis

Oral rehydration therapy (ORT) treats cholera and other diseases involving diarrhea; using osmosis to save lives. Cholera kills by dehydrating (osmosis-driven diarrhea and vomiting) the body.

Cholera is transmitted through water and food supplies contaminated by the bacterium, *Vibrio cholerae*. Direct transmission

Fig. 1.11: Osmosis

between two people is very rare. The cholera bacterium produces a toxin, which stimulates cells lining the upper section of the small intestine (duodenum) to secrete chloride ion (accompanied by Na^+, K^+ and some bicarbonate) into the intestinal lumen.

The excess NaCl and KCl in the intestine raises the osmotic pressure and this sucks water into the intestinal lumen. Water loss by diarrhea can be five or more liters per day, if untreated 50 to 75 percent of cholera patients will die from dehydration and loss of dissolved salts (Na^+, K^+, Cl^-, and HCO_3^-). Cholera and other types of diarrhea are the major killers of small children in developing countries (Fig. 1.12).

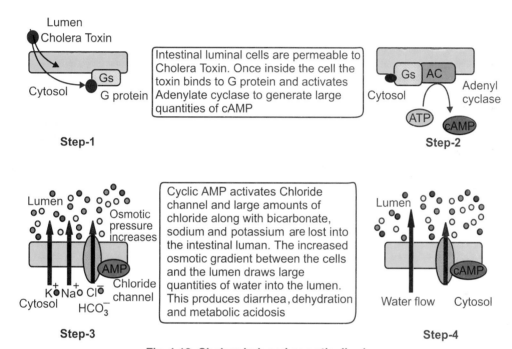

Fig. 1.12: Cholera induced osmotic diarrhea

Step 1: Cholera toxin crosses the membrane of an intestinal cell and permanently activates a G protein.

Step 2: The G protein activates the enzyme adenyl cyclase, which then starts to produce the 2nd messenger, cyclic AMP (cAMP).

Step 3: The cyclic AMP activates a chloride channel and large amounts of Cl^-, bicarbonate; Na^+ and K^+ are secreted into the intestinal lumen. This raises the lumen osmotic pressure.

Step 4: There is now a large osmotic pressure gradient between the cells and the lumen, and this causes large amounts of water to flow into the lumen. This produces diarrhea, metabolic acidosis and dehydration.

Other infections, such as pertussis (whooping cough), produce toxins which act in a similar manner to cholera toxin. The key to treating cholera and similar diseases is to replace the water and salts that have been lost. A patient may go from a coma to an alert state in minutes when he is rehydrated. The most effective method of rehydration takes advantage of a special Na^+ glucose co-transport mechanism (protein) found in cells of the small intestine. The protein works only when glucose and Na^+ are present at the same time in the gut; both substances must bind to the protein at the same time. Oral rehydration therapy (ORT) consists in giving the patient solutions to drink, which have both Na^+ and glucose; Bicarbonate and K^+ are also added to replace salts that are lost by diarrhea.

The Na^+ glucose co-transport protein (Fig. 1.13) binds Na^+ and glucose in the lumen. Both substances must be present in the lumen at the same time. The co-transport protein rotates and releases Na^+ and glucose into the intestinal cells. This raises the osmotic pressure within the cell and sucks water back into the body by osmosis. ORT is labor intensive, but the ingredients are very cheap.

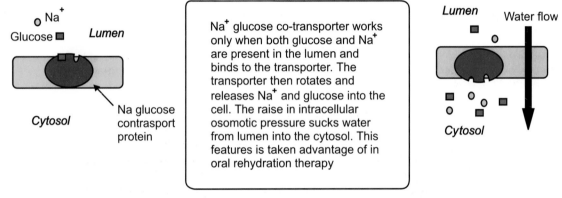

Fig. 1.13: Sodium glucose transporter mechanism

The diarrhea of cholera may last 5 to 6 days; ORT must be maintained during this time and up to 50 liters of solution must be supplied. The solutions use readily available ingredients and cost less than Rs1 per liter, making the method ideal for developing countries. ORT cuts the cholera death rate from 50 to 1 percent. ORT is credited with saving the lives of 1 million children *every year.*

Cells Swell in Hypotonic Solutions and Shrink in Hypertonic Ones

Osmosis often produces significant volume changes, causing swelling or shrinking of cells. If the external solution balances the osmotic pressure of the cytoplasm it is said to be isotonic. If the external solution is more dilute than the cytoplasm it is hypotonic, and if the external solution is more concentrated it is hypertonic.

A. *The animal cell* keeps the intracellular solute concentration low by pumping out ions (Fig. 1.14)
B. *The plant cell* is saved from swelling and bursting by its tough wall
C. *The protozoan* avoids swelling by periodically ejecting the water that moves into the cell.

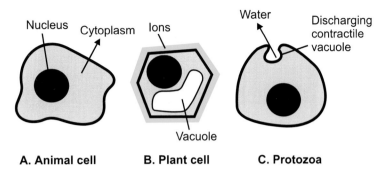

Fig. 1.14: Osmotic swelling

In Facilitated Diffusion Special Proteins help move Substances Across Membranes

Protein transport molecules help to carry many substances across membranes.

In the Figure 1.15, an extracellular molecule (glucose) is shown binding to the transport protein; the transport protein then rotates and releases the molecule inside the cell.

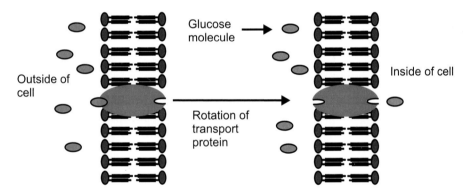

Fig. 1.15: Facilitated diffusion

Examples: There are five different glucose transporters (GLUT) proteins, and two co-transport (Na+ and glucose co-transporters that are used for secondary active transport).

There are eight different types of aquaporins (water channels).

Properties of Facilitated Diffusion

ATP energy not required for facilitated diffusion but cannot cause net transport of molecules from low to high concentration, which would require input of energy. Transport rate reaches a maximum when all of the protein transporters are being used (saturation). These systems are very specific: allows cell to select substances taken up and are sensitive to inhibitors that react with protein side chains.

Active Transport Uses Energy to Pump Molecules Against a Concentration Gradient

Pumps are proteins that use energy to carry substances across the cell membrane and can transport substances from a low concentration to a high concentration ("uphill" transport) and require energy in the form of ATP. Examples: the Na^+/K^+ pump, the Ca^{++} pump, etc.

Properties of Active Transport

Transport rate reaches a maximum when all of the protein transporters are being used (saturation). Very specific: allows cell to select substances taken up and sensitive to inhibitors that react with protein side chains. System is of ancient origin: found in all organisms and is extremely important in physiology: about one-third of our basal metabolism is used in active transport of various substances.

Many Molecules Enter Cells by Secondary Active Transport

It combines active transport and facilitated diffusion. Sodium gradient is produced by the Na^+ pump (active transport). The concentration gradient thus produced is used to produce secondary transport of sugars and amino acids (facilitated diffusion). Some sugar and amino acid transporters must bind Na^+ as well as the sugar or amino acid (coupled transport) simultaneously. Both Na^+ and the organic molecule must be present at the same time and on the same side of the membrane, since there is more Na^+ outside the cell, sugars and amino acids get transported mainly from the outside to the inside. The sugar and amino acid transporters do not use ATP directly, but ATP is required to set up the Na^+ gradient.

Examples: Glucose transport across the wall of the gut. Cells regulate permeability by adding and removing membrane transport proteins. If a molecule is moved across the cell membrane by a protein transporter or pump; adding more transporters or pumps will increase the transport rate, whereas removing transporters or pumps will decrease the transport rate. Often transport proteins are stored in vesicles until they are needed (Fig. 1.16).

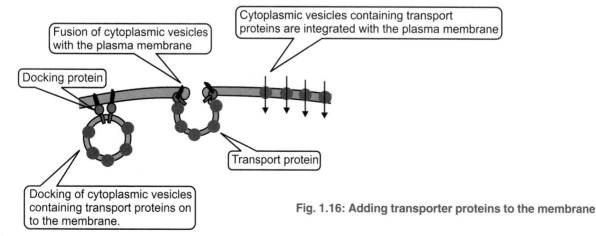

Fusion of cytoplasmic vesicles with the plasma membrane

Cytoplasmic vesicles containing transport proteins are integrated with the plasma membrane

Docking protein

Transport protein

Docking of cytoplasmic vesicles containing transport proteins on to the membrane.

Fig. 1.16: Adding transporter proteins to the membrane

The transporters are down regulated, back into vesicles, when they are not needed. In other cases, new transporters must be synthesized when needed. The body uses hormones to regulate membrane transport in this way. Examples:

Hormone	Transporter	Permeability regulation
Insulin	GLUT 4	Insulin causes glucose transport molecules to be inserted into muscle and adipose tissue cells. Glucose is then taken up into those tissues, lowering the blood glucose concentration.
Antidiuretic hormone (ADH)	Aquaporin 2	ADH causes aquaporin 2 proteins to be added to the kidney collecting duct membrane. The result is water conservation.
Aldosterone	Na pump	Aldosterone causes cells in the distal tubules and the collecting duct of the kidney to make more Na pump molecules. The final result is that it retains more Na and secretes more K into the urine.

Endocytosis can bring Macromolecules into the Cell

In endocytosis, the cell membrane bends inward (invaginates), forming a vesicle containing extracellular fluid, which can bring in large molecules such as proteins. The macromolecules are usually digested by lysosomes (Fig. 1.17).

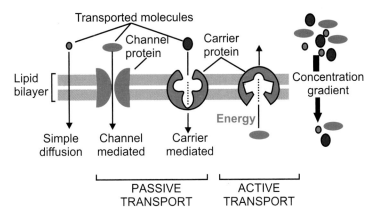

Fig. 1.17: Comparison of passive and active transport

Chemistry Review

2

All Matter Including Biological Matter is Made of Atoms

Atoms are like a planetary system with negatively charged electrons circling around positively charged nucleus. In electricity, opposite charges attract one another and like charges repel, similarly all atoms are formed by the attraction of oppositely charged particles called electrons (–) and protons (+).

Nucleus has protons with positive (+) charge and neutrons with neutral (0) charge. Almost all the mass of an atom is located in the protons and neutrons of the nucleus. The atomic number of an element denotes the number of protons in its nucleus. The number of protons determines the type of atom, e.g. carbon has 6 protons, nitrogen has 7, and so on.

Orbits Electrons with negative charges and a very small mass are organized in a series of orbits around the nucleus called shells. Chemical reactions involve the electrons, especially those in the outer shell. The charges in an uncharged atom must balance; it means the number of electrons must equal the number of protons.

Isotopes If you change the number of neutrons in the nucleus of an atom you are able to produce different isotopes of an element. Some but not all isotopes are radioactive. Schematic diagram of 3 isotopic forms of carbon is shown in Figure 2.1, in which six electrons are arranged around the nuclei in two shells (inner shell has two electrons and outer shell has four electrons).

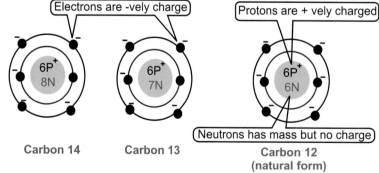

| Electrons are -vely charge | Protons are + vely charged |

6P⁺ 8N — Carbon 14

6P⁺ 7N — Carbon 13

6P⁺ 6N — Carbon 12 (natural form)

Neutrons has mass but no charge

Since all three atoms have 6 protons all are Carbon atoms, but each differ from one another with regard to number of neutrons they possess, hence they are the different isotopic forms of Carbon.

Fig. 2.1: Three isotopic forms of carbon

Nuclei in all the three isotopic forms have six protons; this makes them carbon atoms, but each of them has different number of neutrons that make them different isotopic forms of carbon.

Carbon 12 with six neutrons is the most common isotope of carbon (over 99%) in nature.

Carbon 13 with seven neutrons is a rare natural isotope.

Carbon 14 with eight neutrons is a radioactive isotope produced in the atmosphere by cosmic rays and explosion of atom bombs.

Isotope number is the sum of the protons and neutrons in an atom, which is its relative atomic mass.

Carbon 14 has a higher mass, and weighs more than its other isotopic form carbon 12.

The chemical properties of different isotopes of a given atom will be almost identical, but differ in some of their physical properties. Isotopes are frequently used as "tracers" in the field of research and medicine.

There are about 110 Different Types of Elements

Adding a proton to the nucleus of an atom changes it to another type of atom. When a proton is added to an atom an electron must also be added to maintain its electro-neutrality.

There are about 110 different types of atoms (elements) in nature, each differ from one another with regard to the number of protons they possess. Out of which only about 30 elements are required for life.

Carbon atoms hold the center stage in organic chemistry and biochemistry. Various atoms shown in blue in Table. 2.1 make up about 97.5 percent of body weight. The atoms shown in black in Table 2.1 usually form small water-soluble molecules that tend to form ions in solution and make up almost 2.5 percent of the body weight. There is some overlap: occasionally the atoms on the right are found in macromolecules, and sometimes the atoms on the left produce small water-soluble compounds.

Table 2.1

C	Carbon	Na	Sodium
H	Hydrogen	K	Potassium
O	Oxygen	Ca	Calcium
N	Nitrogen	Mg	Magnesium
P	Phosphorus	Cl	Chlorine
S	Sulfur	Fe	Iron
		I	Iodine

Atoms Combine to Make Molecules

All interactions between atoms are electrical attractions between charges. Ionic and covalent bonds hold atoms together to form molecules, whereas weak bonds (hydrogen, van der Waals and other types) hold molecules together.

Atoms Make Bonds by Donating or Sharing Electrons (Table 2.2)

Ionic bonds Suppose, sodium (Na) gives one of its electrons to chloride (Cl); the Na will now have a (+) charge and the Cl will have a (–) charge, and these charged atoms are referred to as ions. The opposite charged Na^+ and Cl^- attract each other to form NaCl (common table salt) by forming a chemical bond. Positively charged ions are designated as cations (e.g. Na^+) and negatively charged ions are designated as anions (e.g. Cl^-).

Covalent bonds Each of the atoms involved in covalent bond formation donates one or more electrons to the bond, the bonding electrons spend most of their time between the two atoms attracting both nuclei and pulling them together. If each atom donates 2 electrons to a bond a double bond is formed that is stronger and more rigid than single bonds. A triple bond is formed when each atom donates 3 electrons to the bond.

Hydrogen bonds When a hydrogen ion is sandwiched between two atoms (usually nitrogen and oxygen) it forms a hydrogen bond that is much weaker (about 25 times) than covalent or ionic bonds. Hydrogen bonds occur between molecular groups with permanent dipoles.

van der Waals and other weak bonds These are weak forces especially important between chains of carbon atoms that can bond together like atoms, although weak, numerous bonds between the chains can add up to produce significant cohesion that determine physical state of compounds: gas, liquid or solid. Such forces occur when one atom induces a temporary dipole in another atom.

Neutral molecules such as water with covalent bonds have an uneven distribution of charge with a positive end and a negative end. Such a molecule is called a dipole.

If you take water as an example (Fig. 2.2) The black lines represent covalent bonds and the red lines are hydrogen bonds. Water is a polar molecule. Although water molecule is electrically neutral the electrons are unevenly distributed so that there is a partial negative charge (δ^-) on the oxygen and partial positive charges (δ^+) on the hydrogen.

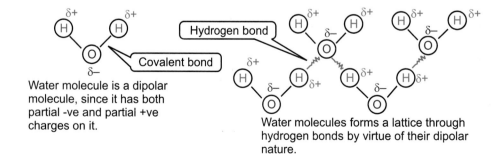

Water molecule is a dipolar molecule, since it has both partial -ve and partial +ve charges on it.

Water molecules forms a lattice through hydrogen bonds by virtue of their dipolar nature.

Fig. 2.2: Formation of hydrogen bonds between polar molecules

Table 2.2

Type of bonds	Characteristics	Biological importance
Covalent	Bonding electrons shared between 2 atoms.	This type of bond holds together the long chains of macromolecules. These molecules do not split apart in water.
Ionic	Complete transfer of electron from one atom to another. Oppositely charged atoms attract one another.	Compounds with ionic bonds split into ions in water. Ions conduct electricity. Gives specialized cells (nerve, muscle) excitable properties.
Hydrogen	Weaker than covalent or ionic bonds. Formed between hydrogen covalently bonded to O or N and a second O or N. The second O or N may be on the same molecule or on another nearby molecule. Occur because H, O and N atoms in molecules usually have partial charges on them, forming dipoles.	Water: makes water molecules stick together. Responsible for many of the strange properties of water. Proteins: cause protein chains to spiral and bend, giving unique shapes. DNA: hold together the 2 chains to form the double helix. Allow chains to "unzip" for replication and transcription.
Van der Waals	Weak bonds that can form where one atom induces a temporary dipole in another atom	Important in holding like molecules together. Often determine the solid, liquid or gas state of a compound. Saturated fats are solid at room temperature because they have more van der Waals attractions than unsaturated fats, which are liquid.
Other weak bonds	Attractions between permanent dipoles of molecules	Help to determine the shapes of molecules.

The bonding electrons are not completely transferred to the oxygen, which would make an ionic bond; they are only shifted so that they are closer to the oxygen than to the hydrogens. The asymmetry of charge creates a tiny dipole; dipolar molecules are attracted to other polar and charged molecules, forming weak bonds such as hydrogen bonds. Each water molecule can form as many as four hydrogen bonds (two with the oxygen, and one each with the hydrogens).

Some Examples of Bonds Between Atoms

The electronic structure of an atom determines the number of bonds it can make.

Some examples are:

H can make only a single bond.

O can make 2 single bonds or 1 double bond.

C can make a total of 4 bonds: 4 single bonds, 1 double and 2 single bonds, or 2 double bonds.

Carbon has a special place in biology, since it can bond to other carbon atoms to form long chains, branched chains, and rings that makes possible the formation of giant molecules with many complex shapes.

Carbon compounds with the same chemical composition may have different structures (isomers) and chemical properties.

Example: C_2H_6O can exist with two different structures ethyl alcohol, and dimethyl ether. Although the chemical composition of these two molecules is the same, the atoms in these two molecules are attached in different patterns.

Ethyl alcohol (CH_3CH_2OH), the alcohol present in beer and wine is very soluble in water and has a boiling point of 78.5^0 C, whereas dimethyl ether (CH_3-O-CH_3) has low solubility in water and a boiling point of only -24°C.

Biological Molecules Interact with those of Opposite Shape (Complementarity)

Complementarity: frequently biological molecules that interact have opposite shapes so that they fit tightly together. For example enzymes and substrates fit together like a lock and key, hormones bind to specific receptor molecules with the right shape. Two strands of DNA molecules fit together precisely to make a double helix: the genetic code is based upon complementarity between nucleotide bases. In immune reactions, antibodies have shapes that exactly match the antigens that they bind. In medicine therapeutic, drugs are often designed to be complementary to a biological molecule such as an enzyme or receptor. In reactions between two complementary molecules, the molecules are not rigid, but bend to the shape of their partner (induced fit).

Christian de Duve expresses such complementarity this way:

"The two partners are not rigid. When they embrace, they mold themselves to each other to some extent. Furthermore, the embrace leads to binding. Its degree of intimacy is such that electrostatic interactions and other short-range physical forces act strongly enough to prevent the association from being disrupted by thermal jostling." (from Vital Dust. Life as a Cosmic Imperative, NY: HarperCollins, 1995).

Because of the tight, fit complementary molecules form very strong bonds of high selectivity.

Carbon Compounds can Exist as Mirror Image Isomers (Enantiomers)

Many carbon compounds have a central carbon to which are attached four different groups. Such compounds can exist as mirror images molecules of each other (Fig. 2.3). In the laboratory, such mirror image isomers usually have identical chemistry, but within the cells the chemistry will be very different. Both sugars and amino acids exist as mirror image isomers. Our bodies can use only one set of these isomers. We use the D-sugars for energy but cannot use L-sugars at all. In case of amino acids, we use the L-forms, but not the D-forms.

Mirror image isomers in solution rotate the plane of polarized light; *d* and *l* refer to the direction to which the plane of polarized light is rotated (right or left respectively).

The preference for D-sugars and L-amino acids is found in all organisms on earth and is evidence that we have a common evolutionary origin. The preference comes about because reactions inside cells use enzymes. Only one type of isomer can dock with the enzyme because it is complementary, whereas the other cannot bind to the enzyme since it is not complementary.

Diagram of two mirror image isomers A and B, and a potential binding site on the surface of an enzyme are shown diagrammatically (Fig. 2.3). The central carbon atom is shown white. The colored balls represent different chemical groups attached to the central carbon. They must bind to the similarly colored complementary sites on the enzyme. Find out which isomer can attach all its three groups to the enzyme?

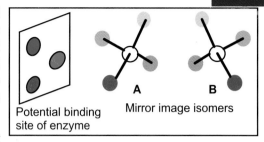

Pharmaceutical application: drugs are usually a mixture of mirror image isomers. Often only one isomer is active and sometimes the inactive isomer has bad side effects.

Fig. 2.3: Enantiomers

Numbers of Atoms and Molecules are Measured in Terms of Moles

In our daily living, we have devised convenient units for dealing with numbers of objects. When we speak of eggs we talk about dozens (12), when dealing with paper we use units of reams (500), similarly in chemistry we use mole as a convenient unit.

Mole = 600,000,000,000,000,000,000,000 atoms (count the zeros), This number is an approximation and has been rounded off.

Mole = 6×10^{23} atoms. An exponential system is preferred to avoid writing all those zeros.

1 mole of N (14 protons and neutrons) weighs 14 grams. In biochemistry, it is often convenient to speak of millimoles (abbreviated mM): 1 millimole = mole/1000   OR   1000 millimoles = 1 mole.

How Chemical Formulas and Reactions are Written

Subscripts: The number of atoms in a molecule is indicated by a subscript (no subscript means a single atom); CO_2 means that carbon dioxide contains one carbon atom and two oxygen atoms.

Prefixes: The prefixes indicate the number of molecules taking part in a reaction. The prefixes for the oxidation of one molecule of glucose show that six molecules of oxygen are consumed to form six molecules each of carbon dioxide, and water.

$$C_6H_{12}O_6 + 6O_2 \longrightarrow 6\,CO_2 + 6\,H_2O$$

Arrows show the direction in which the reaction proceeds.

$$A + B \longrightarrow C$$

It means that reactants A and B react to produce product C.

All chemical reactions proceed in both directions (A + B $\leftrightarrow$ C), but a unidirectional arrow is often used to focus attention on the reaction direction favored under the circumstances.

Conservation of Matter

It holds that equations must balance.

Matter is not created or destroyed in a chemical reaction, so the number of atoms in the products must equal the number of atoms in the reactants.

Example: In the oxidation of glucose reaction shown above there are 18 oxygen, 12 hydrogen and 6 carbon atoms on each side of the equation.

Rates and Equilibrium States of Chemical Reactions are determined by Concentrations of the Reactants (Law of Mass Action)

Consider a simple reaction in which two substances A and B, react to form a third substance, C:

$$A + B \longrightarrow C$$

The rate at which C is formed (in moles/second) will be proportional to the concentrations of A, B and C

Rate = Kf [A][B] – Kb[C]

[A], [B] and [C] = concentrations of A, B and C, respectively; Kf = rate constant of forward reaction, Kb = rate constant of backward reaction

Forward reaction rate = Kf [A] [B]

Backward reaction rate = Kb[C]

This relationship is a fundamental law of chemistry, called the

Law of Mass Action

Note that if you double the concentration of either A or B, the rate of the forward reaction will double.

Usually concentrations are given in moles/liter

Example: if you have 3 moles of NaCl dissolved in 6 liters of water the concentration is:

3 moles/6 liters = 0.5 moles/liter = 500 mM/liter

Why are chemical reaction rates proportional to concentration?

Molecules must collide to react and number of collisions per second is proportional to the concentration of reactants.

Other factors affect reaction rates by changing the rate constants:

At high temperature molecules have more energy and causes molecules to move faster producing more collisions, and are more likely to react with each other.

A chemical reaction proceeds until forward and backward reactions are equal, at that point the reaction is at equilibrium and concentrations do not change.

At equilibrium: Kf [A][B] = Kb[C]

Ke = Kf / Kb = [A] [B] / [C]

The equilibrium constant (Ke) is the forward rate constant (Kf) divided by the backward rate constant (Kb)

Note: at equilibrium [C] = [B] / [C] / Ke; thus both the rates of reaction, and equilibrium concentrations are determined by concentrations of reactants.

STEREOCHEMISTRY

Stereochemistry is the study of molecules in three dimensions.

The major factor influencing inorganic chemical reactions is temperature. Whereas in biological reactions that are driven by enzymes (enzymes are able to make reactions kinetically favorable at room temperature) the shape of the molecules is more important. The deciding factor for biological reaction is the fit between the substrate(s) and the binding site(s) on the enzyme.

The following discussion will emphasize on three main concepts of stereochemistry: **symmetry**, **handedness**, and **chirality**.

Symmetry

You are already familiar with the concept of symmetry. An object is bilaterally symmetrical if it can be bisected with a line or a plane, and the two sides are identical but mirror images of each other. If you could fold the object along the plane of symmetry, the two sides would overlap perfectly. In addition to bilateral symmetry, an object can have symmetry that is best seen when divided into three parts, or five parts, etc. Some examples of symmetrical objects are circles, butterflies, and the letter E (Fig. 2.4). A starfish is also symmetrical but has five-fold symmetry.

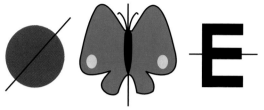

Fig. 2.4: Symmetrical objects

An object that is not symmetrical is called asymmetric. Examples of asymmetric objects are: spirals, and the number 2 (Fig. 2.5).

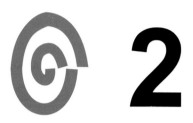

Fig. 2.5: Asymmetrical objects

Handedness

Just as your left and right hands are mirror images of each other, many chemical compounds can exist in two mirror image forms. For example, when the amino acid alanine is synthesized in the laboratory, a mixture of the two possible structures is formed. However, when alanine is produced in a living cell, only one of the two forms is seen.

The naturally occurring form of alanine is called L-alanine, and its mirror image is called D-alanine. Comparison of the 20 common amino acids will show that only the "L" form is used in protein synthesis. The enzymatic machinery used in protein synthesis has an asymmetric binding site the amino acids must fit into. Your right hand would not fit properly into a left-handed glove, and an amino acid of the wrong shape would not fit into an enzyme. Of all the naturally occurring amino acids in proteins, only Glycine—NH_2-CH_2-$COOH$—has a plane of symmetry (along its "spine").

Chirality

Chirality is a special case of asymmetry. A molecule is said to be chiral if there is no internal plane of symmetry and its mirror image are not super imposable (Fig. 2.6). Even after rotating one of the molecules it remains different from its stereoisomer.

In the study of carbohydrates, we often refer to a chiral carbon molecule. A carbon molecule is said to be chiral if it has four different substituents or 'R' groups (Fig. 2.6). To distinguish between the two possible arrangements of four substituents around a chiral carbon molecule, a system of nomenclature was developed.

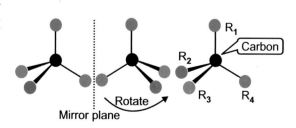

Fig. 2.6: Chiral molecule

Chart 2.1

Functional groups	Class of molecules	Formula	Example
Hydroxyl —OH	Alcohols	R—OH	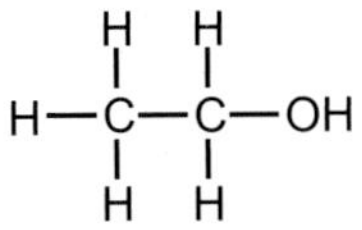 Ethanol
Carbonyl —COH	Aldehydes	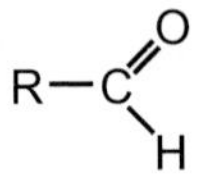	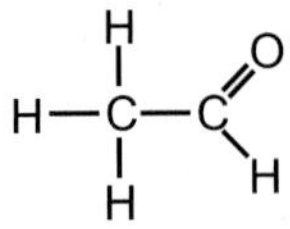 Acetaldehyde
CO	Ketones		Acetone
Carboxyl –COOH	Carboxylic Acids	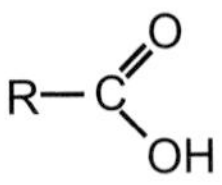	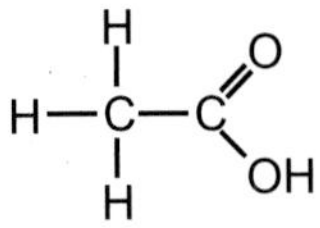 Acetic Acid
Amino –NH$_2$	Amines		Methylamine
Phosphate –OPO$_3$$^{-2}$	Organic phosphates		3–Phosphoglyceric acid
Sulfhydryl ~~SH	Thiols	R—SH	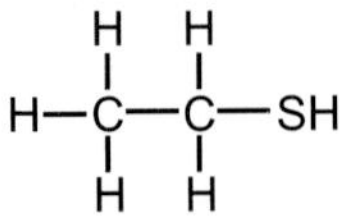 Mercaptoethanol

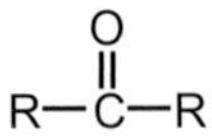

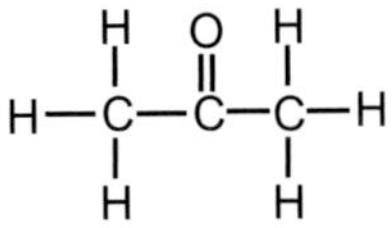

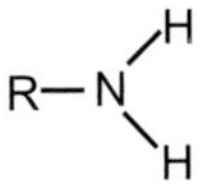

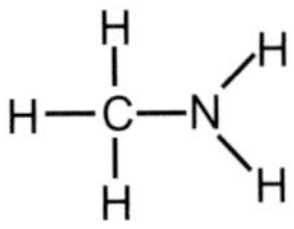

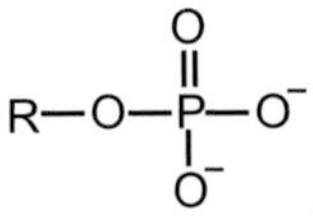

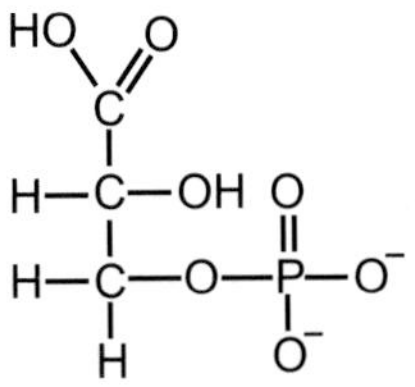

Stereoisomers (Optical Isomers)

A chiral molecule and its mirror image molecule are called stereoisomers or enantiomers. Pairs of stereoisomers are sometimes indistinguishable in chemical reactions, but can be distinguished by examining a physical property of the molecule. A pure solution of a stereoisomer will rotate the plane of plane-polarized light. The other enantiomer will rotate polarized light the same number of degrees, but in the opposite direction. For this reason, stereoisomers are also called optical isomers. A solution that contains a mixture of the two optical isomers will not change the plane of plane polarized light, because the effects of the two isomers cancel each other out.

FUNCTIONAL GROUPS

Chart 2.1 delineates most common chemical functional groups. These functional groups will turn up in later chapters in the biological molecules we study. We recommend studying this chart so you can recognize the functional groups when they appear. R stands for any group of atoms—C, H, N, and S—that is attached by a covalent bond to a chemical functional group.

Introduction to Biological Macromolecules

3

Living Organisms are not in Equilibrium with their Surroundings

Chemical reactions run their courses until there is no further change; this is called equilibrium. In biology, equilibrium means death. Continuous input of energy is required to prevent biological processes reaching equilibrium. To counteract the trend toward equilibrium cells continually burn fuel molecules (sugar, fat, and amino acids) and use the energy released to make ATP. Cells use energy in the form of ATP for many activities, including building macromolecules (giant molecules) from small building blocks.

Without energy input from ATP, cells breakdown into small building-block molecules and die (reach state of equilibrium). Each time a bond is formed to make macromolecule water is removed (dehydration), and when macromolecules breakdown spontaneously they take up water (hydrolysis) this is what happens in digestion.

Generalized Picture of Energy Relationships

Cells exist in a stable relationship with the environment called steady state.

Steady-state 1: production of fresh water from seawater using energy from sun (non-living steady-state).

Steady-state 2: production of macromolecules from small molecules using ATP energy.

Steady-state 3: production of sugars and other carbon compounds from CO_2 and water using light energy (living steady-state).

In these steady states, the system is pushed away from equilibrium by the continuous inflow of energy from outside. More than 99 percent of the energy for life comes from the Sun via photosynthesis.

Adenosine Triphosphate (ATP) is the Energy Currency of the Cell

Animal cells cannot directly use most forms of energy. Most cellular processes require energy stored in the bonds of a molecule adenosine triphosphate (ATP), hence ATP is referred to as the energy currency of the cell (Fig. 3.1).

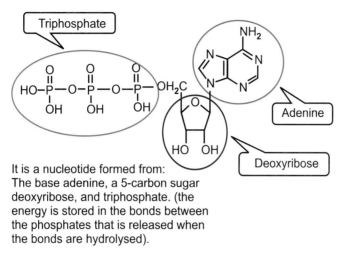

It is a nucleotide formed from:
The base adenine, a 5-carbon sugar
deoxyribose, and triphosphate. (the
energy is stored in the bonds between
the phosphates that is released when
the bonds are hydrolysed).

Fig. 3.1: Structure of ATP

Cells are Designed to use Chemical Energy Rather than heat Energy

The cell is not a heat engine; it runs at a constant low temperature.

Energy storage: Body cannot store much ATP (ATP interferes with many chemical reactions); most of the body's energy is stored in the form of fats (triglycerides) and polysaccharides (glycogen). Cell produces energy as needed by oxidizing ("burning") the stored energy rich molecules (triglycerides and glycogen). Some of the energy is dissipated as heat, but most of it is trapped in the phosphate bonds of ATP, and some electrical energy is also stored as ion gradients.

Cells Contain Four Major Types of Giant Molecules and Polymers

They are proteins, polysaccharides (complex sugars), nucleic acids, and lipids (fats). Biological polymers are made from about 60 small building blocks.

Proteins are Made Up of Exactly 20 Different Amino Acids

Basic amino acid structure: It has an α-amino (NH2) group, an α-carboxyl (COOH) group and a variable side chain (R group).

The 20 amino acids have different side groups (designated as R). In proteins, the amino acids are linked head to tail by peptide bonds (Fig. 3.2).

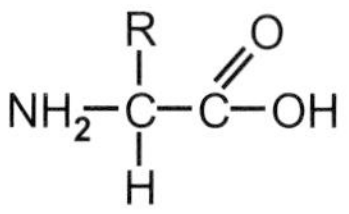

Basic Amino Acid Structure Note the amino (NH_2), carboxyl (COOH) and hydrogen groups (H), which are found on all amino acids. the difference in amino acids are in the 20 different types of R groups.

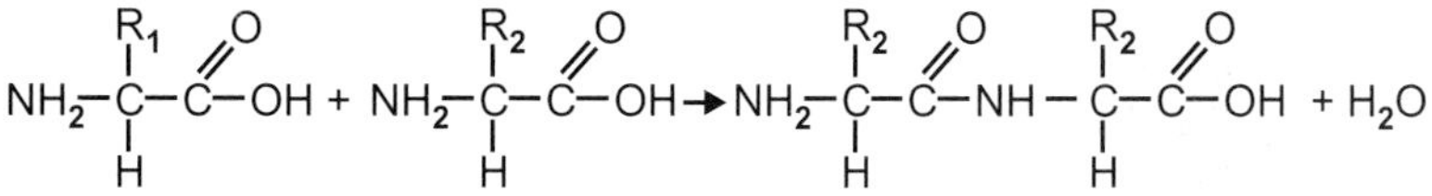

Fig. 3.2: Basic structure of amino acid and peptide bond

Formation of a Peptide Bond Two amino acids can combine, with the carboxyl of one attaching to the amino group of the other (head to tail). Water is removed. This process also requires energy in the form of ATP

Proteins differ from one another in two ways: The size (typical protein has 200 to 1000 amino acids), and sequence of amino acids. Some amino acids are charged or have a polar structure (hydrophilic), some amino acids are neutral and nonpolar (hydrophobic). Hydrophobic proteins are found mostly in membranes.

Proteins do Most of the Work of the Cell

Each cell has thousands of different types of proteins; each specialized to do a certain job.

Some proteins are structural: They control cell shape and bind cells together. Example: collagen binds all of the cells of the body together.

Protein enzymes control the chemical reactions of the cells.

Protein pumps move things across the cell membrane.

Proteins give mobility ("Molecular motors"): example: contractile proteins of muscles, flagella and cilia.

Antibodies defend the body against pathogenic organisms and foreign bodies.

Receptors are required for signaling in endocrine and nervous systems.

Nucleic Acids are the Molecules of Heredity

Nucleic acids are made of five different nucleotide bases, sugars and phosphate groups. The two major types of nucleic acid are DNA and RNA. Both have genetic code, which specifies the sequence of amino acids in proteins. DNA is archival copy of genetic code kept protected in the nucleus.

RNA is working copy of genetic code used to translate a specific gene into a protein in the cytoplasm.

The bases make up the genetic code; the phosphate and sugar make up the backbone.

RNA is a molecule with a single strand.

DNA has two strands (double stranded helix) held together by hydrogen bonds between the bases A = T and G=C because: A always forms two hydrogen bonds with T, and G always forms three hydrogen bonds with C.

Lipids form Cell Membranes and Energy Storage Depots

Lipids are a group of heterogeneous molecules, which are insoluble in water and metabolized by cells. They have high oil/water partition coefficients (Fig. 3.3).

The oil/water partition coefficient is the partition of a substance between oil and water, which is a measure of the extent to which a substance is soluble in oil or water. Hydrophobic substances have high oil/water partition coefficients. In the body, hydrophobic molecules tend to accumulate in fat tissue, hence hydrophobic drugs cross cell membranes faster than water-soluble drugs.

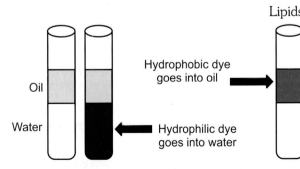

Oil

Water

Hydrophobic dye goes into oil

Hydrophilic dye goes into water

Fig. 3.3: Oil-water partition coefficient illustrated with colored dyes

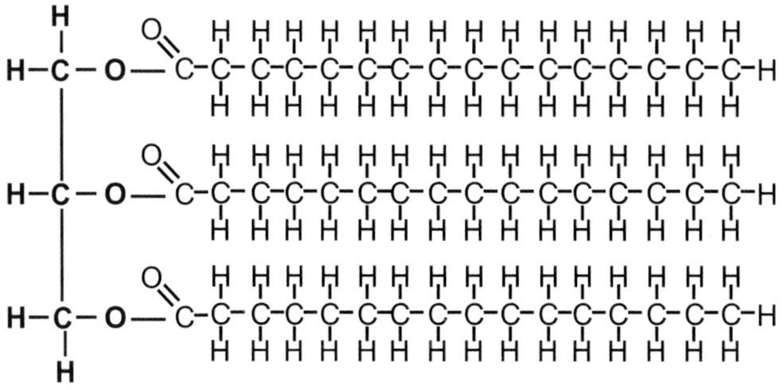

TRIGLYCERIDE (TRIACYLGLYCEROL)
Triglyceride has a glycerol back-bone (in blue)
to which are esterified three fatty acids.
Triglycerides are the main storage form of
energy in the body. Each gram of triglyceride
yields about 9 calories of energy.

Fig. 3.4: Structure of triglycerol

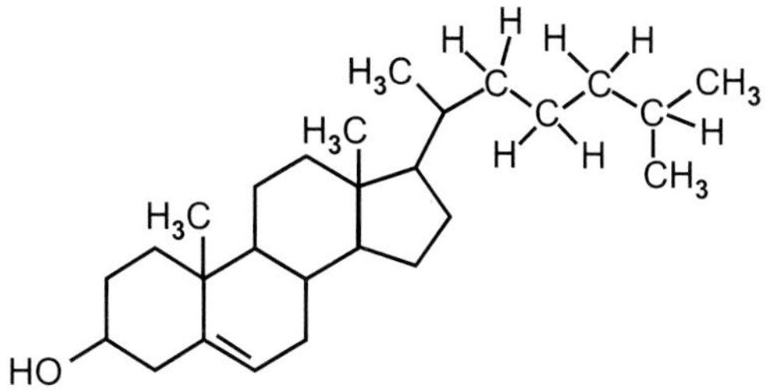

This steroid molecule is cholesterol.
It has a cyclopentenophenanthrene
ring structure to which is attached a
hydrocarbon side chain.

Fig. 3.5: Structure of steroid

Triglycerides are the storage form of fat in the body. It is also called at times as neutral fat. It is composed of glycerol and three fatty acids (Fig. 3.4).

Phospholipids form cell membranes, composed of two fatty acids, glycerol, phosphate and a polar groups. They are structurally similar to triglycerides, but polar groups linked via a phosphogroup replace one of the three fatty acids.

Steroids: have a cyclopentenophenanthrene ring structure (Fig. 3.5). Examples are cholesterol, and some hormones. Cholesterol is required to produce stable cell membranes. It is also a precursor for several hormones produced in the testes, ovaries and adrenal glands, e.g. sex hormones, cortisone and aldosterone. Too much cholesterol will promote atherosclerosis.

Polysaccharides are Used for Structure and Energy Storage

Polysaccharides are polymers made of sugar molecules linked together by glycosidic bonds.

Glycogen is the storage form of carbohydrates in animals. It is polymer of glucose molecules.

Starch is the storage form of carbohydrates in plants. It is polymer of glucose molecules (Fig. 3.6).

Some sugars are attached to membrane proteins (example: ABO blood groups).

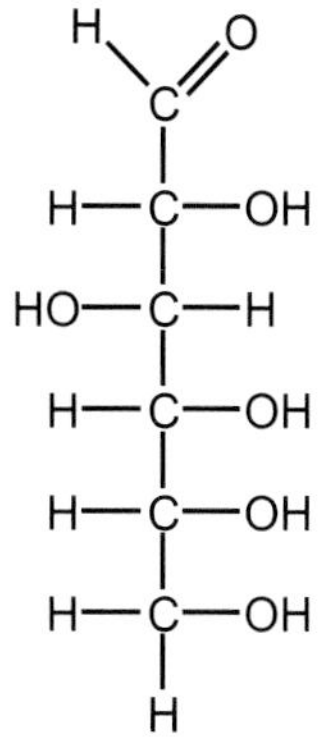

GLUCOSE IS A 6-CARBON SUGAR
Glucose is the major energy source for the body.
Glucose is burned by glycolysis & Krebs cycle to
make ATP. The brain is very sensitive to the blood
glucose concentration, because it cannot use fats for
it's energy needs. Blood glucose levels are regulated
by hormones.

Fig. 3.6: Structure of glucose

Chemistry of Amino Acids and Proteins

4

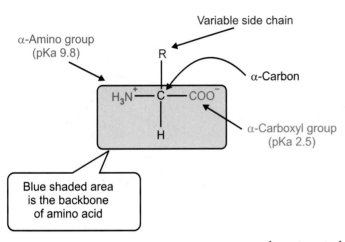

α-Amino group (pKa 9.8)

Variable side chain

R

α-Carbon

α-Carboxyl group (pKa 2.5)

$H_3N^+ - C - COO^-$

H

Blue shaded area is the backbone of amino acid

Fig. 4.1: Structure of an α-amino acid

AMINO ACIDS

Amino acids are the building blocks of proteins. The general structure of amino acid includes an α-amino group, an α-carboxylate group, and a variable side chain (R group). The α-amino group has a pKa of 9.8 therefore ionized (+ vely charged) at physiological pH. The α-corboxylate group has a pKa value of 2.5 therefore ionized (-vely charged) at physiological pH (Fig. 4.1).

Ionization constant (pK) is the pH at which the group is half deprotonated, i.e. at any pH less than its pK the group is fully protonated (+ ve charged), and at any pH above its pK the group is fully deprotonated (- ve charged). Hence, the amino acid backbone at pH 7 is in zwitterions form (Fig. 4.2).

Acid-Base Properties of the Amino Acids

The α-COOH and α-NH_2 groups, as well the acidic and basic R-groups in amino acids are capable of ionizing. As a result of their ionizability the following ionic equilibrium reactions may be written:

$$R\text{-}COOH \rightleftharpoons R\text{-}COO^- + H^+$$
$$R\text{-}NH_3^+ \rightleftharpoons R\text{-}NH_2 + H^+$$

The equilibrium reactions as written, demonstrate that amino acids contain at least two weakly acidic groups. However, the carboxyl group is a far stronger acid than the amino group. At physiological pH (around 7.4) the carboxyl group will be unprotonated and the amino group will be protonated. An amino acid with no ionizable R-group would be electrically neutral at this pH. This species is termed a **zwitterion**.

Like typical organic acids, the acidic strength of the carboxyl amino and ionizable R-groups in amino acids can be defined by the association constant K_a or more commonly the negative logarithm of K_a, the pK_a. The **net charge** (the algebraic sum of all the charged groups present) of any amino acid, peptide or protein, will depend

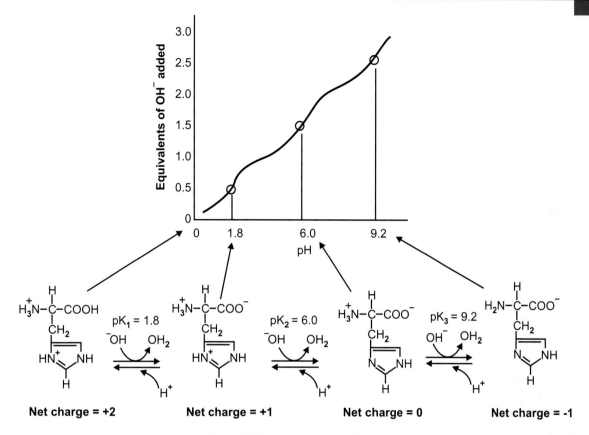

Fig. 4.2: Titration curve of histidine

on the pH of the surrounding aqueous environment. As the pH of a solution of an amino acid or protein changes so too does the net charge on amino acid or protein present in it. This phenomenon can be observed during the titration of any amino acid or protein. The net charge of an amino acid or protein is zero, at a pH equivalent to its isoelectric **point (pI).**

Optical Properties of the Amino Acids

A tetrahedral carbon atom with four distinct substituted groups is said to be **chiral**. The only amino acid not exhibiting chirality is glycine since its "R-group" is a hydrogen atom. Chirality describes the handedness of a molecule that is observable by its ability in solution to rotate the plane of polarized light either to the right (**dextrorotatory**) or to the left (**laevorotatory**) (Fig 4.3). All of the amino acids in proteins exhibit the same absolute steric configuration as **L-glyceraldehyde**. Therefore, they are all L-α-amino acids. Although D-amino acids exist in nature they are never found in proteins, but are often found in polypeptide antibiotics. The aromatic R-groups in aromatic amino acids have an absorbance maximum in the range of 280 nm. The ability of proteins to absorb ultraviolet light is predominantly due to the presence of the tryptophan, which strongly absorbs ultraviolet light.

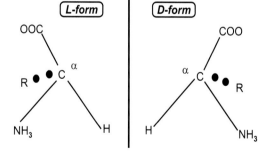

Fig. 4.3: L-and D-forms of amino acid

Functional Significance of Amino Acid R-groups

Amino acids differ from each other only in "R" groups they possess. In solution, it is the nature of the R-groups of amino acids that dictate structure-function relationships of peptides and proteins. The hydrophobic amino acids will generally be encountered in the interior of proteins shielded from direct contact with water. Conversely, the hydrophilic amino acids are generally found on the exterior of proteins as well as in the active site of enzymes protein. Indeed, it is the very nature of R-groups of certain amino acids that allow enzyme reactions to occur.

The imidazole ring of histidine allows it to act as either a proton donor or acceptor at physiological pH. Hence, it is frequently found in the active site of enzymes. Equally important is the ability of histidines in hemoglobin to buffer H^+ ions formed during ionization of carbonic acid in red blood cells. It is this property of hemoglobin that allows it to exchange O_2 and CO_2 at the tissues or lungs, respectively.

The primary alcohol of serine and threonine as well as the thiol (-SH) of cysteine allow these amino acids to act as nucleophiles during enzymatic catalysis. Additionally, the thiol of cysteine is able to form a disulfide bond with other cysteines:

Cysteine-SH + HS-Cysteine $\longleftrightarrow$ Cysteine-S-S-Cysteine

This simple disulfide formed by two cysteine molecules is identified as cystine. The formation of disulfide bonds between cysteines present within proteins is important to the formation of structural domains in a large number of proteins. Disulfide bonding between cysteines in different polypeptide chains of oligomeric proteins plays a crucial role in ordering the structure of complex proteins. Example: the insulin receptor.

CLASSIFICATION OF AMINO ACIDS

Amino acids are variously classified, but a useful classification in terms of function and chemistry would be based on the solubility and acid-base property of "R" groups (Figs 4.4 to 4.7).

Classification of Amino Acids based on Properties and Structures of Side Chains (R-groups).

1. Aliphatic (R-groups consist of carbons and hydrogens)

Glycine - R = H, smallest amino acid with no chiral center.

Alanine - R = CH_3 (methyl group)

Valine - R = branched and hydrophobic; important in protein folding.

Leucine - R = 4-carbon branched side chain.

Isoleucine - R = 4-carbon branched side chain with two chiral centers.

Backbone of amino acids is shown in blue

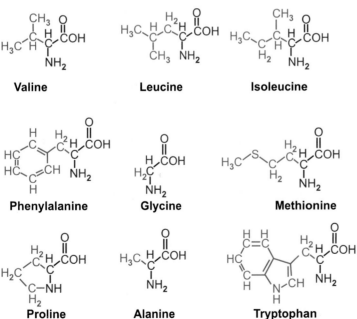

Fig. 4.4: Hydrophobic amino acids

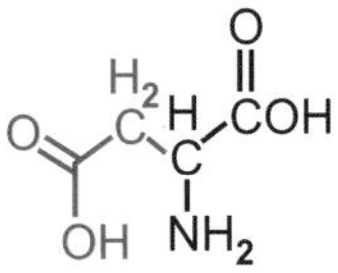

Aspartate

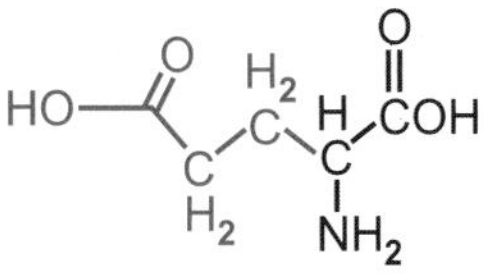

Glutamate

Fig. 4.5: Polar acidic amino acids

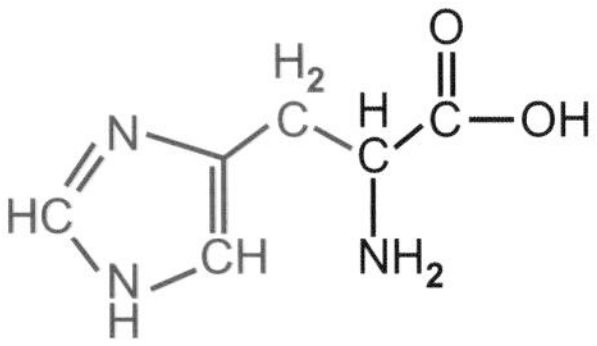

Histidine

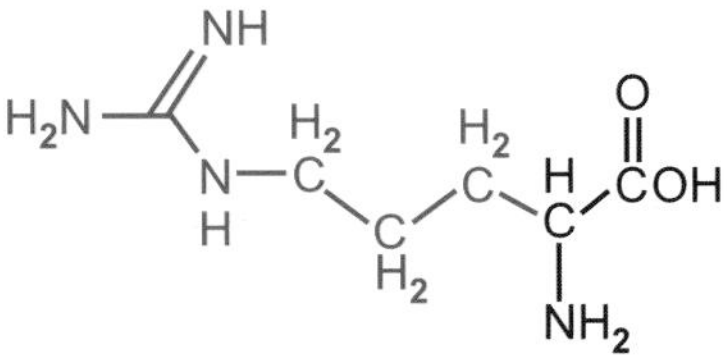

Arginine

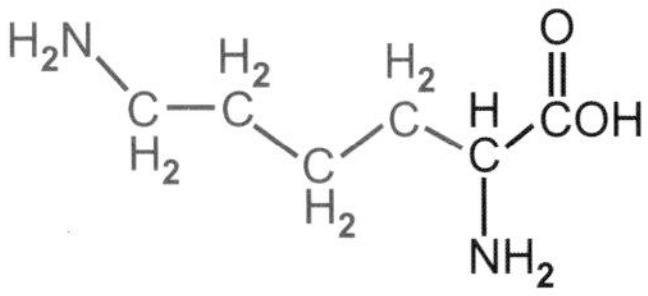

Lysine

Fig. 4.6: Polar basic amino acids

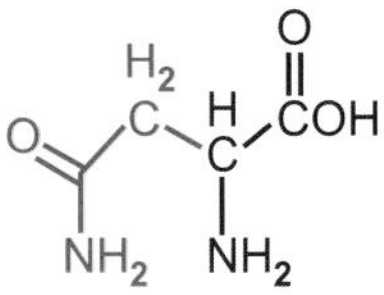

Asparagine

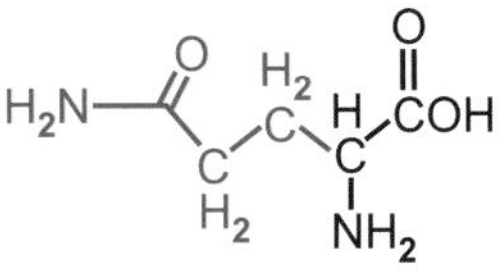

Glutamine

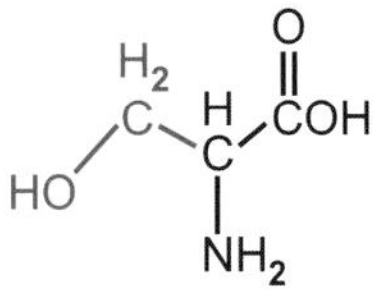

Serine

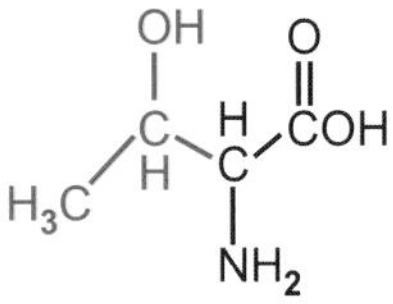

Threonine

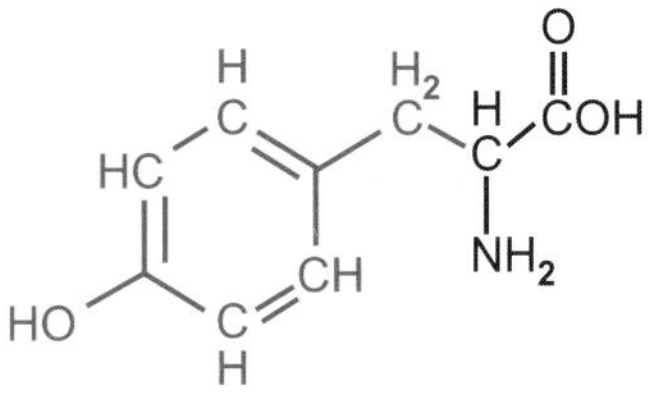

Tyrosine

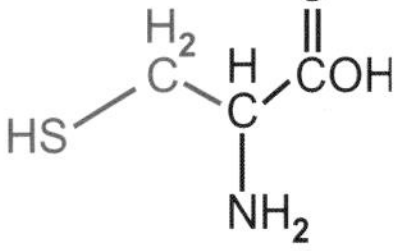

Cysteine

Fig. 4.7: Polar uncharged amino acids

Proline - R = ring; puts bends or kinks in proteins; amino group is part of the ring.

2. Aromatic (R-groups have phenyl ring). Absorb UV light at 280 nm; this property is made use off for quantitating proteins in solution.

   Phenylalanine – R= phenyl ring, which is hydrophobic.

   Tyrosine –R= Phenol ring is hydrophobic, but not as much as phenyl alanine because of presence of hydroxyl group.

   Tryptophan – R = indole ring.

3. Sulfur-containing R-groups

   Methionine- R has – sulfur, which is internal (hydrophobic).

   Cysteine - R has sulfur, which is terminal, highly reactive; can form disulfide bonds

4. Aliphatic side chains with alcohols

   Serine – R has β-hydroxyl group that makes it hydrophilic.

   Threonine – R has β-hydroxy, β-methyl group.

5. Basic R-groups

   Histidine – R has imidazole ring, which is hydrophilic– ring nitrogen is positively charged at neutral pH.

   Lysine –R has 4-carbon side chain with an amino group at ε (epsilon) carbon.

   Arginine – R has a guanido group that acts as a strong base.

6. Acidic R-groups and amide derivatives

   Aspartate -R has carboxyl group at β-carbon, confer negative charges on proteins.

   Glutamate –R has carboxyl group at γ-carbon, confer negative charge on proteins.

   Asparagine - R has amide of aspartate, side groups uncharged but polar.

   Glutamine – R is amide of glutamate, side group uncharged but polar.

   "Amide groups can form H bonds with atoms of other polar amino acids."

Essential vs. Nonessential Amino Acids

Both essential and nonessential amino acids are equally important for growth and development of an organism. Whenever we refer to an amino acid as essential, it only means it is not synthesized by the organism and need to be supplied in the diet. The amino acids arginine, methionine and phenylalanine are considered essential for reasons not directly related to lack of synthesis; arginine is synthesized by mammalian cells but at a rate that is insufficient to meet the growth needs of the body and the majority that is synthesized is cleaved to form urea, methionine is required in large amounts to produce cysteine if the latter amino acid is not adequately supplied in the diet. Similarly, phenylalanine is needed in large amounts to form tyrosine if the latter is not adequately supplied in the diet.

Nonessential amino acids	Essential amino acids
Alanine, Asparagine, Aspartate, Cysteine, Glutamate, Glutamine, Glycine, Proline, Serine, Tyrosine	Arginine, Histidine, Isoleucine Leucine, Lysine, Methionine Phenylalanine, Threonine, Tryptophan, Valine

pK Values of "R" Groups and Backbone of Amino Acids

Acid/Base Group	Approximate pKa
α-amino	9.8
α-carboxylate	2.5
Side chain amino group of lysine and arginine	11.5
Side chain carboxylate of glutamate and aspartate	4.4
Imidazole ring of histidine	6.5
Sulfhydryl group of cysteine	8.5
Alcohol groups of serine and threonine	0 1and 14
Phenol group of tyrosine	10

These ionizable groups change their protonation according to the pH of the surrounding solution.

At any pH more than 1.0 unit above or 1.0 unit below their pK, the group will be completely in one state. It means these groups can undergo protonation or deprotonation within a pH unit of 1.0 on either side of its pKa value.

It is only the imidazole groups of histidyl residues in proteins that act as buffer at physiological range of pH because of its pKa value of 6.5.

Isoelectric Point (pI)

It is the pH at which an amino acid is electrically neutral (the sum of the negative charges equals the sum of the positive charges).

All those amino acids having only two ionizable groups, the pI is the average of the sum of pK1 and pK2.

In case of those having three ionizable groups, the pI is the average of the sum of two nearest pKs.

Properties of "R" Groups in Amino Acids

- *Optical activity:* all amino acids except glycine are optically active, since they have an asymmetric carbon.
- *Light absorption property:* phenylalanine, tyrosine and tryptophan, which have aromatic ring on their side chain, absorb light at 280 nm.
- Amino acids having –OH group on their side chain forms *esters with phosphoric acid* and *O-glycosidic bond* with carbohydrate.
- Amino acids glutamine and asparagines having amide groups on their side chain form *N-glycosidic* bond with carbohydrates.
- The amino group on the side chain of lysine form *Schiff's base (aldimine)* with aldehyde groups of other molecules.
- Sulfhydryl group of cysteine forms *disulfide bond* with sulfhydryl group of another cysteine molecule.

- The imidazole group of histidine, which is fully deprotonated at physiological pH, *acts as a Base*.
- Cyclic structures of proline side chain cause constrains to shape and are *helical breakers* in proteins.
- Methyl group of active methionine (SAM) participate in *transmethylation reaction*.

PEPTIDE BOND

The condensation reaction between α-carboxyl carbon of one amino acid and the α-amino nitrogen of the other amino acid with elimination of a water molecule forms a peptide bond. Series of such condensation reactions lead to the polymerization of amino acids into peptides and proteins. Peptides are small amino acid polymers consisting of few amino acids. Proteins are polypeptides of greatly divergent length. The simplest peptide, a *dipeptide* has only one peptide bond formed between two amino acids.

The peptide bond is slightly shorter than a standard single bond, reflecting the partial delocalization of **pi electrons** from the carbonyl group into orbital shared with the **lone pair** electrons of the amide nitrogen. This **partial double-bond character** inhibits rotation around the peptide bond; thus, the four atoms bound to the carbonyl carbon and amide nitrogen form a plane (Fig. 4.8).

A polypeptide chain may be considered as a series of planes with two angles of rotation between each plane (Fig. 4.9).

Allowed values of angles Phi and Psi are severely restricted by steric interference (Fig. 4.8). Owing to steric interference between consecutive side groups on a polypeptide chain, the *trans* conformation of the peptide bond is strongly favored over the *cis* conformation (Fig. 4.10).

Peptide bonds are rigid planar structures– confer space and shape limitations. Bonds on either side of peptide bond can rotate, which is important in both α-helix and β-sheet. The peptide bond is in trans confirmation. The N and C of peptide bond are polar but uncharged.

Polypeptides has 10 to 2000 amino residues.

Backbone structure is the peptide-linked structure (not the side chain), begins with an α-amino group and ends with an α-carboxylate group.

Proteins contain regions (domains) rich in either hydrophobic or hydrophilic residues.

By convention amino acid sequence is read starting from N-terminal end to C-terminal end.

Examples of Proteins

i. Collagen has 3 polypeptide chains, each with 1052 amino acid residues and similar sequence. The unit is described as homotrimeric.

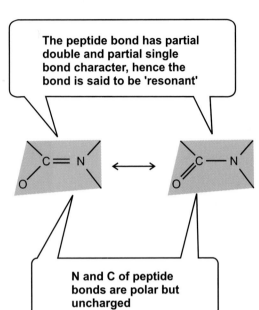

Fig. 4.8: Partial double-bond character of peptide

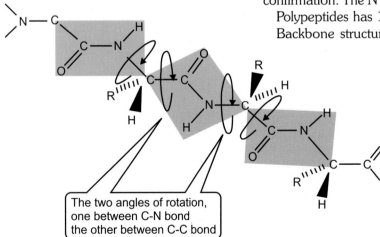

Fig. 4.9: Angles of rotation in a peptide bond

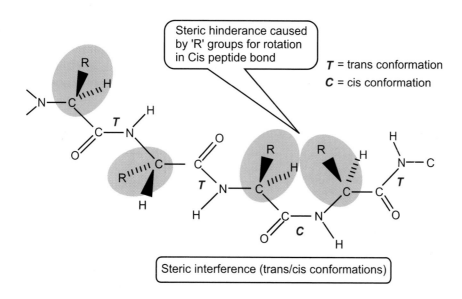

Fig. 4.10: Cis and trans conformation in polypeptide chain

ii. Alcohol dehydrogenase has 2 subunits, each with 374 amino acid residues and similar sequence. The unit is described as homodimeric.
iii. Insulin has 2 chains with dissimilar amino acid content and sequence hence called heterodimeric.
iv. Glucagons has 1 chain, is called monomeric.

Examples of Peptides

The ability of glutathione (γ-glutamylcysteinylglycine) a tripeptide to undergo reversible oxidation-reduction process is important for many biological functions.

Antibiotics such as gramicidin, bacitricin and actinomycin are also peptides.

Hormones such as vasopressin, oxytocin, angiotensin, TRH, bradykinin and kallidin are all peptides.

Proteins have Diversity – How?

Proteins have diversity due to the possible diversity in its amino acid sequence, and post-translational modifications the proteins undergo.

Diversity in amino acid sequence is possible as a consequence to the statistical potential, where a choice of 20 amino acids are available for each position in protein, and due to the presence of two copies for each gene in eukaryotes (humans have 23 types of chromosomes and one pair of each type – a total of 46 chromosomes). This makes it possible to have 2 slightly different versions of each gene – one on each chromosome, which leads to production of 2 slightly different versions of the same protein. Example: Sickle cell anemia where the difference between the mutant protein and the normal protein is one amino acid. An individual can have 2 normal copies, or 1 normal and 1 mutant, or 2 mutant copies.

Diversity due to post-synthetic modification is possible because many of the amino acids in a protein chain undergo chemical modifications after protein synthesis, to enhance their activity. Such a modification is called post-translational or post-synthetic modification of protein. Examples are:

i. Hydroxyproline and hydroxylysine found in collagen are formed by hydroxylation of prolyl and lysyl residues of collagen fiber. Inadequate hydroxylation of prolyl and lysyl residues due to vitamin C deficiency causes scurvy.

ii. γ-carboxyglutamate found in prothrombin and some other proteins involved in blood clotting is formed by γ-carboxylation of glutamyl residues. An inadequate carboxylation of glutamyl residues in prothrombin as a result of vitamin K deficiency causes hemorrhage.

iii. Addition of carbohydrate groups on secreted proteins such as hormones and antibodies makes them more hydrophilic (water-soluble).

iv. Addition of fatty acids and farnesyl groups makes protein more hydrophobic.

v. Phosphoserine and phosphotyrosine found in intracellular proteins are involved in growth and cell division.

vi. Selective cleavage of synthesized proteins that are secreted as inactive precursors makes them active proteins. Examples: fibrinogen to fibrin, chymotrypsinogen to chymotrypsin, and HIV proteins arise from selective cleavage.

FUNCTIONS OF PROTEINS

Proteins are the products of expression of genetic information. Chemically they are linear, unbranched polypeptide chains of amino acids, wherein the amino acids are linked by peptide bonds formed between α-carboxyl of one amino acid and the α-amino group of another amino acid.

Proteins are involved in diverse activities of the living such as:

1. Catalysts in metabolic pathways. Example: enzymes.
2. Transporters and storage. Example: oxygen is transported by hemoglobin. Iron is stored as ferritin.
3. Structural component. Example: collagen.
4. Coordinated motion. Example: movement of flagella and cilia, microtubule movement during mitosis, and muscle contraction.
5. Decoding of genetic information. Example: protein biosynthesis (translation and gene expression).
6. Control of growth and differentiation. Example: promoters and repressors.
7. Immune protection. Example: antibodies.
8. Nerve impulse generation and transmission. Example: receptors.

PROTEIN STRUCTURE

Protein structure has three-dimensional (3D) shape. The 3D shape of protein is important for its function. The 3D shape of protein is the result of different levels of structural organization of polypeptide chain. The protein molecules can have four levels of structural organization – *primary, secondary, tertiary* and *quaternary*.

Primary structure is the content and sequence of amino acids held together by peptide bonds in a polypeptide chain.

Secondary structure is the spatial arrangement of amino acids near to each other in the linear sequence of α-helix, β-pleated sheet, or collagen helix, stabilized by mostly noncovalent bonds such as hydrogen bonds.

Tertiary structure is the spatial arrangement of amino acids that are far from each other in the linear sequence of peptide chain, which cause further folding and bending of the chain.

Quaternary structure is the ordered aggregation of two or more subunits by noncovalent bonds to provide a functional unit.

PRIMARY STRUCTURE

The sequence of amino acids in a polypeptide chain is dictated by DNA sequence in the gene that codes for the specific protein.

The ordered sequence enables secondary, tertiary and quaternary structures of the protein.

Alterations in DNA sequence (mutations) alter the amino acid sequence, which in turn alter the folding and function of protein. Example: sickle cell anemia.

Proteins from different species with same function have conserved structure (homology). Example: 38 out of 105 residues in cytochrome C from 34 species are invariant and many other residues have conservative substitutes (Glu for Asp). *What conclusion?*

The invariant residues must be vital to the function of this enzyme.

SECONDARY STRUCTURE

The polypeptide chain can fold only in one of the three common ways, i.e. α-helix, β-sheet and collagen helix. The primary sequence of amino acid residues determines which way the peptide chain will fold.

The α-helix (Fig. 4.11)

Peptide backbone is coiled in such a way the hydrophilic side chains (R-groups) stick out, where as hydrophobic R-groups face the interior of helical structure.

Helix is right handed tightly coiled rod-like structures.

All the CO and NH on amino acyl residues are 4-apart on the main chain and are hydrogen bonded.

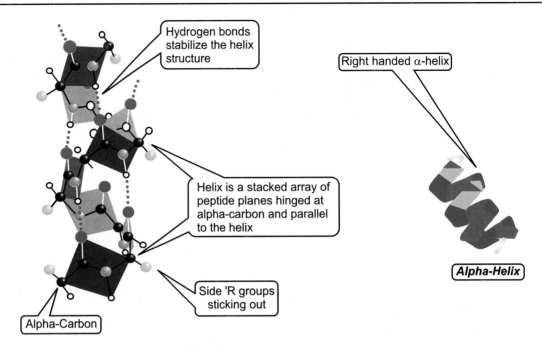

Fig. 4.11: *Alpha-helix*

- Therefore residues 4 apart in the main chain are physically clos€ to each other, but residues 2 apart are on the apposite side of th€ helix and physically distant from each other.
- Distance between each amino acyl residue is 1.5 Angstroms (0.1! nm).
- Number of α-helix in a protein molecule is variable.
- Length of α-helix can be short rods as seen in myoglobi (8 helices) or long rods as seen in α-keratin and fibrin.

Hair – keratin

Hair is made up of three α-helices twisted together to form a protofibri 11 such protofibrils fit together to form a microfibril, which in turn form a macrofibril. Many such macrofibrils are in the hair fiber. I the larger structure, each α-helix is stabilized by disulfide bonds forme€ between interchain cysteinyl residues.

β-pleated Sheets (Fig. 4.12)

Named so, since it is the second structure to be discovered.

These are sheet-like structures formed by nearly fully extendec polypeptide chains placed side by side; distance between amino acy residues is 3.5 Angstrom.

The strands are held together by H-bonds formed between CC and NH groups on different strands, which run parallel or antiparalle to each other (Fig. 1.13).

The most common amino acid in fibrin is Gly, which allow clos contact between H-bonded strands, whereas hydrophobic group

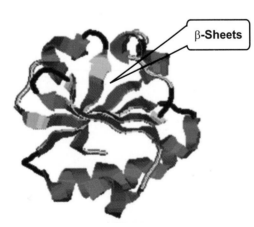

Fig. 4.12: Ribbon model of beta-pleated structure

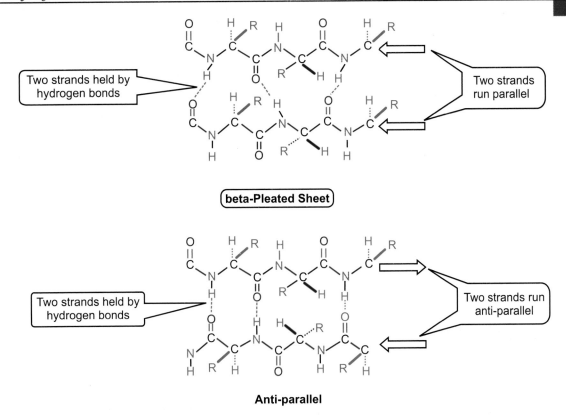

Fig. 4.13: Beta pleated structure of protein

cause distortions and disorders in the structure that allows little stretchiness.

Collagen Helix

Collagen is the protein found in connective tissues, they are very long (300 nm) and strong, rod-like triple helical structures. Their amino acid sequence is unique. One-third is Gly residue which is small and fits inside the cable like structure, the other one-third is Pro, which forms hairpin-like turns in β-turns. The H-bonding between C=O of amino acid **n** to the N-H of the amino acid **n+3** is not possible because of bulky proline in between that breaks the helical structure (Fig. 1.14).

Uncommon amino acids found in collagen are hydroxylysine and hydroxyproline that form covalent bonds between the adjoining strands in the larger structure.

TERTIARY STRUCTURE

Secondary and tertiary structures (Fig.1.15) cannot be demarcated by definition since these levels overlap each other. The hydrophobic bonds along with van der Waals forces are of primary importance in maintaining tertiary structure. Most proteins contain a mixture of α-helix and β-sheet connected by relatively flexible areas that facilitate

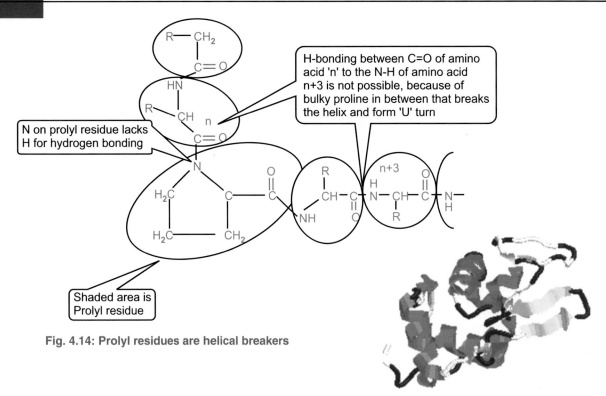

Fig. 4.14: Prolyl residues are helical breakers

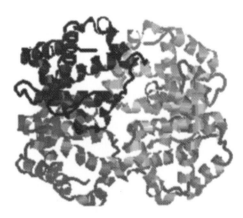

Fig. 4.15: Tertiary structure

further folding of the chain, in such a way the hydrophobic 'R' groups face the interior and hydrophilic 'R' groups face the exterior of the folded protein molecule (the exception being 2 His residues involved in heme binding in myoglobin).

Proteins form lobes or domains, which are globular clusters of α-helix and β-pleats. Domains have specific functions to provide binding sites for small molecules such as NAD, ATP, GTP, and cAMP.

Membrane proteins involved in transporting polar molecules (calcium, glucose) have bundles of α-helices whose internal structure is usually rich in polar residues.

QUATERNARY STRUCTURE

Quaternary structure of protein (Fig. 4.16) is the assembly of two or more polypeptide chains by noncovalent bonds to provide a functional unit. Such an assembly has biological advantages:

- Repair of protein is easier by replacing only the damaged subunit.
- Each subunit is coded by smaller gene.
- Enables easy 3D positioning of *active site amino acid residues* more easily.
- Contributes to *ease of control* of the protein activity, as seen in hemoglobin

Forces that stabilize native conformation of protein

- *Ionic bonds* contributes to lesser extent.
- *van der Waals forces* (dipole-dipole interaction).

Four polypeptide chains in association with each other to provide a biologically functional unit.

Fig. 4.16: Quaternary structure

- *Permanent dipoles* (polar groups C=O and N-H) in core of proteins provide significant contribution to stability.
- *London dispersion forces (-CH₃...CH₃ -)* are transient dipoles between nonpolar side chain groups. Large number of such interactions inside proteins is the major influence on folding.
- *Hydrogen bonding* is usually between N-H to O=C, sometimes S-H to O=C, often H-bond networks in proteins in which a single N-H is H-bonded to multiple O=C, has also major influence on folding.
- *Hydrophobic bonds:* nonpolar substances minimize contact with water and have major influence on folding.
- *Disulphide bonds,* stabilizes 3D structure, especially in an oxidizing environment (in plasma).

PROTEIN DENATURATION

Loss of 3D native structure (except primary structure) of protein that leads to randomized conformation is called denaturation.

Unfolding of one part of a protein's structure destabilizes the rest and promotes further unfolding.

What are the Factors that Disrupt 3D Structure?

Heat, pH extremes, ionic solutions, high concentration of alcohol, and detergents disrupts native conformation of proteins.

STRATEGY FOR PROTEIN SEQUENCING

The basic strategy to determine the content and sequence of amino acids in a protein are:

Determine the Amino Acid Composition

In order to know which amino acids and how many of each amino acid are there in a polypeptide we must break the peptide bonds. This can be accomplished with strong acids (6N HCl) or strong bases or by exhaustive enzymatic digestion. By performing an acid hydrolysis or base hydrolysis we obtain a minimum length for the polypeptide. This information is useful for determining what cleavages to use in divide and conquer step. These procedures destroy several amino acids, so we must be cautious with our estimates.

Break all Disulfide Bonds

Disulfide cross-links complicate the determination of amino acid sequences and usually are cleaved by reduction or oxidation before sequence analysis.

Amino-terminal Sequence Determination

Prior to sequencing peptides, it is necessary to eliminate disulfide bonds within peptides and between peptides. Several different chemical reactions can be used in order to permit separation of peptide strands and prevent protein conformations that are dependent upon disulfide bonds. The most common treatments are to use either 2-*mercaptoethanol* or *dithiothritol*. Both of these chemicals reduce disulfide bonds. To prevent reformation of the disulfide bonds the peptides are treated with *iodoacetic acid* that alkylate the free sulfhydryls. There are three major chemical techniques for sequencing peptides and proteins from the N-terminus. These are *Sanger, Dansyl chloride and Edman techniques*.

Sanger's reagent: This sequencing technique utilizes the compound, 2,4-*dinitrofluorobenzene* (DNF), which reacts with the N-terminal residue under alkaline conditions. The derivatized amino acid can be hydrolyzed and labeled with a dinitrobenzene group that imparts a yellow color to the amino acid. Separation of the modified amino acids (DNP-derivative) by electrophoresis and comparison with the migration of DNP-derivative standards allows for the identification of the N-terminal amino acid.

Dansyl chloride: Like DNF, dansyl chloride reacts with the N-terminal residue under alkaline conditions. Analysis of the modified amino acids is carried out similarly to the Sanger method except that the dansylated amino acids are detected by fluorescence. This imparts a higher sensitivity into this technique over that of the Sanger method.

Edman degradation: The utility of the Edman degradation technique is that it allows for additional amino acid sequence to be obtained from the N-terminus inward. Using this method it is possible to obtain the entire sequence of peptides. This method utilizes *phenylisothiocyanate* to react with the N-terminal residue under alkaline conditions. The resultant phenylthiocarbamyl derivatized amino acid is hydrolyzed in anhydrous acid. The hydrolysis reaction results in a rearrangement of the released N-terminal residue to a phenylthiohydantoin derivative. As in the Sanger and Dansyl chloride methods, the N-terminal residue is tagged with an identifiable marker; however, the added advantage of the Edman process is that the remainder of the peptide is intact. The entire sequence of reactions can be repeated over and over to obtain the sequences of the peptide. This process has subsequently been automated to allow rapid and efficient sequencing of even extremely small quantities of peptide.

Enzyme	Source	Specificity
Carboxypeptidase A	Bovine pancreas	Will not cleave when C-terminal residue is Arg, Lys, or Pro, or if Pro residues are next to terminal residues
Carboxypeptidase B	Bovine pancreas	Will not cleave when C-terminal residue is Arg, Lys or when Pro residue is next to terminal residue
Carboxypeptidase C	Citrus leaves	Cleaves all free C-terminal residues, pH optima is 3.5
Carboxypeptidase Y	Yeast	Cleaves all C-terminal residues, but slowly at Gly residue

Protease Digestion

Due to the limitations of the Edman degradation technique, peptides longer than 50 residues cannot be sequenced completely. The ability to obtain peptides of this length from larger proteins is facilitated by the use of **endopeptidases** that cleave proteins at specific sites. The resultant smaller peptides can be chromatographically separated and sequenced by Edman degradation technique.

Enzyme	Source	Specificity	Additional points
Trypsin	Bovine Pancreas	Cleaves Peptide bond C-terminus to Arg, Lys but not if next to Pro	Highly specific for positively charged residues
Chymotrypsin	Bovine pancreas	Cleaves peptide bonds C-terminal to Phe, Tyr, Trp but not if next to Pro	Prefers bulky hydrophobic residues, cleaves slowly at Asn, His, Met, and Ile
Elastase	Bovine pancreas	Cleaves peptide bonds C-terminal to Ala, Gly, Ser, Val, but not if next to Pro	
Thermolysin	Bacillus thermo-proteolyticus	Cleaves peptide bonds N-terminal to, Ile, Met, Phe, Trp, Tyr, Val but not if next to Pro	Prefers small neutral residues, can cleave at Ala, Asp, His, Thr
Pepsin	Bovine gastric mucosa	Cleaves peptide bond N-terminal to Leu, Phe, Trp, Tyr but when next to Pro	Exhibits little specificity, requires a low pH
Endo-peptidase V8	*Staphylococcus aureus*	Cleaves peptide bond C-terminal	

Carboxy-terminal Sequence Determination

No reliable chemical techniques exist for sequencing the C-terminal amino acid of peptides. However, few *exopeptidases* have been identified that cleave peptides at the C-terminal residue, which can then be analyzed chromatographically and compared to standard amino acids. These classes of exopeptidases are called *carboxypeptidases*.

Chemical Digestion of Proteins

The most commonly used chemical reagent that cleaves peptide bonds by recognition of specific amino acid residues is *cyanogen bromide (CNBr)*. This reagent specifically cleaves methionine residues from the C-terminal side of polypeptide chain. The number of peptide fragments that result from CNBr cleavage is equivalent to one more than the number of methionine residues in the protein.

The most reliable chemical technique for C-terminal residue identification is *hydrazinolysis*. A peptide is treated with **hydrazine (NH$_2$-NH$_2$)** at high temperature (90°C) for an extended length of time (20-100hr). This treatment cleaves all of the peptide bonds yielding amino-acyl hydrazides of all the amino acids except the C-terminal residue, which can be identified chromatographically compared to amino acid standards. Due to the high percentage of hydrazine induced side reactions this technique is only used on carboxypeptidase resistant peptides.

Divide and Conquer

Break the polypeptide into fragments by cleaving at specific amino acids. Several cleavage methods are available, each, of which have different specificity (cleave at different amino acid).

Repeat steps 3 and 4 to determine sub-sequence and create "overlapping".

The initial cleavage is made as specific as possible to generate large peptide fragments. These fragments can be positioned relative to one another after treatment of the original polypeptide by a second cleavage procedure that generates fragments whose sequence extend across the initial cleavage points (referred to as overlapping peptides). The amino acid sequence of each overlap peptide orders two or more of the original fragments.

Reconstruct the original protein from the overlapping peptides and information gained from the original protein; we should be able to construct a unique sequence for the protein or polypeptide of interest. The overlaps should be at least two amino acids in length.

Locate the Disulfide Bonds

Primary structure analysis of a cysteine-containing protein is incomplete until the location of disulfide bonds established. The location of these bonds can be assigned using a multistep process.

PROTEIN SEPARATION TECHNIQUES

Size Exclusion Chromatography (Fig. 4.17)

This chromatographic technique is based upon the use of a porous gel in the form of insoluble beads placed into a column. As a solution of proteins is passed through the column, small proteins can penetrate into the pores of the beads and, therefore, are retarded in their rate of travel through the column. The larger proteins a protein is the less likely it will enter the pores. Different beads with different pore sizes can be used depending upon the desired protein size separation profile.

Ion Exchange Chromatography

Each individual protein exhibits a distinct overall net charge at a given pH. Some proteins will be negatively charged and some will be positively charged at the same pH. This property of proteins is the basis for ion exchange chromatography. Fine cellulose resins are used that are either negatively (cation exchanger) or positively (anion exchanger) charged (Fig. 4.18). Proteins with opposite charge to that of the resin are retained, as the proteins solution is passed through

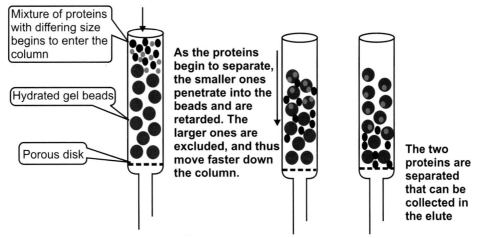

Fig. 4.17: Size exclusion chromatography

the column. The bound proteins are then eluted by passing a solution of ions bearing a charge opposite to that of the column. By utilizing a gradient of increasing ionic strength, proteins with increasing affinity for the resin are progressively eluted.

Example of anion exchanger is diethylcellulose, which has positive charge.

Example of cation exchanger is carboxymethylcellulose, which has negative charge.

Affinity Chromatography

Proteins have high affinities for their substrates, co-factors, prosthetic groups, receptors, or their antibodies. This affinity can be exploited in the purification of proteins. A column of beads bearing the high affinity compound can be prepared and a solution of protein passed through the column. Then passing a solution of unbound soluble high affinity compound through the column elutes the bound proteins.

High Performance Liquid Chromatography (HPLC)

In column chromatography, the separation capability of the column is enhanced by having more tightly packed smaller size resin. In gravity flow columns, the limitation is the column packing and the time the protein solution takes to pass through the column. In HPLC, fine diameter resins are tightly packed to impart increased resolution, and to overcome the flow limitations the solution of proteins are pumped through the column under high pressure. HPLC columns can be used for size exclusion or charge separation.

An additional separation technique commonly used with HPLC is to utilize hydrophobic resins to retard the movement of nonpolar proteins. The proteins are then eluted from the column with a gradient of increasing concentration of an organic solvent. This latter form of HPLC is termed reversed-phase HPLC.

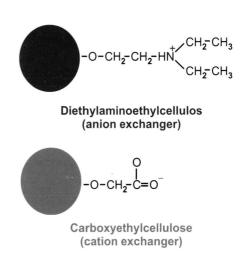

Diethylaminoethylcellulos (anion exchanger)

Carboxyethylcellulose (cation exchanger)

Fig. 4.18: Ion exchange cellulose materials

Electrophoresis of Proteins

Proteins can also be characterized according to size and charge by separation in an electric field (electrophoresis) within solid sieving gels made from polymerized and cross-linked acrylamide. The most commonly used technique is termed SDS (sodium dodecyl sulfate) polyacrylamide gel electrophoresis (SDS-PAGE). The gel is a thin slab of acrylamide polymerized between two glass plates. This technique utilizes a negatively charged detergent (sodium dodecyl sulfate) to denature and solubilize proteins. SDS denatured proteins have a uniform negative charge such that all proteins will migrate through the gel in the electric field based solely upon size. The larger the protein size the more slowly it will move through the matrix of the polyacrylamide. After electrophoretic separation, the migration distance of unknown proteins relative to known standard proteins is assessed by various staining or radiographic detection techniques.

The use of polyacrylamide gel electrophoresis is also used to determine the isoelectric charge of proteins (pI). This technique is termed *isoelectric focusing*. Isoelectric focusing utilizes a thin tube of polyacrylamide made in the presence of a mixture of small positively and negatively charged molecules termed ampholytes. The ampholytes have a range of pIs that establish a pH gradient along the gel when current is applied. Proteins will therefore cease to migrate in the gel when they reach the point where the ampholytes have a pH equal to the pI of the proteins.

Centrifugation of Proteins

Proteins will sediment through a solution in a centrifugal field dependent upon their mass. Analytical centrifugation measures the rate that proteins sediment. The most common solution utilized is a linear gradient of sucrose (generally from 5-20%). Proteins are layered atop the gradient in an ultracentrifuge tube then subjected to centrifugal fields in excess of 100,000-xg. The sizes of unknown proteins can then be determined by comparing their migration distance in the gradient with those of known standard proteins.

CLINICAL SIGNIFICANCE OF MUTANT PROTEINS

Several examples of diseases related to abnormal (mutant) proteins are presented below.

Sickle Cell Anemia

The substitution of a hydrophobic amino acid (Valine) for an acidic amino acid (glutamate) in the β-chain of hemoglobin results in sickle cell anemia also called as hemoglobin S (HbS) disease. This change of a single amino acid alters the structure of hemoglobin molecules in such a way that the deoxygenated hemoglobin polymerize and precipitate within the erythrocyte leading to their characteristic sickle shape.

Collagens are the most abundant proteins in the body. Alterations in collagen structure arising from abnormal genes or abnormal processing of collagen proteins results in numerous diseases, including Larsen syndrome, scurvy, osteogenesis imperfecta and Ehlers-Danlos syndrome.

Ehlers-Danlos Syndrome

Ehlers-Danlos syndrome is actually the name associated with at least ten distinct disorders that are biochemically and clinically distinct, yet all these disorders manifest structural weakness in connective tissue as a result of defective collagen structure.

Osteogenesis Imperfecta

Osteogenesis imperfecta encompasses more than one disorder. At least four biochemically and clinically distinguishable maladies have been identified as osteogenesis imperfecta, all of which are characterized by multiple fractures and resultant bone deformities.

Marfan's Syndrome

Marfan's syndrome manifests itself as a disorder of the connective tissue and was originally believed to be the result of abnormal collagens. However, recent evidence has shown that Marfan's syndrome results from mutations in the extracellular protein *fibrillin*, which is an integral constituent of the noncollagenous microfibrils of the extracellular matrix.

Familial Hypercholesterolemia

Familial hypercholesterolemia is the result of genetic defects in the gene encoding the receptor for low-density lipoprotein (LDL). These defects result in the synthesis of abnormal LDL receptors that fail to bind LDLs, or that bind LDLs but the receptor/LDL complexes are not properly internalized and degraded. This results in elevated serum cholesterol and plaque formation.

Oncogen

A number of proteins can contribute to cellular transformation and carcinogenesis when their basic structure is disrupted by mutations in their genes. These genes are termed ***proto-oncogenes***. For some of these proteins, all that is required to convert them to the ***oncogenic*** form is a single amino acid substitution. The cellular gene ***c-Ras*** is observed to sustain single amino acid substitutions at positions 12 or 61 with high frequency in colon carcinomas. Mutations in c-Ras are most frequently observed genetic alterations in colon cancer.

PLASMA PROTEINS

Plasma is the watery part of whole blood obtained after removing the cellular components by use of anticoagulants.

Almost 8 to 10 percent of plasma is composed of proteins, and organic and inorganic components. Protein component of plasma varies from 6 to 8 g/dl, which is the balance between rate of synthesis and their degradation, and relative amount of water and protein in vascular compartment. Hence a change in total plasma protein does not mean an abnormality in protein metabolism.

Almost all the plasma proteins are synthesized in the liver with the exception of immunoglobulins, which are synthesized by plasma cells. Plasma proteins are heterogenous with regard to their origin and function. All the proteins are glycoproteins, probably with the exception of nascent albumin.

Proteins being colloidal in aqueous solution exert osmotic pressure and help maintain intravascular fluid volume and blood pressure.

Hypoproteinemia can result from hemodilution, or decreased synthesis of albumin or immunoglobulins albumin synthesis.

Hyperproteinemia can result from dehydration, and increased synthesis of immunoglobulins.

A fall in albumin is invariably compensated with a rise in immunoglobulins. A large percent change in any one of the many proteins, may not cause a detectable change in the total plasma protein concentration, since normal range of plasma proteins is very wide.

Functions of Plasma Proteins

- Regulation of water distribution between intravascular and extra-vascular compartments, by exerting colloidal osmotic pressure.
- Plasma proteins play an important role in regulation of acid-base balance.
- Transport of water-insoluble molecules, such as lipids, unconjugated bilirubin, and drugs in aqueous blood.
- Blood clotting and fibrinolysis (hemostasis).
- Immune response of the individual is the combined function of immunoglobulins, complements and acute-phase proteins. Concentration of acute phase proteins in plasma may get elevated by 50 to 10000 folds under stressful conditions such as tissue damage, infections, and malignancies.

Major components of serum proteins on electrophoretic separation		
Fraction	*Major protein*	*Concentration in g/dl*
Albumin	Albumin and prealbumin	3.5 to 5 g/dl
α1-globulin	α1-antitrypsin	
α2-globulin	α2-macroglobulin	
β-globulin	LDL, transferrin, and complement (C3)	2.1 to 4.2 g/dl
γ-globulin	Immunoglobulins	

Serum proteins can be separated by electrophoresis into five major fractions. They are albumin, α-1-globulin, α-2-globulin, β-globulin, and γ-globulin (Fig. 4.19).

Albumin has a half-life of 20 days and is synthesized in the liver. Serum albumin levels are decreased (hypoalbuminemia) in nephrotic

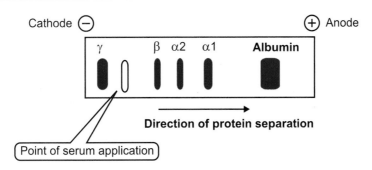

Cathode ⊖   ⊕ Anode

Direction of protein separation

Point of serum application

Fig. 4.19: Electrophoretic separation of serum

syndrome, liver diseases, dilution of blood, redistribution of water between compartments, increased catabolism as in chronic diseases, and loss of albumin as seen in burns, and enteropathy.

The disorders associated with albumin levels are bisalbuminemia (more than one chemical variant), analbuminemia (genetic disorder where albumin is absent), and elevated albumin as a result of dehydration and loss of protein-free fluid.

Consequences of hypoalbuminemia are:
• decreased osmotic pressure and edema, and
• binding and transport of various blood constituents are affected.

In hypoalbuminemia the administration of warfarin and salicylates together, cause an increase in the free form of warfarin that can cause bleeding. Similarly administration of salicylates in jaundice results in an elevation of free form of unconjugated bilirubin that can lead to kernicterus.

Acute-phase proteins are involved in initiation and control of inflammatory reaction, along with complements, immunoglobulins, and cellular components. Examples are C-reactive protein (CRP), and alpha-1-antitrypsin (α-1-AT).

C-reactive protein is so named because it binds to C-polysaccharide found in the capsule of pneumococci. CRP complexes with phospholipids released during tissue damage, and activate complement pathways. Serum levels of CRP are elevated very early in acute infections, and tissue damage.

Alpha-1-antitrypsin controls inflammatory response by inhibiting proteases in particular elastase. Alpha-1-antitrypsin is deficient in emphysema patients. The molecular basis of emphysema in tobacco smokers is the inability of α-1-AT to bind and inactivate elastase (in tobacco smokers the –S-CH$_3$ of methionine residues in α-1-AT are oxidized to the level of sulfoxide, thereby it fails to bind elastase).

Immunoglobulins

Immunoglobulins are synthesized in B lymphocytes (plasma cells). The immunoglobulin is schematically represented as a 'Y' shaped molecule (Fig. 4.20). The molecule is composed of four polypeptide chains; two each are designated as heavy and light chains, linked by disulfide bonds.

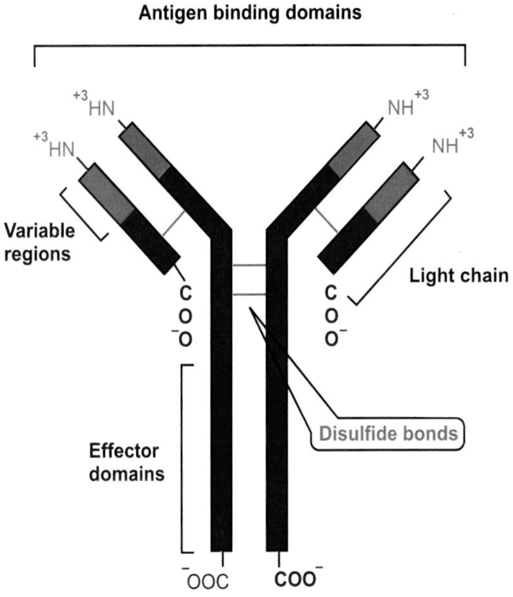

Antigen binding domains

Variable regions

Light chain

Disulfide bonds

Effector domains

Fig. 4.20: Schematic diagram of IgG

The light chains are of kappa or lambda type, but never a mixture of both. The heavy chains are of one of the five types (α, μ, γ, ε, or δ) that determine the class of immunoglobulin. The immunoglobulins are designated as IgA, IgM, IgG, IgE, and IgD respectively.

The amino terminal end of both light chain and heavy chain has variable amino acid sequence that is designated as variable region, which binds antigen. The binding of antigen induces a conformational change in the constant region (effector domain) of heavy chain that facilitates binding of complement to the effector domain of the molecule.

Class of immunoglobulin	Function
IgA	It is a dimmer, belonging to secretory class. It protects the body surface and activates alternate pathway of complement system.
IgM	It is a pentamer, formed as a primary response to antigens. It activates classical pathway of complement system and protects bloodstream.
IgG	It is a monomer, formed as a secondary response to antigens. It activates classical pathway of complement system, neutralizes toxins, and protects extravascular compartment. It crosses placental barrier.
IgE	It is a monomer always bound to mast cells. Binding of antigen to IgE results in release of mediatros and hypersensitivity reaction.
IgD	Function not known.

Chemistry of Carbohydrates

5

Carbohydrates are among the most abundant molecules on earth. Carbohydrates are carbon compounds that contain large quantities of hydroxyl groups. Even the simplest carbohydrates have an aldehyde or a ketone moiety. All carbohydrates can be classified as **monosaccharides, oligosaccharides** or **polysaccharides**. Oligosaccharides are made of 2 to 10 monosaccharide units linked by glycosidic bonds. Polysaccharides are much larger, made of hundreds of monosaccharide units linked by glycosidic bonds. The presence of the hydroxyl groups allows carbohydrates to interact with the aqueous environment and to participate in hydrogen bonding, both within and between chains. Derivatives of the carbohydrates can contain nitrogens, phosphates or sulfur compounds. Carbohydrates can also combine with lipid to form glycolipids, or with protein to form glycoproteins.

Functions

1. Yield energy (ATP) to drive metabolic processes (e.g. oxidation of glucose).
2. Energy-storage molecules (e.g. glycogen, and starch).
3. Structural constituent of cell walls and exoskeletons of some organisms (e.g. cellulose, and chitin).
4. Carbohydrates are the components of coenzymes (ribose is the component of FAD) and nucleic acids (ribose and deoxyribose are the constituents of RNA and DNA).

Carbohydrate Nomenclature

The predominant carbohydrates encountered in the body are structurally related to the **aldotriose** (glyceraldehydes) and to the **ketotriose** (dihydroxyacetone). All carbohydrates contain at least one asymmetrical (chiral) carbon and are therefore optically active. In addition, carbohydrates can exist in either of two conformations as determined by the orientation of the hydroxyl group about the asymmetric carbon farthest from the carbonyl carbon (the one adjacent to the terminal primary alcohol). With a few exceptions, carbohydrates of physiological significance exist in the **D-conformation**. The mirror-image conformations, called *enantiomers* are in the **L-conformation** (Fig. 5.1).

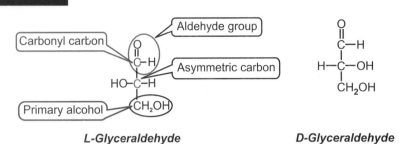

L-Glyceraldehyde   *D-Glyceraldehyde*

Fig. 5.1: D and L isomers of glycerose

Classification

Carbohydrates are described based on the number of monomers they contain.

1. Monosaccharides are single sugar unit $(CH_2O)_n$ where n = 3 to 6; one sugar molecule
2. Oligosaccharides are polymers of 2 to 20 monosaccharide units.
3. Polysaccharides are polymers of greater than 20 monosaccharide units.
4. Glycoconjugates are derivatives of carbohydrates; carbohydrates attached to proteins (glycoprotein), lipids (glycolipid), or peptide chains (glycosaminoglycans).

MONOSACCHARIDES

The monosaccharides found in humans are further classified based on the number of carbons they contain, and the type of carbonyl group (-C=O) in their backbone structures. Majority of monosaccharides contain four to six carbon atoms.

The aldehyde and ketone moieties of monosaccharides with five and six carbons react spontaneously with alcohol groups present in neighboring carbons to form intramolecular **hemiacetals** or **hemiketals** respectively. This results in the formation of five- or six-membered rings. Because the five-membered ring structure resembles the organic molecule **furan**, derivatives with this structure are termed **furanoses.** Those with six-membered rings resemble the organic molecule **pyran** and are termed **pyranoses.** These structures are depicted in either **Fischer** or **Haworth-style,** and also in **chair** and **boat-form** (Fig. 5.2).

The numbering of the carbons in carbohydrates starts from the carbonyl carbon for aldoses, or the carbon nearest to carbonyl for ketoses. The ring forms can open and re-close allowing rotation to

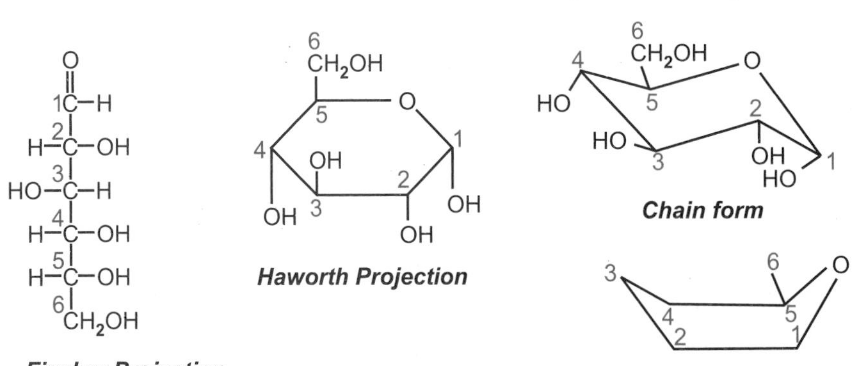

Fischer Projection

Haworth Projection

Chain form

Boat form

Fig. 5.2: Glucose structure depicted in different forms

occur about the carbon bearing the reactive carbonyl to yield two distinct configurations (α-glucose has the -OH group below the plane of the ring, and β-glucose has the -OH group above the plane of the ring) of the hemiacetals and hemiketals. The carbon about which this rotation occurs is the **anomeric carbon** and the two forms are termed **anomers**. The anomeric carbohydrates can change spontaneously between the α and β configurations. This process is known as **mutarotation** (Fig. 5.3).

When glucose molecule is drawn in the Fischer projection, the configuration places the hydroxyl attached to the **anomeric carbon** to the right. When drawn in the Haworth projection the α configuration places the hydroxyl downward. The chair form and

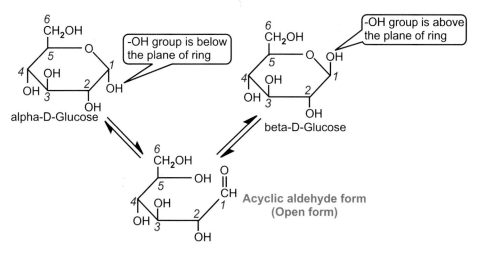

Fig. 5.3: Mutarotation of glucose and the formation of alpha and beta anomers

the boat form more correctly describe the spatial relationship of the atoms in the furanose and pyranose ring structures (Fig. 5.4). The chair form is the more stable of the two. Constituents of the ring that project above or below the plane of the ring are **axial** and those that project parallel to the plane are **equatorial**. In the chair conformation, the orientation of the hydroxyl group about the anomeric carbon of α-D-glucose is axial and in β-D-glucose it is equatorial.

Epimerism of Sugars

When two or more sugars are similar to each other in their chemical formula, but differ from each other with regard to the orientation of hydroxyl group arround a single carbon atom they are called epimers. For example, D-glucose, D-mannose, and D-galactose have same chemical formula, but D-glucose and D-mannose are a pair of epimers, since the difference between the two is only with regard to

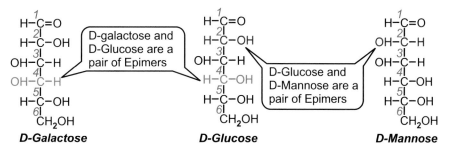

Fig. 5.4: Epimers of D-glucose

orientation of –OH group at carbon-2. Similarly D-glucose and D-galactose are a pair of epimers, since they differ from each other with regard to the orientation of –OH group at carbon-4.

Derivatives of monosaccharides

1. *Sugar phosphates* are the active forms of sugars in which they enter metabolic pathways.
2. *Deoxy sugars:* The hydroxyl group on C-2 is replaced by hydrogen atom, e.g. conversion of ribose to deoxyribose (deoxyribose is a structural component of DNA).
3. *Amino sugars:* In amino sugars, an amino group replaces one of the hydroxyl groups (OH).
4. *Sugar alcohols:* Polyhydroxy alcohols are derived from sugars by substituting their carbonyl oxygen by a hydroxyl group, e.g. glyceraldehydes to glycerol, and ribose to ribitol (replace "-ose" with "-itol").
5. *Sugar acids:* Carbonyl carbon or highest carbon is oxidized to a carboxylate group, e.g glucose to gluconate or glucuronate (important constituent in many polysaccharide).
6. Ascorbic acid is derived from D-glucuronate (enzyme required for this conversion is absent in primates; hence Vit C must be supplied in the diet).

DISACCHARIDES

The linking of two monosaccharides by glycosidic bond yields a disaccharide. A covalent bond formation between the hydroxyl group at anomeric carbon of a cyclic sugar, and the hydroxyl of a second sugar or another alcohol containing compound is designated as **glycosidic bond**, and the resultant molecule is a **glycoside**. Physiologically important disaccharides are sucrose, lactose and maltose.

Sucrose

Sucrose is the sugar present in sugar cane and sugar beets. It is composed of glucose and fructose linked through an α-(1,2) β-glycosidic bond (Fig. 5.5).

Lactose

Lactose is found exclusively in the milk of mammals. It is composed of galactose and glucose linked by a β-(1→ 4) glycosidic bond (Fig. 5.6).

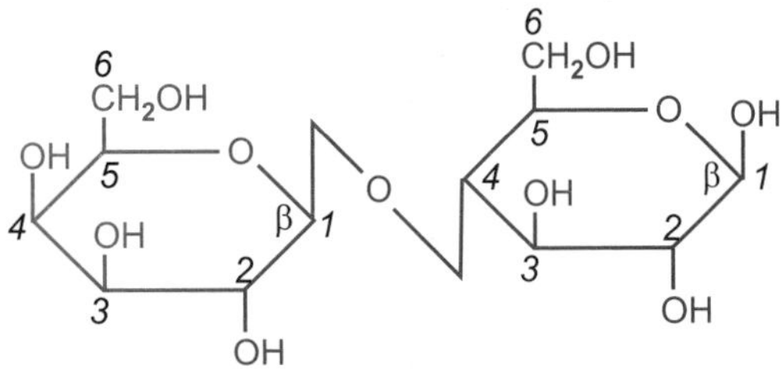

Maltose

Maltose is the major degradation product of starch. It is composed of two glucose monomers linked by an α-(1→ 4) glycosidic bond (Fig. 5.7).

Cellobiose is a plant polysaccharide, where 2 molecules of β-D-glucose are linked by 1→ 4 glycosidic bond.

Trehalose is a nonreducing disaccharide formed by α(1 → 1) glycosidic linkage between 2 molecules of α-D-glucose

Fig. 5.5: Sucrose (α-D-glucopyranosyl (1→2) β-D-fructofuranoside)

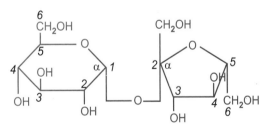

Fig. 5.6: Lactose (β-D-galactopyranosyl (1→4) β-D-glucopyranoside)

Reducing and Nonreducing Sugars

All monosaccharides and most disaccharides have a reactive carbonyl group or anomeric carbon that can be oxidized. Examples: glucose, maltose, cellobiose, and lactose.

Reducing sugars can be detected by their ability to reduce Cu^{2+} to Cu^+ in Benedict's reagent (color changes from blue to red in presence of reducing sugars).

Nonreducing sugars fail to reduce copper in Benedict's solution, since both anomeric carbons are in a glycosidic bond (e.g. sucrose)(Fig. 5.8).

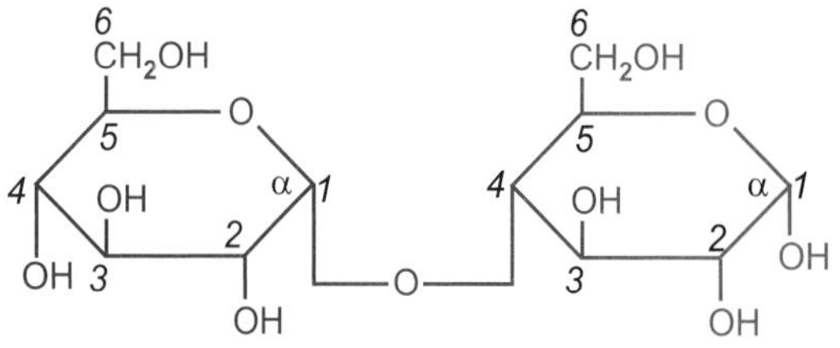

Fig. 5.7: Maltose (α-D-glucopyranosyl-(1→4) α-D-glucopyranoside)

POLYSACCHARIDES

Most of the carbohydrates found in nature occur in the form of high molecular weight polymers called **polysaccharides**. The monomeric building blocks used to generate polysaccharides can be varied. However, the predominant monosaccharide found in polysaccharides is D-glucose. When polysaccharides are composed of only one type of monosaccharide, they are termed **homopolysaccharides**. Those polysaccharides composed of more than one type of monosaccharide are termed **heteropolysaccharides**. Often polysaccharides are classified based on their biological role: Starch is storage form of

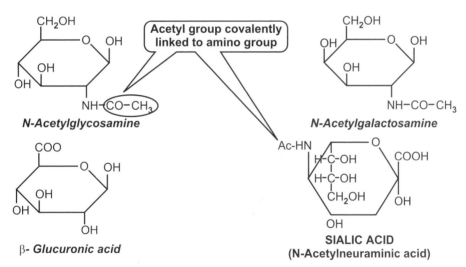

Fig. 5.8: Glucuronic acid and amino sugars

carbohydrate in plant; glycogen is storage form of carbohydrate in animals. Bacteria have both starch and glycogen.

Starch

Starch is a mixture of amylose and amylopectin. Amylose is an unbranched polymer of 100-1000 α-D-glucose molecules in (1→ 4) glycosidic linkages. Amylopectin is a branched polymer of α-D-glucose with (1 → 4) linkages in the linear part, and (1→ 6) linkage at branch points (Fig. 5.9). The branches are present once every 25 residues; side chains are 15-25 residues long. The enzyme α-**amylase** is an endoglycosidase found in human saliva and plants that randomly

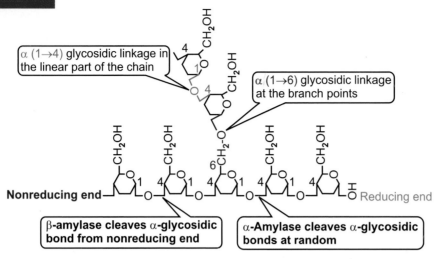

α (1→4) glycosidic linkage in the linear part of the chain

α (1→6) glycosidic linkage at the branch points

Nonreducing end

Reducing end

β-amylase cleaves α-glycosidic bond from nonreducing end

α-Amylase cleaves α-glycosidic bonds at random

Fig. 5.9: Structure of amylopectin and glycogen

hydrolyzes the α (1→ 4) glycosidic bonds of amylose and amylopectin. The enzyme β-**amylase** is an exoglycosidase found in higher plants that hydrolyzes maltose residues from nonreducing ends of amylopectin (Fig. 5.9).

Glycogen

Glycogen is the major form of stored carbohydrate in animals. This crucial molecule is a highly branched and compact homopolymer of β-D-glucose, with (1 → 4) linkages in the linear part and (1→ 6) linkage at branch points. The branches are present once every 8-10 residues; branches containing as many as 50,000 glucose residues that result in the coiling of polymer chains. This compactness allows large amounts of carbon energy to be stored in a small volume, with little effect on cellular osmolarity.

Cellulose and Chitin are Structural Polysaccharides

Cellulose

Cellulose is the structural carbohydrate of plants. It is a straight chain homoglycan of β-D-glucose with (1→ 4) glycosidic linkages. The chain length ranges from 300-15,000 glucose residues. The β-glycosidic linkages are not hydrolyzed by human digestive enzymes (α-amylase). Thus it is an important source of fiber content (nondigestible polysaccharide) in the diet. Extensive H-bonding within and between cellulose chains makes bundles or fibrils that are rigid.

Chitin

Chitin is the structural carbohydrates found in invertebrates, which forms the shell and exoskeleton of insects and crustaceans. It is a linear polymer that consists of N-acetyl-D-glucosamine residues joined by β-(1 → 4) linkage. Lots of H-bonding between adjacent strands makes it rigid and hard.

GLYCOCONJUGATES

Glycoconjugates are heteroglycans that are of three types.

1. **Proteoglycans** are complexes of polysaccharides called glycosaminoglycans and core proteins. They are found in extra-cellular matrix of connective tissues. Glycosaminoglycans are unbranched heteroglycans of repeating disaccharide units made of amino sugar (D-galactosamine or D-glucosamine) and β-uronic acid, e.g. hyaluronic acid (Fig. 5.10) found in cartilage and synovial fluid.

2. **Peptidoglycans** are found in cell wall of bacteria. It is composed of alternating residues of N-acetylglucosamine and N-acetylmuramic acid joined by α-(1→ 4) linkages.

3. **Glycoproteins** are proteins to which oligosaccharides are attached. Carbohydrate chain length varies from 1-30 residues, e.g. enzymes, hormones, structural proteins, and transport proteins found in eukaryotic cells. Oligosaccharides are attached to proteins with one of the two configurations:
   1. O-linked - carbohydrate bonded to -OH of serine or threonine
   2. N-linked - carbohydrate (usually N-acetylglucosamine) linked to asparagines.

CARBOHYDRATES SERVE AS INFORMATION-RICH MOLECULES

1. **Asialoglycoprotein receptors** are present in liver cells. The circulating glycoproteins without sialic acid groups attached to it (aged proteins) are recognized by these receptors and the proteins get internalized for removal. Presence of sialic acid residues attached to glycoproteins such as antibodies and peptide hormones, prevent them from being internalized by hepatocytes. Presence of sialic acid on terminal galactose on these proteins marks the passage of time; when they are removed (usually by the protein itself), the glycoproteins are removed from circulation.

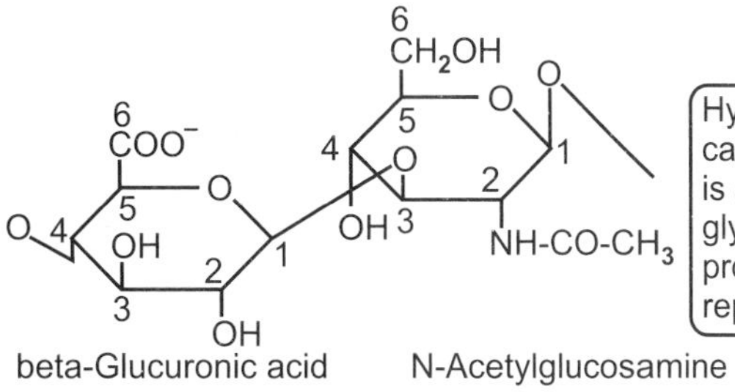

beta-Glucuronic acid   N-Acetylglucosamine

Hyaluronic acid found in cartilage & synovial fluid is an example of glycosaminoglycan (part of proteoglycan) made of repeating disaccharide unit.

Fig. 5.10: Hyaluronic acid

2. **Lectins** are carbohydrate-binding proteins of plant origin that contain 2 or more binding sites for carbohydrate units found on cell membranes of *erythrocytes* and other cells. By virtue of this lectins cross-link or agglutinate erythrocytes and other cells.

3. **Many viruses and bacteria** gain entry into host cells via carbohydrates displayed on cell surface. Influenza virus contains a hemagglutinin protein that recognizes sialic acid residues on cells lining respiratory tract and binds to it. *Neisseria gonorrhoeae* infects human genital and oral epithelial cells because of recognition of cell surface carbohydrates by the glycoproteins on the cell surface of *N. gonorrhoeae*.

4. **Interaction of sperm with ovulated eggs** Ovulated eggs contain zona pellucida, an extracellular coat made of O-linked oligosaccharides. Sperm cells have receptor for these carbohydrates. Binding of sperm to egg causes release of proteases and hyaluronidase, which dissolve zona pellucida to allow entry of sperm into the ovum.

5. **Selectins** are carbohydrate-binding adhesion proteins that mediates binding of neutrophils and other leukocytes to sites of injury in the inflammatory response.

6. **Homing receptor of lymphocytes** Homing is phenomenon in which lymphocytes tend to migrate to lymphoid sites from which they were originally derived. Carbohydrates on lymphocyte surface and endothelial lining of lymph nodes mediate this phenomenon.

Chemistry of Lipids

6

MAJOR BIOLOGICAL ROLES OF LIPIDS

Lipids are heterogeneous bio-organic molecules, which are sparingly soluble in water but are freely soluble in organic solvents (ether and chloroform). Living cells are able to metabolize lipids.

Lipids have four major biological functions, they are:

1. Lipids are the structural components of biological membranes, e.g. phospholipids and cholesterol.
2. They are the major storage form of energy in the body, e.g. triacylglycerol.
3. Some of the vitamins and hormones are lipids, e.g. vitamin D2, D3, and steroidal hormones.
4. Amphipathic bile acids (catabolic product of cholesterol) aid digestion and absorption of lipids.

MAJOR LIPID CLASSES

1. Simple lipids
    a. Fats and oils (acyl glycerols)
    b. Waxes (Cetyl alcohols)

2. Compound lipids
    a. Phospholipids
       i. Glycerophospholipids, e.g: Cephalin, Lecithin
       ii. Sphingophospholipid, e.g: Sphingomyelin
    b. Glycolipids
       i. Cerebroside
       ii. Ganglioside
       iii. Sulfatide
    c. Lipoproteins e.g: HDL, LDL, VLDL, and Chylomicrons

3. Derived lipids
    a. Derived from lipids, e.g: Fatty acids, Glycerol
    b. Precursors of lipids, e.g: Terpens, Squalene

4. Steroids
    Ring nucleus made of cyclopentenophenanthrene, e.g: Cholesterol, Steroid hormones

FATTY ACIDS

Fatty acids are long-chain hydrocarbon molecules having carboxylate group at one end. The numbering of carbon atoms in fatty acids starts from carboxyl carbon. The carbon atom adjacent to the carboxyl carbon is referred to as α-carbon. Carbon atom No. 3 is β-carbon and the methyl carbon at the end is designated as ω-carbon. At physiological pH, the carboxylate group is ionized; hence fatty acids are negatively charged in body fluids.

Fatty acids have two major functions in the body, one is they are the structural components of membrane lipids (e.g. component of phospholipids); secondly they are the components of storage form of lipids (e.g. component of triacylglycerols).

Fatty acids that lack carbon-carbon double bonds are termed **saturated fatty acids**, and those that have double bonds are termed **unsaturated fatty acids**. Various conventions are in use to indicate the number and position of the double bonds, e.g. Δ^9 indicate a double bond between carbon 9 and 10 of the fatty acid. A widely used convention is to indicate the number of carbons, the number of double bonds, and the position of the double bond, e.g. oleic acid C18:1;Δ^9, and linolenic acid C18:2;$\Delta^{9,12}$.

Saturated fatty acids of less than eight carbon atoms are liquid at physiological temperature, whereas those with more than ten are solid. The presence of double bonds in fatty acids significantly lowers the melting point relative to a saturated fatty acid with same number of carbon atoms.

Most of the body's requirement of fatty acids is met by dietary source. Although the body is capable of synthesizing various fatty acids that are needed, the two unsaturated fatty acids **linoleic acid** and **linolenic acid** (having unsaturated bonds beyond carbons 9 and 10) are not synthesized and are considered **essential fatty acids**. These fatty acids are essential, in the sense they must be provided in the diet (of plant origin). Deficiency of essential fatty acids along with zinc causes **acrodermatitis enteropathica** and **Phrynoderma**.

Physiologically Relevant Fatty Acids

14:0	$CH_3(CH_2)_{12}COOH$ **Myristic acid**	Often found attached to the N-terminal membrane-associated cytoplasmic protein.
16:0	$CH_3(CH_2)_{14}COOH$ **Palmitic acid**	End product of mammalian fatty acid synthesis.
18:2; $\Delta^{9,12}$	$CH_3(CH_2)_4(CH=CHCH_2)_2(CH_2)_6COO$ **Linoleic acid**	Essential fatty acid
18:3; $\Delta^{9,12,15}$	$CH_3CH_2(CH=CHCH_2)_3(CH_2)_6COOH$ **Linolenic acid**	Essential fatty acid
20:4; $\Delta^{5,8,11,14}$	$CH_3(CH_2)_3(CH_2CH=CH)_4(CH_2)_3COOH$ **Arachidonic acid**	Precursor for Eicosanoid synthesis

Geometric Isomerism

The orientation of atoms or groups around the axis of double bond makes molecules a pair of geometric isomers. If the atoms or groups are on one side of the axis of double bond, the compound is

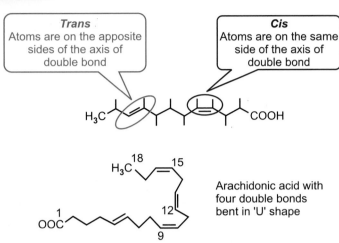

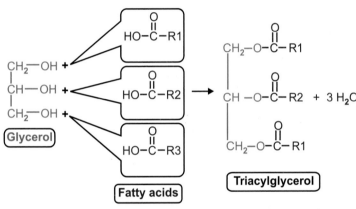

Fig. 6.1: Trans and cis isomers of fatty acids

Fig. 6.2: Basic structure of triacyl glycerol

designated as **cis** form; if they are positioned on apposite sides, it is designated as **trans** form. Nearly all the naturally occurring unsaturated fatty acids are in cis configuration. Arachidonate with four double bonds in cis form is bent and **U-shaped** (Fig. 6.1).

BASIC STRUCTURE OF TRIGLYCERIDE

Triacylglycerides are composed of a glycerol backbone to which three fatty acids are esterified. (R, R1, R2) (Fig. 6.2).

BASIC STRUCTURE OF PHOSPHOLIPIDS

The basic structure of phospholipid is very similar to that of the triacylglycerides except that C-3 (sn3) of the glycerol backbone is esterified to phosphoric acid. This molecule is termed **Phosphatidic acid** (Fig. 6.3), which forms the building block of the phospholipids.

The phosphatidate in turn is linked to one of the bases shown in Figure 6.4 to form phospholipids. The possible X-substitutions (Fig. 6.3) in the basic structure of phospholipid areethanolamine (**phosphatidylethanolamine**), serine (**phosphatidylserine**), glycerol (**phosphatidylglycerol**), choline (**phosphatidylcholine**, also called **lecithins**), myo-inositol (**phosphatidylinositol**, myinositol can have a variety in the numbers of inositol alcohols that are phosphorylated generating **polyphosphatidylinositols**), and phosphatidylglycerol (**diphosphatidylglycerol** more commonly known as **cardiolipins**).

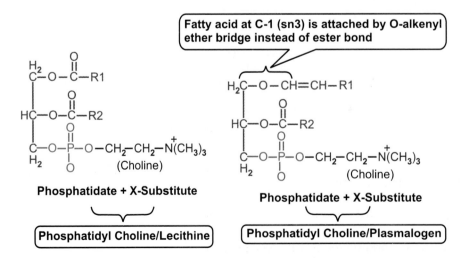

Fig. 6.3: Structure of lecithine and plasmalogen

BASIC STRUCTURE OF PLASMALOGENS

Plasmalogens are complex membrane lipids found in brain and muscle. Plasmalogens resemble phosphatidylcholine (Fig.6.3). The major difference is that the fatty acid at C-1 (*sn1*) of glycerol backbone contains either an *O*-alkyl or *O*-alkenyl ether species. One of the most potent biological molecules **platelet-activating factor** (PAF) is a choline plasmalogen in which the C-2 (*sn2*) position of glycerol is esterified with an acetyl group instead of a long chain fatty acid.

Sphingomyelin is a unique form of a phospholipid in which phosphocholine moiety is esterified to ceramide (Fig. 6.5). Ceramide is an amino alcohol (sphingosine) to which fatty acid is attached by amide bond.

BASIC STRUCTURE OF SPHINGOLIPIDS

Sphingolipids are composed of a backbone of sphingosine, which is derived itself from glycerol. Sphingosine is N-acylated (amide bond) by a variety of fatty acids generating a family of molecules referred to as **ceramides**. Sphingolipids are predominant lipids in the myelin sheath of nerve fibers. **Sphingomyelin** is an abundant sphingolipid generated by substitution of the bases. The other major classes of sphingolipids (besides the sphingomyelins) are the **glycosphingolipids** generated by substituting the base with carbohydrates to the *sn1* carbon of the sphingosine backbone of a ceramide. There are four major classes of glycosphingolipids. They are:

Cerebrosides have a single carbohydrate moiety, principally galactose (Fig. 6.6).

Sulfatides have sulfated galactose (esters of galactocerebrosides).

Globosides have two or more sugars.

Gangliosides are similar to globosides but they also contain sialic acid (NANA / NAGA).

STEROIDS

All the steroids have a cyclic nucleus phenanthrene to which is attached a cyclopentane ring. This uniformly saturated parent ring structure is designated as cyclopenteno-perhydrophenanthrene. It is a rigid and planar structure. Classical example of steroid is cholesterol, which is the precursor of biologically important steroids such as 7-dehydrocholesterol,

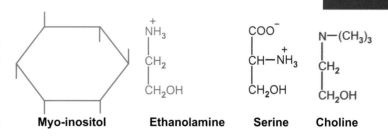

Fig. 6.4: Common bases found in phospholipids

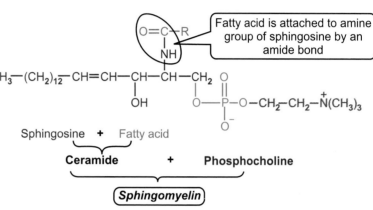

Fig. 6.5: Structure of sphingomyelin

Fig. 6.6: Cerebroside (R=H)/cerebroside sulfate (R=SO$_4$)

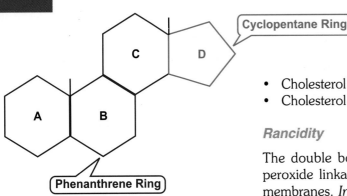

Fig. 6.7: Cyclopentanoperhydrophenanthrene ring structure

mineralocorticoids, glucocorticoids, male and female sex hormones, and bile acids (Fig. 6.7).

• Cholesterol is the major component of cell membranes in animals.
• Cholesterol modulates fluid state of membrane.
• Cholesterol is a poor conductor of electricity.

Rancidity

The double bonds in fatty acids when exposed to oxygen, form peroxide linkage and generates free radicals, which damages cell membranes. *In vivo*, heme compounds and lipoxygenase found in platelets catalyze peroxidation reactions. The effective free radical scavengers in biological system are glutathione, beta-carotenes and tocopherols (Fig. 6.8).

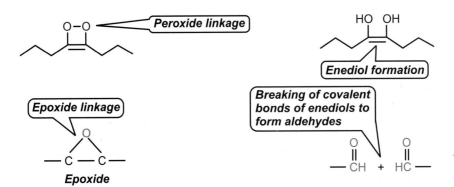

Fig. 6.8: Oxidative rancidity of fatty acids

PROPERTIES OF LIPID AGGREGATES

The polar heads (hydrophilic) of lipids interact with water, whereas the nonpolar tails (hydrophobic) keep away from water (Figs 6.9 and 6.10). The fatty acids form small micelles of monolayers, whereas phospholipids with double tails form bilayers (Fig. 6.11).

FEATURES OF LIPID BILAYER

Lipid bilayers are impermeable to most polar substances (ions, glucose, etc) but permit passage of water. Lipid bilayers are 2-D fluids in which the sideway or lateral movements of molecules within the leaflet is very fast, but the transverse movement across to apposite leaflet is slow. Membrane fluidity is a feature of importance for biological membrane. The membrane fluidity depends on temperature. At higher temperature membrane is fluid since acyl tails are randomly arranged. At lower temperature it is solid since acyl tails are organized. Phase transition from liquid to gel and gel to solid with a change in temperature, depends on the **acyl chain length** (with increasing acyl chain length van der Waals interaction increases, and more energy is needed to pull apart acyl chains, hence solid even at higher temperature), **degree of saturation** (with increasing number of

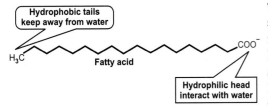

Fig. 6.9: Polar and nonpolar parts of fatty acid

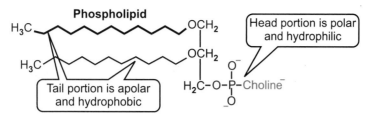

Fig. 6.10: Polar and nonpolar parts of phospholipid

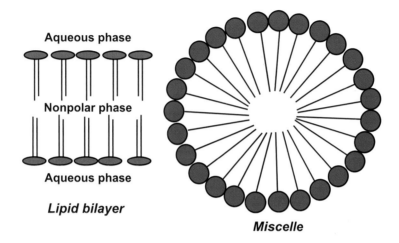

Fig. 6.11: Lipid bilayer and miscelle

double bonds steric hindrance prevent close packing of acyl chains and van der Waals interaction decreases, hence liquid even at lower temperature) of acyl chains and **amount of cholesterol** (an increased cholesterol content inhibits crystallization of acyl chains by fitting between them and prevent gel formation even at colder temperatures) in membrane.

Factors	Change in transition Temperature	Explanation	
Increased acyl chain length	Increase	Increased van der Waals interaction	More energy needed to pull apart Acyl chains
Increased unsaturation	Decrease	Steric hindrance prevent close packing of acyl chains, hence van der Waals interaction is decreased	Less energy needed to pull apart acyl chains
Increased cholesterol content	Broadens range	Inhibits crystallization of acyl chains by fitting between them. Prevents gel/solid formation at colder temperature	

BIOLOGICAL MEMBRANES

Biological membranes are composed of proteins associated with lipid bilayer (phospholipids, glycolipids and cholesterol). The proteins are specific to particular membranes and they have specific tasks to perform such as cell-cell recognition, signaling, channels, pumps and enzymes (Fig. 6.12).

In 1972, Singer and Nicholson postulated that biological membranes resemble proteins floating in a 2D lipid (***Fluid Mosaic Model of membrane structure***). Biological membranes act as permeability barrier and solvent for integral membrane proteins. These proteins could be peripheral, integral or transmembrane. **Integral proteins** are embedded through or within membrane tightly bound by hydrophobic forces, peripheral are attached to membrane. Membrane proteins are amphiphiles, they have both polar and nonpolar regions hence are asymmetrically arranged, i.e. attached to one side, but located within the membrane. Both proteins and lipids are glycosylated (ex: Ganglioside). Lipids are asymmetrically distributed; most common externally exposed lipids are sphingomyelin and phosphatidylcholine. Lipids exposed to the interior are phosphatidylethanolamine. Integral proteins and lipids rapidly diffuse within the plane of the membrane. **Lateral mobility** of a lipid is fast but **Flip-flop of lipids** (from one half of a bilayer to the other) is very **slow**. Flip-flop would require the polar head-group of a lipid to

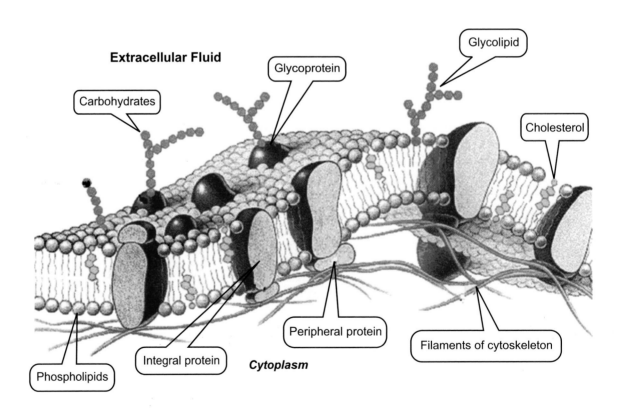

Fig. 6.12: Cell membrane structure

traverse the hydrophobic core of the membrane. **Flippase** enzymes catalyze flip-flop in membranes where lipid synthesis occurs. Otherwise, flip-flop of lipids is rare. The two leaflets of a membrane bilayer tend to differ in their lipid composition

Flip-flop of integral proteins does not occur All copies of a given type of integral protein have the same orientation relative to the two sides of the bilayer membrane.

Glycosaminoglycans and Proteoglycans

7

GLYCOSAMINOGLYCANS

The most abundant heteropolysaccharides in the body are the **glycosaminoglycans (GAGs)**. These molecules are long unbranched polysaccharides made of repeating disaccharide units (Fig. 7.1).

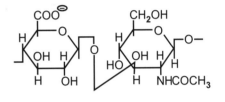

Hyaluronates
Composed of b-d-Glucuronate
and N-acetyl glucosamine
Linkage is b (1®3)

Dermatan Sulfates
Composed of L-Iduronate (many are sulfated)
and 4-sulfated N-acetyl glucosamine
Linkage is b (1®3)

Chondroitin 4-and 6-Sulfates
Composed of D-glucuronate and
4-or-6-sulfate N-acetyl galactoseamine
Linkage is b (1®3)

Heparin and Heparan Sulfates
Composed of 2-sulfated glucuronate or iduronate
and 6-sulfated N-sulfo-D-glucosamine
Linkage is a (1®4)
(heparins are more sulfated than Heparans)

Keratan Sulfates
Composed of of b-D-Galactose and
6 sulfated N-acetylglucosamine
Linkage is a (1®4)

Fig. 7.1: Structures of glycosaminoglycans

The disaccharide units contain either of the two modified sugars **N-acetylgalactosamine (GalNAc)** or **N-acetylglucosamine (GlcNAc),** and an uronic acid such as **glucuronate** or **iduronate**. Glycosaminoglycans are located primarily on the cell surface in the extracellular matrix (ECM). Glycosaminoglycans in solution are extensively negatively charged molecules with extended conformation that imparts high viscosity and low compressibility to the solution. These properties make GAG an ideal lubricating fluid in the joints. At the same time, the rigidity of GAG provides structural integrity to cells. The specific GAGs of physiological significance are hyaluronic acid, dermatan sulfate, chondroitin sulfate, heparin, heparan sulfate, and keratan sulfate. Hyaluronic acid is unique among the GAGs in that it does not contain any sulfate and is not found covalently attached to proteins as a proteoglycan. It, however, forms noncovalent complexes with proteoglycans in the extracellular matrix. Polymers of hyaluronic acid are very large (with molecular weights of 100,000-10,000,000) and can displace large volumes of water. This property makes them excellent lubricators and shock absorbers.

Features of Glycosaminoglycans		
GAG	**Localization**	**Comments**
Hyaluronate	Synovial fluid, vitreous humor, ECM of loose connective tissue	Large polymers, shock absorbing
Chondroitin sulfate	Cartilage, bone, heart valves	Most abundant GAG
Heparan sulfate	Basement membranes, components of cell surfaces	Contains higher acetylated glucosamine than heparin
Heparin	Component of intracellular granules of mast cells lining the arteries of the lungs, liver and skin	More sulfated than heparan sulfates
Dermatan sulfate	Skin, blood vessels, heart valves	
Keratan sulfate	Cornea, bone, cartilage aggregated with chondroitin sulfates	

PROTEOGLYCANS

The majority of GAGs in the body are linked to core proteins to form **proteoglycans** that are also called **mucopolysaccharides**. The protein cores of proteoglycans are rich in serine and threonine residues, which allows multiple GAG attachments. The GAG molecules extend perpendicularly from the core protein in a brush-like structure. The linkage of GAGs to the protein core involves a specific trisaccharide composed of two galactose residues and a xylulose residue (**GAG-GalGalXyl-O-CH$_2$-protein**). The trisaccharide linker is coupled to the protein core through an O-glycosidic bond to a serine residue in the protein (Fig. 7.2). Some forms of keratan sulfates are linked to the protein core through an N-asparaginyl bond.

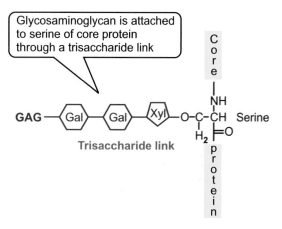

Fig. 7.2: O-glycosidic bonds in proteoglycans

Clinical Significance

Proteoglycans and GAGs perform numerous vital functions within the body, some of which still remain to be studied. One well-defined function of heparin (one of the glycosaminoglycan) is its role in preventing coagulation of the blood. Heparin is abundant in granules of mast cells that line blood vessels. The release of heparin from these granules in response to injury and its subsequent entry into the serum leads to an inhibition of blood clotting by a mechanism well elucidated. Free heparin, complexes with and activates antithrombin III, which in turn inhibits all the serine proteases of the coagulation cascade. This phenomenon has been clinically exploited in the use of heparin in anti-coagulant therapies (Fig. 7.3).

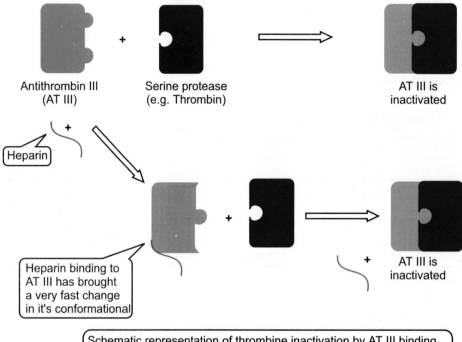

Antithrombin III (AT III)

Serine protease (e.g. Thrombin)

AT III is inactivated

Heparin

Heparin binding to AT III has brought a very fast change in it's conformational

AT III is inactivated

Schematic representation of thrombine inactivation by AT III binding. Heparin is believed to accelerate AT III binding to thrombin by bringing about a conformational change in AT III

Fig. 7.3: Schematic representation of thrombin inactivation by AT III binding

Several genetically inherited diseases, e.g. the lysosomal storage diseases, result from defects in the lysosomal enzymes responsible for the metabolism of complex membrane-associated GAGs. These specific diseases, termed mucopolysaccharidoses (MPS) (in reference to the earlier term, mucopolysaccharide, used for glycosaminoglycans) lead to an accumulation of GAGs within cells. There are at least 14 known types of lysosomal storage diseases that affect GAG catabolism; some of the more commonly encountered examples are Hurler's syndrome, Hunter's syndrome, Sanfilippo syndrome, Maroteaux-Lamy syndrome and Morquio's syndrome. All of these disorders, excepting Hunter's syndrome, are inherited in an autosomal recessive manner.

Diseases of Glycosaminoglycan (Mucopolysaccharides) Metabolism

Syndrome	Enzyme defect	Affected GAG	Symptoms
Hurler's	α-L-iduronidase	dermatan sulfate, heparan sulfate	corneal clouding, dystosis multiplex, organomegaly, heart disease, dwarfism, mental retardation; early mortality
Scheie's	α-L-iduronidase	dermatan sulfate, heparan sulfate	corneal clouding; aortic valve disease; joint stiffening; normal intelligence and lifespan
Huler/Scheie	α-L-iduronidase	dermatan sulfate, heparan sulfate	intermediate between I H and I S
Hunter's	L-iduronate-2-sulfatase	dermatan sulfate, heparan sulfate	mild and severe forms, only X-linked MPS, dystosis multiplex, organomegaly, facial and physical deformities, no corneal clouding, mental retardation, death before 15 except in mild form then survival to 20-60
Sanfilippo A	Heparan N-sulfatase	heparan sulfate	profound mental deterioration, hyperactivity, skin, brain, lungs, heart and skeletal muscle are affected in all 4 types of MPS-III
Sanfilippo B	α-N-acetyl-D-glucosa-minidase	heparan sulfate	phenotype similar to III A
Sanfilippo C	Acetyl CoA: α-glucosa-mine acetyltransferase	heparan sulfate	phenotype similar to III A
Sanfilippo D	N-acetylglucosamine-6-sulfatase	heparan sulfate	phenotype similar to III A
Morquio A	Galactose-6-sulfatase	keratan sulfate, chondroitin 6-sulfate	corneal clouding, odontoid hypoplasia, aortic valve disease, distinctive skeletal abnormalities
Morquio B	β-Galactosidase	keratan sulfate	severity of disease similar to IV A
Maroteaux-Lamy	N-acetylgalactosamine-4-sulfatase also called arylsulfatase B	dermatan sulfate	3 distinct forms from mild to severe, aortic valve disease, dystosis multiplex, normal intelligence, corneal clouding, coarse facial features
Sly	β-Glucuronidase	heparan sulfate, dermatan sulfate, chondroitin 4-, 6-sulfates	hepatosplenomegaly, dystosis multiplex, wide spectrum of severity, hydrops fetalis

Collagen

8

The extracellular matrix (ECM) is a complex structural entity surrounding, and supporting cells that are found within mammalian tissues. The extracellular matrix is often referred to as the connective tissue and is composed of three major classes of biomolecules:

Structural proteins are collagen and elastin.

Specialized proteins are fibrillin, fibronectin, and laminin.

Proteoglycans are composed of a protein core to which are attached long chains of repeating disaccharide units of glycosamino-glycans (GAGs) forming extremely complex high molecular weight components of the extracellular matrix.

COLLAGENS

Collagens are the most abundant proteins found in the animal. They are essential structural components of all connective tissues such as cartilage, bone, tendons, ligaments, fascia and skin.

Collagen is the major protein component of extracellular matrix. There are at least 12 types of collagens. Types I, II and III are the most abundant and form fibrils of similar structure. Type IV collagen forms a two-dimensional reticulum and is a major component of the basal lamina. Collagens are synthesized predominantly by fibroblasts but epithelial cells also synthesize these proteins.

The fundamental higher order structure of collagens is a long and thin rod-like protein. Type I collagen for instance is 300 nm long, 1.5 nm in diameter and consists of three coiled subunits composed of two α1 chains and one α 2 chain (Fig. 8.1). Each chain consists of 1050 amino acids wound around each other in a characteristic **right-handed triple helix** There are 3 amino acids per turn of the helix and every third amino acid is a glycine (Gly - X - Y)n where X is often proline (Pro) and Y is often hydroxyproline. The bulky pyrollidone rings of prolyl residues are on the outside of the triple helix.

Lateral interactions of triple helices of collagens result in the formation of fibrils roughly 50 nm diameter. The packing of collagen is such that the adjacent molecules are displaced approximately 1/4 of their length (67 nm), what is described as quarter staggered arrangement. This staggered array produces a striated effect that can be seen under electron microscope.

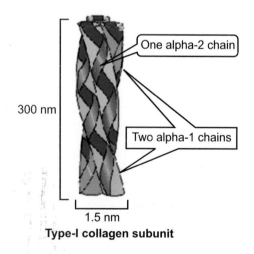

One alpha-2 chain

Two alpha-1 chains

300 nm

1.5 nm

Type-I collagen subunit

Fig. 8.1: Three alpha-helix chains wound around each other in a right-handed triple helix

Collagens are synthesized as longer precursor proteins called **procollagens**. Type I procollagen contains an additional 150 amino acids at the N-terminus and 250 amino acids at the C-terminus. These pro-domains are globular and form multiple intrachain disulfide bonds. The disulfide bonds stabilize the proprotein and allow the triple helical section to form. Collagen fibers begin to assemble in the endoplasmic reticule and Golgi complexes, where signal sequence is removed and numerous modifications take place in the collagen chains:

1. Specific proline residues are hydroxylated by **prolyl 4-hydroxylase** and **prolyl 3-hydroxylase**.
2. *Specific lysine residues are hydroxylated by **lysyl hydroxylase**. Both the prolyl hydroxylases are absolutely dependent upon vitamin C as co-factor.*
3. O-linked glycosylations occur in Golgi during transit.

Following completion of processing the procollagens is secreted into the extracellular space where extracellular enzymes remove the pro-domains. The collagen molecules then polymerize to form collagen fibrils. Accompanying fibril formation is the oxidation of certain lysine residues by the extracellular enzyme **lysyl oxidase** forming reactive aldehydes. These reactive aldehydes form specific cross-links between chains, thereby stabilizing the staggered array of the collagens in the fibril.

Types of Collagen

Types	Chains	Structural details	Localization
I	$[\alpha1(I)]_2[\alpha(I)]$	300nm, 67nm banded fibrils	skin, tendon, bone, etc.
II	$[\alpha1(II)]_3$	300nm, small 67nm fibrils	Cartilage, vitreous humor
III	$[\alpha1(III)]_3$	300nm, small 67nm fibrils	Skin, muscle, frequently with type I
IV	$[\alpha1(IV)]_2[\alpha2(IV)]$	390nm C-term globular domain, nonfibrillar	All basal lamina
V	$[\alpha1(V)][\alpha2(V)][\alpha3(V)]$	390nm N-term globular domain, small fibers	Most interstitial tissue, assoc. with type I
VI	$[\alpha1(VI)][\alpha2(VI)][\alpha3(VI)]$	150nm, N+C term. Globular domains, microfibrils, 100nm banded fibrils	Most interstitial tissue, assoc. with type I
VII	$[\alpha1(VII)]_3$	450nm, dimer	Epithelia
VIII	$[\alpha1(VIII)]_3$	Not known	Some endothelial cells
IX	$[\alpha1(IX)][\alpha2(IX)][\alpha3(IX)]$	200nm N-term. Globular domain, bound proteoglycan	Cartilage, assoc. with type II
X	$[\alpha1(X)]_3$	150nm C-term. Globular domain	Hypertrophic and mineralizing cartilage
XI	$[\alpha1(XI)][\alpha2(XI)][\alpha3(XI)]$	300nm, small fibers	Cartilage
XII	$\alpha1(XII)$	Not known	Interacts with types I and III

Clinical Significance of Collagen Disorders

Collagens are the most abundant proteins in the body. Alterations in collagen structure as a result of mutated genes or abnormal processing of collagen results in numerous diseases, e.g. Larsen syndrome, scurvy, osteogenesis imperfecta and Ehlers-Danlos syndrome. **Ehlers-**

Danlos syndrome is actually the name associated with at least ten distinct disorders that are biochemically and clinically distinct yet all of them manifest structural weakness in connective tissue. **Osteogenesis imperfecta** also encompasses more than one disorder. At least four biochemically and clinically distinguishable disorders have been identified all of which are characterized by multiple fractures and resultant bone deformities. **Marfan's syndrome** manifests itself as a disorder of the connective tissue and was believed to be the result of abnormal collagens, however, recent evidence has shown that Marfan's results from mutations in the extracellular protein **fibrillin**, which is an integral constituent of the non-collagenous microfibrils of the extracellular matrix.

Clinical Significance of Collagen Disorders

Disorder	Collagen Defect	Symptomatology
Ehlers-Danlos IV	Decrease in type III	Arterial, intestinal and uterine rupture, thin easily bruised skin
Ehlers-Danlos V	Decreased cross-linking	Skin and joint hyperextensibility
Ehlers-Danlos VI	Decreased hydroxylysine	Poor wound healing, musculo-skeletal deformities, skin and joint hyperextensibility
Ehlers-Danlos VII	N-terminal pro-peptide not removed	Easily bruised skin, hip dislocations, hyperextensibility
Osteogenesis imperfecta	Decrease in type I	Blue sclera, bone deformities
Scurvy	Decreased hydroxyproline	Poor wound healing, deficient growth, capillary weakness

LAMININ

All basal laminae contain a common set of proteins and GAGs. These are **type IV collagen, heparan sulfate, proteoglycans, entactin** and **laminin**. The basal lamina is often referred to as the **type IV matrix**. The cells that rest upon it synthesize each of the components of the basal lamina. Laminin anchors cell surfaces to the basal lamina. **Laminin** is a large family of 18 isoforms. It is a cross-shaped glycoprotein, which is formed by three polypeptides two β chains, and one α chain. It has multiple binding sites (for collagen-IV, cells, and heparan sulfate), which makes it a major interlinker forming networks and anchoring cells to basal laminae (Fig. 8.2). The laminins are primarily restricted to basal laminae, where it is the most abundant linking glycoprotein. It is widely distributed in vertebrates, but also has been detected in invertebrates like insects and sea urchins. Like fibronectin, laminin has many functions

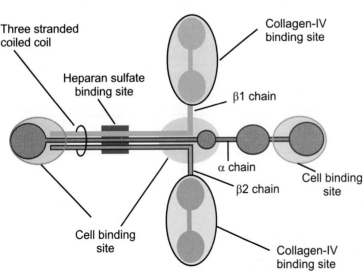

Fig. 8.2: Schematic diagram of basal laminin

along with its roll in cross-linking and anchoring extracellular structures to the cell surface.

Representative matrix types produced by vertebrate cells

Collagen	Anchor	Proteoglycan	Cell-Surface receptor	Cells
I	Fibronectin	Chondroitin and Dermatan sulfates	Integrin	Fibroblasts
II	Fibronectin	Chondroitin sulfate	Integrin	Chondrocytes
III	Fibronectin	Heparan sulfate and Heparin	Integrin	Quiescent hepatocytes, epithelial; assoc. fibroblasts
IV	Laminin	Heparan sulfate and Heparin	Laminin receptors	All epithelial cells, endothelial cells, regenerating hepatocytes
V	Fibronectin	Heparan sulfate and Heparin	Integrin	Quiescent fibroblasts
VI	Fibronectin	Heparan sulfate	Iitegrin	Quiescent fibroblasts

FIBRONECTIN

The role of fibronectins is to attach cells to a variety of extracellular matrices. Fibronectin attaches cells to all matrices except type IV that involves laminin as the adhesive molecule. Fibronectins are dimers of two similar peptides. Each chain is 60-70 nm long and 2 to 3 nm thick. At least 20 different fibronectin chains have been identified that arise by alternative RNA splicing of the primary transcript from a single fibronectin gene. Fibronectins contain at least six tightly folded domains each with a high affinity for a different substrate such as heparan sulfate, collagen (separate domains for types I, II and III), fibrin and cell-surface receptors. The cell-surface receptor-binding domain contains a consensus amino acid sequence, arginine, glycine, aspartic acid, and serine.

Hemoglobin is an Allosteric Protein

9

Vertebrates must supply and deliver a constant amount of oxygen to tissues for aerobic respiration. This is achieved by having a well-developed circulatory system that delivers oxygen to cells, and efficient oxygen-carrying molecules (hemoglobin and myoglobin) to overcome oxygen's low solubility in water.

The ability of hemoglobin or myoglobin to bind oxygen is the function of heme groups (prosthetic group) they carry. Heme consists of a protoporphyrin ring (organic part), and an iron atom occupying the center of it. The iron atom in heme can form 6 bonds; four with nitrogens of protoporphyrin and two on either side of plane with histidyl residue. Iron atom can be in ferrous (reduced) or ferric (oxidized) state. Ferrohemoglobin and ferromyoglobin are the **reduced forms** (Fe^{+2}), whereas ferrihemoglobin and ferrimyoglobin are **oxidized forms** (Fe^{+3}). Only ferrous (Fe^{+2}) state can transport oxygen.

Salient Features of Hemoglobin

1. Hemoglobin molecule is extremely compact
2. Alpha-helical (eight helices, named A, B, C, ...H) conformation constitutes 75 percent of the globin molecule.
3. Four of the helices are terminated by proline residue.
4. Main-chain peptide groups are planar.
5. Little empty space inside the molecule; interior of hemoglobin molecule is lined almost entirely by nonpolar aminoacyl residues, amphipathic amino acids are oriented such that their hydrophilic portions face exterior. The only polar amino acids in the interior of hemoglobin molecule are two histidyl residues, which are part of heme binding site.
6. Heme is located in the pocket formed by helices E and F of myoglobin molecule (Fig. 9.1).

Iron atom is bonded to histidine in F8 (histidine); the oxygen-binding site on iron is located on other side of heme plane (E7). Binding of oxygen to heme must occur in a bent, end-on orientation. Free heme exposed to oxygen gets rapidly oxidized to Fe^{+3}, which cannot bind oxygen. Heme in hemoglobin and myoglobin is much

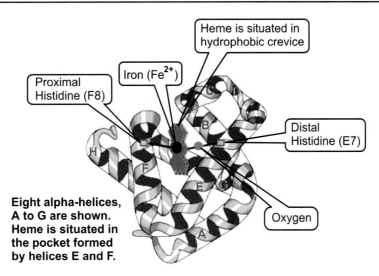

Fig. 9.1: Myoglobin structure

less susceptible to oxidation because the globin part allows heme to bind oxygen reversibly.

Carbon monoxide is a poison because it combines with ferromyoglobin (Fe^{+2}) and ferrohemoglobin (Fe^{+2}) to block oxygen transport.

Carbon monoxide's (CO) affinity to bind heme is about 200 times stronger than that of oxygen. If CO is allowed to interact with isolated iron porphyrins, the iron, carbon, and oxygen atoms will form a linear array.

If CO is allowed to interact with myoglobin or hemoglobin; CO axis is bent, similar to oxygen binding because of steric hindrance from His E7 that greatly weakens the interaction of CO with heme. Breakdown of heme within cells produce CO, which block about 1% of binding sites on hemoglobin and myoglobin. If affinity were close to that of isolated heme, it would cause massive poisoning. The globin of myoglobin and hemoglobin modulates the functioning of heme. Hemoglobin consists of 4 polypeptide chains, 2 of one type and 2 of another ($\alpha_2 \beta_2$), held together by noncovalent bonds. Each polypeptide contains a heme group and oxygen-binding site. Embryos and fetuses have zeta chains (ζ) and epsilon (ε) chains; zeta chains are replaced by alpha (α), epsilon chains are replaced with gamma (γ), then beta (β) chains.

The three-dimensional structure of myoglobin is very similar to α and β chains of hemoglobin.

Hemoglobin is more Intricate than Myoglobin

1. Hemoglobin is involved in transport protons (H^+), carbon dioxide (CO_2), and oxygen (O_2).
2. Hemoglobin is an allosteric protein.
3. Binding of oxygen to hemoglobin is cooperative.
4. Affinity of hemoglobin for oxygen and CO_2 is pH dependent.
5. BPG (2,3-bisphosphoglycerate) also regulates oxygen dissociation from hemoglobin.

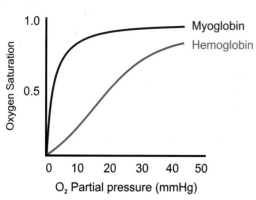

Fig. 9.2: Oxygen dissociation curve

Oxygen Dissociation Curves for Myoglobin and Hemoglobin differs

1. Saturation of myoglobin is higher than hemoglobin at all oxygen pressure (Fig. 9.2). It means myoglobin has higher affinity for oxygen than does hemoglobin (P_{50} for myoglobin is 1 torr; P_{50} for hemoglobin is 26 torr).
2. Oxygen dissociation curve of myoglobin is hyperbolic and that of hemoglobin is sigmoidal. Binding of oxygen to hemoglobin is cooperative (seen in Hill plot); such cooperativity enables hemoglobin to deliver nearly twice as much oxygen it delivers under typical physiological conditions if binding sites were independent.

Effect of pH on oxygen binding: Decrease in pH shifts oxygen dissociation curve to the right (hemoglobin's affinity for oxygen is decreased).

Effect of CO_2 concentration on oxygen binding: An increase in carbon dioxide concentration lowers hemoglobin's affinity for oxygen.

An increase in H^+ and CO_2 concentrations actually **promotes** the release of oxygen from oxyhemoglobin. These effects together are known as the **Bohr effect** (Fig. 9.3).

Effect of BPG: An increase in BPG concentration lowers oxygen affinity of hemoglobin by a factor of 26, thereby hemoglobin unloads more of its oxygen at the tissue level. BPG works by binding to deoxyhemoglobin, but not oxyhemoglobin.

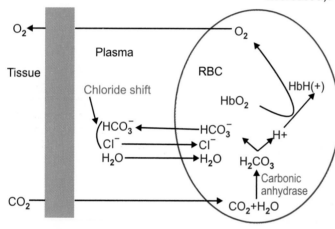

Representation of the delivery of O_2 to the tissues and transport of CO_2 from the tissues to the blood. The opposite process occurs at the alveoli of the lungs when O_2 is taken up and the CO_2 is expelled. All the processes of the transport of CO_2 and O_2 are not shown, such as the formation and ionization of H_2CO_3 in the plasma. The latter is a major mechanism for the transport of CO_2 to the lungs. Phosphate and proteins buffer the H^+ produced in the plasma by the ionization of carbonic acid. Additionally, some 15 percent of the CO_2 is transported from the tissues to the lungs as hemoglobin carbonate.

Fig. 9.3: Transport of CO_2 and the Bohr effect

Differences between Fetal and Adult Hemoglobin

Hemoglobin F ($\alpha_2\gamma_2$) vs. hemoglobin A ($\alpha_2\beta_2$)

Fetal hemoglobin has higher affinity for oxygen than does adult hemoglobin, which optimizes transfer of oxygen from maternal to fetal circulation.

Also, hemoglobin F binds BPG less strongly than does hemoglobin A, which makes hemoglobin F to have higher affinity for oxygen, but in the absence of BPG fetal hemoglobin actually has lower affinity for oxygen than does adult hemoglobin.

Structural Basis of Allosteric Effects

The allosteric properties of hemoglobin arise from interactions between its subunits.

The functional unit of hemoglobin is a tetramer with 2 alpha and 2 beta chains.

The 3D conformation of oxyhemoglobin and deoxyhemoglobin are very different.

1. Oxygenated Hb molecule is more compact.

2. Binding of oxygen to hemoglobin results in a large conformational change at two of the four contact points ($\alpha_1\beta_2$ and $\beta_1\alpha_2$).
3. The $\alpha_1\beta_1$ pair rotates relative to other pair of protein chains (Fig. 9.4).

The $\alpha_1\beta_2$ contact region is designed to act as a switch between two alternative structures. All mutations at this interface diminish oxygen binding; mutations elsewhere have no effect. Oxyhemoglobin is R (relaxed) form and deoxyhemoglobin is T (taut) form, which has lower affinity.

In deoxyhemoglobin, the iron atom is out of porphyrin plane and pulled toward proximal histidine (F8) and heme group appears domed-shaped toward His F8. Binding of oxygen to iron atom pulls it into porphyrin plane and heme appear more planar.

Proximal histidine (F8) is pulled along with iron atom and becomes less tilted, which shifts F helix, these shifts are transmitted to subunit interfaces, where they break interchain salt links to form R form.

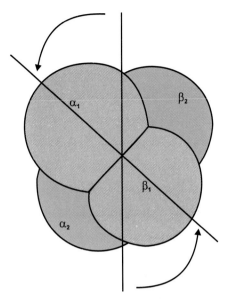

During transition of the T form to the R form of hemoglobin, there occurs a rotation of one pair of rigid subunits ($\alpha_1\beta_2$) through 15 degrees relative to the other rigid paid of subunits ($\alpha_2\beta_2$). The axis of rotation is eccentric, and the $\alpha_1\beta_1$ pair also shifts towards the axis somewhat. In the diagram $\alpha_1\beta_2$ pair is blue and held fixed, while the grey shaded $\alpha_1\beta_1$ pair rotates and shifts.

Fig. 9.4: Transition between oxyhemoglobin ('R' or relaxed) and deoxyhemoglobin ('T' or relaxed)

How does BPG Lower Oxygen Affinity of Hemoglobin?

BPG with four negative charges binds to symmetry axis of deoxyhemoglobin molecule in its central cavity, which contains eight positively charged amino group residues of beta chains. Binding of BPG stabilizes deoxyhemoglobin structure by cross-linking β chains through additional salt bridges that causes shift in equilibrium toward T form. When oxygen binds to hemoglobin, the shift in conformation causes the central cavity to become too small and BPG gets expelled.

How does CO_2 Lower Oxygen Affinity of Hemoglobin?

Much of the CO_2 is transported as bicarbonate in RBCs, the H^+ formed is taken up by deoxyhemoglobin in the Bohr effect.

$$CO_2 + H_2O \longrightarrow HCO_3^- + H^+$$

To a lesser extent CO_2 is bound to hemoglobin as carbamate

$$R\text{-}NH_2 + CO_2 \longrightarrow R\text{-}NH\text{-}C\text{-}O^- + H^+$$

Carbamate forms salt bridges that stabilize T form and lowers affinity for O_2.

Uptake of H^+ helps to buffer the pH of metabolically active cells, but it also affects the pKs of some amino acids. The only amino acid affected this way is His 146, which acquires a greater affinity for H^+ because of more negatively charged local environment (location of Asp 94).

There are two Models for Allosteric Interactions

1. Sequential Model

Each subunit of hemoglobin can exist in either T or R form.

Binding of ligand to a subunit alters its conformation, but not that of its neighbors, that means the subunit must have ligand binding to switch from T to R form. Conformational change of the one subunit can increase or decrease the binding affinity of other subunits.

2. *Concerted or MWC Model (Monod, Wyman, and Changeux)*

The hemoglobin subunits interconverts between T and R form; all subunits must be in T or R form; no hybrids (RT) are allowed. Ligands bind with low affinity to T form, and with high affinity to R form. Binding of ligand to each subunit increases the probability that all subunits are in R form.

HEMOGLOBINOPATHIES

More than 300 types of abnormal hemoglobin molecules with altered functions have been identified, which are the result of genetic mutations.

The genetic mutation can alter the structure and function of hemoglobin by one of the four possible mechanisms:

1. *Altered exterior* can affect solubility of hemoglobin, e.g. hemoglobin S (sickle cell anemia)
2. *Altered active site* can affect oxygen binding, because of a change in the primary structure of globin near the oxygen-binding site, e.g. hemoglobin M in which iron atom is permanently in ferric state, and patients are cyanotic. The homozygotic state is probably lethal.
3. *Altered tertiary structure*–the polypeptide chain is prevented from folding into normal conformation.
4. *Altered quaternary structure* can lead to a loss of allosteric properties and usually have abnormal oxygen affinity. The $\alpha_1\beta_2$ contact region is the most commonly affected.

THALASSEMIAS

Thalassemias are a group of disorders in which the normal hemoglobin is produced but in quantities lower than usual. The thalassemias are a complex group of disorders because of the genetics of hemoglobin production and the structure of the hemoglobin molecule. Chain that is affected is designated in the name: e.g. α-thalassemia (α-chains are affected), β-thalassemia (β-chains are affected). Such changes can be produced in a variety of ways:

1. Gene coding for specific hemoglobin chain is missing
2. Gene is present, but RNA synthesis or processing is impaired, e.g. TATA box (promoter sequence) is mutated.
3. Synthesis of mRNA is in abnormal quantities.

Types of Hemoglobins

Hemoglobin A

This is the designation for the normal hemoglobin found in humans.

Hemoglobin F

This is the hemoglobin produced by fetuses before birth. Fetal hemoglobin arises from a gene different from that, which produces hemoglobin. The genes for hemoglobin F and hemoglobin A are closely related. Hemoglobin F production falls dramatically after birth, although some people continue to produce small amounts of hemoglobin F for their entire lives.

Hemoglobin S

The hemoglobin produced by the "sickle gene". The "sickle gene" arose by a mutation in the gene that produces normal hemoglobin A. Hemoglobin S is the hemoglobin found in patients with sickle cell disease.

Hemoglobin C

This is abnormal hemoglobin produced by a mutation of the normal hemoglobin A gene. This hemoglobin is found most commonly in people of African ancestry.

Hemoglobin E

This hemoglobin variant is found commonly in people of Asian descent. This variant hemoglobin produces few if any problems. A significant exception is the co-inheritance of hemoglobin E and beta thalassemia.

Sickle Syndromes

The sickle syndromes are a group of disorders with the common feature of having at least one gene that produces hemoglobin S. The members of this family are:

Sickle Cell Disease

This refers to a condition in which a person has inherited two genes for hemoglobin S, one from each parent. This is the most common of the sickle syndromes. The condition formerly was referred to as sickle cell anemia. This term has been largely replaced in standard usage, since it emphasizes the anemia, which is the least important manifestation of this potentially devastating condition. The severity of sickle cell disease varies tremendously. Some patients have almost no symptoms, while others are virtually incapacitated. Although we have some clues as to the cause of the variable expression of the disorder, most of the heterogeneity is unexplained. The hemoglobin of these patients can be analyzed by hemoglobin electrophoresis. These patients have primarily hemoglobin S in their red blood cells, with small amounts of the other two hemoglobins in some cases. Most importantly, these patients have no normal hemoglobin.

Sickle/beta-thalassemia

In this condition, the patient has inherited a gene for hemoglobin S from one parent and a gene for beta-thalassemia from the other. The severity of the condition is determined to a large extent by the quantity of normal hemoglobin produced by the beta-thalassemia gene. (Thalassemia genes produce normal hemoglobin, but invariably in reduced amounts). If the gene produces no normal hemoglobin, $beta^0$-thalassemia, the condition is virtually identical to sickle cell disease. Some patients have a gene that produces a small amount of normal hemoglobin, called $beta^+$-thalassemia. The severity of the condition is dampened when the $beta^+$-thalassemia gene produces significant quantities of normal hemoglobin. Sickle/beta-thalassemia is the most common sickle syndrome seen in people of Mediterranean descent (Italian, Greek, Turkish). Beta-thalassemia is quite common in this region, and the sickle cell gene occurs in some sections of these countries. Hemoglobin electrophoresis of hemolysate from a patient with sickle/$beta^0$-thalassemia shows no normal hemoglobin. Patients with sickle/$beta^+$-thalassemia have an amount of normal hemoglobin that depends on the level of function of the $beta^+$-thalassemia gene.

Hemoglobin SC Disease

Patients with hemoglobin SC disease have inherited a gene for hemoglobin S from one parent, and a gene for hemoglobin C from the other. Hemoglobin C is abnormal hemoglobin that can interact with hemoglobin S to produce some of the abnormalities seen in patients with sickle cell disease. On average, patients with hemoglobin SC disease have milder symptoms than patients with sickle cell disease. This is only an average, however, some people with hemoglobin SC disease have a condition that is equally severe as that of any patient with sickle cell disease. A number of other syndromes that involve hemoglobin S exist. They are less common than the above-mentioned disorders in most cases.

Other Hemoglobinopathies

Hemoglobin E is one of the most common hemoglobin variant. This gene is most common in people of S.E. Asian ancestry, e.g. Cambodian, Vietnamese, and Thai. The combination of hemoglobins E and A is benign. People with two hemoglobin E genes have mild anemia and few other manifestations. The combination of hemoglobin E and beta-thalassemia produces a clinically severe condition with marked anemia. The condition is much like thalassemia intermedia.

SICKEL CELL ANEMIA

Sickle cell anemia is a classic example of a genetic mutation that results in an abnormal hemoglobin molecule.

Patients with sickle cell anemia are homozygous (both the genes are defective) for the gene. Those that receive one abnormal gene from only one parent are heterozygous and are called carriers, who are usually asymptomatic.

The name sickle cell comes from the observation that red cells from patients with this disease will sickle on a microscope slide when oxygen concentration is reduced.

Deoxygenated sickle cell hemoglobin has an abnormally low solubility and forms fibrous precipitate. People with "sickle cell" gene are designated Hb S to distinguish it from Hb A.

Biochemical studies have revealed that isoelectric point of sickle-cell hemoglobin is higher than normal hemoglobin in both oxygenated and deoxygenated forms that implies that there is a difference in the number or kind of ionizable side groups in the two hemoglobins.

There are between 2 and 4 more net positive charges per molecule in sickle cell hemoglobin than normal hemoglobin.

Using protein fingerprinting (selective cleavage of a protein into small peptides followed by separation in two dimensions, electrophoresis and chromatography) revealed that one of the spots was different.

Hemoglobin S contains valine instead of glutamate at position 6 of β-chain that places a nonpolar residue on the outside of hemoglobin S. This does not affect oxygen affinity and allosteric properties but does reduce solubility of deoxygenated form of hemoglobin.

Valine side chain interacts with complementary sticky patch on another hemoglobin molecule, which is exposed in deoxygenated, but not oxygenated form, for this reason sickling occurs when there is a high concentration of deoxygenated form of hemoglobin S. Precipitate that is formed actually consists of fibers that are the deoxygenated form of hemoglobin S. If the transport time to the lungs is greater than the time it takes to form a nucleation site, then sickling occurs. Sickling is self-propagating because sickle cells block blood vessels, setting up area of low oxygen concentration.

High incidence of sickle gene is seen in areas of Africa where malaria is endemic. Heterozygotes are actually protected from the most lethal form of malaria. By accelerating the destruction rate of infected RBCs.This is an example of **balanced polymorphism** - an allele that is highly deleterious in homozygote persists because heterozygous state is advantageous.

Defective gene can be detected in fetal cells using restriction endonuclease and Southern blotting. The cells used for this test can come from chorionic villi obtained at about 8 weeks gestation. While screening for genetic defects one can also use PCR to amplify fetal DNA.

Heme Metabolism

10

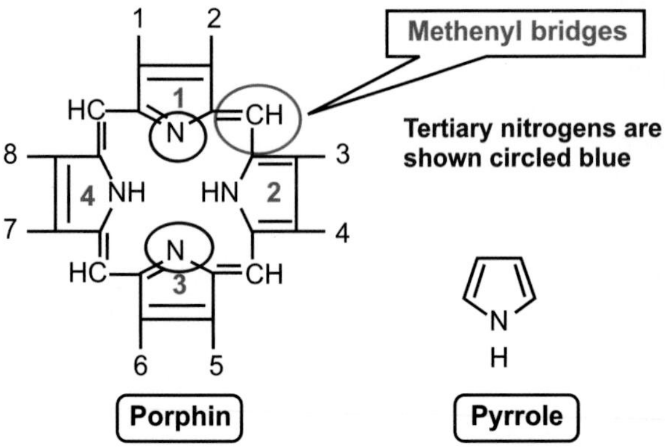

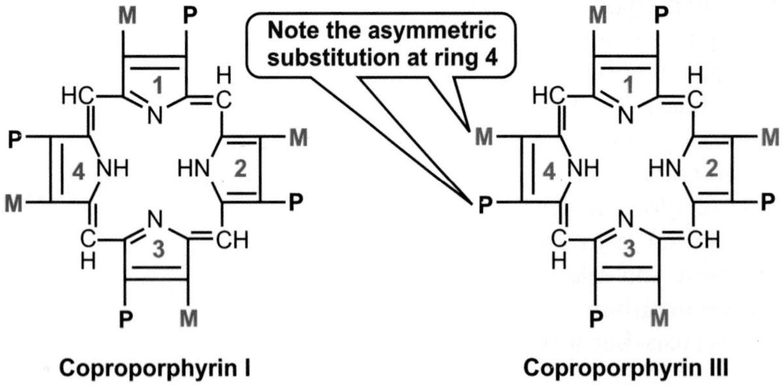

Fig. 10.1: Coproporphyrin I and Coproporphyrin III

PORPHYRINS

Porphyrins may be considered as derivatives of Porphin (Fig. 10.1). They are cyclic compounds formed by the linkage of 4 pyrrole rings through methenyl bridges (Fig. 10.1). Substitution of hydrogen atoms numbered 1 to 8 by various groups can produce large number of isomers. Two of the nitrogen atoms at the center of the ring are tertiary nitrogens. The characteristic property of porphyrins is the formation of metaloporphyrins with cationic metal ions bound to the nitrogen atoms of pyrrole rings. Biologically functional porphyrins contain only one of the two metals such as iron, and magnesium. The iron porphyrin is called heme, and the magnesium-porphyrin is called chlorophyll.

In nature, the metalloporphyrins form the prosthetic group of biologically important conjugated proteins such as, hemoglobin, myoglobin, cytochromes, peroxidases, catalase, and tryptophan pyrolase.

It is important to know that hemoglobin and myoglobin are involved in transport of oxygen and carbon dioxide; hence the iron in heme (Fig. 10.2) of these proteins is always in reduced form (ferrous Fe^{2+}). Whereas cytochromes are involved in transfer of electrons; hence the iron in heme of cytochromes oscillates between ferrous (Fe^{2+}) and ferric (Fe^{3+}) form.

Classification

All the naturally occurring porphyrins belong to type I or type III. When all the substituted side groups are arranged symmetrically they are called type I porphyrins, if the symmetry is lost at ring 4, they are called type III porphyrins. Type III porphyrins are the most abundant in nature.

In biological system, we come across only three kinds of porphyrins: uroporphyrin III, coproporphyrin III and protoporphyrin III.

Chemistry of Porphyrins

- The presence of two tertiary nitrogens in the ring structure, make these compounds act as weak bases.
- Those compounds that possess a carboxyl group on side chains act also as weak acids.
- Their isoelectric points ranges from pH 3 to 4.5, and within this pH range they can easily be precipitated from aqueous solutions.
- The intermediary molecules encountered, in the biosynthesis of protoporphyrin starting from aminolevulinic acids, have increasing hydrophobicity because of loss of carboxylic groups on the side chains.
- The more hydrophilic molecule uroporphyrin is excreted in the urine, whereas the more hydrophobic molecules are secreted in the bile and feces.
- The various porphyrinogens are reduced and colorless, whereas the various porphyrins are colored and fluoresce red under UV light.
- They absorb light maximally at 400 nm. This band is called **Soret band.**

BIOSYNTHESIS OF HEME

Although the two most prominent fates of amino acids are incorporation into protein and oxidative degradation, the biosynthesis of numerous physiologically important compounds require the availability of amino acids and their constituent nitrogen. Aside from importance of heme as the prosthetic group of hemoglobin, and a small number of enzymes, it is important because a number of genetic disease states are associated with its biosynthesis and deficiencies of the enzymes required in the process.

Some of these disorders are readily diagnosed, because abnormally colored heme intermediates appear in the circulation, the urine, feces, and in other tissues such as teeth and bones. Some disorders of heme biosynthesis are more insidious such as the various porphyrias.

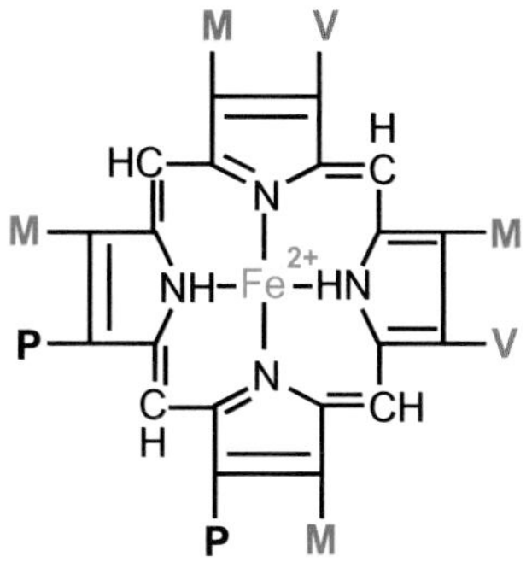

Heme is the prosthetic group of hemoglobin, myoglobin, cytochromes, and tryptophan pyrolase. The structure of heme of hemoglobin is shown in Figure 10.2.

The heme ring system is synthesized from active form of **glycine** (glycine in Schiff base with PLP), and active **succinate** (succinyl-CoA).

Synthesis of heme begins in the *mitochondria*, catalyzed by **δ-aminolevulinate synthase** (ALA synthase). A molecule each of

M	-CH$_3$	Methyl
A	-CH$_2$-COO$^-$	Acetate
P	-CH$_2$-CH$_2$-COO$^-$	Propionate
V	-CH$_2$=CH$_2$	Vinyl

Fig. 10.2: Heme

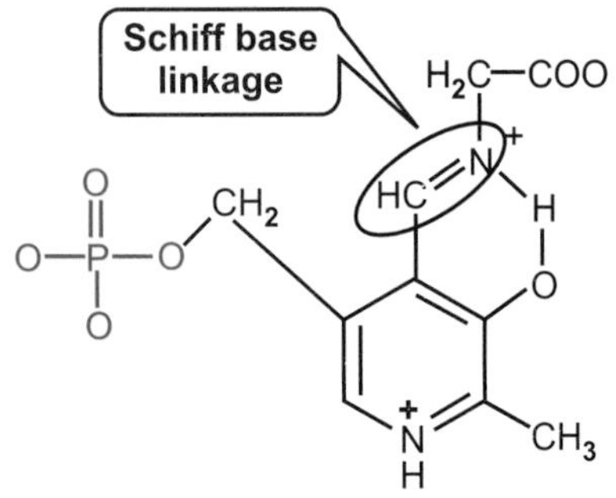

activated glycine and succinyl-CoA condenses, with concomitant decarboxylation, to form δ-aminolevulinic acid (ALA).

Pyridoxal phosphate (PLP) serves as coenzyme for ALA synthase, which is evolutionarily related to transaminases. Condensation between glycine and succinyl-CoA takes place, while the amino group of glycine is in Schiff base linkage to the aldehyde group of PLP (Fig. 10.3). Coenzyme A and the carboxyl group of glycine are lost following the condensation reaction (Fig. 10.4).

ALA synthase catalyzed reaction is the committing step in the heme synthesis pathway, and is the rate-limiting enzyme for the overall reactions of the pathway. The amount, and activity of the enzyme is regulated, through control of transcription, repression of translation by heme, and its translocation into the mitochondria.

The next reaction takes place in the *cytosolic compartment*

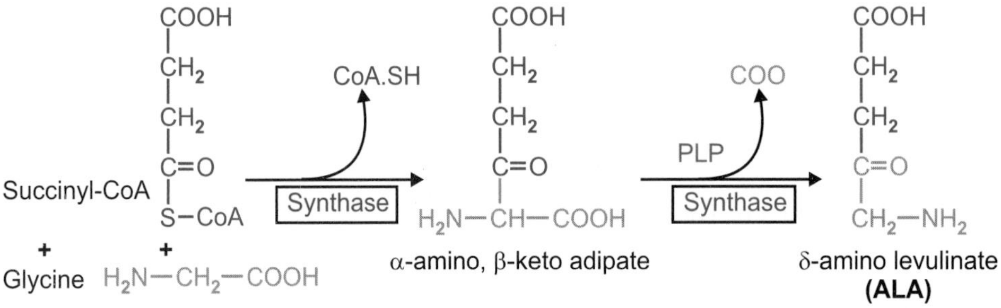

Fig. 10.3: Glycine PLP schiff base (aldamine)

Fig. 10.4: Synthesis of ALA

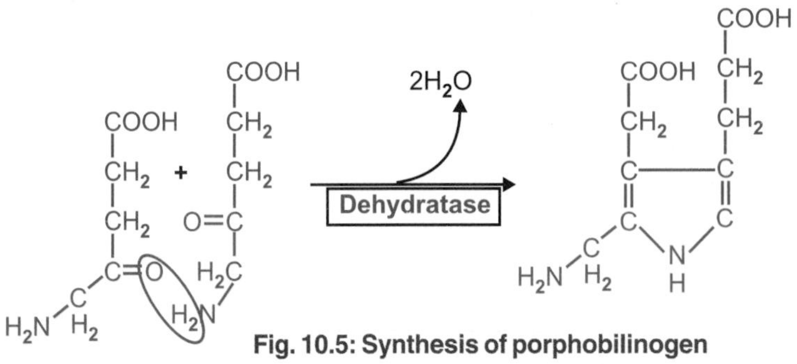

Fig. 10.5: Synthesis of porphobilinogen

(Fig. 10.5), where porphobilinogen synthase, which is also called **ALA dehydratase,** catalyzes the condensation of two molecules of δ-aminolevulinate, to form the pyrrole ring of porphobilinogen (PBG).

There is evidence that the amino N of a lysine residue of *PBG synthase* reacts with the keto C of one δ-aminolevulinate (ALA) to form an **Schiff base** linkage, which has a role in promoting cyclization during interaction with the second ALA.

Each homo-octomeric complex of PBG synthase binds eight **zinc** ions (Zn^{++}), four of which are essential for activity. The Zn^{++}-binding sites, which include cysteine S ligands, can also bind **lead** (Pb^{++}), leading to enzyme inhibition. Elevated levels of ALA in blood may cause some of the neurological effects of **lead poisoning**. High levels of ALA can result also from hereditary deficiency of some enzymes of the heme synthesis pathway.

ALA is toxic to the brain for the reasons; ALA resembles the structure of GABA (γ-aminobutyric acid, a neurotransmitter), and auto-oxidation of ALA generates reactive oxygen species (oxygen radicals).

A linear hydroxymethylbilane is formed in the next step by condensation of four molecules of porphobilinogen (PBG) catalyzed by **Porphobilinogen deaminase** (PBG deaminase) also called **Uroporphyrinogen I synthase.** Successive condensations of PBG initiated in each case by elimination of the amino group. Porphobilinogen deaminase enzyme has a **dipyrromethane** prosthetic group, linked at the active site via S of cysteine (Fig.10.6). The enzyme catalyzes formation of its own dipyrromethane prosthetic group by condensation of two molecules of PBG.

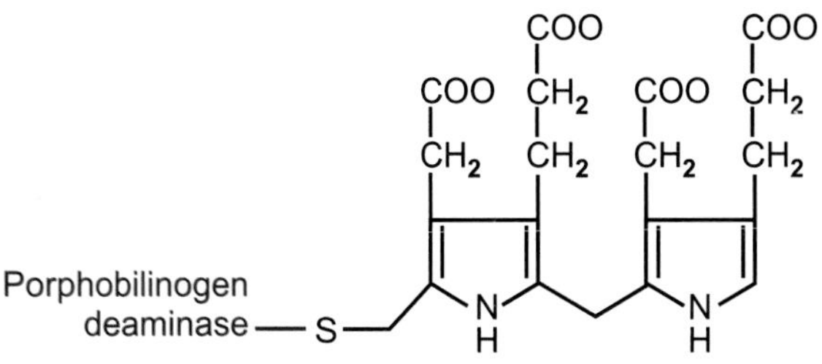

Fig. 10.6: Dipyromethane

Once four PBGs have condensed, prior to hydrolysis of the link to the enzyme's dipyrromethane, the enzyme has a bound hexapyrrole, derived from 6 PBG. Porphobilinogen deaminase is organized in three domains. Predicted interdomain flexibility may accommodate the growing polypyrrole in the active site cleft.

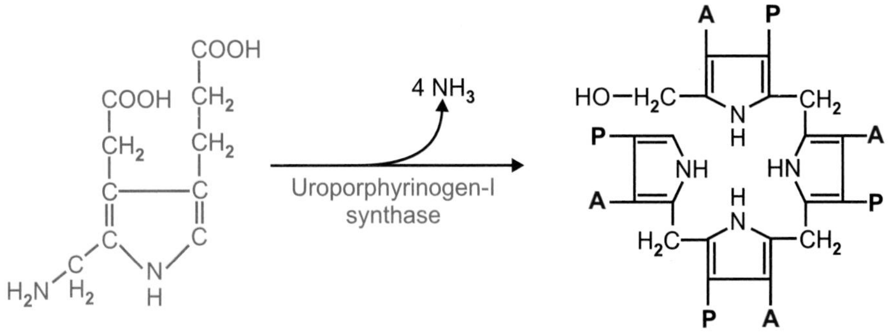

4 molecules of porphobilinogen

Hydroxymethylbilane

Fig. 10.7: Hydroxymethylbilane

Hydrolysis of the link to the dipyrromethane moiety yields free **hydroxymethylbilane** (Fig.10.7). Cyclyzation of hydroxymethylbilane forms uroporphyrinogen-I.

Uroporphyrinogen-I synthase along with **uroporphyrinogen III cosynthase** (uroporphyrinogen isomerase) converts the uroporphyrinogen-I to uroporphyrinogen-III, and flipping over one of the pyrroles, to yield an **asymmetric** tetrapyrrole.

Note the distribution of **acetyl** and **propionyl** side chains (Fig. 10.8). This rearrangement is thought to proceed via a spiro intermediate. The active site is located in a cleft between the two domains of the uroporphyrinogen-III synthase enzyme. The structural flexibility inherent in this arrangement is proposed to be essential to catalysis.

Uroporphyrinogen-III is the precursor for synthesis of **vitamin B_{12}, chlorophyll**, and **heme** in organisms that produce these compounds.

Conversion of uroporphyrinogen-III to protoporphyrin-III (above) occurs in several steps (Fig. 10.8). These steps include:

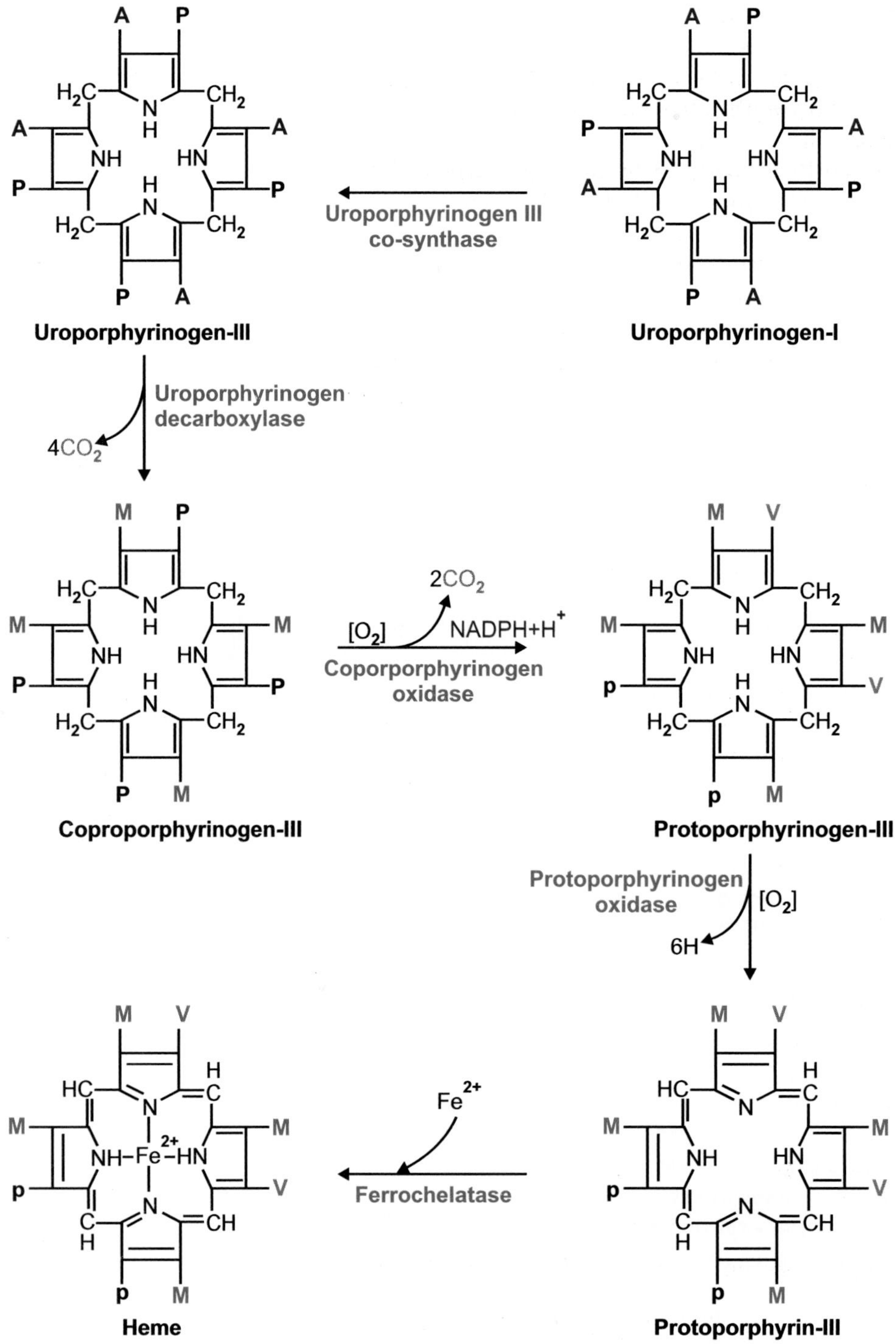

Fig. 10.8: Synthesis of heme

1. Decarboxylation of all four acetyl side chains of uroporphyrinogen-III, to the level of methyl groups is catalyzed by **uroporphyrinogen decarboxylase** to yield coproporphyri-nogen-III that enters mitochondria.

2. **Oxidative decarboxylation** of two of the four 'propionyl' side chains of coproporphyrinogen III, to the level of vinyl groups is catalyzed by **coproporphyrinogen oxidase,** to yield protoporphyrinogen-III.

3. Protoporphyrinogen-III is oxidized to **protoporphyrin-III**, wherein the methylene bridges are oxidized to methenyl bridges, and two of the ring nitrogens are oxidized to the level of tertiary nitrogen. The reaction is catalyzed by **protoporphyrinogen oxidase** that requires oxygen.

4. Fe^{++} is added to protoporphyrin-III via **ferrochelatase (heme synthase)** to yield heme. Fe^{++} may bind to a conserved histidine residue in the enzyme, prior to being transferred to proto-porphyrin-III.

HEME CATABOLISM (BILE METABOLISM)

Most of the heme in human body is within erythrocytes, whose life-span is about 120 days. There is thus a turnover of about 6 g of hemoglobin per day, which presents two problems:

1. The hydrophobic porphyrin ring needs to be made hydrophilic to facilitate excretion.

2. Iron must be conserved for new heme synthesis.

Normally, cells of the reticuloendothelial system engulf heme from senescent erythrocytes and other hemoproteins. The globin is recycled or broken down to amino acids that are recycled or catabolized as required. Oxidation of heme and ring opening is

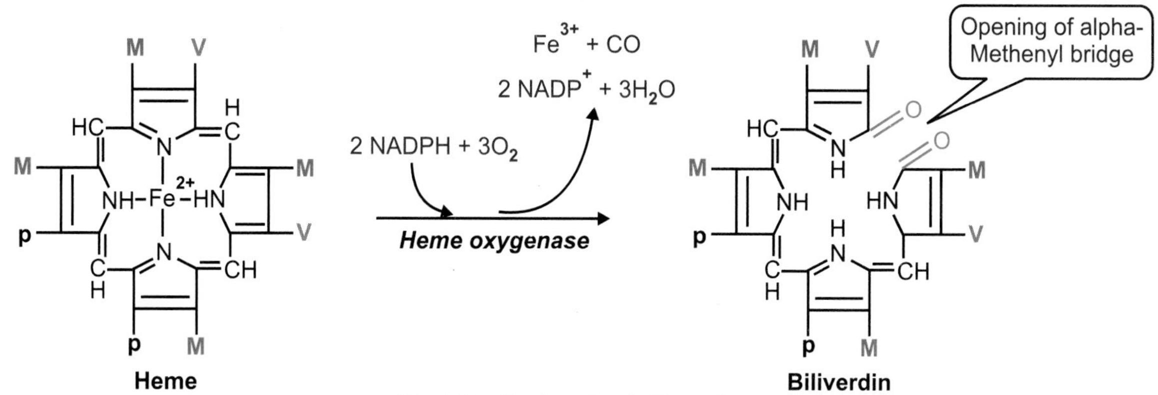

Fig. 10.9: Synthesis of biliverdin

catalyzed by **heme oxygenase,** an enzyme of endoplasmic reticulum (Fig. 10.9).

The oxidation step requires heme as a substrate, and any hemin (Fe^{3+}) is first reduced to heme (Fe^{2+}) prior to oxidation by **heme oxygenase.** The oxidation of a specific carbon (alpha-methenyl bridge) of heme opens up the ring and forms the linear tetrapyrrole **biliverdin**, with release of ferric iron (Fe^{3+}), and carbon monoxide (CO). This is the only reaction in the body that is known to produce CO. Most of the CO is exhaled through the lungs. The CO content

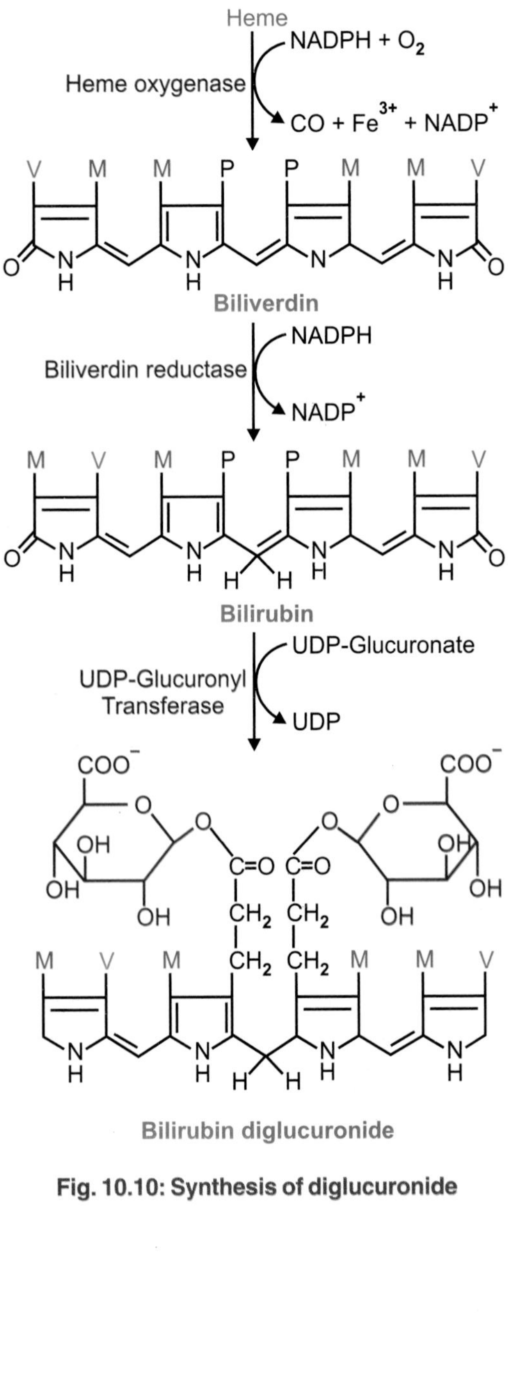

Fig. 10.10: Synthesis of diglucuronide

of expired air is a direct measure of **heme oxidase** activity in the individual.

In the next reaction, a second bridging methenyl (between rings III and IV) is reduced by **biliverdin reductase,** producing **bilirubin** (Fig. 10.10).

Bilirubin has significantly less conjugated double bonds than biliverdin that causes a change in the color of the molecule from blue-green (biliverdin) to yellow-red (bilirubin). The latter catabolic changes in the structure of tetrapyrroles are responsible for the progressive changes in color of a hematoma, or bruise, in which the damaged tissue changes its color from an initial dark blue to a red-yellow, and finally to a yellow color before all the pigment is transported out of the affected tissue.

Peripherally arising bilirubin is sparingly soluble in water, and is transported in blood bound to albumin. At the sinusoidal surface of hepatocyts, albumin bound bilirubin is taken up by carrier mediated system, and within the hepatocyte bilirubin is transported bound to ligandin. Drugs such as aspirin, sulfa drugs, and certain antibiotics, displace bilirubin from their binding-sites on albumin.

In hepatocytes, **UDP glucuronyl transferase** sequentially transfers two molecules of glucuronic acid, from UDP-glucuronate to bilirubin, to form bilirubin monoglucuronate and bilirubin diglucuronate (Fig.10.10). Alternately an enzyme dismutase facilitates transfer of glucuronate molecule from one molecule of bilirubin monoglucuronate to another molecule of bilirubin monoglucuronate to form bilirubin diglucuronate. The addition of glucuronate groups make bilirubin water-soluble, and facilitates its excretion in the bile as the bile pigments.

UDP-glucuronyl transferase is an inducible enzyme, whose activity can be induced by a number of enzymes including phenobarbitone.

Conjugated bilirubin is secreted by hepatocytes, by an active transport system, into the canaliculi against concentration gradient. The transport system that secretes bilirubin into the bile can be induced by those same drugs, which induces glucuronyl transferases.

When the conjugated bilirubin reaches the large intestine, the glucuronides are removed by specific bacterial glucuronidases. The free bilirubin is subsequently reduced to colorless compounds called urobilinogen by bacterial enzymes. Small quantities of urobilinogen is reabsorbed and re-excreted through the liver that constitutes intrahepatic urobilinogen cycle. Under conditions where a large quantity of bilirubin is reaching intestine or there is an intrference with intrahepatic cycle, can lead to increased excretion of urobilinogen in urine.

Most of the colorless urobilinogen formed in the colon is oxidized to colored urobilins by the action of bacterial enzymes.

Abnormally high rate of erythrocyte lysis, or liver damage with bile duct obstruction, cause an accumulation of bilirubin and its precursors in the circulation; the result is **hyperbilirubinemia**, and the cause of abnormal body pigmentation is known as **jaundice**. Under normal conditions, intestinal bacteria act on bilirubin to produce the final porphyrin products **urobilinogens** and **urobilins** that are found in the feces and urine. Bilirubin and its catabolic products are collectively designated as **bile pigments**.

CLINICAL ASPECT OF HEME METABOLISM

Clinical problems associated with heme metabolism are of two types.
1. Disorders that arise from defects in the enzymes of heme biosynthesis are termed **porphyrias**, which cause an elevation of intermediates of heme synthesis pathway in the serum and urine.
2. Disorders that arise from defects in bilirubin metabolism (product of heme catabolism) lead to **hyperbilirubinemia (Jaundice)**.

PORPHYRIAS

Porphyrias are heterogeneous group of both inherited and acquired disorders of heme synthesis. These disorders are classified as erythroid, hepatic, and hepatoerythropoietic classes, depending upon the principal site of expression of the enzyme defects. Eight different porphyrias have been identified. With the exception of the reaction catalyzed by **ALA synthase**, defects in each of the other enzymes of heme synthesis have been identified. The most commonly occurring porphyria is **acute intermittent porphyria (AIP)**, which is caused by a defect in **porphobilinogen deaminase**, (PBG deaminase). This enzyme is also called **hydroxymethylbilane synthase** or **uroporphyrinogen synthase**.

All of the porphyrias lead to excretion of intermediaries of heme biosynthesis that turn the urine red, and when deposited in the teeth turn them reddish brown. Accumulation of these byproducts in the skin renders it extremely sensitive to sunlight causing ulceration and disfiguring scars. Increased hair growth is also a symptom of the porphryias leading to appearance of fine hairs over the entire face and on the extremities.

Neurological syndrome These are characteristically precipitated by drugs such as phenobarbitones, resulting in abdominal pain, peripheral neuropathy, and mental disturbance. These neurovisceral and psychiatric symptoms occur only in those porphyrias where there is over production of ALA and PBG. The depleted heme production might affect tryptophan pyrolase levels, leading to accumulation of tryptophan and **5-HTA** (affect viscera and behavioral mood).

Photosensitivity It is directly related to elevated production and accumulation of porphyrin that has characteristic light absorption properties, which generate **singlet oxygen** (free radical) that in turn causes peroxidation of lipids in the lysosomal membranes and release of **lysozymes**.

Inherited porphyrias They exhibit variable expressivity. Drugs, hormones and liver diseases precipitate exacerbation of asymptomatic patient.

Porphyria	Enzyme defect	Symptoms
Erythropoietic		
Congenital erythropoietic porphyria, CEP	Uroporphyrinogen-III Cosynthase	Photosensitivity
Erythropoietic protoporphyria, EPP	Ferrochelatase	Photosensitivity
Hepatic		
ALA dehydratase deficiency porphyria, ADP	ALA dehydratase	Neurovisceral
Acute intermittent porphyria, AIP	PBG deaminase	Neurovisceral
Hereditary coproporphyria, HCP	Coproporphyrinogen oxidase	Neurovisceral, some photosensitivity
Variegate porphyria, VP	Protoporphyrinogen oxidase	Neurovisceral, some photosensitivity
Porphyria cutanea tarda, PCT	Uroporphyrinogen decarboxylase	Photosensitivity
Hepatoerythropoietic		
Hepatoerythropoietic porphyria, HEP	Uroporphyrinogen decarboxylase	Photosensitivity, some neurovisceral

HYPERBILIRUBINEMIA (JAUNDICE)

Bilirubin is potentially a toxic waste product of heme catabolism. The body eliminates bilirubin by transporting it to the liver bound to albumin in the serum (Fig. 10.11). In the hepatocytes, bilirubin is conjugated with two molecules of glucuronate, which renders it water-soluble. The diglucuronate conjugate is then excreted in the bile.

Persons with extreme elevation in unconjugated bilirubin are prone to develop bilirubin **encephalopathy**, also referred to as **kernicterus**. Accumulation of bilirubin in the plasma and tissues results in **jaundice**.

Jaundice or icterus is the classical manifestation of hepatic diseases, where there is accumulation of bilirubin in the body fluids that causes yellow discoloration of plasma, skin, mucous membrane and

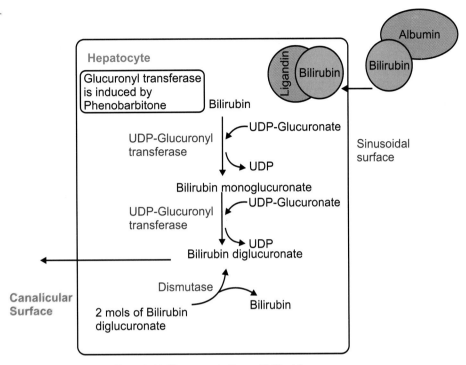

Fig. 10.11: Transportation of bilirubin

conjunctiva. Jaundice is clinically apparent when serum bilirubin levels are in excess of 2 to 3 mg/dl (normal range of serum total bilirubin is 0.25 to 1.0 mg/dl).

Jaundice is variously classified based on:
i. Type of bilirubin in plasma
   a. Unconjugated hyperbilirubinemia
   b. Conjugated hyperbilirubinemia
ii. Presence or absence of bilirubin in urine
   Only conjugated bilirubin can appear in urine.
   a. Choluric jaundice (regurgitation hyperbilirubinemia)
   b. Acholuric jaundice
iii. Site of cause of hyperbilirubinemia
   a. Prehepatic jaundice
   b. Hepatic jaundice
   c. Posthepatic jaundice

From clinical point of view, classification based on type of bilirubin is much more informative than the other two classifications.

Under physiological conditions almost all the bilirubin found in serum is the unconjugated type that is on its way to the liver from the reticuloendothelial tissues for conjugation and secretion (unconjugated bilirubin 0.2 to 0.7 mg/dl, and conjugated bilirubin 0.1 to 0.4 mg/dl).

Causes of Unconjugated Hyperbilirubinemias

- Increased production of bilirubin due to increased hemolysis.
- Decreased delivery of unconjugated bilirubin to liver due to congestive cardiac failure.

- Decreased uptake of unconjugated bilirubin across hepatocytes, e.g. Gilbert's syndrome.
- Decreased conjugation of bilirubin, e.g. in neonates where conjugation system is still not developed, and Crigler-Najjar syndrome, an inherited disorder where glucuronyl transferase is deficient or absent.

Causes of Conjugated Hyperbilirubinemias

- Decreased secretion of conjugated bilirubin into canaliculi as seen in hepatitis, hepatocellular diseases, toxicity due to certain drugs, and Dubin Johnson disease due to a defect in the hepatic secretion of conjugated compounds, which can be diagnosed by bromsulphthalein excretion test.
- Decreased drainage of biliary secretions into the GI tract due to an obstruction in the biliary system, as seen in intrahepatic obstruction caused by inflammation, and extrahepatic obstruction due to gallstones and tumors of head of the pancreas.

Van den Bergh Reaction

This test consists of two parts, the direct and indirect reactions.

The direct reaction This test is essentially a test for determining total bilirubin. When serum is treated with diazo reagent under acidic conditions (Ehrlich's diazo reagent), the bilirubin reacts to form a purple colored azobilirubin.

Three different responses may be obtained:

  i. Immediate direct reaction, in which there is an immediate rapid color development that is maximal by the end of 4 min. This is due to the presence of conjugated bilirubin.
  ii. Delayed direct reaction, in which the color begins to appear from 5 to 30 min after mixing the serum and reagent, and then the color develops slowly to a maximum. This is due to unconjugated bilirubin.
  iii. No direct reaction may be observed.

The indirect reaction This test is essentially to determine total serum bilirubin. The term arose because proteins were precipitated before addition of diazo reagent.

Urine Findings in Jaundice

Bilirubin is not a normal urinary constituent. Whenever bilirubin happens to appear in the urine, it is always the conjugated bilirubin due to conjugated hyperbilirubinemia.

Bilirubin that enters the GI tract through biliary secretions is reduced to urobilinogens by bacterial action, and small quantities are absorbed into the blood and excreted into urine by the kidneys. It means under physiological conditions only trace amounts of urobilinogens are found in the urine. Urinary urobilinogens are elevated in hemolytic jaundice, since large quantity of conjugated bilirubin is entering GI tract through biliary secretions.

Bile salts are not normal urinary constituents, but are found in urine, in obstructive jaundice.

Mineral Metabolism

11

Metabolically important minerals are grouped under two classes. They are:

i. **Nutritionally important minerals** are those, which are required in quantities more than 100 mg/day, examples are: sodium, potassium, chloride, calcium, phosphorus and magnesium.

ii. **Trace elements** are those, which are required in quantities less than 100 mg/day, examples are: cobalt, copper, iodine, iron, manganese, molybdenum, zinc, selenium, and fluorides.

Most minerals with the exception of sodium and potassium form salts with other compounds that are relatively insoluble and not readily absorbed. Specific carrier proteins are often required for mineral absorption; the synthesis of these proteins serves an important mechanism for control of mineral levels in the body. Specific proteins are also required for transport and storage of many minerals. Most minerals are excreted in urine, and many are also secreted into digestive juice and bile.

Mineral deficiencies are rare among those individuals, whose diet includes sufficient variety of foods. Deficiencies are usually secondary to malabsorption, chronic bleeding, renal disease or other clinical problems. Toxicity is usually noticed when control of absorption fails in some way.

COPPER

The earliest manifestation of copper deficiency in experimental animals was found to lead to anemia, defective wool keratinization, abnormal bone formation, and arterial and cardiac aneurysm. Other features among the offspring born to animals subjected to severe copper deficiency include neurological problems such as ataxia, seizures and episodic apnea, which are believed to be due to a lack of myelination, leading to a reduced nerve cell formation during embryonic development. The identification of intermediary pathways of various cuproenzymes has provided an increased understanding of the pathophysiological basis for these abnormalities. An increasing number of disorders associated with copper deficiency have been recognized in humans, which are strikingly similar to those observed in animal experiments. Important copper containing enzymes include cytochrome C oxidase, tyrosinase, dopamine hydroxylase, monoamine oxidase, diamine oxidase, superoxide dismutase, lysyl oxidase and ceruloplasmine ferroxidase.

Metabolism of Copper

A small molecular weight protein keeps copper soluble in saliva and gastric juice. In the intestinal mucosal cells, copper is associated with metallothionine and is transported in the plasma bound to histidine and albumin. Copper content in the body is almost exclusively maintained by biliary excretion, and only trace amounts of copper are excreted in the normal urine.

Daily requirement of copper is 0.5 to 3 mg.

Copper Deficiency in Anemia

In humans, nutritional copper deficiency leads to hypochromic anemia and neutropenia. The anemia appears to be related to iron mobilization due to a combined defect of **ceruloplasmin ferroxidase** activity and intracellular iron utilization.

Copper in Superoxide Dismutase (SOD)

In human blood, copper is distributed equally in erythrocytes and plasma. In erythrocytes, copper is loosely bound to amino acids. Almost 60 percent of copper in the blood is tightly bound to a copper-zinc-dependent enzyme known as *superoxide dismutase* (CuZnSOD), which is a powerful antioxidant. A similar antioxidative enzyme is dependent on the trace mineral manganese (MnSOD). The role of superoxide dismutases is to protect cells against free-radical injury, similar to *glutathione peroxidase.*

Copper in Bone and Arterial Defects

Menkes' kinky or steely hair syndrome is an X-linked disorder affecting copper transport across the serosal aspect of the mucosal cell causing copper deficiency, it was first described in 1962 as a syndrome seen in infants characterized by poor growth, white brittle hair with peculiar twisting, arterial defects, focal cerebral degeneration and mental retardation. Severe copper deficiency in infants leads to pathological bone fractures that are similar to seen in **'battered child syndrome'**. These defects are related to decreased activity of a copper-dependent enzyme, **lysyl oxidase**, which is vital for the cross-linking of collagen.

Copper in Cardiovascular and Lung Disorders

Cardiovascular disorders and emphysema-like lung condition observed in some copper deficiency states appear to be caused by an impairment of cross-linking of elastin and collagen due to depression of *lysyl oxidase* activity. The peroxidative damage that is frequently seen in lung and cardiovascular systems is directly related to an excessive free radical formation due to a reduced superoxide dismutase (CuZnSOD) activity.

Wilson's Disease

It is an inherited autosomal recessive defect, in the incorporation of copper into newly synthesized apocerruloplasmin to form *cerruloplasmin*. In addition, the liver fails to excrete copper into the bile that results in increased copper deposition, particularly in liver, lenticular nucleus of brain (*hepatolenticular degeneration*), and decement's membrane of the cornea (*Kayser-Fleischer rings*). Markedly increased excretion of copper in urine is noticed in individuals suffering from this disorder. Chelation of the excess copper by *penicillamine* can reverse some of the organ damage.

Copper Poisoning and Toxicity

Most of us seem to suffer from a low-level copper toxicity. One of the most prominent sources of copper is acidic food that is cooked in copper pans. Cigarette smoking is also a prominent source of excessive copper accumulation. Similarly oral contraceptives are notorious in raising the body's copper burden.

High body copper burden can be responsible for such diverse disorders as hypotension, heart disease, pre-menstrual tension, postpartum depression, paranoid and hallucinatory schizophrenias, childhood hyperactivity and autism.

MOLYBDENUM

Molybdenum (Mo) is a transition metal that forms oxides and is a component of pterin coenzyme essential for the activity of xanthine oxidase, sulfite oxidase, and aldehyde oxidase. Genetically conditioned sulfite oxidase deficiency was described in 1967 in a child with mental retardation, convulsions, opisthotonus, and lens dislocation. This disorder was due to the child's inability to form the molybdenum coenzyme despite the presence of adequate molybdenum. The principal sources of molybdenum are organ meats, whole-grain cereals, and legumes, which provides about 100 to 500 μg/day. Safe, adequate intake of molybdenum is 75 to 250 μg/day for adults and 25 to 75 μg/day for children aged 1 to 6 years.

IODINE

The primary function of iodine (I) in the body is to provide a substrate for the synthesis of the thyroid hormones, *thyroxin (T_4)* and *triiodothyronine (T_3)*, which are crucial for normal growth and development. About 80 percent of the body's iodine pool, i.e. about 15 mg is found in thyroid gland. Iodide, the ionic form of iodine is rapidly absorbed from the GI tract and distributed in extracellular water. Fasting plasma concentration of iodide is about 1 μg/L (7.88 nmol/L). In adults, about 80 percent of the iodide ingested and absorbed is trapped by the thyroid gland through an ATP-dependent iodide pump.

Iodide occurs in soil and seawater and is oxidized by sunlight to iodine, which is vaporized into the air. The iodide concentration in seawater is 50 to 60 μg/L. Iodine deficiency is found in humans, living at higher altitudes and in countries where salt is not fortified with iodide. In iodine-deficient areas, the iodide concentration in drinking water is less than 2 μg/L, whereas in areas close to the sea, the drinking water contains 4 to 10 μg/L.

The usual intake of iodide in healthy persons is 100 to 200 μg/day, mostly from iodized salt (70 μg/g).

Deficiency Diseases

Iodine deficiency results when iodide intake is less than 20 μg/day. In moderate iodine deficiency, the thyroid gland, under the influence of thyroid-stimulating hormone (TSH), hypertrophies to concentrate iodide, resulting in a colloid goiter. Most of these cases remain euthyroid.

Severe iodine deficiency may cause *endemic myxedema* among adults, and *endemic cretinism* among infants. Several metabolic disturbances in thyroid hormone synthesis can cause both adult and infantile hypothyroidism. Severe maternal iodine deficiency retards fetal growth and brain development. Endemic cretinism may occur in one of two forms neurologic or myxedematous, depending on the interplay of iodine deficiency and genetics.

Infants with iodine deficiency are given L-thyroxin (3 μg/kg/day) for a week plus 50 μg of iodide to quickly restore an euthyroid state. Iodide supplementation is continued. Plasma TSH levels are monitored until they are in the normal range, i.e. less than 5 μIU/mL. Deficient adults are given iodide at a dose of 1500 μg/day for several weeks to restore the iodine content of the depleted gland and permit thyroxin synthesis.

Iodine Toxicity

When iodide intake is 20 times greater than the daily requirement, it results in chronic iodine toxicity. Increased uptake of iodine by the thyroid may lead to inhibition of thyroid hormone synthesis (*Wolff-Chaikoff effect*) and eventually causes iodide goiter or myxedema. At very high doses of iodide, a brassy taste, increased salivation, gastric irritation, and acne form skin lesions may occur.

FLUORIDE

Ionic form of fluorine (F) is fluoride, which is widely distributed in nature. Most of the body's fluorine is found in bones and teeth.

Main source of fluorine is drinking water but rich sources are saltwater fish and tea.

Deficiency

Fluoride is essential for the prevention of dental caries and possibly osteoporosis. Fluoridation of water that contains less than the ideal level of 1 ppm significantly reduces the incidence of dental caries.

Toxicity

Individuals living in areas where drinking water contains more than 10 ppm are commonly affected with fluorosis (excess accumulation of fluorine in teeth and bones). Fluorosis is most evident in permanent teeth that develop during high fluorine intake. Deciduous teeth are affected only when intake is very high. The earliest changes are chalky-white, irregularly distributed patches on the surface of the enamel; these patches become stained yellow or brown, producing the characteristic mottled appearance. Severe fluorosis weakens the enamel and cause surface pitting. Prolonged high intake of fluorine in adults, results in bony changes characterized by osteosclerosis, exostoses of the spine, and genu valgum.

MANGANESE

Manganese (Mn) is a component of several enzyme systems, including manganese-specific *glycosyltransferase, phosphoenol pyruvate carboxykinase, diamine oxidase* and *superoxide dismutase.* It is also essential for normal bone structure.

Rich sources of manganese include unrefined cereals, green leafy vegetables, and tea.

The usual intake of this mineral is 2 to 5 mg/day, and only 5 to 10 percent of it is absorbed.

Manganese deficiency has not been documented in the clinical literature.

Manganese toxicity is usually limited to people who work in manganese mines and refinery; prolonged exposure causes neurological symptoms resembling parkinsonism or Wilson's disease.

SELENIUM

Selenium is a vital part of the enzyme **glutathione peroxidase**, which functions with vitamin E as an antioxidant to protect cells from free radical damage. *Glutathione peroxidase* metabolizes hydro-peroxides formed from polyunsaturated fatty acids. Selenium is also a part of the enzymes that de-iodinate thyroid hormones. It also helps to eliminate heavy metals like lead, mercury, cadmium and aluminum. Generally, selenium functions as an **antioxidant** that works in **conjunction with vitamin E**. Plasma levels of selenium ranges from 8 to 25 μg/dl, depending on selenium intake.

Dietary Sources of selenium are wheat germ, brazil nuts and nutritional yeast. Whole grains and seafood are also good sources. Selenium content of foods depends on the level of selenium in the soil.

Deficiency

Selenium deficiency is rare among humans. However, selenium deficiency is noticed in association with **Keshan disease,** an endemic viral cardiomyopathy affecting children and young women in China.

Toxicity

At high doses (more than 900 μg/day), selenium produces a toxic syndrome called selenosis, consisting of dermatitis, loose hair, diseased nails, and peripheral neuropathy, associated with plasma levels of selenium in excess of 100 μg/dl.

Function

Mild deficiency of selenium results in decreased immune function and increased risk of cancer. More pronounced deficiency causes Keshan disease, a severe heart disease of children and young women. Selenium deficiency has also been linked to Kashin-Beck disease, an arthritic condition and to heart disturbances and muscle weakness.

Deficiency

Selenium deficiency occurs with malnutrition and in areas where the soil has very low selenium levels. Selenium toxicity can occur with daily intake of 900 μg, and is characterized by depression, nervousness, irritability, nausea, vomiting, skin rash, garlic smelling breath (Selenomethionine) and loss of hair and fingernails.

Daily Requirement

For infants 10 to 15 μg, children in the age group of 1 to 10 years 20 to 30 μg, adults 40 to 70 μg, during pregnancy 65 μg and lactating women 75 μg.

Therapeutic Dose

Therapeutic administration of 200 μg daily is given in the following conditions.

Prevention of cancer, prevention of heart disease and high blood pressure, immune system enhancement, and respiratory syncytial virus infection.

ZINC

The body contains 2 to 3 g of zinc (Zn), which is found mainly in bones, teeth, hair, skin, liver, muscle, leukocytes, and testes. Normal serum zinc level is about 100 μg/dl. One-third of it is attached loosely to albumin, and about two-third is firmly bound to globulins. There are more than 100 zinc metalloenzymes, including a large number of nicotinamide adenine dinucleotide (NADH) dehydrogenases, *zinc-insulin complex for storage of insulin* in β-cells of islets of Langerhans, *RNA and DNA polymerases*, and *DNA transcription factors* as well as alkaline phosphatase, superoxide dismutase, and carbonic anhydrase. Dietary intake of zinc in healthy adults varies from 6 to 15 mg/day, and only about 20 percent of it is absorbed.

Good sources of zinc are meat, liver, eggs, and seafood (especially oysters).

Daily requirement for adults is about 0.2 mg/kg/day.

Deficiency

The signs and symptoms of zinc deficiency include anorexia, growth retardation, delayed sexual maturation, hypogonadism and hypospermia, alopecia, immune disorders, dermatitis, night blindness, impaired taste (hypogeusia), and impaired wound healing. The first signs of zinc deficiency in marginally nourished children are suboptimal growth, anorexia, and impaired taste. Some patients with cirrhosis suffer from zinc deficiency because the liver fails to retain zinc.

Biochemical changes associated with zinc deficiency include decreased levels of plasma zinc (less than 70 μg/dL), alkaline phosphatase, alcohol dehydrogenase in the retina (which accounts for night blindness), plasma testosterone, impaired T lymphocyte function, decreased collagen synthesis (resulting in poor wound healing), and decreased RNA polymerase activity in several tissues.

Maternal zinc deficiency may cause anencephaly in the fetus. Secondary deficiency occurs in liver disease, malabsorption states, and during prolonged parenteral nutrition.

Acrodermatitis enteropathica is a rare autosomal recessive disorder, which results from malabsorption of zinc. The defect involves the failure to synthesize a transport protein that enables zinc absorption in the intestine. Symptoms usually begin after an infant is weaned from breast milk. This disorder is characterized by psoriasiform dermatitis, hair loss, paronychia, growth retardation, and diarrhea. Complete remission is achieved by oral administration of 30 to 150 mg/day of zinc sulfate.

Toxicity

Ingesting zinc in excess of 200 mg/day, usually by consuming acidic food or drink from a galvanized container, can cause toxicity characterized by vomiting and diarrhea. Doses of zinc ranging from 100 to 150 mg/day interfere with copper metabolism and cause hypocupremia, microcytic erythrocytes, and neutropenia. *Metal fume fever,* also called *brass-founders' ague* or *zinc shakes,* is an industrial hazard caused by inhaling zinc oxide fumes that results in neurological damage.

The discovery of zinc "finger proteins" has led to a better understanding of how cells replicate and divide. Their role in behavior is not yet clear, but could be involved in the transport or availability of zinc. Recent research has shown zinc to be far more important than previously believed and low levels of zinc are associated with behavior disorders.

The copper/zinc ratio appears to be more decisively important than either of the individual metals alone. Zinc deficiency often results in elevated blood levels of copper, due to the dynamic competition of these metals in the body. Elevated blood copper has been associated with episodic violence, hyperactivity, learning disabilities and depression.

Treatment of Zinc Deficiency

Indiscriminant dosages of zinc to persons who do not need it can cause anemia and imbalanced trace metals. Treatment of mild or moderate zinc depletion can take months to complete. Some cases of severe zinc depletion require a year or more to resolve. Achievement of a proper zinc balance is slowed by growth spurts, injury, illness, or severe stress. In addition, persons with malabsorption or type-A blood respond to treatment more slowly.

Zinc deficient individuals usually respond well to inexpensive supplementation with zinc and augmenting nutrients. Zinc deficiency can be corrected, but not cured. Zinc deficiency, requires life long treatment. Fortunately, it is a simple, low cost, safe treatment.

IRON

Metabolism

Iron metabolism depends on body's iron status. As an essential nutrient, there is no mechanism of excreting any excesses iron that may accumulate in the body. The total iron content of an adult, weighing 70 Kg is about 3.7 g, almost 69 percent of this is present in hemoglobin, the rest (almost 29%) is stored as ferritin, and the remainder is in myoglobin, cytochromes, other hemoproteins, and the iron-sulfur proteins of respiration. Iron is always found in bound form because free iron is chemically very reactive, e.g. it binds nonspecifically to many proteins, with deleterious consequences to their structures, acts catalytically in assorted oxidation reactions such as peroxidation of unsaturated fatty acids in cellular membranes. Since iron is in bound form it does not get excreted. Iron is lost from the body only by processes such as: bleeding, sloughing of cells, menstrual flow and transfer to a developing fetus. The only mechanism by which, the body's iron content gets regulated is by absorption.

Absorption

The form in which iron is presented to the digestive tract affects absorption of iron, and inorganic iron ions change their oxidation state during the process of absorption (Fig. 11.1).

The two major forms of dietary iron are **heme iron** found primarily in red meats that is most easily absorbed, and the **other forms of iron** is bound to organic constituent of the food. These interactions are disrupted during cooking of food and increase bioavailability of iron. Some iron-rich foods are poor sources of the mineral because other compounds render it nonabsorbable. The classic example is spinach. It contains iron, but it also contains considerable oxalate, which chelates iron and renders it nonabsorbable. Phytates, present in whole grains that have not been subjected to fermentation by yeast (e.g., during bread making), have a similar effect.

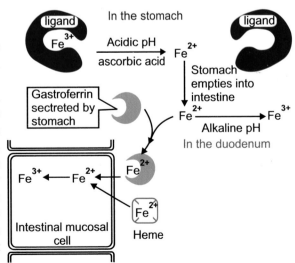

Fig. 11.1: Iron absorption events in stomach and duodenum

Iron ions undergo two important changes of oxidation state during digestion and absorption. The first change occurs in the stomach. Here iron (III) is reduced to iron (II). This reduction is favored by the low pH (Fig. 11.1). Reducing agents, such as ascorbic acid assist this process. Reduction is important because iron (II) dissociates from ligands more easily than iron (III). The second change occurs in the alkaline pH of duodenum where Fe^{2+} is oxidized to Fe^{3+}. In the bicarbonate rich alkaline environment of duodenum, heme is absorbed directly by the mucosal cells. The mucosal cells absorb iron bound to gastroferrin (protein secreted by stomach) as Fe^{2+} form. Within the cells, the iron dissociates from it, and the free iron (II) ions are oxidized to iron (III). The mucosal cells of intestine take up iron in substantial amounts under all circumstances of nutritional iron status.

Iron Storage

Iron is stored in intestinal mucosal cells (Fig.11.2), and mostly in the liver as ferritin or hemosiderin. Ferritin is a protein with a capacity to bind about 4500 iron (III) ions per protein molecule. This is the major form of iron storage. When the storage capacity for iron in ferritin is exceeded, iron complexes with phosphate and hydroxides. This is called **hemosiderin,** which is the physiologically available form. As the burden of iron increases beyond normal levels, excess hemosiderin is deposited in the liver and heart. This can reach a point when the function of these organs is impaired, and death ensues.

Several conditions can lead to excess iron deposition in the body. Idiopathic hemochromatosis is a condition in which control of iron absorption is defective, and the excess iron absorbed is deposited as hemosiderin that disrupts cellular or organ architecture. Multiple transfusions can also lead to hemochromatosis. This is a serious problem for persons with beta-thalassemia, a disease in which hemoglobin is not made normally, and is supplemented by repeated blood transfusion as needed.

Treatment of excess iron storage involves artificial removal of iron by bleeding, which is the treatment of choice for idiopathic hemochromatosis. In beta-thalassemia, bleeding would be inappropriate since ability of the body to synthesize hemoglobin is compromised. In this case, *chelators (deferoxamine)* are administered which bind iron, and the complex of chelator with iron is excreted in the urine. Although deferoxamine is effective, it is an inconvenient process of overnight infusion. Treatment becomes critical as the patients reach their teenage years, a period of life associated with rebelliousness and feelings of invulnerability. These patients are not receptive to the treatment.

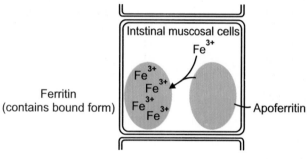

Iron is stored in muscosal cells and is lost when the cells die and slough

Fig. 11.2: Iron is stored as ferritin in intestinal mucosal cells

Iron Transport

Iron, stored in intestinal mucosal cells and the liver may be transferred into the blood for transport to other tissues (Fig. 11.3). The storage form of iron (Fe^{3+}) must be reduced to iron (Fe^{2+}) in order to cross

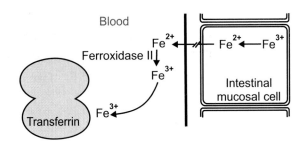

Fig. 11.3: Iron uptake into the blood

the plasma membrane. In the blood, iron (Fe^{2+}) is reoxidized to iron (Fe^{3+}) by ferroxidase-II. Iron (Fe^{3+}) is carried by the serum protein, transferrin. Transferrin contains two sites that bind iron (Fe^{3+}) tightly. Normally about 1/9 of the transferrin molecules have iron bound at both sites about 4/9 of them have iron bound at one site and about 4/9 have no iron bound. This means that transferrin is normally only about 1/3 saturated with iron, and there is a substantial unsaturated plasma iron binding capacity (Fig. 11.4). An unexpected influx of iron can be handled easily.

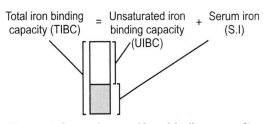

Fig. 11.4: Serum iron and iron binding capacity

The iron binding capacity of serum is of clinical interest. It is accounted for almost entirely by transferrin. There are three components to the iron binding capacity of serum.

i. Serum iron is the concentration of iron present, which is about 100 micrograms of iron per 100 milliliters of blood.

ii. Total iron binding capacity (TIBC) is the maximum amount of iron that can be bound, which is about 300 micrograms per 100 milliliters.

iii. The unsaturated iron binding capacity (UIBC) is the difference between the TIBC and the serum iron, which is normally about 200.

Iron binding capacity is used in the differential diagnosis of certain diseases (Fig. 11.5). In conditions associated with increased need for iron, such as iron deficiency or late pregnancy, TIBC is increased, but saturation is decreased from the normal 33 percent.

In hemochromatosis, TIBC is low, but it is saturated.

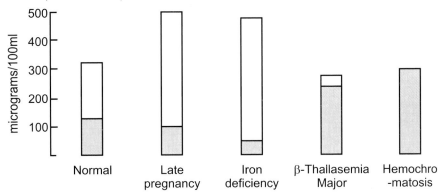

Fig. 11.5: SI and TIBC in various physiological and pathological conditions

Certain other clinical conditions are associated with their own characteristic patterns of TIBC and percent saturation.

Regulation of Iron Uptake

Iron uptake is regulated at the basal membrane of the intestinal mucosal cells. These cells make an iron-binding protein, apoferritin. In the iron-depleted state, little apoferritin is made, and the iron passes through the cells freely and enters the plasma. And, more apoferritin is synthesized. In replete state, more apoferritin is synthesized and iron is trapped in the cells as ferritin; ferritin can bind up to 3000 iron atoms per molecule of protein. As the mucosal cells slough, the iron is lost into the intestinal lumen with no absorption.

Diagnostic Significance of Disorders of Iron Metabolism in Ischemic Heart Disease (IHD)

Iron excess can induce lipid peroxidation and promotion of ischemic myocardial injury. The exact mechanisms of such damage are still not very clear.

The elevated serum ferritin concentration is considered as a diagnostic marker of risk for IHD, and possibly related to the damage of myocardial tissue. The elevated levels of stored iron, as assessed by elevated serum ferritin concentration can be a case for secondary prevention of IHD by using cardio-protective medicine (trimetazidine or preductal).

MAGNESIUM

Intestinal absorption of magnesium is hampered by increased dietary content of proteins, calcium and phosphate. Most of the magnesium filtered at the glomeruli is reabsorbed by the renal tubules.

Total body content of magnesium is about 24 g, of which 50 percent is found in bone, and the remaining is in soft tissue and muscle.

Good natural sources of magnesium are green leafy vegetables and unrefined cereals.

Plasma concentration of magnesium ranges from 1.6 to 2.4 mg/dl (0.7 to 1.0 mmol/L).

Daily requirement is about 100-350 mg/day.

Functions of Magnesium

i. It maintains structural integrity of ribosomes, nucleic acids and proteins.
ii. Influences permeability and electrical properties of membrane. Deficiency causes hyperexcitability.
iii. Mg-ATP complex is the substrate for enzymes requiring ATP. All those enzymes of nucleotide synthesis, lipid synthesis, glycolysis, and protein biosynthesis that require ATP also require magnesium. Magnesium is chelated between the β and γ phosphates of ATP and diminishes the dense ionic character

of ATP, so that it can approach and bind reversibly to specific sites on the enzyme.

Magnesium deficiency is seen in malabsorption, diarrhea from any cause, protein-calorie malnutrition, and alcoholism. Neuriritis, in alcoholics is due to combined deficiency of thiamin and magnesium. In chronic renal failure, magnesium is retained, but in renal tubular acidosis and diabetes mellitus, magnesium is lost in the urine. Diuretics as well lead to magnesium loss in the urine.

Calcium and Phosphate

12

CALCIUM

Almost 99 percent of the body's calcium is in the form of hydroxyapatite. Both bone and teeth contain the mineral hydroxyapatite (calcium phosphate with some hydroxyl groups) associated with a cartilage (protein) matrix. The skeleton system is main storage depot for calcium. Blood calcium is maintained at an optimal level of 8.5-10.5 mg/dl (2.1-2.6 mmol/L) by adding or removing calcium. About 50 percent of the blood calcium is in the ionized form.

Teeth and Bone Composition

	Mineral	Organic & water	Notes
Pulp	0%	100%	Innermost layer of teeth. Contains connective tissue, blood vessels, and nerves.
Dentin	70%	30%	Main tooth structure. Middle layer. Similar to bone in structure. Secreted by odontoblasts lining pulp cavity.
Enamel	97%	3%	Hard outer surface of tooth. Secreted by ameloblast cells.
Cementum	61%	39%	Lines the root of the tooth and helps hold it in the socket. Secreted by the periodontal-membrane.
Bone	65%	35%	Secreted by osteoblasts and broken down by osteoclasts. These processes occur continuously (remodeling).

Structure of Bone

Compact bone in the shafts of long bones is organized into Haversian systems. Cylindrical rings of bone have cavities with osteocyte (bone cells), and central canal with blood vessels. Long bones (femur, humerus, radius, ulna, tibia, fibula, etc.) have a shaft and heads (epiphyses) at each end. Epiphyseal plates (soft and with no calcium) allow bone to grow in length till they are sealed at puberty with no further growth.

Bone is a Dynamic Tissue because of Osteoblasts and Osteoclasts

Osteoblasts deposit minerals whereas osteoclasts remove minerals. These two types of cells work together to constantly remodel bone. If bone is subjected to weight bearing stress it will remodel into reinforced stronger bone. If bone is not weight bearing it will decalcify and become weaker (disuse atrophy seen in patients with long bed rests).

Functions of Ionized Calcium

About half the serum calcium is in ionized form and the rest is bound to proteins.

i.   Ionized serum calcium is required for secretion of hormones into blood.
ii. Flow of ionized calcium into cytoplasm triggers contraction of skeletal and heart muscles.
iii. Calcium is one of the hormone "second messengers".
iv. Ionized calcium is also required for blood coagulation, membrane formation, membrane and capillary permeability, nerve impulse transmission, and release and activation of enzymes.

Regulation of Calcium Metabolism

Calcium levels in serum and within the cells are precisely regulated and maintained at a few millimoles/liter. Such a fine control is possible by the combined and coordinated action of PTH, calcitriol, and calcitonin on bones, intestine and kidney.

About 50 percent of serum calcium is protein bound (30% to albumin and 20% to γ-globulin). Only the ionized form of calcium is biologically active, which can also complex with anions such as citrate, phosphate and bicarbonate. In acidosis, calcium bound to proteins gets displaced and also mobilized from bone, hence plasma calcium is elevated. In alkalosis, the events are reversed and ionized calcium in plasma is lowered that leads to tetany. If plasma calcium is too low nerves become more excitable, but transmission may be blocked at synapses; the net effect is muscular spasms, which can be fatal if they involve respiratory muscles.

Intracellular calcium is stored in sarcoplasmic and endoplasmic reticulum. Depolarization of membrane results in influx of calcium into the cytoplasm. It is later restored by calcium sequestration by *calsequestrin*. Intracellular calcium levels are kept low by active transport: cytoplasmic calcium is maintained at a concentration thousand times lower than serum calcium (about 0.1 micromoles/liter), which is necessary because high levels of cytoplasmic calcium can kill cells since they activate enzymes that hydrolyze proteins and other cell components.

Hormone	Production	Function
Parathyroid hormone	A peptide with 84 amino acids. Synthesized and secreted by parathyroid glands.	Elevates blood calcium level by promoting calcium resorption from bone, and intestinal absorption of calcium. It also reduces renal secretion of calcium.
Calcitriol	Made in steps at three different organs: skin, liver and kidney.	Elevates blood calcium level by promoting intestinal absorption of calcium
Calcitonin	Apeptide made of 32 amino acids. Synthesized by cells of thyroid gland.	Reduces blood calcium. Inhibits bone resorption by decreasing osteoclast activity.

Other Hormones Affecting Calcium Metabolism

Estrogens promote bone growth. When estrogens are reduced at menopause, osteoporosis is accelerated.

Testosterone stimulates growth of bone and cartilage.

Growth hormone promotes growth of bone and cartilage; it also increases intestinal absorption of calcium.

Parathyroid Hormone

Parathyroid hormone is synthesized as a "prohormone" of 110 amino acids, which is later, converted to the active hormone of 84 amino acids in the endoplasmic reticulum and Golgi apparatus by limited proteolysis.

Parathyroid hormone is a peptide hormone that causes an elevation of blood calcium levels by acting on three organs:
- *Bone:* stimulates osteoclasts that breakdown bone to release calcium.
- *Intestine:* increases absorption of calcium from intestine by enhancing the synthesis of calcium binding protein.
- *Kidney:* stimulates calcium reabsorption from the renal tubules.

Calcitriol (active form of Vitamin D)

Calcitriol is made in three steps by different organs (Fig. 12.1):

- 7-dehydrocholesterol is converted to vitamin D3 (cholecalciferol) in the skin by the action of ultraviolet light.

- Cholecalciferol is then hydroxylated in the liver (stimulated by PTH) to yield 25-hydroxycholecalciferol.

- Which is further hydroxylated in the kidney (stimulated by PTH) to yield calcitriol (1, 25-dihydroxycholecalciferol). The main effect of calcitriol is to increase intestinal absorption of calcium.

Calcitonin

Calcitonin is synthesized by the C cells of the thyroid gland as a large peptide "prohormone", which is then cut down to the 32 amino

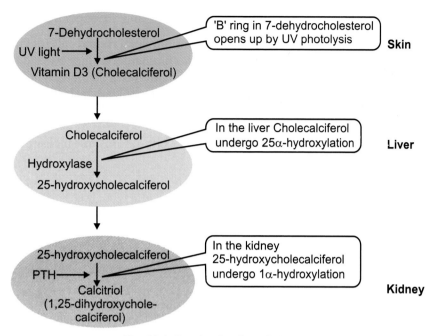

Fig. 12.1: Synthesis of calcitriol

acids calcitonin. It stimulates osteoblasts, but inhibits osteoclasts. It promotes calcification of bone by removing calcium from serum, thereby lowers serum calcium (opposing action of PTH).

Osteoporosis

In old age, bones get decalcified (osteoporosis) and become more susceptible for fractures.

Osteoporosis is secondary to reduced levels of sex hormones, which is much more common in postmenopausal women since they live longer (more time to decalcify).

PHOSPHATE

Inorganic phosphate is absorbed in intestine by active transport against electrochemical gradient. Ratio of calcium: phosphate in diet affects absorption of both. Optimal dietary ratio is 1:1. Excess of one mineral increases excretion of the other. Two-third of the phosphate is secreted in urine, and one-third is excreted in feces.

Though 80 to 85 percent of body's phosphate are found in the bone, the remaining 10 to 15 percent play important biological roles in association with other macromolecules. It is a component of structural molecules such as nucleic acids, proteins (phosphoproteins), lipids (phospholipids) and carbohydrates (mucopolysaccharides).

It is also a component of very important intracellular buffering system. Component of coenzymes (NAD, NADH, FAD and FMN), and energy transfer system (ATP, GTP, etc). Phosphates are also involved in signal transduction (phosphorylation and dephosphory-lation of enzymes).

Plasma phosphorus levels: 2.5 to 4.5 mg/dl.

Regulation of Plasma Phosphorus

Parathyroid hormone (PTH) and calcitriol mobilize phosphorus from bone whenever plasma levels are low and *vice versa*. Under normal physiological conditions, 85 percent of filtered phosphates are reabsorbed by renal tubules, which can be inhibited by PTH. Urinary phosphorus levels are low in glomerular damage, but are high in tubular damage.

Calcium and phosphorus metabolism is regulated reciprocally.

Water and Electrolytes

13

BODY FLUIDS

Almost 60 percent of body weight is contributed by water, which is distributed in three compartments:

  i.   Intracellular compartment (cytoplasm) is 67 percent,
  ii. Extracellular compartment (outside the cell /interstitial) is 25 percent, and
  iii. Intravascular compartment (plasma) is 8 percent, separated by semipermeable membranes (capillary wall separates plasma and the interstitial fluid, whereas cell membrane separates the cytoplasm and interstitial fluid). The dissolved ions in the body fluids are potassium, sodium, calcium, magnesium, chlorine, bicarbonate, and proteins. Ions, molecules, and water present in different compartments are exchanged by: simple diffusion, passage through channels, facilitated diffusion, and active transport (Na-K pump).

FLUID SHIFTS

Fluid may shift from one compartment to the other as the result of disease or injury. The accumulations of fluids in a tissue or in a body cavity are called third space compartment, e.g. liver disease may lead to significant accumulations of fluid in the peritoneal cavity which, represents a fluid loss as it is trapped.

Factors Controlling Fluid Exchanges

  i.   Diffusion
  ii. Filtration
  iii. Hydrostatic pressure, and
  iv. Osmotic (oncotic) pressure.

Diffusion It is the movement of water, small molecules, and ions, from areas of higher concentration to areas of lower concentration across semipermeable membrane.

Filtration It is the net flow of water across a water permeable membrane due to overall effect of pressure on sides of a membrane, e.g. fluid is filtered out of capillaries in response to changes in hydrostatic and oncotic pressure (osmotic pressure).

Hydrostatic pressure (HP) It is the fluid pressure, e.g. blood pressure in the capillaries, and pressure exerted by interstitial fluid. Hydrostatic pressure in plasma is due to difference in blood pressure at arterial end of capillaries (30 mm Hg) and venous end of capillaries (10 mm Hg), which forces fluid out of capillaries into the interstitial fluid. Negative hydrostatic pressure (-6 mm Hg) in interstitial space is created by draining of interstitial fluid into lymphatic system, which pulls the fluid out of capillaries.

Osmotic (oncotic) pressure It is the drawing force resulting from the pressure created by presence of protein dissolved in cytoplasm, plasma, and interstitial fluid. The pressure created by net movement of water across a membrane (osmosis) is directly proportional to solute concentration, thus osmotic pressure is dependent on the concentration of proteins, urea, glucose, amino acids, and electrolytes.

Factors Contributing for Edema

Various liver diseases that result in decreased protein synthesis lead to edema. Inhalation of noxious gases, inflammation (pneumonia), or respiratory burns may increase the permeability of pulmonary capillaries with loss of proteins and fluid. Cause of pulmonary edema in these cases may be a combination of factors.

Causes for Edema

  i. Malnutrition
 ii. Capillary wall damage
iii. Obstructed lymph flow
 iv. Fluid accumulation in the lungs
  v. Left ventricle heart failure
 vi. Congestive heart failure
vii. Glomerulonephritis
viii. Nephrotic syndrome, and
 ix. Infusion of rapid and large volumes of blood or salt solution.

Fluid imbalance may result in either *cellular dehydration* or *cellular hydration*.

Cellular dehydration: e.g. in diabetes mellitus, increased glucose concentrations in extracellular fluids will draw water out of the cells by creating an osmotic pull.

Cellular hydration: sodium ions predominate in extracellular fluid thus sodium plays a major role in determining osmotic pressure. Low sodium levels caused by diuretics, vomiting and low sodium intake can lead to low sodium in extracellular fluid, and an intracellular osmotic pull on water. If low sodium levels are combined with excess water intake it will lead to exaggerated cell hydration.

Effects of Imbalance on Compartments

Intravascular (plasma) compartment is the first most likely to be affected by fluid volume changes.

Interstitial and intracellular compartments are less likely to be affected and thus represent fluid reservoirs. Sudden loss or gain of fluids, affect only intravascular compartments. In hemorrhage, both compartments share losses or gains equally if they occur over a period of hours.

Regulation of Fluid Intake

Thirst is a powerful regulator of fluid consumption. Thirst center in the hypothalamus is stimulated by:
   i. Cellular dehydration: as a result of inadequate intake of water or increased extracellular solute concentration.
   ii. Decreased salivary production, dry sensation of the mucosa of the mouth and pharynx, and
   iii. Increased blood osmotic pressure stimulates osmoreceptors in the hypothalamus, which in turn stimulate the thirst center of the hypothalamus.
   iv. Decreased blood volume (decreased blood pressure) stimulates the release of renin by the kidney, which promotes synthesis of angiotensin II that in turn affects the thirst center of the hypothalamus.

Regulation of Fluid Loss

Fluid loss is adjusted by antidiuretic hormone (ADH)/vasopressin, atrial natriuretic peptide (ANP), and aldosterone. ADH and aldosterone decrease fluid losses from kidney whereas ANP causes diuresis. If the body is dehydrated, blood pressure falls, and glomerular filtration is decreased thus water is conserved.

HYDRATION

Causes of Overhydration

   i. Psychiatric disorder of compulsive water drinking (psychogenic polydipsia) 10-15 liters/day.
   ii. Forced water ingestion as a form of punishment (child abuse.)
   iii. Increased ADH (vasopressin) secretion, which promotes water retention (reabsorption) by increasing permeability of the collecting ducts in the kidney and vasoconstriction of arterioles.
   iv. Other causes such as head injuries, lung cancers, pneumonia, CNS diseases, and encephalitis. Some types of tumors secrete substances with ADH-like activity.

Effects of Overhydration

If blood has excessive fluid, the blood pressure raises, glomerular filtration increases thus excess fluid is eliminated. Fluid excess initially affects the extracellular compartments. Increased fluid volume can result in cerebral, pulmonary or generalized edema usually the result of inadequate renal output rather than fluid intake. If the retained water is hypotonic as compared to plasma the effect is to dilute the extracellular fluid, this causes a decrease in osmolality.

When interstitial fluid is dilute as compared to intracellular fluid, water is drawn into the cells by osmotic pull resulting in increased cellular volume and changes in cell function, which is most apparent in CNS tissue.

If the total body water is increased by *IV infusion of an isotonic solution* the result will be an increased extracellular volume with little or no effect on cellular volume.

Infusion of a hypertonic solution results in diffusion of both solute and water into the interstitial fluid, the increased concentration of solutes created in interstitial fluid causes an osmotic drawing force pulling water out of the cell.

DEHYDRATION

Causes of Dehydration

i. Excessive sweating (sweat is hypotonic) leading to hypernatremia.
ii. Insensible fluid loss from the skin or lungs due to various causes.
iii. Diuresis, solute cleared from the blood by the kidney and not reabsorbed remains in the glomerular filtrate; this high solute concentration creates an osmotic pull that draws water in that direction, which results in increased urine output and water loss as seen in diabetes mellitus. Mannitol (polysaccharide) a nonreabsorbable solute is sometimes used in cerebral edema to creates an osmotic pull on water and promoting water loss
iv. Diabetes insipidus due to deficiency of ADH, cause excessive urine of low specific gravity and thirst.

Effects of Dehydration

Dehydration effects of a fluid deficit depend on the volume, rate of loss, and amount of electrolytes lost with water. Effects of hypotonic fluid loss (water loss exceeds solute loss) have a concentrating effect resulting in increased osmolality and hypernatremia (increased Na^+ concentration). Water is drawn out of cells into the extracellular compartment leading to cell volume depletion and release of ADH and aldosterone. ADH helps renal water reabsorption, and aldosterone favors both sodium and water reabsorption.

Elderly individuals have a decreased renal capacity to reabsorb water significantly when fluid intake is limited, due to decreased diet or insensible fluid loss as in fever. They are also susceptible to water intoxication, when ADH secretion is increased due to stress of surgery, pneumonia, and meningitis.

Infants have less renal concentrating ability than an adult since they have a greater surface area compared to body weight.

ELECTROLYTE BALANCE

The principle cation in the extracellular fluid is sodium (Na^+). The anions that accompany sodium are chloride (Cl^-) and bicarbonate (HCO_3^-). The three together are considered an indicator of total solute concentration of plasma osmolality of which, sodium ions are osmotically important in determining water movements. A discussion of sodium must also include chlorine, bicarbonate, hydrogen ions, and potassium. Serum calcium is also important electrolytes in the living system.

SODIUM

Sodium Principles

i. Sodium ions do not cross cell membranes as quickly as water does.
ii. Cells pump sodium ions out of the cell by using sodium-potassium ATPase pump.
iii. Increases in extracellular sodium ion levels do not change concentration of intracellular sodium.

HYPERNATREMIA

Normal range of serum sodium is approximately 137-143 mEq/liter. Hypernatremia refers to an elevated serum sodium level of 145-150 mEq/liter.

In hypernatremia, water is osmotically drawn out of cells, which results in cellular dehydration and increased volume of extracellular fluid.

Response of CNS to Hypernatremia

The tight junctions between capillary endothelial cells in the CNS restrict diffusion from capillaries into the interstitium of the brain. An increased level of sodium ions in the blood results in an osmotic gradient, which shifts water from the interstitium and cells of the brain into the capillaries. This results in shrinking of brain and dilatation of capillaries that could lead to possible rupture, resulting in cerebral hemorrhage, blood clots, and neurological dysfunction. There is an unknown mechanism that protects the brain from shrinkage. Within 24 hours, intracellular osmolality of brain cells increases in response to extracellular hyperosmolality. The idiogenic osmoles are contributed by release of *potassium* and *magnesium* from cellular binding sites, and *amino acids* from protein catabolism, which accumulate inside brain cells. These idiogenic osmoles create an osmotic force that draws water back into the brain and protects cells from dehydration.

Causes of Hypernatremia

The causes of hypernatremia are water loss, and sodium ion overload, which in most cases are due to water deficit as a result of loss, or inadequate intake. Infants without access to water or increased insensible water loss can be very susceptible to hypernatremia.

Water Loss

Inadequate ADH, or renal insensitivity to ADH, results in large urinary fluid loss. Increased fluid loss can also occur due to osmotic diuresis (high solute loads are delivered to the kidney for elimination) in diabetes mellitus, which results in loss of fluids as well solutes. The other cause is high protein feedings by a stomach tube that create high urea levels in the glomerular filtrate, which produce an osmotic gradient and result in increased urinary output.

Sodium Overload

Sodium overload is less frequent than water loss. Rapid infusion of hypertonic sodium ion solutions can lead to excess sodium intake, similarly administration of aldosterones or hyperaldosteronism promotes sodium and water retention by the kidney, which may result in mild hypernatremia.

Treatment of Hypernatremia

The primary objective in most cases is to decrease sodium concentrations by re-hydration, but the point of concern is when and how rapid the re-hydration should occur.

If hypernatremia has been left untreated for 24 hours or more, the brain would have responded by producing idiogenic osmoles to re-hydrate brain cells, if this adaptation has occurred and treatment involves a rapid infusion of dextrose e.g. there is danger of cerebral edema with fluid being drawn into brain tissues, in such situation treatment is best handled by giving slow infusions of glucose solutions, which dilutes high plasma sodium. Ideally the goal is to avoid fluid overload and to remove excess sodium, this can be achieved by administering diuretics, which induce sodium and water diuresis. However, if kidney function is not normal peritoneal dialysis may be required.

HYPONATREMIA

Serum sodium level lower than normal (137–143 mEq/liter) is defined as hyponatremia that implies an increased ratio of water to sodium in extracellular fluid, which results in a shift of water into cells.

Hyponatremia is produced by a loss of sodium ions or water excess, which could be due to ingestion or renal retention of fluids.

Response of CNS to Hyponatremia

In order to protect against cerebral edema, brain cells lose osmoles and create a higher extracellular solute concentration, which draws water out of the brain tissue.

General Response to Hyponatremia

ADH secretions are suppressed, which favors increase in urinary output.

Symptoms of Hyponatremia

Symptoms of hyponatremia are primarily neurological due to net flux of water into the brain. Sodium ion levels of 125 mEq/liter are enough to begin the onset of symptoms, but sodium ion levels of less than 110 mEq/liter bring on seizures and coma.

Dilutional Effects

- Isotonic fluid loss indirectly causes hyponatremia. Any volume loss stimulates thirst and leads to increased water ingestion thus isotonic fluid loss can cause hyponatremia not because of sodium loss but because of increased water intake.
- Antidiuretic hormone secretion enhances water retention.
- Acute or chronic renal failure can lead to hyponatremia since the kidney fails to excrete water.
- When potassium ions are lost they are replaced by diffusion of intracellular potassium into extracellular fluid. Electrical balance is maintained by the diffusion of sodium ions into the cells in exchange for potassium ions, thus hyponatremia may ensue.
- Diuretic therapy is the common cause of hyponatremia, loss of sodium and potassium often occurs in addition to fluid loss.

POTASSIUM

Hyperkalemia

Normal range of serum potassium is 3 to 5 mEq/liter, as compared to intracellular levels of 140 to 150 mEq/liter; this high intracellular level is maintained by active transport by the sodium-potassium pump.

Hyperkalemia is an elevated serum potassium level in excess of 5 mEq/L. A consequence of hyperkalemia is an increase in H^+ ions in body fluids and acidosis. A change in either potassium or hydrogen ion levels causes a compartmental shift of the other. When hyperkalemia develops potassium ions diffuse into the cell this causes a movement of H^+ ions out of the cell to maintain a neutral electrical balance, as a result the physiological response to hyperkalemia causes acidosis, the reverse occurs in hypokalemia. The body is protected from harmful effects of an increase in extracellular H^+ ions (acidosis) by binding H^+ ions to proteins (Pr^-) inside the cells, which causes a shift of potassium ions out of the cells.

To summarize: Hyperkalemia causes acidosis, and acidosis causes hyperkalemia.

Symptoms of Hyperkalemia

Hyperkalemia causes muscle weakness and paralysis. It can also cause arrhythmias and heart conduction disturbances.

Causes for Hyperkalemia

I. *Increased input of potassium* due to intravenous KCl infusion, use of K^+ containing salt substitutes, hemolysis of RBC due to increased erythrocyte fragility or mismatched blood transfusions with release of K^+, or release K^+ from damaged and dying cells (burns, crush injuries, ischemia).

II. *Impaired excretion of potassium* due to:
- *Cellular-extracellular shifts:* Insulin deficiency predisposes an individual to hyperkalemia. Cellular uptake of K^+ ions is enhanced by insulin, aldosterone and epinephrine, which protects from extracellular K^+ overload. Insulin deficiency represents decreased protection, if an excess of potassium ions challenges the body. In the absence of aldosterone, there is loss of Na^+ in the urine and renal retention of potassium.
- *Hyperkalemic periodic paralysis:* It is an inherited disorder in which serum K^+ level rise periodically caused by a shift of K^+ from muscle to blood in response to ingestion of potassium or exercise, reasons for such shifts are not clear and the attacks are characterized by muscle weakness.
- *Renal insufficiency:* Aldosterone has a primary role in promoting conservation of Na^+ and secretion of K^+ by the nephrons of the kidney. Addison's disease is characterized by aldosterone deficiency thus the kidney is unable to secrete potassium at a normal rate. In oliguric renal failure, the kidney has lost the ability to secret potassium.
- *Spiranolactone:* It is a diuretic that is antagonistic to the effects of aldosterone (absorption of sodium and secretion of potassium I the kidney), it causes some rise in serum K^+ levels by interfering with K^+ secretion in the kidneys. Such increases may not be significant but individuals taking the diuretic are at risk if potassium is administered.

Treatment of Hyperkalemia

Treatment is based on:
1. Counteract effects of K^+ ions at the level of the cell membrane.
2. Promote K^+ ion movements into cells.
3. Remove K^+ ions from the body.

Infusion of calcium gluconate or NaCl solutions immediately counteracts the effects of K^+ ions on the heart but effective for only 1-2 hours.

Sodium bicarbonate ($NaHCO_3$) reverses hyperkalemic effects on the heart and also raises the pH of body fluids if acidosis is a factor.

Insulin-glucose infusion is effective in about 30 minutes and has duration of action of up to 6 hours. Insulin promotes the shift of K^+ ions into cells and glucose prevents insulin-induced hypoglycemia.

Kayexalate (cation exchange resin) removes K^+ ions from the body by exchanging K^+ for Na^+, the exchange time is about 45 minutes and is effective for up to 6 hours.

Peritoneal dialysis or hemodialysis effectively clears the blood of high K^+ levels as well causes of hyperkalemia.

HYPOKALEMIA

Serum potassium level that is below normal (< 3 mEq/liter) is defined as hypokalemia.

Serum potassium concentrations decrease when there is an intracellular flux of potassium, or potassium ions are lost from the gastrointestinal or urinary tract. Alkalosis causes hypokalemia, and hypokalemia causes alkalosis. Alkalosis is defined as a decrease of hydrogen ions or an increase of bicarbonate in extracellular fluids, which is opposite of acidosis. Alkalosis elicits a compensatory response that causes movement of intracellular H^+ ions into extracellular fluids. The H^+ ions are exchanged for K^+ (potassium moves into cells) thus serum concentrations of K^+ are decreased and alkalosis causes hypokalemia. Conversely when K^+ ions are lost from the cellular and extracellular compartments sodium and hydrogen ions enter cells in a ratio of 2:1 as replacement. This loss of extracellular H^+ causes alkalosis. Renal function is altered by hypokalemia. Sodium ions are reabsorbed into the blood when potassium ions are secreted into the urine by renal tubules, if adequate numbers of K^+ are not available for this exchange hydrogen ions are secreted instead, hypokalemia promotes renal loss of H^+ ions and thus results in alkalosis.

Treatment of Hypokalemia

Hypokalemia is treated by replacement of potassium either by oral potassium salt supplements and diet, or intravenous administration of potassium salt solution. If the primary pathology is renal loss of potassium, spiranolactone (diuretic) is to be administered.

CALCIUM HOMEOSTASIS

Calcium plays an important role in muscle contraction, transmission of nerve impulse, hormone secretion and blood clotting. The normal range for serum calcium is 9-10.5 mg/dl (4.5-5.3 mEq/liter).

- *Calcitriol* is involved in maintaining serum calcium levels. Calcitriol enhances serum calcium levels by:
  1. Directly promoting bone resorption with the release of chemical salts
  2. Potentiating the effects of parathormone (PTH) on bone reabsorption
  3. Increasing absorption of Ca^{++} ions from the intestine
  4. Reabsorption by the kidney tubules
- *Parathormone (PTH)* secreted into the bloodstream by the parathyroid glands is an essential part of the calcium homeostasis. PTH has the following actions:
  1. Increases calcium ion absorption from the intestine and enhances the synthesis of the active form of vitamin D.
  2. Favors reabsorption of calcium and excretion of phosphate (PO_4^{-3}) by kidney tubules.
  3. Enhances bone reabsorption with the release of calcium.
  PTH secretion is **stimulated** by decreased level of serum calcium, and **inhibited** by increased serum levels of calcium.
- *Calcitonin* is a hormone secreted by the thyroid gland, which decreases serum calcium level by:

1. Interfering with bone resorption.
2. Favoring calcium uptake by bones.
3. Promoting excretion of calcium by the kidney.

Effects of calcitonin are weak compared to PTH.

HYPERCALCEMIA

Serum calcium level of above 10.5 mg/dl is defined as hypercalcemia.

High levels of calcium interfere with nerve impulse, and muscle contraction. At high levels calcium may precipitate out of body fluid to form calcinosis and renal stone formation.

Causes for Hypercalcemia

Causes for hypercalcemia are:
- Overactive parathyroid glands,
- Hyperthyroidism increases bone resorption
- Large doses of vitamin D
- Immobilization: confinement to bed for weeks at a time causes bone reabsorption to occur at a more rapid rate than bone formation
- Some malignancies secrete hormones that cause bone resorption
- Milk-alkali syndrome: excessive and prolonged ingestion of milk and alkaline antacids (sodium bicarbonate and calcium carbonate) for peptic ulcer results in metabolic acidosis because of increased levels of plasma bicarbonate
- Alkalosis promotes hypercalcemia, by promoting renal reabsorption of calcium, and decreasing the capacity of bone to take up additional calcium.

Treatment

Intravenous or oral administration of *phosphate* decreases plasma calcium levels by interfering with bone resorption. *Calcitonin* reduces activities of bone destroying cells (osteoclasts). *Glucocorticoids* inhibit intestinal absorption of calcium and some *diuretics* promote excretion of calcium by the kidneys.

Infusion of *saline* (NaCl) or *sodium sulfate_(Na$_2$SO$_4$)* increases urinary calcium excretion.

HYPOCALCEMIA

Serum calcium level less than 9 mg/dl is defined as hypocalcemia. Physiological response to low calcium serum levels is increased secretion of PTH, which increases serum calcium by favoring resorption of bone, absorption of calcium from intestine, and renal reabsorption of calcium.

Causes of Hypocalcemia

Causes of hypocalcemia are:
- Inadequate vitamin D
- Nutritional deficiencies

- Impaired intestinal absorption (ex: partial gastrectomy)
- Liver or kidney dysfunction, which interferes with formation of active form of vitamin D
- Inadequate exposure to sunlight reduction in formation of active vitamin D in the skin
- Intestinal or bone unresponsiveness to action of vitamin D
- Loss of parathyroid glands or loss of function
- Use of certain drugs (phenobarbitone) over long periods, which affects the formation of active form of vitamin D.

Treatment

Intravenous or oral administration of calcium gluconate or calcium chloride solutions. Vitamin D may also be given.

RENAL REGULATION OF SALT AND WATER

Accumulation of Extracellular Water Volume can Cause Hypertension and Edema

Almost two-third of the body volume is water, excess water in a body region leads to swelling, which can be harmful or even fatal (i.e., brain swelling). Blood pressure is proportional to the amount of water in the circulatory system. If the water volume is too low, blood pressure falls to push adequate amounts of blood through organs, if water volume is too high it will cause high blood pressure and can lead to hemorrhage and strokes.

Sensory Receptors Monitor Salt and Water Status

Osmoreceptors found in hypothalamus, kidney, and adrenal cortex respond to changes in osmotic pressure.

Similarly *stretch receptors* found in hypothalamus, carotid sinus, aortic arch, and walls of atria respond to stretch caused by changes in blood pressure.

Amount of Na^+ in the Extracellular Space Controls Extracellular Water

If you drink a liter of water, the kidneys will produce large amounts of urine and eliminate water to keep the plasma volume constant. Pure water lowers the osmotic pressure of the plasma and inhibits ADH (Antidiuretic hormone) release.

If you drink a liter of saline, urine production is low and the water is retained for a much longer period of time due to the osmotic pressure of the saline. The saline solution raises the plasma osmotic pressure, which triggers ADH release over a long period of time, till the Na^+ in the saline solution gets excreted and this will take water with it by osmosis.

Water Regulation is much Faster than Na^+ Regulation

The kidney can adjust extracellular water by making either concentrated or dilute urine. If there is too much extracellular water the kidney will correct the situation by making large volume of dilute urine with low specific gravity. If the person is dehydrated, the kidney will compensate by producing small volume of urine with high specific gravity.

The Kidney has an Osmotic Gradient from Cortex to Medulla

The outer layer of the kidney is isotonic (about 300 mOsm/L) with the blood. The innermost layer (medulla) is very hypertonic (about 1200 mOsm/L).

Osmotic gradient is produced by a countercurrent mechanism located in the loop of Henle. The countercurrent mechanism is based upon the Na^+ pump. A very high concentration is built up in the medulla by pumping large quantities of Na^+ into the interstitial fluid in the medulla.

Concentration and Volume of Urine is Controlled by the Osmosis in the Renal Collecting Ducts

The concentration of the urine is adjusted in the collecting ducts that pass through renal medulla, which has a very high osmotic pressure. If the tubules are permeable, water will be sucked out of the tubules by osmosis. This produces small amounts of concentrated urine.

As the urine passes into the collecting duct it first passes through a region of isotonic osmotic pressure (300 mOsm/L) and then through a region of hypertonic osmotic pressure (up to 1200 mOsm/L). If the collecting duct has low water permeability the dilute urine in the tubule passes through with little reabsorption of water. This produces large amounts of dilute urine (diuresis).

If the collecting duct has high water permeability much of the water will be reabsorbed from the collecting duct, into the interstitial fluid. This produces small amounts of concentrated urine (anti-diuresis).

Kidney Osmosis is Regulated by Insertion of Water Pores into the Collecting Ducts by ADH

The permeability of the collecting duct is determined by aquaporin-2 (water pores), which is under the control of antidiuretic hormone secreted from the posterior pituitary. The cells lining the collecting duct synthesize aquaporin molecules, which are stored in vesicles called endosomes and are inserted when needed. In the presence of ADH, aquaporins are inserted into the luminal face of the cell membranes lining the tubule, which facilitate water reabsorption from the tubule. If ADH is low the channels are removed from the membranes (down-regulation).

High ADH Levels Conserve Water and Urine Gets Concentrated

Dehydration elevates the blood osmotic pressure. Under these conditions osmoreceptors in the hypothalamus are stimulated that result in secretion of large amounts of ADH from posterior pituitary.

The ADH causes insertion of aquaporins into the collecting ducts; thereby more water will be reabsorbed, preventing further dehydration.

Low ADH Levels Produce Large Volume of Diluted Urine

If a person has recently consumed a lot of water the ADH secretion will be low, water channels will be down regulated from the collecting duct and less water will be reabsorbed. The excess water is removed by increased urine production.

Diabetes Insipidus is the Result of Defects of ADH Mechanism

Diabetes insipidus is a condition where there is continuous production of large amounts of urine (5-10 L/day) with very low specific gravity.

Failure of ADH Mechanism can Happen in Two Ways

- Posterior pituitary does not secrete enough ADH. Blood ADH will be low.
- Kidney does not respond to ADH (nephrogenic diuresis). Blood ADH will be normal.

Aldosterone synthesizes sodium pump molecules that allow kidneys to adjust Na^+ level.

The kidney can also adjust urine Na^+ concentration by reabsorption in the distal tubule.

This activity is under control of aldosterone, which is released from the adrenal cortex mainly in response to a lowered blood pressure. Aldosterone acts by turning on genes, responsible for synthesis of Na^+ pump molecules.

Renin and Angiotensin are also Involved in Na^+ Retention

Hypovolemia and low blood pressure cause the juxtaglomerular cells of the kidney to secrete an enzyme called renin into the blood (Fig.13.1). Renin converts a protein called angiotensinogen (produced by the liver) into angiotensin-I, which in turn is converted to angiotensin-II by *Angiotensin converting enzyme* (ACE) that is found in capillary walls (ACE inhibitors are used to lower blood pressure). Angiotensin-II causes the adrenal cortex to secrete more aldosterone into the blood, which in turn causes distal renal tubular cells of the kidney to produce more Na^+ pumps. More Na^+ is pumped out of the distal tubule and enters the blood that results in Na^+ retention.

Angiotensin-II Raises the Blood Pressure by Several Other Activities

Angiotensin-II stimulates the hypothalamus to increase thirst and ADH secretion. It stimulates the cardiovascular center in the medulla to increase the cardiac output and also causes vasoconstriction of arterioles.

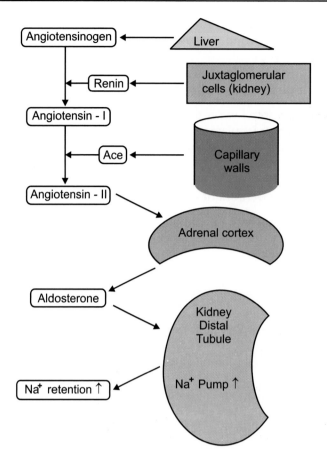

Fig. 13.1: Summary of renin-angiotensine-aldosterone mechanism

Both Sodium and Water are Lost by the Action of Atrial Natriuretic Peptide (ANP)

When the blood volume is too high the atria are stretched more than normal as blood enters the heart, which causes the release of ANP by atrial cells.

ANP inhibits aldosterone, renin and ADH secretion, which increases glomerular filtration rate and causes the body to lose both Na^+ and water, to restore the blood volume to normal.

Acid-Base Regulation

14

IONIC EQUILIBRIUM REVIEW

As water is the medium of biological systems one must consider the role water in the dissociation of ions from biological molecules. Water is essentially a neutral molecule but will ionize to a small degree. This can be described by a simple equilibrium equation:

$$H_2O \rightleftharpoons H^+ + OH^- \qquad \textbf{Eqn. 1}$$

This equilibrium can be calculated for any reaction:

$$K_{eq} = [H^+][OH^-]/[H_2O] \qquad \textbf{Eqn. 2}$$

Since the concentration of H_2O is very high (55.56M) relative to that of the $[H^+]$ and $[OH^-]$, it is generally removed from the equation.

By multiplying both sides by 55.56, we arrive a new term, K_w:

$$K_w = [H^+][OH^-] \qquad \textbf{Eqn. 3}$$

This term is referred to as the ion product in pure water, to which no acids or bases have been added:

$$K_w = 1 \times 10^{-14} \, M^2 \qquad \textbf{Eqn. 4}$$

As K_w is constant, if one considers the case of pure water to which no acids or bases have been added:

$$[H^+] = [OH^-] = 1 \times 10^{-7} \, M \qquad \textbf{Eqn. 5}$$

This term can be reduced to reflect the hydrogen ion concentration of any solution. This is termed the pH, where:

$$pH = -\log [H^+] \qquad \textbf{Eqn. 6}$$

pK_a

Acids and bases can be classified as proton donors and proton acceptors, respectively. This means that the conjugate base of a given acid will carry a net charge that is more negative than the corresponding acid. In the study of biologically relevant compounds, various weak acids and bases are encountered, e.g. the acidic and basic amino acids, nucleotides, phospholipids, etc.

Since weak acids and bases in solution do not fully dissociate, there is equilibrium between the acid and its conjugate base. This equilibrium can be calculated and is termed the **equilibrium constant = K$_a$**. This is also sometimes referred to as the dissociation constant as it pertains to the dissociation of protons from acids and bases.

In the reaction of a weak acid:

$$HA \rightleftharpoons A^- + H^+ \qquad \text{Eqn. 7}$$

The equilibrium constant can be calculated from the following equation:

$$K_a = [H^+][A^-]/[HA \qquad \text{Eqn. 8}$$

As in the case of the ion product: $pK_a = -\log K_a$ **Eqn. 9**

Therefore, in obtaining the -log of both sides of the equation describing the dissociation of a weak acid we arrive at the following equation:

$$-\log K_a = -\log [H^+][A^-]/[HA] \qquad \text{Eqn. 10}$$

Since as indicated above $-\log K_a = pK_a$ and taking into account the laws of logarithms:

$$pK_a = -\log [H^+] -\log [A^-]/[HA] \qquad \text{Eqn. 11}$$
$$pK_a = pH -\log [A^-]/[HA] \qquad \text{Eqn. 12}$$

From this equation it can be seen that the smaller the pK_a value the stronger is the acid. This is due to the fact that the stronger an acid the more readily it will give up H^+ and, therefore, the value of [HA] in the above equation will be relatively small.

Henderson-Hasselbalch Equation

By rearranging the above equation we arrive at the Henderson-Hasselbalch equation:

$$pH = pK_a + \log [A^-]/[HA] \qquad \text{Eqn. 13}$$

It should be obvious now that the pH of a solution of any acid (for which the equilibrium constant is known) can be calculated knowing the concentration of the undissociated acid [HA], and its conjugate base [A^-].

At the point of the dissociation where the concentration of the conjugate base [A^-] = to that of the acid [HA]:

$$pH = pK_a + \log [1] \qquad \text{Eqn. 14}$$

The log of $1 = 0$. Thus, at the mid-point of a titration of a weak acid:

$$pK_a = pH \qquad \text{Eqn. 15}$$

In other words, pK_a is that pH at which an equivalent distribution of acid and conjugate base (or base and conjugate acid) exists in solution.

BUFFERING

It should be noted that around the pK_a the pH of a solution does not change appreciably even when large amounts of acid or base are added. This phenomenon is known as **buffering**. In most biochemical studies, it is important to perform experiments in a solution of a buffering agent that has a pK_a near the pH optimum for the experiment.

Clinical Significance of Blood Buffering

The pH of blood is maintained in a narrow range 7.35-7.45. Relatively small changes in this pH value of blood can lead to severe metabolic consequences. Therefore, **blood buffering** is extremely important in order to maintain homeostasis. Although the blood contains numerous cations (e.g., Na^+, K^+, Ca^{2+} and Mg^{2+}) and anions (e.g., Cl^-, PO_4^{3-} and SO_4^{2-}), that can play a role in buffering, *the primary buffers in blood are hemoglobin in erythrocytes, and bicarbonate ion (HCO_3^-) in the plasma. Buffering by hemoglobin is accomplished by ionization of the imidazole ring of histidines in this protein.*

The formation of bicarbonate ion in blood from CO_2 and H_2O, allows the transfer of relatively insoluble CO_2 from the tissues to the lungs, where it is expelled. The major source of CO_2 in the tissues comes from the oxidation of ingested carbon compounds. Carbonic acid is formed from the reaction of dissolved CO_2 with H_2O. The relationship between carbonic acid and bicarbonate ion formation is shown in equations 16 and 17.

$$CO_2 + H_2O \rightleftharpoons H_2CO_3 \qquad \textbf{Eqn. 16}$$

$$H_2CO_3 \rightleftharpoons H^+ + HCO_3^- \qquad \textbf{Eqn. 17}$$

This reaction (Eqn.16) catalyzed by **carbonic anhydrase** occurs predominately in the erythrocytes, since nearly all of the CO_2 leaving tissues via the capillary endothelium is taken up by erythrocytes. Ionization of carbonic acid (Eqn.17) then occurs spontaneously, yielding bicarbonate ion. Carbonic acid is a relatively strong acid with a pK_a of 3.8. However, carbonic acid is in equilibrium with dissolved CO_2. Therefore, the equilibrium equation for the sum of equations 16 and 17 requires a conversion factor, since CO_2 is a dissolved gas. This factor has been shown to be approximately 0.03 times the partial pressure of CO_2 (PCO_2). When this is entered into the Henderson-Hasselbalch equation:

$$\textbf{pH} = \textbf{6.1} + \textbf{log } [HCO_3^-/(0.03)(PCO_2)] \qquad \textbf{Eqn. 18}$$

Where the apparent pKa of 6.1 for bicarbonate formation, has been introduced into equation 18.

The PCO_2 in the peripheral tissues is approximately 50 mmHg, whereas in the blood entering the peripheral tissues it is approximately 40 mmHg. This difference results in the diffusion of CO_2 from the tissues into the blood in the capillaries of the periphery. When the CO_2 is converted to H_2CO_3 within the erythrocytes and then ionizes, the hydrogen ions (H^+) are buffered by hemoglobin. The production of H^+ ions within erythrocytes and their subsequent buffering by hemoglobin results in a reduced affinity of hemoglobin for oxygen. This leads to a release of O_2 to the peripheral tissues, this phenomenon is termed the **Bohr effect**.

As CO_2 from the tissues enters the plasma, a minor amount is converted to carbonic acid, which then ionizes to release H^+. In the plasma, proteins and phosphates predominantly buffer H^+ ions. As the concentration of bicarbonate ions rises in erythrocytes, an osmotic imbalance occurs. The imbalance is relieved as bicarbonate ion leaves the erythrocytes in exchange for chloride ions from the plasma. This phenomenon is known as the **chloride shift** (Fig.14.1). Therefore, the majority of the bicarbonate ion formed from CO_2 leaves the peripheral tissues and is transported by the plasma to the lungs.

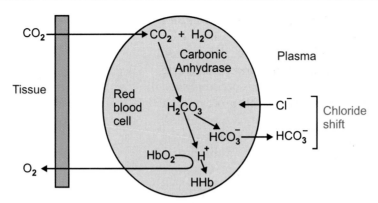

Fig. 14.1: Carbon dioxide transport in blood and hemoglobin buffering

Around 15 percent of CO_2 transport, from the tissues to the lungs occurs through a reversible combination with unionized amino groups (-NH_2) of hemoglobin forming what is termed hemoglobin carbamate.

Hemoglobin-NH_2 + CO_2 ⇌ Hemoglobin-NH-COO⁻ + H⁺

The formation of hemoglobin carbamate reduces the affinity of hemoglobin for O_2, thus in tissues where the concentration of CO_2 is high, dissociation of bound oxygen is favored. When the erythrocytes enter the lungs where the partial pressure of O_2 is high, the process is reversed.

The partial pressure of O_2 (PO_2) in the pulmonary alveoli is higher than the PO_2 of the entering erythrocytes that contain predominantly deoxygenated hemoglobin. This increased PO_2 leads to oxygenation of hemoglobin and release of H⁺ ions from the hemoglobin. The released H⁺ ions combine with the bicarbonate ions to form H_2CO_3. Cellular **carbonic anhydrase** then catalyzes the reverse of reaction 17, leading to release of CO_2 from erythrocytes. Owing to the PCO_2 gradient (described above), the CO_2 diffuses from the blood to the alveoli where it is expelled.

The significance of bicarbonate as a physiological buffer is because of the fact, that if excess acid is added to the blood, the bicarbonate ion concentration declines and the level of CO_2 increases. The CO_2 then diffuses from capillaries in the pulmonary alveoli and is expelled. As a consequence, when H⁺ ion concentration is elevated, bicarbonate ion acts as a buffer until all of the hydrogen ion is consumed. Conversely, when excess base is added to the blood, CO_2 is consumed to form carbonic acid and replaced by metabolic reactions within the body.

If blood is not adequately buffered, it results in **metabolic acidosis** or **metabolic alkalosis**. These physiological states can be reached if a metabolic defect results in the inappropriate accumulation or loss of acidic or basic compounds. These compounds may be ingested, or they may accumulate as metabolic by-products such as acetoacetic acid and lactic acid. Both of these will ionize, thereby increasing the level of H⁺ ions that will in turn remove bicarbonate ions from the blood and alter blood pH. The predominant defect in acid or base elimination arises when the excretory system of the kidneys is impaired. Alternatively, if the lungs fail to expel accumulated CO_2 adequately and CO_2 accumulates in the body, the result will be **respiratory acidosis**. If a decrease in PCO_2 within the lungs occurs, as during hyperventilation, the result will be **respiratory alkalosis**.

Ampholytes, Polyampholytes, pI and Zwitterion

Many substances in nature contain both acidic and basic groups as well as many different types of these groups in the same molecule. (e.g. proteins). These are called **ampholytes** (one acidic and one basic group) or **polyampholytes** (many acidic and basic groups). Proteins contain many different amino acids some of which contain ionizable side groups, both acidic and basic. Therefore, a useful term for dealing with the titration of ampholytes and polyampholytes (e.g. proteins) is the **isoelectric point (pI)**. This is described as the pH at which the effective net charge on a molecule is zero.

For the case of a simple ampholyte like the amino acid glycine, the pI, when calculated from the Henderson-Hasselbalch equation, is shown to be the average of the pK for the α-COOH group and the pK for the α-NH$_2$ group: $pI = [pK_{a\text{- (COOH)}} + pK_{a\text{- (NH3)}^+}]/2$.

For more complex molecules such as polyampholytes, the pI is the average of the pK_a values that represent the boundaries of the zwitterionic form of the molecule. The pI value, like that of pK, is very informative as to the nature of different molecules. A molecule with a low pI would contain a predominance of acidic groups, whereas a high pI indicates predominance of basic groups.

Solvation and Hydration Shells

Depending on the pH of a solution, macromolecules such as proteins, which contain many charged groups, will carry substantial net charge, either positive or negative. Cells of the body and blood contain many **polyelectrolytes** (molecules that contain multiple same charges, e.g. DNA and RNA) and **polyampholytes** that are in close proximity. The close association allows these molecules to interact through opposing charged groups. The presence, in cells and blood, of numerous small charged ions (e.g. Na^+, Cl^-, Mg^{2+}, Mn^{2+}, K^+) leads to the interaction of many small ions with the larger macroions. This interaction can result in a **shielding** of the electrostatic charges of like-charged molecules. This electrostatic shielding allows macroions to become more closely associated than predicted based upon their expected charge repulsion from one another. The net effect of the presence of small ions is to maintain the solubility of macromolecules at pH ranges near their pI. This interaction between solute (e.g. proteins, DNA, RN/A, etc.) and solvent (e.g. blood) is termed **solvation** or **hydration**. The opposite effect to solvation occurs when the salt (small ion) concentration increases to such a level as to interfere with the solvation of proteins by H_2O. This results from the H_2O forming **hydration shells** around the small ions.

ROLE OF KIDNEYS IN ACID-BASE BALANCE

From a biochemical standpoint, the kidneys serve important roles in the regulation of plasma acid-base balance and the elimination of nitrogenous wastes.

Sodium Bicarbonate Reabsorption

Regulation of plasma acid-base balance is primarily effected within the kidney through control over HCO_3^- reabsorption and H^+ secretion (Fig. 14.2). Secretion of H^+, in excess of its capacity to react with HCO_3^- in the tubular lumenal fluid, requires the presence of other buffers.

The generation of HCO_3^- and H^+ occurs by dissociation of **carbonic acid (H_2CO_3)**, formed in the tubule cells from H_2O and CO_2, through the action of **carbonic anhydrase**. Secretion of H^+ into the lumen of the tubule is accompanied by an exchange for Na^+. The reabsorption of Na^+ into the tubule cells occurs by an antiport mechanism during the exchange for H^+. The reduction in the intracellular Na^+ concentration is accomplished by Na^+/K^+-ATPase pump (an active transport process), which pumps the excess intracellular Na^+ into the interstitial fluid. The intracellular HCO_3^- then diffuses from the tubule cell into the interstitial fluid.

The capacity of the kidney to secrete H^+ is regulated by the maximal H^+ gradient that can form between the tubule and lumen and still allow transport mechanisms to operate. This gradient is determined by the pH of the urine, which in humans is near 4.5. The capacity to secrete H^+ would be rapidly reached if it were not for the presence of buffers within the interstitial fluid. The H^+ secreted into the tubular lumen can undergo three different fates depending upon the concentration of the three primary buffers of the interstitial fluid. These buffers are HCO_3^-, HPO_4^{2-} and NH_3. Reaction of H^+ with HCO_3^- forms H_2O and CO_2 that diffuse back into the tubule cell. The net result of this process is the regeneration of HCO_3^- within the tubule cell. This process is termed reabsorption of sodium bicarbonate. The reabsorption of sodium bicarbonate takes place primarily within the proximal convoluted tubules.

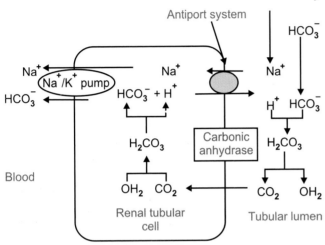

Fig. 14.2: Reabsorption of bicarbonate by renal tubular cells

PHOSPHATE BUFFERING

As the concentration of HCO_3^- in the tubular lumen depletes, the H^+ concentration keeps increasing that results in a drop in the pH of the tubular fluid. The pH of the tubular fluid gradually approaches the pK_a for he dibasic/monobasic phosphate buffering system (pK_a = 6.8). The excess H^+ reacts with dibasic phosphate (HPO_4^{2-}) forming monobasic phosphate ($H_2PO_4^-$). The $H_2PO_4^-$ so formed is not reabsorbed and its excretion results in the net excretion of H^+ (Fig. 14.3). The greatest extent of $H_2PO_4^-$ formation occurs within the distal convoluted tubules and the collecting ducts.

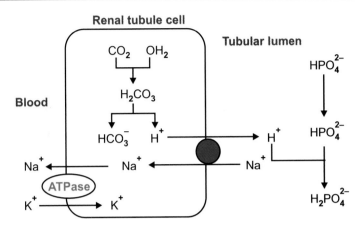

Fig. 14.3: Phosphate buffering in the renal tubule

AMMONIA SECRETION

Buffering of H^+ is also accomplished by reaction with NH_3 to form ammonium ion, NH_4^+. Because the pK_a of NH_4^+ is 9.3 excretion of acid in this form can be accomplished without lowering the pH of the urine. Additionally important is the fact that excretion of acid in the form of NH_4^+ occurs without depleting Na^+ or K^+. Two principal reactions within tubule cells result in the generation of NH_3, conversion of glutamine to glutamate and conversion of glutamate to α-ketoglutarate (Fig. 14.4). These reactions are catalyzed by **glutaminase** and **glutamate dehydrogenase**, respectively down its concentration gradient out of the tubule cell into the tubular fluid. There it reacts with H^+ to yield NH_4^+, which is excreted in the urine.

Glutamine $\rightarrow$ Glutamate + NH_4^+

Glutamate $\rightarrow$ α-ketoglutarate + NH_4^+

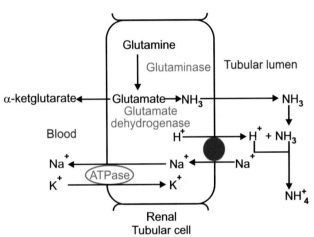

Fig. 14.4: Ammonia buffering in the renal tubule

BASE EXCESS

The "Buffer Base" is the total of all the anionic buffer components in the blood such as bicarbonate, sulfates, and phosphates. The base excess is the amount of deviation of the patient's buffer base from normal, in other words, how much extra-basic (anionic) chemicals the patient has in his blood, expressed in milliequivalents per liter (mEq/L).

The base excess is also defined as the amount of acid (in mEq/L) that would have to be added to the patient's blood to bring it to normal pH of 7.4.

Base excess can be a negative value. If the patient were acidotic, acid would have to be taken away to bring the pH to normal. In this case, for example, a base excess of -8 would mean that 8 mEq/L of base would have to be added to bring the patient's blood to normal pH.

Although many physicians use the difference between the patient's bicarbonate and an average bicarbonate of 24 as an indication of the patient's need for bicarbonate replacement, the base excess is a more accurate measure because it also takes into account other buffers such as phosphate and hemoglobin. It remains accurate in cases where the buffering capacity of hemoglobin is decreased due to anemia.

DIAGNOSIS OF ACID-BASE DISTURBANCE

Check Arterial Blood Gas (ABG) Values pH, $PaCO_2$, HCO_3^-.

In alkalosis pH is greater than 7.4.

In acidosis pH is less than 7.4.

A pH of 7.4 corresponds to a 20:1 ratio of HCO_3^- and H_2CO_3. The concentration of HCO_3^- is 24 mEq/L and H_2CO_3 is 1.2 mEq/L. Acidosis is a decrease in pH below 7.35, which means a relative increase of H^+ ions. The pH may fall as low as 7.0 without irreversible damage but any fall less than 7.0 is usually fatal. This may be caused by an increase in H_2CO_3 or a decrease in HCO_3^-, both lead to a decrease in the ratio of 20:1.

Alterations in pH due to changes primarily attributable to PCO_2 are classified as *respiratory* (Respiratory acidosis and Respiratory alkalosis).

Alterations in pH due to changes primarily attributable to HCO_3 are classified as *metabolic* (metabolic acidosis and metabolic alkalosis).

METABOLIC ACIDOSIS

Clinical Causes of Metabolic Acidosis

Tissue metabolism normally produces about 12,500 mEq of acid per day. This acid is in the form of CO_2, which is removed from the body in expired air. If aerobic metabolism ceases, tissues fail to completely oxidize sugar to CO_2. This results in lactic acid accumulation, since it cannot be expired through the lungs as CO_2 is, it causes metabolic acidosis. In untreated diabetes, normal sugar metabolism is deranged due to lack of insulin. In this case, acid buildup is due to acetoacetic and betahydroxybutyric acids, the products of fatty acid breakdown.

When dietary proteins are metabolized, their sulfate and phosphate groups form sulfuric and phosphoric acid. These acids amount to only about 150 mEq per day, however, they must be excreted from the body through the slow process of kidney filtration. If the kidneys fail, acidosis results after several days. Ingestion of acidifying salts, and loss of bicarbonate through chronic diarrhea, are less common causes of metabolic acidosis.

Typical ABG values in metabolic acidosis: pH = 7.21, $PaCO_2$ = 40, HCO_3 = 15.6.

Compensation for Metabolic Acidosis

As the blood becomes more acidic, the brain's respiratory centers are stimulated that causes increased depth and rate of breathing.

This lowers the content of CO_2 in the blood, and decreases its acidity.

The kidney then begins to remove the excess acid. As the plasma is filtered, acid anions enter the urine. In the kidney tubules, hydrogen ion is secreted. For each hydrogen ion that enters the urine, an ion each of sodium and bicarbonate return into the plasma. In this way, acid is eliminated from the body.

Typical ABG values in compensated metabolic acidosis: pH = 7.34, $PaCO_2$ = 28, HCO_3 = 14.7.

METABOLIC ALKALOSIS

Causes of Metabolic Alkalosis

Fruits are the normal source of alkali in the diet. They contain the potassium salts of weak organic acids. When the anions are metabolized to CO_2 and removed from the body, alkaline potassium bicarbonate and sodium bicarbonate remain. Metabolic alkalosis may be found in vegetarians and fad dieters who are ingesting a low-protein, high fruit diet.

A more common way to get alkali into the body is ingestion of sodium bicarbonate for gastritis, which is probably the most common cause of symptomatic metabolic alkalosis. If acid is eliminated from the body, it has the same effect as adding alkali. Persons with protracted vomiting of acidic content of stomach will often develop metabolic alkalosis. Typical ABG values in metabolic alkalosis: pH = 7.51, $PaCO_2$ = 39, HCO_3 = 30.4.

Compensation for Metabolic Alkalosis

As a short-term rapid mechanism respiratory rate is decreased, which leads to an accumulation of CO_2 in serum (The carbon dioxide is transported as hydrogen ion — buffered by hemoglobin — and bicarbonate). This lowers the pH towards normal, partially compensating for the additional alkali present in the blood.

Then begins the slow but effective process of eliminating bicarbonate through the kidney. Hydrogen ions are transported from the filtered urine back into plasma, leaving behind sodium ions and bicarbonate. Alkaline sodium bicarbonate is thus eliminated.

Typical ABG values in compensated metabolic acidosis: pH = 7.45, $PaCO_2$ = 46, HCO_3 = 31.2.

RESPIRATORY ACIDOSIS

Causes of Respiratory Acidosis

When ventilation is inadequate there is buildup of carbon dioxide. This is usually observed in the absence of adequate respiratory effort, such as depression of respiratory center due to narcotics or barbiturates. When respiration ceases due to cardiac arrest, it results in immediate respiratory acidosis.

Respiratory acidosis can also result when there is obstruction to airway, due to severe asthma and foreign body in the airway, which leads to carbon dioxide buildup.

Typical ABG values in respiratory acidosis: pH = 7.21, $PaCO_2$ = 55, HCO_3 = 22.

Compensation of Respiratory Acidosis

Respiratory changes can occur within seconds or minutes, but metabolic changes take hours to days. Compensation for respiratory acidosis must occur through elimination of acid through the kidney, as discussed above under metabolic acidosis. Compensation is seen only in chronic respiratory problems, such as severe obstructive pulmonary disease.

Typical ABG values in compensated respiratory acidosis: pH = 7.34, $PaCO_2$ = 56, HCO_3 = 29.5.

RESPIRATORY ALKALOSIS

Causes of Respiratory Alkalosis

Hyperventilation causes respiratory alkalosis. The most common cause of hyperventilation is psychological.

The other causes of hyperventilation may be due to abnormal stimulation of ventilation due to disease. Changes in the lung due to pulmonary embolism, asthma, or pulmonary edema often trigger increased respiratory rate that results in respiratory alkalosis.

Aspirin poisoning causes central stimulation of respiration that leads to respiratory alkalosis, which is a separate effect from the metabolic acidosis produced by aspirin.

Typical ABG values in respiratory alkalosis: pH = 7.57, $PaCO_2$ = 24, HCO_3 = 21.5.

Compensation of Respiratory Alkalosis

Compensation of respiratory alkalosis takes hours before metabolic compensation can be seen. The pH is normalized by renal elimination of alkaline sodium hydroxide.

Typical ABG values in compensated respiratory alkalosis: pH = 7.46, $PaCO_2$ = 22, HCO_3 = 15.3.

THERAPY OF RESPIRATORY ACIDOSIS

Theoretically treatment of respiratory acidosis is simple. All that need to be done increase the ventilation of the lungs, which removes carbon dioxide from the bloodstream, and the pH raises.

In the conscious patient with severe asthma or pulmonary edema, a decision must be made whether to await results from conservative therapy, or to take control the airway through intubation and assisted ventilation. You either improve air motion with drugs, or force better air motion with an artificial airway.

In a patient with poor gas exchange due to intrapulmonary causes, increasing ventilatory rate and depth may be only marginally helpful. In this situation, only improvement of the disease process will help.

Some cases of carbon dioxide retention as seen in patients with CHF and emphysema are better left untreated.

THERAPY OF METABOLIC ACIDOSIS

Mild cases of metabolic acidosis are best left alone. Usually no treatment is needed if the pH is above 7.1, and rarely is it needed if the pH is above 7.2, although the patient's level of discomfort and compensating hyperventilation must be considered.

Metabolic acidosis is treated with sodium bicarbonate, given intravenously. There is considerable question, however, how beneficial acidosis treatment is for certain patients.

For the semi-comatose diabetic patient in ketoacidosis, there is no question that bicarbonate will raise the serum pH. But as the acid is neutralized in the blood, CO_2 is formed. The increase in pH decreases respiratory drive, which slows the elimination of this extra carbon dioxide. The CO_2 diffuses into the cerebrospinal fluid, causing a paradoxical lowing of pH around the brain, with deepening of coma. It means, give bicarbonate slowly and maintain the hyperventilatory state, even if bag-valve assist or intubation is required.

For the patient in cardiac arrest, raising the pH has not been shown to improve the ultimate outcome. And alkalosis caused by too much bicarbonate is positively deadly for the arrest victim.

Bicarbonate dosage recommendations vary widely — most sources recommend from 0.1 to 0.3 times the weight of the patient in kilograms times the (negative) base excess (BE) expressed in milliequivalents per liter.

Vitamins and Coenzymes

15

Vitamins are organic molecules that perform a wide variety of functions within the body. The most prominent function is as cofactors in enzymatic reactions. The most distinguishing feature of vitamins in general is that they cannot be synthesized by mammalian cells and, therefore, must be supplied in the diet. The vitamins are of two distinct types, they are:

Water soluble vitamins	Fat soluble vitamins
Thiamin (B_1)	
B_1 deficiency and disease	
Riboflavin (B_2)	**Vitamin A**
B_2 deficiency and disease	Gene control by vitamin A
Niacin (B_3)	Role of vitamin A in vision
B_3 deficiency and disease	Additional roles of vitamin A
Pantothenic acid (B_5)	Clinical Significances of Vitamin A
Pyridoxal, Pyridoxamine, Pyridoxine (B_6)	**Vitamin D**
Biotin	Clinical significances of vitamin D
Cobalamin (B_{12})	**Vitamin E**
B_{12} defciency and disease	Clinical significances of vitamin E
Folic Acid	**Vitamin K**
Folate deficiency and disease	Clinical significance of vitamin K
Ascorbic Acid	

THIAMIN

Thiamin is also known as vitamin B_1. Thiamin is derived from a substituted pyrimidine and a thiazole rings, which are coupled by a methylene bridge. Thiamin is rapidly converted in the brain and liver, to its active form, thiamin pyrophosphate (TPP) by the enzyme, *thiamin diphosphotransferase* (Fig. 15.1a).

TPP is necessary as a cofactor for the reactions catalyzed by *pyruvate* and *α-ketoglutarate dehydrogenase* (Oxidative decarboxylation of α-keto acids), and the *transketolase* catalyzed reactions (in which aldehyde groups are removed) of the pentose phosphate pathway. In each case, thiamin pyrophosphate provides a reactive carbon on the thiazole that forms a carbanion, which is stabilized by the positively charged ring nitrogen of TPP. This carbanion is then free to add to the carbonyl carbon of substrate, for instance-

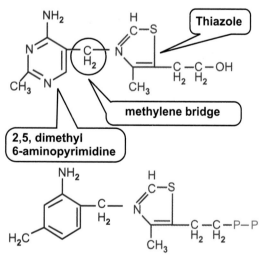

Fig. 15.1a: Thiamin pyrophosphate (TPP)

pyruvate. The *Addition-compound* then decarboxylates to eliminate CO_2 and generate the two resonance forms of ionized hydroxyethyl TPP. Hydroxyethyl TPP being an integral part of pyruvate dehydrogenase complex transfers the acetaldehyde moiety to lipoamide yielding acetyl lipoamide. In the next step, acetyl group of acetyl lipoamide is transferred to SH-CoA to form acetyl-CoA (Fig. 15.1b).

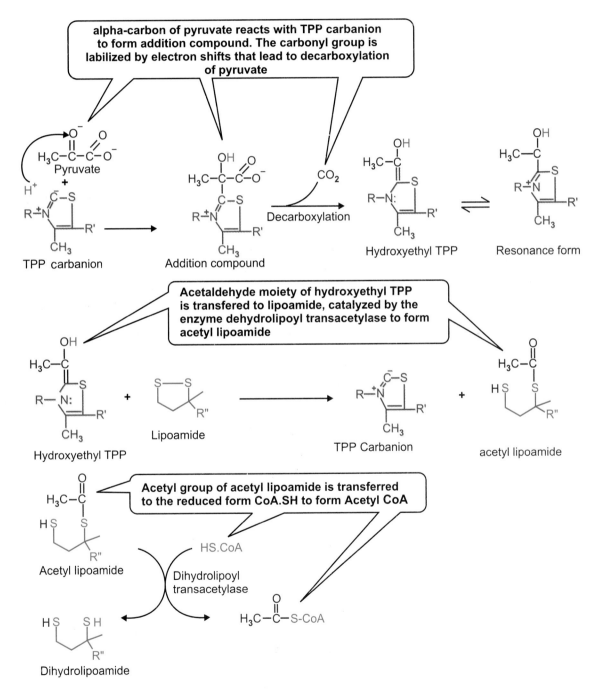

Fig. 15.1b: Thiamin (B_1) biochemical functions

Transketolase reaction is very similar to oxidative decarboxylation described above, but the only difference is the *glyceraldehydes moiety* of *glyceraldehydes thiamin pyrophosphate* is transferred to *a ribose 5-phosphate* to form *sedoheptulose 7-phosphate* rather than to *lipoamide*.

As a result of its role in these reactions, thiamin deficiency leads to a severely reduced capacity of cells to generate energy. The dietary requirement of thiamin ranges from 1.0-1.5 mg/day for normal adults, which is proportional to carbohydrate intake. The thiamin requirement increases with an increased carbohydrate content in the diet.

Clinical Manifestations of Thiamin Deficiency

The earliest symptoms to appear in thiamin deficiency include constipation, anorexia, mental depression, peripheral neuropathy and fatigue. Chronic thiamin deficiency leads to more severe neurological symptoms that include ataxia, mental confusion and loss of eye coordination. Other clinical symptoms of prolonged thiamin deficiency are related to cardiovascular and musculature defects.

Beriberi is a severe thiamin deficiency disease, which is the result of carbohydrate rich and thiamin deficient diet. The symptoms include myocardial failure, which is reversed by thiamin administration. **Wernicke-Korsakoff syndrome** is a thiamin deficiency related disease most commonly found in chronic alcoholics due to their poor dietetic lifestyles. It is characterized by acute encephalopathy followed by chronic impairment of short-term memory. Early treatment with high doses of thiamin and magnesium stabilizes the disease, yet thiamin deficiency alone is not sufficient to cause the syndrome.

Transketolase Defect and Alcohol Induced Encephalopathy

Patients with Wernicke-Korsakoff syndrome appear to have an inborn error of metabolism that is clinically important only when the diet is inadequate in thiamin. Probably this means that the Wernicke-Korsakoff syndrome is a recessive disorder, presumably autosomal recessive. Studies of a nonalcoholic Amish family suggested that the transketolase abnormality may occur in nonalcoholic populations and that it is present in both male and female siblings. This might be expected with autosomal recessive inheritance. Europeans are more vulnerable to this syndrome than are Asians (and probably Africans) on the same thiamin-deficient diet. The syndrome is said to be rare in American blacks.

RIBOFLAVIN (B$_2$)

Riboflavin is also known as **vitamin B$_2$**. Riboflavin consists of a heterocyclic conjugated ring structure called isoalloxazine to which ribitol is attached to (Fig.15.2). The isoalloxazine ring is light sensitive as well thermo-labile. Riboflavin is absorbed by the intestinal mucosal cells, which then undergo phosphorylation by flavokinase to form

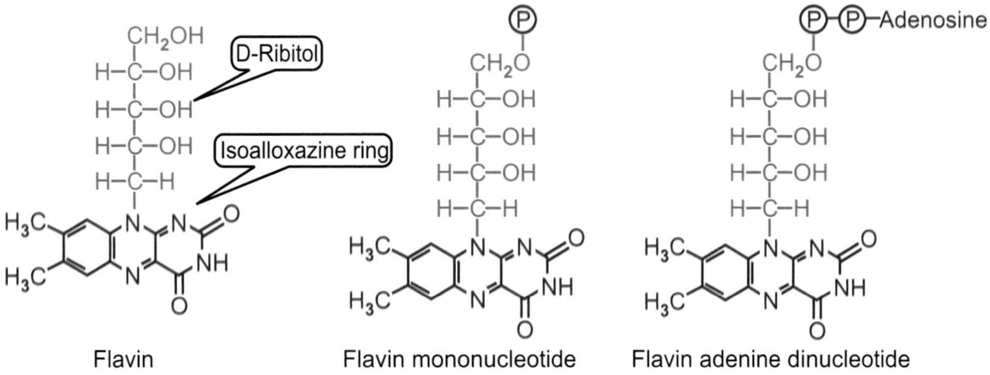

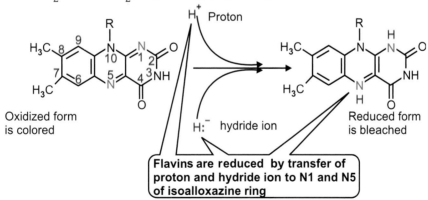

Fig. 15.2: Structures of riboflavins

flavin mononucleotide (FMN) and **flavin adenine dinucleotide (FAD)** (Fig. 15.2). Hence riboflavin is the precursor for the coenzymes FMN and FAD. Those enzymes, which require FMN or FAD as cofactors are, designated flavoproteins. Free riboflavin cannot cross the placenta, but in pregnant animals an estrogen induced carrier protein transports riboflavin across the placenta. Several flavoproteins also contain metal ions and are termed metalloflavoproteins. Both classes of enzymes are involved in a wide range of redox reactions, e.g. **succinate dehydrogenase, xanthine oxides, dihydrolipoate dehydrogenase, and L and D-amino acid oxidases**. During the course of the enzymatic reactions involving the flavoproteins, the protons (H^+) and hydride ion (:H^-) are transferred from substrate to N1 and N5 of the isoalloxazine ring that undergoes reversible reduction to from the reduced forms of FMN and FAD, called $FMNH_2$ and $FADH_2$, respectively (Fig. 15.3).

Fig. 15.3: Reduced and oxidized forms of flavins

The normal daily requirement of riboflavin is 1.2-1.7 mg for normal adults.

Clinical Significances of Flavin Deficiency

Riboflavin deficiencies are rare because of its wide distribution in adequate amounts in various food items such as eggs, milk, meat and cereals. Riboflavin deficiency is often seen in chronic alcoholics due to their poor dietetic habits. Symptoms associated with riboflavin deficiency include, glossitis, seborrhea, angular stomatitis, cheilosis and photophobia.

Riboflavin decomposes when exposed to visible light. This characteristic can lead to riboflavin deficiencies in newborns treated by phototherapy for hyperbilirubinemia.

Riboflavin deficiency is also seen in those individual treated with chlorpromazine (Phenothiazine class of drug) over long periods, since chlorpromazine completely inhibits flavokinase that phosphorylates flavoproteins.

NIACIN

Niacin (nicotinic acid and nicotinamide) is also known as *vitamin B$_3$*. Dietary sources of vitamin B$_3$ are nicotinic acid and nicotinamide. Niacin is absorbed by the intestinal mucosal cells, and then undergoes phosphoribosylation (by 1-pyrophospho-5-phosphoribose), adenylation (by ATP), and amidation (amide group of glutamine)

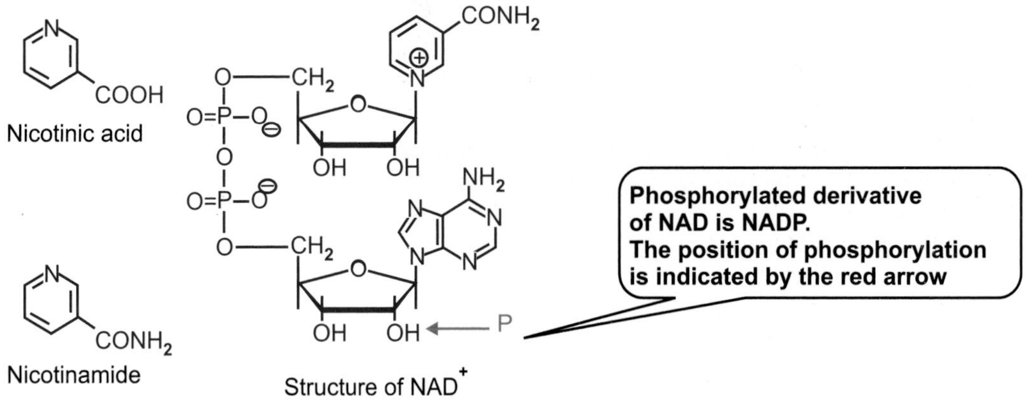

Fig. 15.4 Structure of nicotinic acid, nicotinamide and NAD

reactions to form the active forms of vitamin B$_3$, *nicotinamide adenine dinucleotide (NAD$^+$)* and *nicotinamide adenine dinucleotide phosphate (NADP$^+$)* (Fig. 15.4).

Both NAD$^+$ and NADP$^+$ function as cofactors in numerous reversible oxidation-reduction reactions involving **dehydrogenase**, e.g., **lactate** and **malate dehydrogenases (Fig. 15.5)**.

The effectiveness of pyridine nucleotides as cofactors for oxidation-reduction reactions is the ability of pyridine ring to serve as an electron sink (the hydride or reduced form can exist in multiple resonant forms and therefore is relatively stable).

Most oxidation-reduction enzymes exclusively utilize NAD$^+$ or NADP$^+$. But some use either of the two. As a general guide, all those oxidoreductases involved in catabolism of macromolecules require NAD$^+$ as cofactor, where as all those enzymes involved in reductive synthetic reactions require NADP$^+$ as cofactor.

Niacin is not a true vitamin in the strictest definition since it can be derived from the amino acid tryptophan. However, the ability to utilize tryptophan for niacin synthesis is inefficient (60 mg of tryptophan are required to synthesize 1 mg of niacin). Also, synthesis

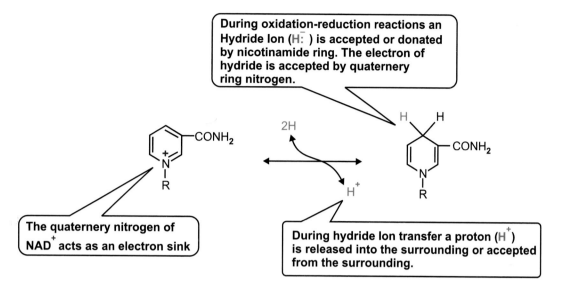

During oxidation-reduction reactions an Hydride Ion (H:⁻) is accepted or donated by nicotinamide ring. The electron of hydride is accepted by quaternery ring nitrogen.

The quaternery nitrogen of NAD⁺ acts as an electron sink

During hydride Ion transfer a proton (H⁺) is released into the surrounding or accepted from the surrounding.

Fig. 15.5: Oxidation-reduction of NAD⁺

of niacin from tryptophan requires vitamins B_1, B_2 and B_6, which would be limiting in them on a marginal diet. The major sources of niacin are tryptophan containing proteins such as, meat, grains and cereals, yeast, milk, and leafy vegetables. Corn is a very poor source of tryptophan. Thus, individuals consuming diets, in which corn is a major source of protein, can suffer from niacin deficiency syndrome called pellagra. The specific diseases of tryptophan metabolism are carcinoid syndrome and Hartnup disease.

The recommended daily requirement for niacin is 13-19 niacin equivalents (NE) per day for a normal adult (One NE is equivalent to 1 mg of free niacin).

Clinical Significances of Niacin and Nicotinic Acid

A diet deficient in niacin (as well as tryptophan) leads to glossitis of the tongue, dermatitis, weight loss, diarrhea, depression and dementia. The severe symptoms, **depression, dermatitis** and **diarrhea**, are associated with the condition known as *pellagra*. Several physiological conditions (e.g. Hartnup disease and malignant carcinoid syndrome) as well as certain drug therapies (e.g. isoniazid) can lead to niacin deficiency. In Hartnup disease, tryptophan absorption is impaired and in malignant carcinoid syndrome tryptophan metabolism is altered resulting in excess serotonin synthesis.

Nicotinic acid (but not nicotinamide) when administered in pharmacological doses of 2 - 4 g/day lowers plasma cholesterol levels and has been shown to be a useful drug in the treatment of hypercholesterolemia. The major action of nicotinic acid in this capacity is a reduction in fatty acid mobilization from adipose tissue. Although nicotinic acid therapy lowers blood cholesterol it also causes depletion of glycogen stores and fat reserves in skeletal and cardiac

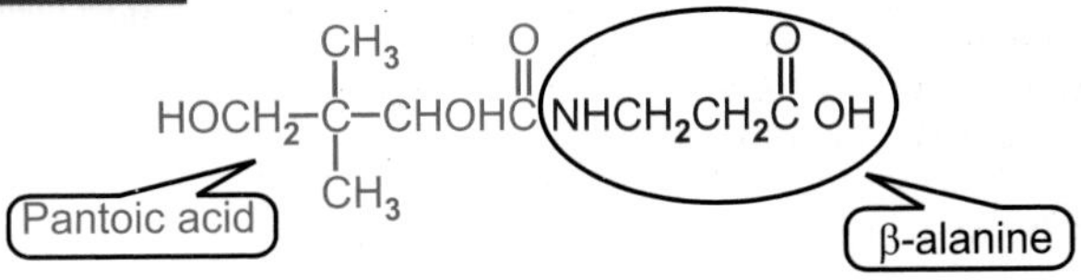

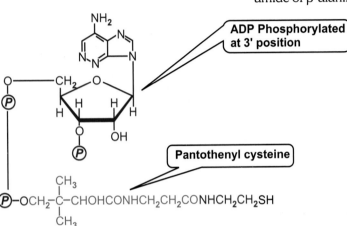

Fig. 15.6: Pantothenic acid

muscle. Additionally, there is an elevation in blood glucose and uric acid production. For these reasons, nicotinic acid therapy is not recommended for diabetics or persons who suffer from gout.

PANTOTHENIC ACID

Pantothenic acid is also known as **vitamin B$_5$**. Pantothenic acid is an amide of β-alanine and pantoic acid (Fig. 15.6). It is widely distributed in foods, particularly abundant in animal tissues and whole-grain cereals and legumes. Pantothenic acid is readily absorbed from the intestine and subsequently phosphorylated by ATP to form 4'-phosphopantothenate.

Pantothenate is required for synthesis of coenzyme A (CoA), and is a component of the acyl carrier protein (ACP) domain of fatty acid synthase. The thiol group of pantothenate acts as a carrier of acyl groups in reactions involving fatty acid synthesis, oxidation, and acetylation reactions. Acetyl Co-A is also required for oxidative phosphorylation reactions in which thiamin pyrophosphate participates. Pantothenate is, therefore, required for the metabolism of carbohydrate via the TCA cycle, all fats and proteins. At least 70 enzymes have been identified as requiring CoA or ACP derivatives for their function (Fig. 15.7).

ADP Phosphorylated at 3' position

Pantothenyl cysteine

Fig. 15.7: Coenzyme A

Deficiency of pantothenic acid is extremely rare due to its widespread distribution. Symptoms of pantothenate deficiency are difficult to assess since they are subtle and resemble those of other B vitamin deficiencies.

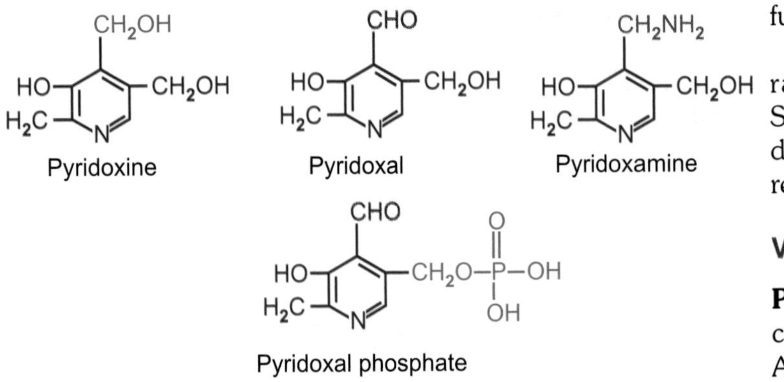

Pyridoxine

Pyridoxal

Pyridoxamine

Pyridoxal phosphate

Fig. 15.8: Pyridoxal phosphate

VITAMIN B$_6$ (PYRIDOXAL)

Pyridoxal, pyridoxamine and **pyridoxine** are collectively known as **vitamin B$_6$** (Fig. 15.8). All three compounds are efficiently converted to their respective phosphate esters (biologically active forms). The ATP requiring enzyme pyridoxal kinase catalyzes this conversion. Only the *Pyridoxal phosphate* and *Pyridoxamine phosphate* functions as cofactors in enzymes involved in *transamination* and *decarboxylation* reactions required for the synthesis and catabolism of amino acids. It also acts as a cofactor for *glycogen phosphorylase* in glycolytic pathway.

Daily requirement for vitamin B$_6$ in the diet is proportional to the level of protein consumption ranging from 1.4 - 2.0 mg/day for a normal adult. During pregnancy and lactation the requirement for vitamin B$_6$ increases approximately 0.6 mg/day.

Pyridoxal phosphate binds to its apoenzyme via an Schiff base between its 4-aldehyde group and ε-amino group of a lysine residue

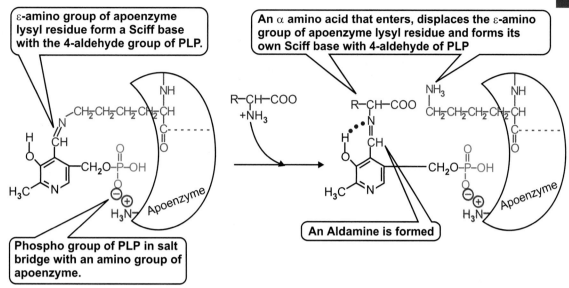

Fig. 15.9: Schiff's base formation between enzyme and substrate

in the enzyme, and an ionic bond (salt bridge) between its phosphate group and the enzyme (Fig. 15.9).

The ability of pyridoxal phosphate (PLP) to form the Schiff base with an amine is of utmost importance for its function as a coenzyme in transamination and decarboxylation reactions. In the absence of substrate, the 4-aldehyde group of PLP remains in the Schiff base linkage with the lysyl residue of the enzyme active site. Upon entry of an amino acid, the α-amino group displaces the ε-amino group of the lysyl residue, forming a new Schiff base; but the coenzyme remains bound to the enzyme by the salt bridge. By a series of electron shifts and rearrangements, the PLP changes to pyridoxamine phosphate as the substrate is oxidatively deaminated to form the corresponding α-keto acid (Fig.15.10). Subsequently, the other α-keto substrate of the transamination reaction forms Schiff base with the pyridoxamine phosphate, and the α-amino group removed from

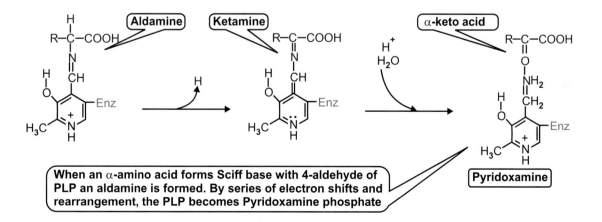

Fig. 15.10: First phase of transamination

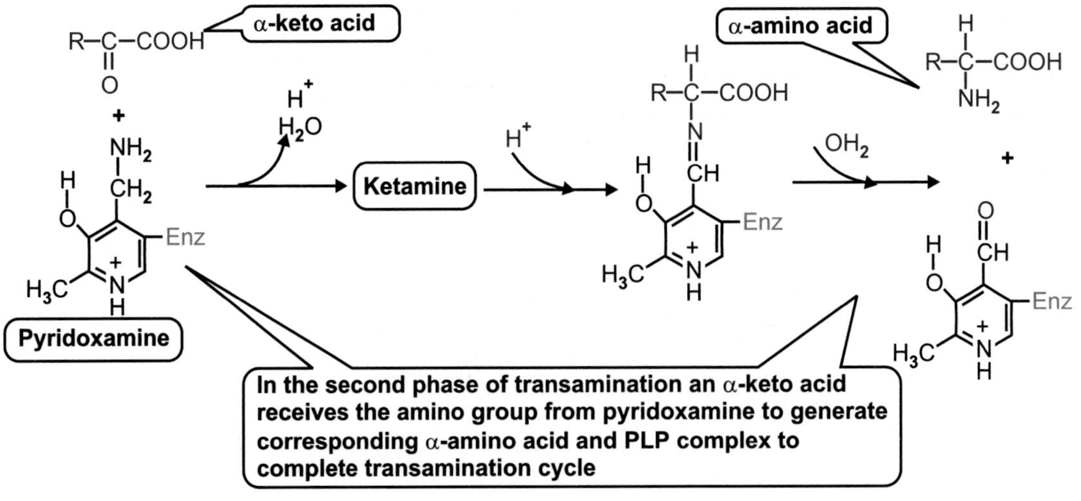

Fig. 15.11: Ketamin formation.

In the second phase of transamination an α-keto acid receives the amino group from pyridoxamine to generate corresponding α-amino acid and PLP complex to complete transamination cycle

the amino acid is transferred to the α-keto acid, completing the transamination cycle (Fig. 15.11).

PLP serves as a coenzyme in decarboxylation reactions of amino acids as well. This reaction is again with the formation of intermediate Schiff base and the rearrangement of electrons and their distribution in resonant structures over the entire PLP molecule that labilizes various groups.

Clinical Significance

Deficiencies of vitamin B_6 are, rare and are usually related to an overall deficiency of all the B-complex vitamins. Isoniazid used in the treatment of tuberculosis, can cause vitamin B_6 deficiency if the individual is a slow acetylator of isoniazide. Penicillamine, used in the treatment of rheumatoid arthritis and cystinurias is the other drugs, that complex with pyridoxal and pyridoxal phosphate resulting in vitamin B_6 deficiency.

BIOTIN

Biotin is found in numerous foods and is also synthesized by intestinal bacteria, and as such deficiency of biotin is rare. Deficiencies are generally seen only after long antibiotic therapies, which deplete the intestinal flora or following excessive consumption of raw eggs. The egg white protein, **avidin**, has high affinity for biotin, hence consumption of raw eggs prevents intestinal absorption of biotin.

Biotin is the cofactor required for enzymes that are involved in carboxylation reactions (Fig. 15.12).

The first step in the carboxylation reactions is the attachment of carboxylate ion to the N_1 of the biotin, which generates an activated intermediate,

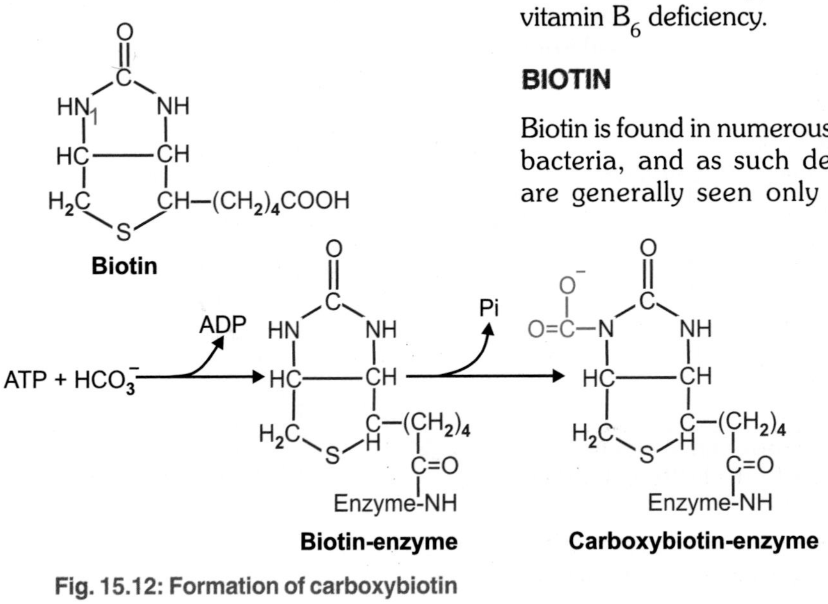

Fig. 15.12: Formation of carboxybiotin

carboxybiotin-enzyme. This energy dependent reaction requires, HCO_3^-, ATP, Mg^{2+}, and an allosteric effector-acyl CoA. The activated carboxyl group is then transferred to the substrate to form carboxy-substrate and biotin holoenzyme is regenerated.

Enzyme	Role
Acetyl-CoA carboxylase	Commits acetate units to fatty acid synthesis by forming malonyl CoA.
Pyruvate carboxylase	The first reaction in the synthesis of glucose from pyruvate (gluconeogenesis). Synthesis of Oxaloacetate from pyruvate.
Propionyl-CoA carboxylase	Conversion of propionate to succinate.
β-methylcrotonyl-CoA carboxylase	Catabolism of leucine and isoprenoid compounds.

Clinical Significance

A single enzyme called *holocarboxylase synthase* is responsible for attaching biotin to the proper lysyl residue of all the carboxylase apoenzyme. A decreased or absence of the activity of holocarboxylase synthase results in the accumulation and excretion in urine of substrates of the biotin-dependent carboxylase enzymes. These metabolites are lactate, β-methylcrotonate, β-hydroxyisovalerate, and β–hydroxypropionate. Children with this deficiency suffer from dermatitis, growth retardation, alopecia, immune deficiency disease and loss of muscular control.

COBALAMIN

Cobalamin is also known as **vitamin B$_{12}$**, composed of a complex tetrapyrrol ring structure (corrin ring) and a cobalt ion in the center. Vitamin B$_{12}$ is synthesized exclusively by microorganisms and is stored in the liver of animals, bound to protein as methycobalamin or 5'-deoxyadenosylcobalamin (Fig. 15.13). The vitamin must be hydrolyzed from protein in order to be active. Following consumption of animal meat, the complex is hydrolyzed in the stomach by gastric acids, or in the intestines by trypsin digestion. The vitamin is then bound by **intrinsic factor**, a protein secreted by parietal cells of the stomach, and carried to the ileum where it is absorbed. Following absorption the vitamin is transported to the liver in the blood bound to **transcobalamin-II**.

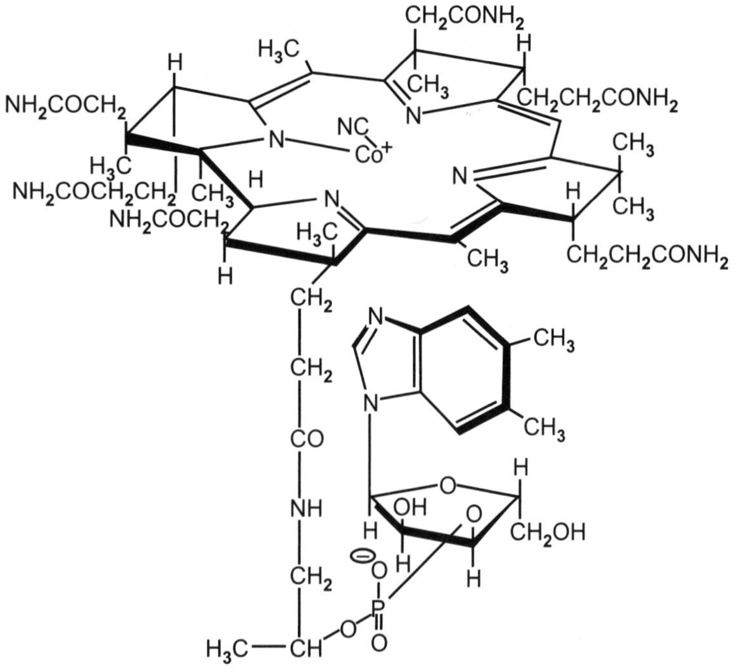

There are only two clinically significant reactions in the body that require vitamin B$_{12}$ as a cofactor.

1. Propionyl-CoA formed during the catabolism of fatty acids with an odd number of carbon atoms, valine, isoleucine and threonine

Fig. 15.13: Deoxyadenosylcobalamin

are converted to succinyl-CoA for oxidation in the TCA cycle. One of the enzymes in this pathway, **methylmalonyl-CoA mutase**, requires vitamin B_{12} as a cofactor in the conversion of methylmalonyl-CoA to succinyl-CoA. The 5'-deoxyadenosine derivative of cobalamin is required for this reaction.

2. The second reaction, requiring vitamin B_{12} catalyzes the conversion of homocysteine to methionine and is catalyzed by **methionine synthase**. This reaction results in the transfer of the methyl group from N^5-methyltetrahydrofolate to hydroxycobalamin, generating tetrahydrofolate (THF) and methylcobalamin.

Clinical Significances of B_{12} Deficiency

The liver can store vitamin B_{12} that will last for periods up to six years; hence deficiencies of this vitamin are rare. Pernicious anemia is a megaloblastic anemia caused by vitamin B_{12} deficiency that develops as a result of lack of intrinsic factor in the stomach, which is required for vitamin B_{12} absorption. Deficiency of vitamin B_{12}, blocks purine and thymidine biosynthesis that is required for DNA synthesis. The block in nucleotide biosynthesis is a consequence of the effect of vitamin B_{12} on folate metabolism. When vitamin B_{12} is deficient essentially all of the folate become trapped, as N^5-methylTHF derivative. This trapping prevents the synthesis of other THF derivatives required for the purine and thymidine nucleotide biosynthesis pathways.

Neurological complications also are associated with vitamin B_{12} deficiency and result from a progressive demyelination of nerve cells. The demyelination is thought to result from the increase in methylmalonyl-CoA, consequent to vitamin B_{12} deficiency. Methylmalonyl-CoA is a competitive inhibitor of malonyl-CoA in fatty acid biosynthesis as well as being able to substitute for malonyl-CoA in any fatty acid biosynthesis that may occur. Since the myelin sheath is in continual flux, the methylmalonyl-CoA induced inhibition of fatty acid synthesis results in the eventual destruction of the sheath. Shunting of methylmalonyl-CoA into fatty acid biosynthesis results in production of branched-chain fatty acids that may severely alter the architecture of the normal membrane structure of nerve cells.

FOLIC ACID

Folic acid is a conjugated molecule consisting of a pteridine ring structure linked to para-aminobenzoic acid (**PABA**) that forms pteroic acid. Folic acid itself is then formed by conjugating, pteroic acid to glutamic acid residues (Fig. 15.14). Folic acid is obtained primarily from yeasts and leafy vegetables as well as animal liver. Animal cannot synthesize PABA nor attach glutamate residues to pteroic acid, thus, requiring folate intake in the diet.

The ingested folic acid, and the one that is stored in liver exist in a polyglutamate form. Intestinal mucosal cells remove some of the glutamate residues through the action of the lysosomal enzyme, **deconjugase.** The removal of glutamate residues makes folate less

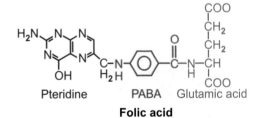

Pteridine   PABA   Glutamic acid

Folic acid

Positions , and $_8$ carry hydrogens in dihydrofolate (DHF)
Positions $_5$ and $_8$ carry hydrogens in tetrahydrofolate (THF)

Fig. 15.14: Structure of folic acid

negatively charged (from the polyglutamic acids) and therefore more capable of passing through the basal lamenal membrane of the epithelial cells of the intestine and into the bloodstream. Within the cells (principally the liver where it is stored) folic acid is reduced to tetrahydrofolate (THF also H_4folate) through the action of **dihydrofolate reductase (DHFR)**, an NADPH-requiring enzyme (Fig. 15.15).

The function of THF derivatives is to carry and transfer various forms of one-carbon units during biosynthetic reactions. The one-carbon units are methyl, methylene, methenyl, formyl or formimino groups. These one-carbon transfer reactions are required in the biosynthesis of serine, methionine, glycine, choline and the purine nucleotides and dTMP.

The ability to acquire choline and amino acids from the diet and to salvage the purine nucleotides makes the role of N^5, N^{10}-methylene-THF in dTMP synthesis the most metabolically significant function for this vitamin. The role of vitamin B_{12} and N^5-methyl-THF in the conversion of homocysteine to methionine also can have a significant impact on the ability of cells to regenerate needed THF (Fig. 15.15).

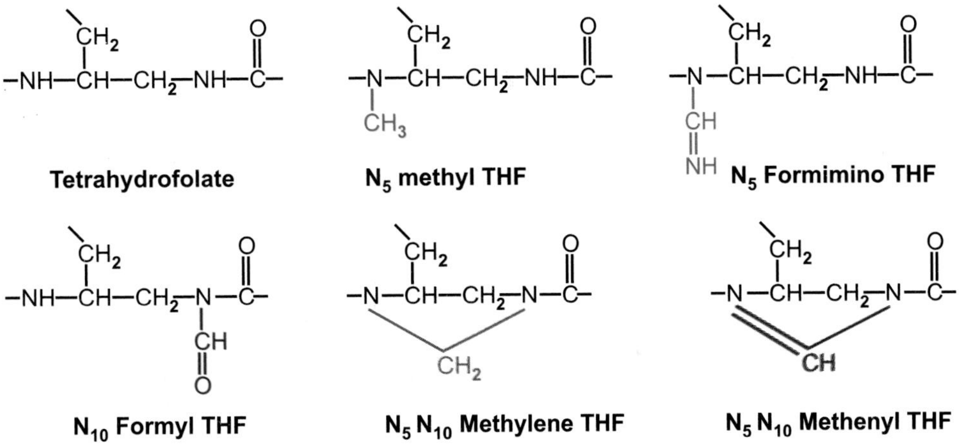

Fig. 15.15: Active centers of tetrahydrofolate (THF) are N^5 and N^{10}

Clinical Significance of Folate Deficiency

Folate deficiency results in complications nearly identical to those described for vitamin B_{12} deficiency. The most pronounced effect of folate deficiency on cellular processes is upon DNA synthesis. This is due to impairment in dTMP (thymidine) synthesis, which leads to cell cycle arrest in S-phase of rapidly proliferating cells, in particular hematopoietic cells. The result is **megaloblastic anemia** similar to vitamin B_{12} deficiency. The inability to synthesize DNA during erythrocyte maturation leads to abnormally large erythrocytes termed **macrocytes.**

Folate deficiencies are rare due to the adequate presence of folate in food. Poor dietary habits as those of chronic alcoholics can lead to folate deficiency. The predominant causes of folate deficiency in non-alcoholics are impaired absorption or metabolism or an increased demand for the vitamin. The predominant condition requiring an increase in the daily intake of folate is pregnancy. This is due to an increased number of rapidly proliferating cells present in the blood. The need for folate will nearly double by the third trimester of pregnancy. Certain drugs such as anticonvulsants and oral contraceptives can impair the absorption of folate. Anticonvulsants also increase the rate of folate metabolism (Fig. 15.16).

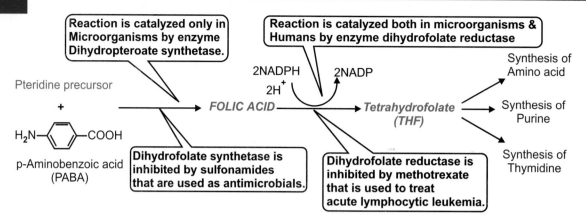

Fig. 15.16: Inhibitors of tetrahydrofolate synthesis

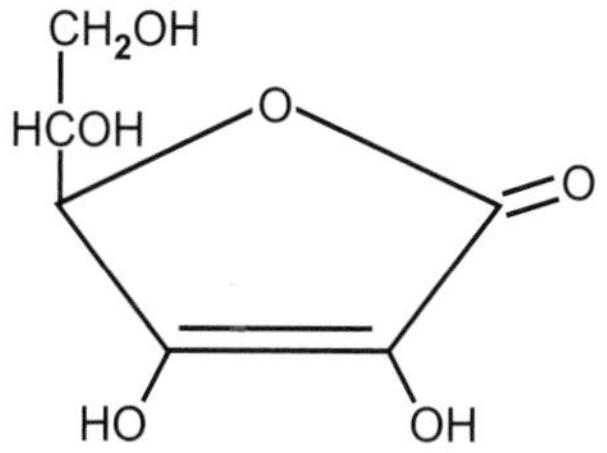

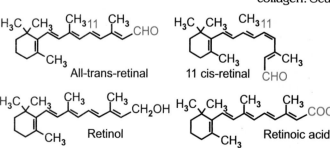

Fig. 15.17: Ascorbic acid

ASCORBIC ACID

Ascorbic acid is more commonly known as *vitamin C* (Fig. 15.17). Ascorbic acid is derived from glucose via the uronic acid pathway. Primates lack the enzyme *L-gulonolactone oxidase* responsible for the conversion of gulonolactone to ascorbic acid. Hence primates require ascorbic acid in their diet.

The active form of vitamin C is ascorbate acid itself. The main function of ascorbate is as a reducing agent in a number of reactions. Vitamin C has the potential to reduce cytochromes a and c of respiratory chain as well as molecular oxygen. The most important reaction requiring ascorbate as a cofactor is the *hydroxylation* of proline residues in collagen. Vitamin C is, therefore, required for the maintenance of normal connective tissue as well as for wound healing since synthesis of connective tissue is the first event in *wound tissue remodeling*. Vitamin C also is necessary for *bone remodeling* due to the presence of collagen in the organic matrix of bones.

Several other metabolic reactions require vitamin C as a cofactor. These include the metabolism of tyrosine and the synthesis of epinephrine from tyrosine and the synthesis of the bile acids. It is also believed that vitamin C is involved in the process of steroidogenesis, since the adrenal cortex contains high levels of vitamin C, which are depleted upon adrenocorticotropic hormone (ACTH) stimulation of the gland. Deficiency in vitamin C leads to the disease **scurvy** due to the role of the vitamin in the post-translational modifications of collagen. Scurvy is characterized by easily bruised skin, muscle fatigue, soft swollen gums, decreased wound healing, hemorrhage, osteoporosis, and anemia. Vitamin C is readily absorbed and so the primary cause of vitamin C deficiency is poor diet and/or an increased requirement.

The primary physiological state leading to an increased requirement for vitamin C is severe stress (or trauma). This is due to a rapid depletion in the adrenal stores of the vitamin. The reason for the

Fig. 15.18: Structure of different forms of vitamin A

decrease in adrenal vitamin C levels is unclear but may be due either to redistribution of the vitamin to areas that need it or an overall increased utilization.

VITAMIN A

Vitamin A consists of three biologically active molecules, **retinol, retinal** (retinaldehyde), and **retinoic acid** (Fig. 15.18).

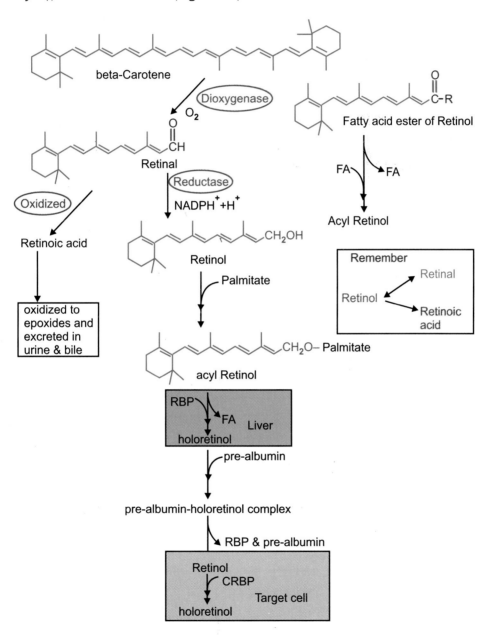

Fig. 15.19: Vitamin A synthesis and functions

Each of these compounds is derived from the plant precursor molecule, β-**carotene** (a member of a family of molecules known as **carotenoids**). Beta-carotene, which consists of two molecules of retinal linked at their aldehyde ends. Beta-carotene is referred to as the provitamin form of vitamin A (Fig.15.19).

Ingested β-carotene is cleaved in the lumen of the intestine by *β-carotene dioxygenase* to yield retinal. Retinal is reduced to retinol by *retinaldehyde reductase*, an NADPH requiring enzyme within the intestines. Retinol is esterified to palmitic acid and delivered to the blood via chylomicrons. The uptake of chylomicron remnants by the liver results in delivery of retinol to this organ for storage as a lipid ester within lipocytes. Transport of retinol from the liver to extrahepatic tissues occurs by binding of hydrolyzed retinol to **aporetinol binding protein (RBP).** The retinol-RBP complex is then transported to the cell surface within the Golgi and secreted. Within extrahepatic tissues retinol is bound to **cellular retinol binding protein (CRBP).** Plasma transport of retinoic acid is accomplished by binding to albumin (Fig. 15.19).

Retinol and Retinoic Acids Control Gene Expression

Within cells both retinol and retinoic acids bind to specific receptor proteins. Following binding, the receptor-vitamin complex interacts with specific sequences in several genes involved in growth and differentiation and affects expression of these genes. In this capacity, retinol and retinoic acids function similar to hormones of the steroid/ thyroid hormone super family of proteins. Retinol and retinoic acids are involved in the earliest processes of embryogenesis including the differentiation of the three germ layers, organogenesis and limb development (Fig. 15.19).

Vision and the Role of Vitamin A

Photoreception in the eye is the function of two specialized cell types located in the retina the rod and cone cells. Both rod and cone cells contain a photoreceptor pigment in their membranes.

The photosensitive compound of most mammalian eyes is a protein called **opsin** to which retinal is bound covalently by schiff's base formed between aldehyde group of retinal and epsilon amino group of lysyl residue of opsin (Fig. 15.20). The photoreceptor of rod cells is specifically called **rhodopsin** or **visual purple.** This compound is a complex between scotopsin and the 11-*cis*-retinal (also called 11-*cis*-retinene) form of vitamin A. Rhodopsin is a serpentine receptor imbedded in the membrane of the rod cell.

Coupling of 11-*cis*-retinal occurs at three of the transmembrane domains of rhodopsin. Intracellularly, rhodopsin is coupled to a specific G-protein called **transducin.**

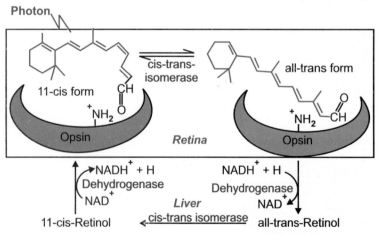

Fig. 15.20: Cis-trans isomerization of retinol

When the rhodopsin is exposed to light, it gets **bleached** and all-trans retinal is released from opsin. Absorption of photons by 11-cis-retinal causes its photoisomerization to all-transretinal, which triggers a series of conformational changes in opsin. One such important conformational intermediate is **metarhodopsin-II**. The release of opsin results in further conformational change in the photoreceptor opsin. This conformational change activates transducin (G-protein), leading to an increased GTP-binding by the α-subunit of transducin. Binding of GTP releases the α-subunit from the inhibitory β- and χ-subunits. The GTP-activated α-subunit in turn

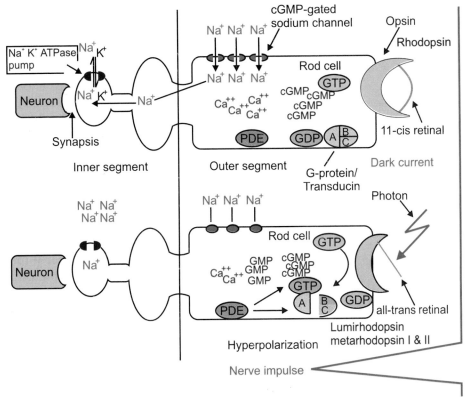

Fig. 15.21: Vitamin A in vision

activates an associated **phosphodiesterase** an enzyme that hydrolyzes cyclic-GMP (cGMP) to GMP. Cyclic GMP is required to maintain the Na^+ channels of the rod cell in the open conformation. The drop in cGMP concentration results in complete closure of the Na^+ channels. Metarhodopsin-II appears to be responsible for initiating the closure of the channels. The closing of the channels leads to hyperpolarization of the rod cell with concomitant propagation of nerve impulses to the brain (Fig. 15.21).

Additional Role of Retinol

Retinol also functions in the synthesis of certain glycoproteins and mucopolysaccharides necessary for mucous production and normal growth regulation. This is accomplished by phosphorylation of retinol to **retinyl phosphate**, which then functions similarly to dolichol phosphate.

Clinical Significances of Vitamin A Deficiency

Vitamin A is stored in the liver and deficiency of the vitamin occurs only after prolonged lack of dietary intake. The earliest symptoms of vitamin A deficiency are **night blindness**. Additional early symptoms include follicular hyperkeratinosis, increased susceptibility to infection and cancer and anemia equivalent to iron deficient anemia. Prolonged lack of vitamin A leads to deterioration of the eye tissue through progressive keratinization of the cornea, a condition known as xerophthalmia.

The increased risk of cancer in vitamin A deficiency is thought to be the result of depletion in β-carotene. Beta-carotene is a very effective antioxidant and is said to reduce the risk of cancers initiated by the production of free radicals. Of particular interest is the potential benefit of increased β-carotene intake to reduce the risk of lung cancer in smokers. However, caution needs to be taken when increasing the intake of any of the lipid soluble vitamins. Excess accumulation of vitamin A in the liver can lead to toxicity, which manifests as bone pain, hepatosplenomegaly, nausea and diarrhea.

VITAMIN D

Vitamin D is a steroid hormone that functions to regulate specific gene expression following interaction with its intracellular receptor. The biologically active form of the hormone is **1,25-dihydroxy vitamin D_3** (1,25-$(OH)_2$ or D_3) also termed **calcitriol**. Calcitriol functions primarily to regulate calcium and phosphorus homeostasis.

Active calcitriol is derived from **ergosterol** (produced in plants) and **7-dehydrocholesterol** (produced in the skin). **Ergocalciferol** (vitamin D_2) is formed by UV irradiation of ergosterol. In the skin, 7-dehydrocholesterol is converted to **cholecalciferol** (vitamin D_3) following UV irradiation. The same enzymatic pathway in the body converts Vitamins D_2 and D_3, to D_2-calcitriol and D_3-calcitriol, respectively. Cholecalciferol (or egrocalciferol) is absorbed from the intestine and transported to the liver bound to a specific **vitamin D-binding protein**. In the liver cholecalciferol is hydroxylated at the 25 position by a specific ***D_3-25-hydroxylase*** generating 25-hydroxy-D_3 [25-$(OH)D_3$] which is the major circulating form of vitamin D. Conversion of 25-$(OH)D_3$ to its biologically active form calcitriol, occurs through the activity of a specific ***D_3-1-hydroxylase*** (which hydroxylates at 1-position) present in the proximal convoluted tubules of the kidneys, in bone and placenta. Hydroxylation of 25-$(OH)D_3$ at the 24-position can also take place by a specific ***D_3-24-hydroxylase*** in the kidneys, intestine, placenta and cartilage (Fig.15.22).

Calcitriol functions in concert with **parathyroid hormone (PTH)** and **calcitonin** to regulate serum calcium and phosphorus levels. PTH is released in response to low serum calcium and induces the production of calcitriol. In contrast, reduced levels of PTH stimulate synthesis of the inactive 24,25-$(OH)_2D_3$. In the intestinal epithelium, calcitriol functions as a steroid hormone in inducing the expression

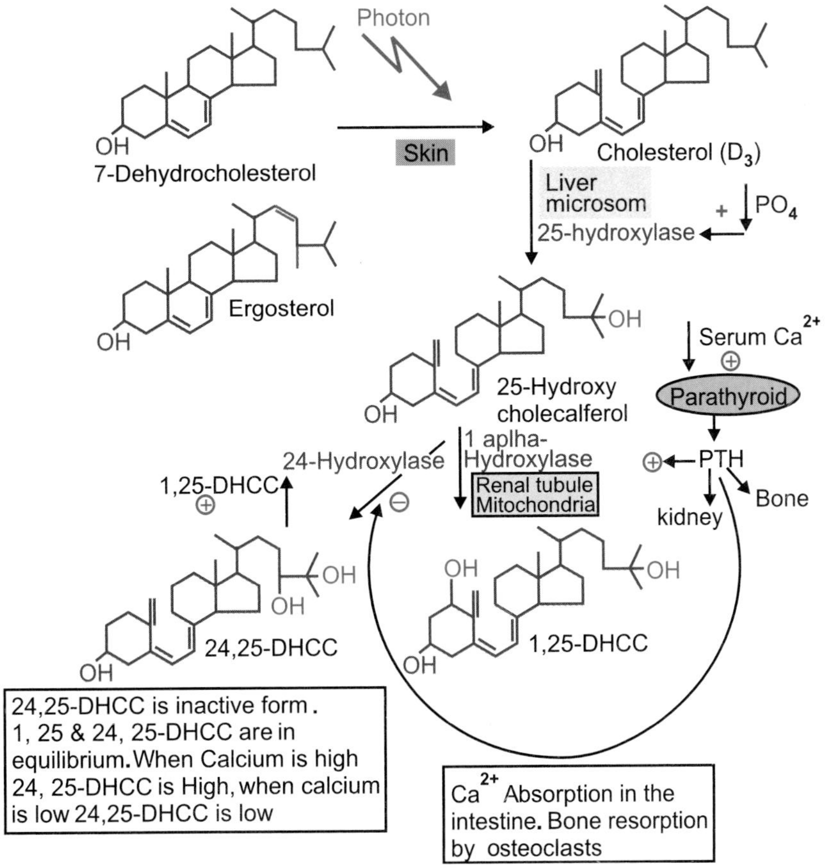

Fig. 15.22: Vitamin D functions

of **calbindin**, a protein involved in intestinal calcium absorption. The increased absorption of calcium ions requires simultaneous absorption of a negatively charged counter ion to maintain electrical neutrality. The predominant counter ion is Pi. When plasma calcium level falls, calcitriol and PTH stimulate bone resorption, and calcium reabsorption by the distal renal tubules. The role of calcitonin in calcium homeostasis is to decrease elevated serum calcium levels by inhibiting bone resorption.

Clinical Significance of Vitamin D Deficiency

Vitamin D deficiencies are rare. The main symptom of vitamin D deficiency in children is **rickets** and in adults is **osteomalacia**. Rickets is characterized improper mineralization during the development of the bones resulting in soft bones. Osteomalacia is characterized by demineralization of previously formed bone leading to increased softness and susceptibility to fracture.

VITAMIN E

Vitamin E is a mixture of several related compounds known as **tocopherols** (Fig.15.23). The α-tocopherol molecule is the most

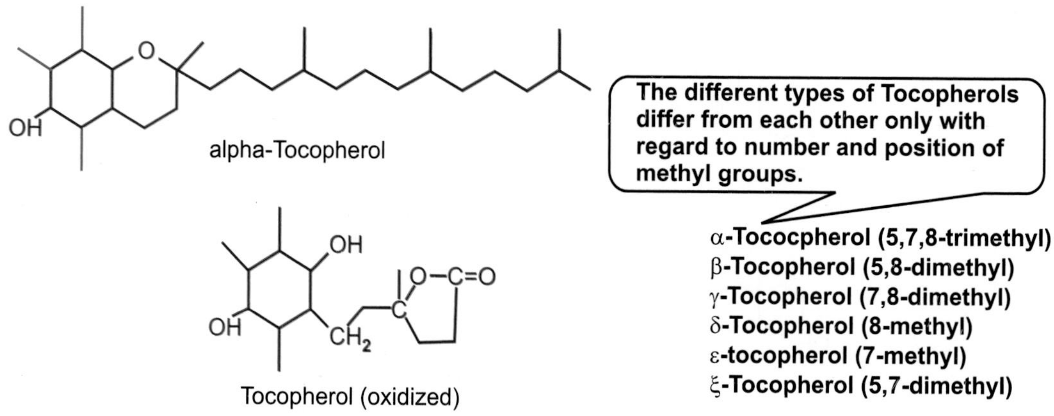

alpha-Tocopherol

The different types of Tocopherols differ from each other only with regard to number and position of methyl groups.

Tocopherol (oxidized)

α-Tococpherol (5,7,8-trimethyl)
β-Tocopherol (5,8-dimethyl)
γ-Tocopherol (7,8-dimethyl)
δ-Tocopherol (8-methyl)
ε-tocopherol (7-methyl)
ξ-Tocopherol (5,7-dimethyl)

Fig. 15.23: Different types of tochopherols

potent of the tocopherols. Vitamin E is absorbed from the intestines, packaged in chylomicrons. It is delivered to the tissues via chylomicron transport and then to the liver through chylomicron remnant uptake. The liver can export vitamin E in VLDLs. Due to its lipophilic nature; vitamin E accumulates in cellular membranes, adipose tissue and other circulating lipoproteins. The major site of vitamin E storage is in adipose tissue.

The major function of vitamin E is to act as a natural **antioxidant** by scavenging free radicals and singlet-oxygen. In particular, vitamin E is important for preventing peroxidation of polyunsaturated membrane fatty acids. The vitamins E and C are interrelated in their antioxidant capabilities. Active α-tocopherol can be regenerated by interaction with vitamin C following scavenge of a peroxy free radical. Alternatively, α-tocopherol can scavenge two peroxy free radicals and then be conjugated to glucuronate for excretion in the bile.

Clinical Significances of Vitamin E Deficiency

No major disease states have been found to be associated with vitamin E deficiency due to adequate levels in the average diet. The major symptom of vitamin E deficiency in humans is an increase in red blood cell fragility. Since vitamin E is absorbed from the intestines in chylomicrons, any fat malabsorption diseases can lead to deficiencies in vitamin E intake. Neurological disorders have been associated with fat malabsorptive disorders and vitamin E deficiency. Vitamin E supplementation is recommended in premature infants fed on formula diets that are low in the vitamin, and individuals consuming a diet high in polyunsaturated fatty acids. Polyunsaturated fatty acids tend to form free radicals upon exposure to oxygen and this may lead to an increased risk of certain cancers.

VITAMIN K

The vitamin K exists naturally as K_1 (phytylmenaquinone) in green vegetables and K_2 (multiprenylmenaquinone) in intestinal bacteria. Menadione is the parent compound (Fig. 15.24).

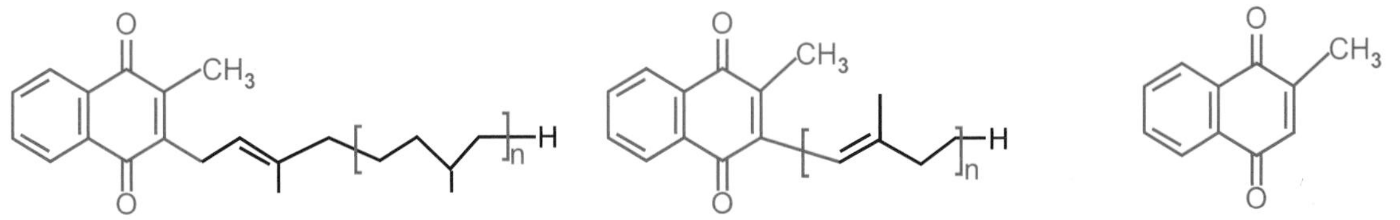

Fig. 15.24: Naturally occurring forms of vitamin K

The major function of vitamin K is in the maintenance of normal levels of the blood clotting proteins, **factors II, VII, IX, X** and **protein C** and **protein S**, which are synthesized in the liver as inactive precursor proteins. Conversion from inactive to active, clotting factor requires a post-translational modification of specific glutamyl residues in these proteins. This modification is a carboxylation reaction that is catalyzed by protein carboxylase, which requires vitamin K as a cofactor. The resultant modified residues are γ-**carboxyglutamate (gla),** which are effective calcium ion chelators (Fig. 15.25).

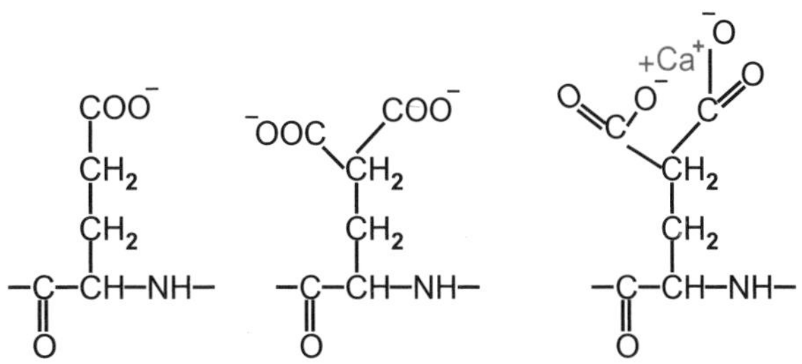

Fig. 15.25: Calcium binding by γ-carboxyglutamate

This process is most clearly understood for factor II, also called **preprothrombin**. Prothrombin upon chelation of calcium interacts with membrane phospholipids and is proteolytically cleaved to **thrombin** by the action of activated factor X (Xa).

During the carboxylation reaction, reduced hydroquinone form of vitamin K is converted to a 2,3-epoxide form. The regeneration of the hydroquinone form requires an *epoxide reductase* and *quinone reductase*. This latter reaction is the site of action of the dicumarol-based anticoagulants such as warfarin (Fig. 15.26).

Clinical Significance of Vitamin K Deficiency

Naturally occurring vitamin K is absorbed from the intestines only in the presence of bile salts and other lipids through interaction with chylomicrons. Therefore, fat malabsorptive diseases can result in vitamin K deficiency. The synthetic vitamin K_3 (Hykinone) is water soluble and absorbed irrespective of the presence of intestinal lipids and bile (Fig. 15.27). Since intestinal bacteria synthesize the vitamin K_2 form, deficiency of the vitamin in adults is rare. However, long-term oral antibiotic treatment can lead to deficiency in adults. The intestine of newborn infants is sterile; therefore, vitamin K deficiency in infants is possible. The primary symptom of deficiency in infants is **hemorrhagic syndrome**.

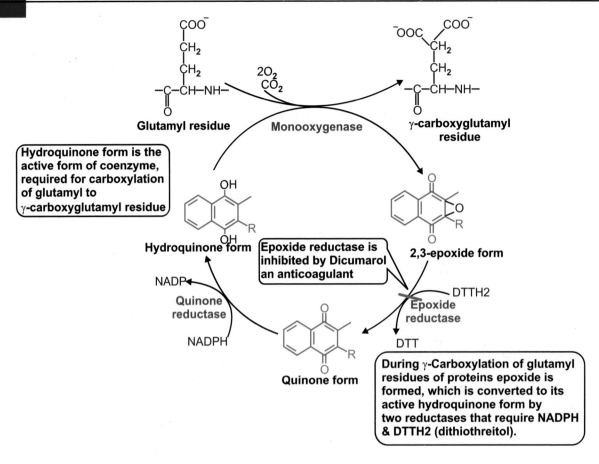

Glutamyl residue
$2O_2$
CO_2
Monooxygenase
γ-carboxyglutamyl residue
Hydroquinone form is the active form of coenzyme, required for carboxylation of glutamyl to γ-carboxyglutamyl residue
Hydroquinone form
Epoxide reductase is inhibited by Dicumarol an anticoagulant
2,3-epoxide form
NADP
Quinone reductase
NADPH
DTTH2
Epoxide reductase
DTT
Quinone form
During γ-Carboxylation of glutamyl residues of proteins epoxide is formed, which is converted to its active hydroquinone form by two reductases that require NADPH & DTTH2 (dithiothreitol).

Fig. 15.26: These reactions takes place in the microsomal fraction of hepatocytes

Dicumarol
Hykinone
(menadione Na bisulfate)

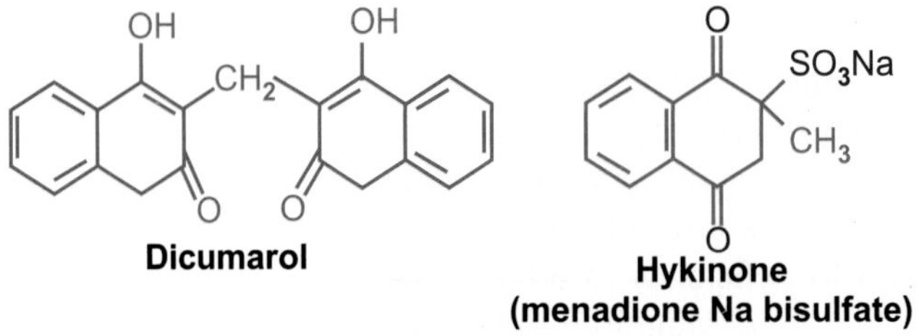

Fig. 15.27: Structures of dicumarol and hykinone

Oxidative Phosphorylation

16

The reducing equivalents generated in the form of NADPH by hexose monophosphate shunt pathway, malic enzyme (linked to $NADP^+$ malate dehydrogenase) and isocitrate dehydrogenase activity in the cytosol are used for reductive synthetic reactions. Whereas NADH generated during oxidation of various metabolites in mitochondria is mostly used for ATP synthesis via oxidative phosphorylation.

Electron transport chain (ETC) and **ATP synthase complex** are integral protein complexes found in the mitochondrial inner membrane. The ETC is composed of a series of protein complexes that catalyze sequential oxidation-reduction reactions (NADH oxidation), which support the phosphorylation of ADP by ATP synthase. These two systems are coupled by proton translocation to develop transmembrane H^+ (proton) gradient.

What are Reduction/Oxidation (Redox) Reactions?

Redox reactions are the transfer of electrons from one chemical species to another. The oxidized plus the reduced form of each chemical species having at least one common intermediate comprise a complete, coupled, redox reaction. An example of a coupled redox reaction is the oxidation of NADH by the electron transport chain:

$$NADH + H^+ + (1/2)\ O_2 \longrightarrow NAD^+ + H_2O$$

For the oxidation of NADH, the standard biological reduction potential is -52.6 kcal/mol. With a free energy change of -52.6 kcal/mol, it is clear that NADH oxidation has the potential for driving the synthesis of a number of ATPs since the standard free energy for the reaction:

$$ADP + P_i \longleftrightarrow ATP \text{ is } +7.3 \text{ kcal/mole.}$$

Direct chemical analysis has shown that for every 2 electrons transferred from NADH to oxygen, 3 equivalents of ATP are synthesized.

ADP Phosphorylation is of Two Types

1. ***Substrate level phosphorylation***: ATP is formed from ADP by phosphate-group transfer from a substrate, without the involvement of ETC.

2. *Oxidative phosphorylation*: Respiration-linked (ETC-linked) phosphorylation of ADP to form ATP in the mitochondria.

NADH generated during glycolysis (in the cytosol) and TCA (in the mitochondria) are funneled to oxidative phosphorylation. Since the NADH binding sites of *NADH dehydrogenase* of complex-I is on the matrix side of the inner impermeable mitochondrial membrane, NADH generated in the cytosol should be transported into the mitochondrial matrix, by special shuttles.

Special Shuttles for NADH Transport

1. *Malate-Aspartate shuttles:* NADH binds to complex I; 1 molecule NADH yields 3 molecules of ATP. (α-ketoglutarate – glutamate).
2. *Glycerol-3-phosphate (Dihydroxyacetone phosphate, gly-3-P dehydrogenase) shuttles:* NADH binds directly to complex III; 1 molecule NADH yields only 2 molecules of ATP.

STRUCTURE AND PROPERTIES OF MITOCHONDRIA

The outer mitochondrial membrane has transmembrane channels called porins that readily allow the passage of small molecules, of molecular weight less than 5000. Whereas the inner mitochondrial membrane is impermeable to most small molecules and ions, including protons (H^+). Hence transport of molecules across inner mitochondrial membrane requires specific transporter proteins.

The enzymes found in the mitochondrial matrix are pyruvate dehydrogenase complex, enzyme of the TCA cycle, enzymes of β-oxidation pathway of fatty acids, and enzymes of amino acids oxidation. The enzymes and the intermediates of cytosolic metabolic pathways are segregated from those of the mitochondrial matrix.

Pyruvate, fatty acids, amino acids and their α-keto derivative are transported into the mitochondrial matrix by special transporters, to access the machinery of the citric acid cycle. Similarly ADP and Pi are specifically transported into the matrix, as the synthesized ATP is transported out.

Electrons are Transported along Respiratory Chain by Three Mechanisms

1. Direct transfer of electron
2. Transfer of electron and hydrogen atom
3. Transfer of hydride ion (**:H⁻**).

NAD-linked dehydrogenase removes two hydrogen atoms from the substrate, as :H⁻ (hydride ion) and H^+ (proton).

Reduced substrate + NAD^+ ⇌ Oxidized substrate + NADH + H^+

Reduced substrate + $NADP^+$ ⇌ Oxidized substrate + NADPH + H^+

NAD^+ can also collect reducing equivalents from NADPH, by NADP-linked dehydrogenase. This reaction is catalyzed by *pyridine nucleotide transhydrogenase.*

$$NAD^+ + NADPH \rightleftharpoons NADH + NADP^+$$

NADH and NADPH are water-soluble electron carriers that associate reversibly with dehydrogenases. NADH is an electron carrier in catabolic reactions and NADPH is an electron carrier in anabolic reaction.

Flavoproteins are proteins to which, a flavin nucleotide (FMN and FAD) is very tightly sometimes covalently bound. The standard potential depends on the protein with which it is associated. Interaction of flavin nucleotide with the functional group of this protein distorts the electron cloud arround FMN/FAD. The flavin nucleotides can accept one or two electron depending on the flavoprotein's reduction potential.

Iron-containing Proteins

Two types of iron-containing proteins are involved in reduction of quinone to hydroquinone.
1. **Cytochromes** are the integral membrane proteins of mitochondrial inner membrane, which hold iron of heme tightly but not covalently. The three classes of cytochromes are **cyt a** (600 nm), **cyt b** (560 nm), and **cyt c** (550 nm). Cyt c is water soluble and associated with the outer surface of the mitochondrial inner membrane through electrostatic interaction.
2. **Iron-sulfur proteins** are paramagnetic in which iron is associated with sulfur atom and cysteine residues of proteins.

Ubiquinone/benzoquinones (CoQ) are small and hydrophobic molecules freely diffusible within the lipid bilayer of the inner mitochondrial membrane. They shuttle reducing equivalents between other less mobile electron carriers in the membrane. It exists in three states of oxidation: ubiquinone (CoQ), semiquinone (CoQH.), and ubiquinol ($CoQH_2$).

Mitochondrial Electron Carriers' Function in Serially Ordered Complexes

Standard reduction potential/redox potential (E_O') for the components of ETC have been determined experimentally. Carriers function in order of increasing reduction potential because e^- tend to flow spontaneously from carriers of lower E_O' to carrier of higher E_O'. The direction of flow of electrons from one redox system to another is shown in Figure 16.2.

$$NADH \rightarrow CoQ \rightarrow Cyt\ b \rightarrow cyt\ c_1 \rightarrow cyt\ c \rightarrow cyt\ a + a_3 \rightarrow O_2$$

If all the carriers are reduced by providing an electron source but no electron acceptor (O_2) and then suddenly introduce O_2 into the system, the carrier at the end of the chain gives up its electron first, the second carrier from the end is oxidized next and so on.

ETC has Four Electron Carrier Complexes

Centrifugation and gentle treatment of inner membrane with detergents allows the resolution of four electron carrier complexes (Fig. 16.1).

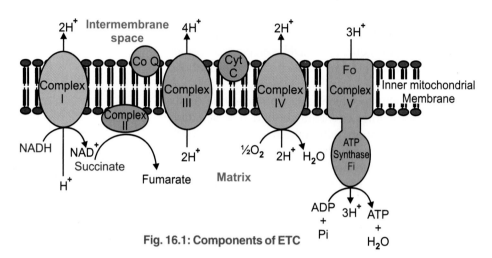

Fig. 16.1: Components of ETC

Complexes I and II catalyzes the e-transfer to ubiquinone (Co.Q), from two different electron donors (NADH and succinate).

Complex III carries electron from ubiquinone to cytochrome c.

Complex IV completes the sequence by transferring electrons from cyt c to O_2.

ATP synthase is often considered as Complex V, has Fo and F1 protein subunits that are involved in pumping proton into the mitochondrial matrix and ATP synthesis (Fig. 16.2).

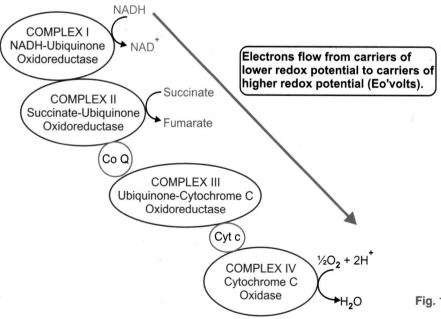

Fig. 16.2: Schematic representation of electron flow in ETC

Complex I is NADH-Ubiquinone Oxidoreductase (NADH Dehydrogenase)

It consists of 25 polypeptide chains and is responsible for transfer of electrons from NADH to ubiquinone. NADH binding site faces matrix, which contains 7 Fe-S centers of at least 2 different types. Inhibitors of electron flow from Fe-S centers to CoQ are amytal (barbiturate), rotenone (insecticide), and piericidine (antibiotic).

$$NADH + H^+ + CoQ \longrightarrow NAD^+ + CoQH2$$

(The actual transfer of electrons from NADH to CoQ passes through FMN of complex II) Flow of electron from complex I to CoQ to complex III is accompanied by flow of H^+ from mitochondrial matrix, into the mitochondrial intermembrane space.

Complex II is Succinate-Ubiquinone Oxidoreductase (Succinate Dehydrogenase)

It is the only membrane bound enzyme of TCA cycle. The enzyme has covalently bound FAD and a Fe-S center with four Fe atoms. Electrons, flow from succinate to FAD to Fe-S centers and then to ubiquinone.

Complex III is Ubiquinol-Cytochrome c Oxidoreductase

This complex is located in inner mitochondrial membrane and contains cytochromes b562, b566, and cyt c1 and iron-sulfur proteins. Cyt b is transmembrane but both cyt c1 and iron-sulfur proteins are on the outer surface of inner membrane of mitochondria. In the process of oxidation of CoQH2 to CoQ, Cyt c gets reduced, and protons are pumped out of mitochondrial matrix into the intermembrane space of the mitochondria.

Complex IV is Cytochrome c Oxidase

It is composed of Cyt a and cyt a3, which contains two heme groups bound to different regions of the same large proteins and also contains two copper ions Cu_A and Cu_B that are crucial to the transport of e^- to O_2. Flow of e^- from cyt c to O_2 through complex IV causes movement of H^+ from matrix into intermembrane space of the mitochondria.

ATP Synthase (Fo F1 Complex) is Regarded as Complex V

It is a transmembrane multiple subunit complex that binds ADP and inorganic phosphate at its catalytic site inside the mitochondrion, and requires a proton gradient for activity in the forward direction. **ATP synthase** is composed of 3 fragments: F_0, which is localized in the membrane; F_1, which protrudes from the inside of the inner membrane into the matrix it has multiple subunits, three α, three β, one γ, one δ and one ϵ (site of ATP synthesis is β subunits) and oligomycin sensitivity—conferring protein (OSCP), which connects F_0 to F_1 (Fig.16.3). In damaged mitochondria permeable to protons,

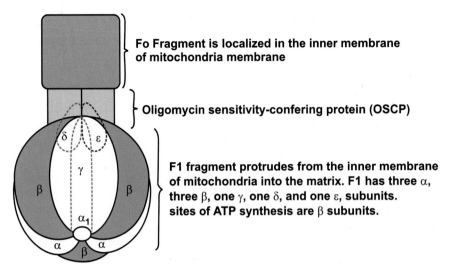

Fo Fragment is localized in the inner membrane of mitochondria membrane

Oligomycin sensitivity-confering protein (OSCP)

F1 fragment protrudes from the inner membrane of mitochondria into the matrix. F1 has three α, three β, one γ, one δ, and one ε, subunits. sites of ATP synthesis are β subunits.

Fig. 16.3: Schematic diagram of ATP synthase

the **ATP synthase** reaction is active in the reverse direction acting as a very efficient ATP hydrolase or ATPase.

OXIDATIVE PHOSPHORYLATION

The free energy available as a consequence of transferring 2 electrons from NADH or succinate to molecular oxygen through ETC is -57 and -36 kcal/mol, respectively. This energy is trapped as high-energy phosphate of ATP by oxidative phosphorylation.

In order for oxidative phosphorylation to proceed, two principal conditions must be met. First, the inner mitochondrial membrane must be physically intact so that protons can only reenter the mitochondrion by a process coupled to ATP synthesis. Second, a high concentration of protons must be developed on the outside of the inner membrane.

The energy of the proton gradient is known as the **chemiosmotic potential**, or **proton motive force (PMF)**. This potential is the sum of the difference, in the concentration of protons across the inner mitochondrial membrane. The 2 electrons from NADH generate a 6-proton gradient. Thus, oxidation of 1 mole of NADH leads to the availability of a free energy of about -31.2 kcal. The energy of the gradient is used to drive ATP synthesis as the protons are transported back down their thermodynamic gradient into the mitochondrion, through the integral membrane protein known as **ATP synthase (or Complex V)**.

Stoichiometry of Oxidative Phosphorylation

For each pair of electrons originating from NADH, 3 equivalents of ATP are synthesized, requiring 22.4 kcal of energy. Thus, with 31.2 kcal of available energy, it is clear that the proton gradient generated by electron transport contains sufficient energy to drive normal ATP synthesis. Electrons from succinate have about two-thirds the energy of NADH electrons: they generate PMFs that are about two-thirds as great as NADH electrons and lead to the synthesis of only 2 moles of ATP per mole of succinate oxidized.

Regulation of Oxidative Phosphorylation

Since electron transport is directly coupled to proton translocation, the flow of electrons through the electron transport system is regulated by the magnitude of the PMF. The higher the PMF the lower the rate of electron transport, and vice versa. Under resting conditions, with a high cell energy charge *(high ATP concentration)*, demand for synthesis of ATP is limited. Although the PMF is high, flow of protons back into the mitochondrion through ATP synthase is minimal. When energy demands are increased, such as during vigorous muscle activity, cytosolic ADP rises and is exchanged with intramitochondrial ATP via the transmembrane adenine nucleotide carrier *ADP/ATP translocase*. Increased intramitochondrial concentrations of ADP cause the PMF to become discharged as protons pour through ATP synthase, regenerating the ATP pool. Thus, while the rate of electron transport is dependent on the PMF, the magnitude of the PMF at any moment simply reflects the energy charge of the cell. *In turn the energy charge of the cell, or ADP concentration, is the one that determines the rate of electron transport by mass action principles.* The rate of electron transport is usually measured by assaying the rate of oxygen consumption and is referred to as the cellular respiratory rate. The respiratory rate is known as the **state 4 rate,** when the energy charge is high, the concentration of ADP is low, and ADP limits electron transport. When ADP levels rise and inorganic phosphate is available, the flow of protons through ATP synthase is elevated and higher rates of electron transport are observed; the resultant respiratory rate is known as the **state 3 rate.** Thus, under physiological conditions mitochondrial respiratory activity cycles between state 3 and state 4 rates.

Inhibitors of Oxidative Phosphorylation

The pathway of electron flow through the electron transport assembly, and unique properties of the PMF, has been determined by use of a number of antimetabolites. Some of these agents inhibit electron transport at specific sites in the electron transport assembly, while others stimulate electron transport by discharging the proton gradient.

For example, *antimycin A* is a specific inhibitor of cytochrome *b*. In the presence of *antimycin A*, cytochrome *b* remains reduced and cannot be oxidized. As expected, cytochrome *c* remains oxidized in presence of *antimycin A*, as do the downstream cytochromes *a* and *a*3.

NAME	FUNCTION	SITE OF ACTION
Rotenone	e⁻ transport inhibitor	Complex I
Amytal	e⁻ transport inhibitor	Complex I
Antimycin A	e⁻ transport inhibitor	Complex III
Cyanide	e⁻ transport inhibitor	Complex IV

Carbon monoxide	e^- transport inhibitor	Complex IV
Azide	e^- transport inhibitor	Complex IV
2,4-dinitrophenol	*Uncoupling agent*	Transmembrane H^+ carrier
Oligomycin	**Inhibits ATP synthase**	OSCP fraction of ATP synthase

An important class of antimetabolites is the *uncoupling agent* such as 2,4-dinitrophenol (DNP). Uncoupling agents act as lipophilic weak acids, associating with protons on the exterior of mitochondria, passing through the membrane with the bound proton, and dissociating the proton on the interior of the mitochondrion. These agents cause maximum respiratory rates but the electron transport generates no ATP, since the translocated protons do not return to the interior through ATP synthase.

Boyer's Mechanism of ATP Synthesis.

1. Three active sites on F1 alternate in catalyzing ATP synthesis. The limiting step is the release of newly synthesized ATP from the enzyme. A conformational transition driven by the proton motive force reduces enzyme's affinity for ATP.
2. Transition induced by the proton motive force may be envisioned as a structural change in α–β positions that orients one of the three α–β pair in a special position relative to the proton channel of Fo. These structural changes may be an allosteric transition in which changes at one α–β pair force compensating changes in the other two pairs.
3. Enzyme must sense difference in proton concentration between the two regions in space (inside the matrix and in the intermembrane space).
4. A proton gradient couples electron flow and phosphorylation.
5. The inherent electrochemical energy due to differences of proton concentration and separation of charges by membrane, the proton motive force represents a part of the energy of oxidation. The proton motive force is subsequently used to drive the F1 catalyzed ATP synthesis, as protons flows passively back into the matrix through pores formed by Fo.

The equation for the synthesis of ATP:

$$ADP + Pi + \{H^+\}\ out \rightleftharpoons ATP + H_2O + \{H^+\}\ in$$

When proton flows spontaneously down their electrochemical gradient, an amount of free energy equal to ΔG becomes available to do work; it is the proton motive force.

ENERGY FROM CYTOSOLIC NADH

When cytosolic NADH is oxidized in the electron transport system via *glycerol-phosphate shuttle* it yields only 2 equivalents of ATP. If NADH is oxidized via the *malate-aspartate shuttle* it yields 3 ATPs.

Glycerol-phosphate Shuttle

The glycerol-phosphate shuttle (Fig. 16.4) is coupled FAD-linked dehydrogenase enzyme in the inner mitochondrial membrane. The shuttle involves two different **glycerol-3-phosphate dehydrogenases**: one is cytosolic that reduces dihydroxyacetone-phosphate to glycerol-3-phosphate, and the other is an integral protein of the inner mitochondrial membrane that acts to oxidize glycerol-3-phosphate to regenerate dihydroxyacetone phosphate. The net result of the process is that reducing equivalents from cytosolic NADH are transferred to the mitochondrial electron transport system. The catalytic site of the mitochondrial *glycerol-3-phosphate dehydrogenase* is on the outer surface of the inner membrane, allowing ready access to the product of the cytosolic **glycerol-3-phosphate dehydrogenase**.

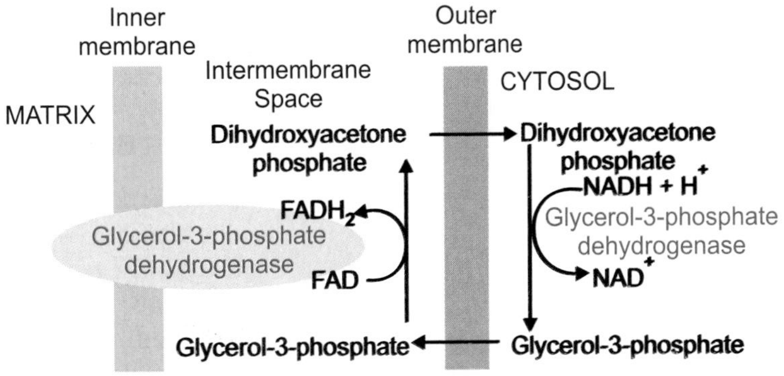

Fig. 16.4: Glycerol-phosphate shuttle

Malate-aspartate Shuttle

In some tissues, such as that of heart and muscle, mitochondrial **glycerol-3-phosphate dehydrogenase** is present in very low amounts, and the *malate-aspartate shuttle* (Fig. 16.5) is the dominant pathway for aerobic oxidation of cytosolic NADH.

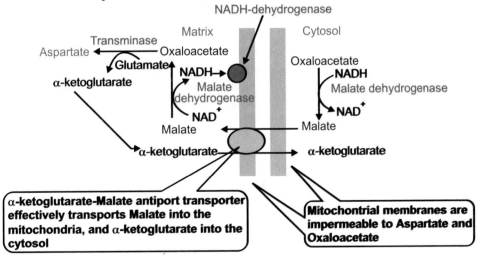

Fig. 16.5: Malate shuttle

The cytosolic **malate dehydrogenase (MDH)** utilizes NADH to reduce oxaloacetate (OAA) to malate. Malate is transported to the interior of the mitochondrion via the α-ketoglutarate/malate antiporter. Inside the mitochondrion, malate is oxidized by the MDH of the TCA cycle, producing oxaloacetate and NADH. In this step, the cytosolic NADH-derived reducing equivalents become available to the **NADH dehydrogenase** of the inner mitochondrial membrane and are oxidized, giving rise to 3 ATPs as described earlier. The mitochondrial transaminase uses glutamate to convert membrane-impermeable oxaloacetate to aspartate and α-ketoglutarate. This provides a pool of α-ketoglutarate for the above-mentioned antiporter. The aspartate that is also produced is translocated out of the mitochondrion.

OTHER BIOLOGICAL OXIDATIONS

Oxidase complexes such as **cytochrome oxidase** transfer electrons directly from NADH and other substrates to oxygen, producing water. *Oxygenase complexes* that catalyze the addition of molecular oxygen to organic molecules are localized in membranes of the endoplasmic reticulum.

There are two kinds of oxygenase complexes, ***monoxygenases*** and ***dioxygenases***. Dioxygenases add two atoms of molecular oxygen (O_2) to carbon and nitrogen of organic compounds. Monoxygenase complexes play a key role in detoxifying drugs and other compounds (e.g., PCBs and dioxin), and in the normal metabolism of steroids, fatty acids and fat-soluble vitamins. Monoxygenases act by sequentially transferring two electrons from NADH or NADPH to one of the two atoms of O_2 to generate H_2O and incorporating the other oxygen atom into an organic compound to form hydroxyl group (R-OH). The hydroxylated products are markedly more water-soluble than their precursors and are much more readily excreted from the body. Monoxygenases are also called as: mixed function oxidases, hydroxylases, and mixed function hydroxylases.

The components of monoxygenase complexes include cytochrome b5, cytochrome P_{450}, and **cytochrome P_{450} reductase**, which contain both FAD and FMN. There are many P_{450} isozymes; found in liver, where the bulk of drug metabolism occurs. Some of these P_{450} isozymes are also found in other tissues, where they are responsible for tissue-specific oxygenase activities. Reducing equivalents for P_{450} arise either from NADH or from NADPH.

Enzymatic reactions involving molecular oxygen usually produce water or organic oxygen in well-regulated reactions having specific products. However, under some metabolic conditions (e.g., reperfusion of anaerobic tissues) unpaired electrons gain access to molecular oxygen in unregulated, non-enzymatic reactions. The products, called **free radicals**, are quite toxic. These free radicals, especially hydroxy radical, randomly attack cell components, including proteins, lipids and nucleic acids, potentially causing extensive cellular damage.

Tissues are armed with enzymes to protect against the random chemical reactions that these free radicals initiate. Several free radical scavenging enzymes have been identified:

Superoxide dismutases (SODs) in animals contain either zinc (Zn^{2+}) or copper (Cu^{2+}), known as CuZnSOD, or CuMnSOD as in the case of the mitochondrial form. These SODs convert superoxide to peroxide and thereby minimizes production of hydroxy radical, which is the most potent of the free radicals. Peroxides produced by SOD are also toxic. They are detoxified by conversion to water via the enzyme **peroxidase**. The best-known mammalian peroxidase is **glutathione peroxidase**, which contains selenium as a prosthetic group.

Glutathione is important in maintaining the normal reduction potential of cells, and provides the reducing equivalents for glutathione peroxidase to convert hydrogen peroxide to water. In red blood cells, the lack of glutathione leads to extensive peroxide attack on the plasma membrane, producing fragile red blood cells that readily undergo hemolysis, as seen in glucose 6-phosphate dehydrogenase (G6PD) deficiency.

Catalase (located in peroxisomes) provides a reductant route for the degradation of hydrogen peroxide.

Free Radical Formation

17

Atoms are most stable in the ground state. An atom is considered to be "ground" when every electron in the outermost shell has a complimentary electron that spins in the opposite direction. By definition a free radical is any atom (e.g. oxygen, nitrogen) with at least one unpaired electron in the outermost shell, and capable of independent existence. A free radical is easily formed when a covalent bond between entities is broken and one electron remains with each newly formed atom.

Free radicals are highly reactive due to the presence of unpaired electron(s). Any free radical involving oxygen can be referred to as *reactive oxygen species* (ROS). Oxygen centered free radicals contain two unpaired electrons in the outer shell. When free radicals steal an electron from a surrounding compound or molecule a new free radical is formed in its place. The newly formed radical tries to return to its ground state by stealing electrons with antiparallel spins from cellular structures or molecules. Thus the chain reaction continues and can be "thousand of events long".

The **electron transport chain** (ETC) found in the inner mitochondrial membrane, utilizes oxygen as the terminal electron acceptor to generate energy in the form of **adenosine triphosphate** (ATP). About two to five percent of total oxygen intake is transformed to superoxide radicals by electron escape. During exercise oxygen consumption increases 10 to 20 fold (35-70 ml/kg/min) that further enhances electron escape from ETC. Thus when calculated 0.6 to 3.5 ml/kg/min of the total oxygen intake during exercise are transformed to free radicals. The site of electron escape in ETC appears to be ubiquinone-cytochrome c.

Lipid Peroxidation

Cell membranes and low-density lipoproteins (LDL) have abundant quantities of **polyunsaturated fatty acids** (PUFAs), which allow for fluidity of cellular membranes. A free radical prefers to steal electrons from PUFA present in the lipid membrane of cells, which initiate a free radical attack on the cell known as lipid peroxidation. Reactive oxygen species target the carbon-carbon double bond of polyunsaturated fatty acids. The double bond on the carbon weakens the carbon-hydrogen bond allowing for easy dissociation of the hydrogen. A free radical will steal the single electron from the hydrogen associated with the carbon at the double bond. In turn this leaves the carbon with an unpaired electron and hence becomes a free radical.

In an effort to stabilize the carbon-centered free radical, molecular rearrangement occurs. The newly arranged molecule is called a **conjugated diene** (CD). The CD then very easily reacts with oxygen to form a peroxy radical. The peroxy radical steals an electron from another lipid molecule in a process called propagation. This process then continues in a chain reaction.

Types of Free Radicals

There are numerous types of free radicals that can be formed within the body. The most common ROS generated by univalent reduction steps of molecular oxygen includes: the **superoxide anion** (O_2^-), the **hydroxy radical** (OH$^•$), **singlet oxygen** ($1/2\ O_2$), and **hydrogen peroxide** (H_2O_2).

$$O_2 \rightarrow O_2^{-}: \ \rightarrow \ OH^• \rightarrow H_2O_2$$

Superoxide anions are formed when molecular oxygen (O_2) acquires an additional electron, leaving the molecule with only one unpaired electron. Within the mitochondria $O_2^-:$, is continuously being formed. The rate of formation depends on the amount of oxygen flowing through the mitochondria at any given time.

Hydroxyl radicals are short-lived, but the most damaging radicals within the body. This type of free radical can be formed from $O_2^-:$, and H_2O_2 via the Haber-Weiss reaction. The interaction of copper or iron with H_2O_2 also produces OH. These reactions are significant as the substrates are found within the body and could interact.

Hydrogen peroxide is produced *in vivo* by many reactions. Hydrogen peroxide is unique in that it can be converted to the highly damaging hydroxyl radical or be catalyzed and excreted harmlessly as water. Glutathione peroxidase is essential for the conversion of glutathione to oxidized glutathione, during which H_2O_2 is converted to water. If H_2O_2 is not converted to water, $½\ O_2$ (singlet oxygen) is formed.

Singlet oxygen, formed during radical reactions is not a free radical but causes further reactions. Singlet oxygen has eight outer electrons existing in pairs leaving one orbital of the same energy level empty. When oxygen is energetically excited one of the electrons can jump to the empty orbital, creating unpaired electrons. Singlet oxygen can then transfer the energy to a new molecule and act as a catalyst for free radical formation. The molecule can also interact with other molecules leading to the formation of a new free radical.

Catalyst

All transition metals, with the exception of copper contain one electron in their outermost shell and can be considered free radicals. Copper has a full outer shell, but loses and gains electrons very easily making itself a free radical. Iron has the ability to gain and lose electrons (i.e. ($Fe^{2+} \leftrightarrow Fe^{3+}$) very easily. This property makes iron and copper, the two common catalysts of oxidation reactions. Iron is major component of red blood cells (RBC). The stress encountered during circulation through capillaries may breakdown RBC releasing free iron. The release of iron can be detrimental to cellular membranes because of the pro-oxidation effects it can have. Zinc exists in one valence (Zn^{2+}) and does not catalyze free radical formation. In fact zinc may actually act to stop radical formation by displacing those metals having more than one valence.

Measurement of Free Radicals

The markers of oxidative stress are measured using a variety of different assays.

When a fatty acid is peroxidized it is broken down to aldehydes, which are excreted. Aldehydes such as ***thiobarbituric acid reacting substances*** (TBARS) have been widely accepted as a general marker of free radical production. The most commonly measured TBARS is ***malondialdehyde*** (MDA). The TBA test has been challenged because of its lack of specificity, sensitivity, and reproducibility. The use of liquid chromatography instead spectrophotometer techniques help reduce these errors. In addition, the test seems to work best when applied to membrane systems such as microsomes. Gases such as pentane and ethane are also created as lipid peroxidation occurs. These gases are expired and commonly measured during free radical research. Lastly, conjugated dienes (CD) are often measured as indicators of free radical production. Oxidation of unsaturated fatty acids results in the formation of CD. The CD formed is measured and provide a marker of the early stages of lipid peroxidation. A newly developed technique for measuring free radical production shows promise in producing more valid results. The technique uses monoclonal antibodies and may prove to be the most accurate measurement of free radicals. However, until further more reliable techniques are established it is generally accepted that two or more assays be utilized whenever possible to enhance validity.

Physiological Effects

Under normal conditions at rest, the antioxidant defense system within the body can easily handle free radicals that are formed. During times of increased oxygen flux (i.e. exercise) free radical production may exceed that of removal, ultimately resulting in lipid peroxidation.

In order to prevent or counter lipid peroxidation and its effects, one need to understand the interrelationship between lipid peroxidation and free radical generation during exercise and stress.

Need for Antioxidant Supplementation

Oxygen consumption greatly increases during exercise, which leads to increased free radical production. The antioxidant defense system in the body counters the increase in free radical production. Oxidative damage occurs only when free radical production exceeds clearance. Free radicals formed during chronic exercise may exceed the protective capacity of the antioxidant defense system, thereby making the body more prone to disease and injury. Therefore the need for antioxidant supplementation is discussed.

Fatigue

A free radical attack usually damages a cell membrane to the point that it must be removed from the system. If free radical formation and attack are not controlled within the muscle during exercise, a large quantity of muscle could easily be damaged. Damaged muscle could in turn inhibit performance by the induction of fatigue.

Recovery

One of the first steps in recovery from exercise induced muscle damage is an acute inflammatory response at the site of muscle damage. Free radicals are commonly associated with the inflammatory response and are hypothesized to be greatest at twenty-four hours after completion of a strenuous exercise. If this theory were valid then antioxidants would play a major role in helping prevent this damage. However, if antioxidant defense systems are inadequate or not elevated during the post-exercise infiltration period, free radicals could further damage muscle beyond that acquired during exercise. This in turn would increase the time needed to recover from an exercise bout.

Importance of Free Radicals

So far we have discussed the negative aspects that are associated with free radical production. However, free radicals are naturally produced by some systems within the body and have beneficial effects that cannot be overlooked. The immune system is the main body system that utilizes free radicals. Foreign invaders or damaged tissue is marked with free radicals by the immune system. This allows for determination of which tissue need to be removed from the body. Because of this, some question the need for antioxidant supplementation, as they believe supplementation can actually decrease the effectiveness of the immune system.

Antioxidant Defenses

Antioxidants protect lipids from peroxidation by radicals. Antioxidants are effective because they are willing to give up their own electrons to free radicals. When a free radical gains the electron from an antioxidant it no longer needs to attack the cell and the chain reaction of oxidation is broken. After donating an electron an antioxidant becomes a free radical by definition. Antioxidants in this state are not harmful because they have the ability to accommodate the change in electrons without becoming reactive. The human body has an elaborate antioxidant defense system. Antioxidants are manufactured within the body and can also be obtained from the food we eat such as fruits, vegetables, seeds, nuts, meats, and oil.

There are two lines of antioxidant defense within the cell. The first line, found in the fat-soluble cellular membrane consists of vitamin E, beta-carotene, and coenzyme Q. Of these, vitamin E is considered the most potent chain breaking antioxidant within the membrane of the cell.

Inside the cell water-soluble antioxidant scavengers are present. These include vitamin C, glutathione peroxidase, superoxide dismutase (SD), and catalase (Fig. 17.1). Only those antioxidants that are commonly supplemented (vitamins E and the mineral selenium) are further discussed.

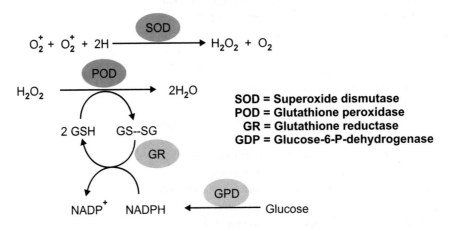

SOD = Superoxide dismutase
POD = Glutathione peroxidase
GR = Glutathione reductase
GDP = Glucose-6-P-dehydrogenase

Fig. 17.1: Enzymes involved in free radical scavenging

Vitamin E and Prevention of Oxidative Stress/Lipid Peroxidation

The effectiveness of vitamin E in preventing exercise-induced oxidative stress (lipid peroxidation) is poorly understood. From human studies the following indicators of oxidative stress have been measured: DNA damage, *creatine kinase* (CK) leakage, *maximum voluntary contraction* (MVC), thiobarbituric acid reacting substances (TBARS) and/or conjugated dienes (CD). Differing indices of oxidative stress along with a multitude of contrasting design variables (i.e. subject conditions, length of study, dose of vitamin, type of exercise) have created confusion when trying to interpret the role vitamin E, in preventing oxidative damage. Creatine kinase is a commonly measured indicator of oxidative stress. The enzyme is considered a hallmark for muscle damage as it leaks from the muscle during periods of injury to muscle cell membrane. Ingestion of 400 I.U. of vitamin E for 48 days reduced the amount of CK leakage in young and old men during recovery from downhill running bouts. The majority of literature suggests that supplementation with vitamin E does protect against lipid peroxidation.

SELENIUM

Selenium is a non-metal that exists in multiple oxidation states (i.e. 2, +4, +6). Within biological systems the element is a constituent of the amino acids found in proteins. Selenium is an essential component of the glutathione peroxidase enzyme system. The importance of selenium in the human diet was discovered in 1979. Chinese scientists showed that children living in selenium-deficient areas were suffering from a cardiomyopathy known as Keshan disease. The symptoms of the disease were reversed when selenium was added to the diet.

Sources

The best sources of selenium are seafoods with the exception of some fishes. Mercury compounds found in some fish bind the selenium thereby making it unavailable to humans. Animal sources of selenium also appear to be higher due to a greater homeostatic control of the element during a wide variety of exposure conditions.

Absorption and Bioavailability

Several forms of selenium enter the body as part of amino acids within proteins. The two most common forms of the element that enter the body are selenomethionine and selenocysteine, which are found mainly in plants and animals respectively. The primary site of absorption is from the duodenum. Selenomethionine is absorbed from the duodenum at a rate close to 100 percent. Other forms of the element are also well absorbed. However, absorption of inorganic forms of the element varies widely due to luminal factors. Selenium absorption is not affected by body selenium status. Absorption of selenium is closely related to multiple nutritional factors that inhibit or promote absorption. Vitamins A, C, and E along with reduced glutathione enhance absorption of the element. In contrast, heavy metals decrease absorption via precipitation and chelation.

Transport

The exact mechanisms of selenium transport are thus far unclear and debatable. Within the blood, free selenium binds to lipoproteins such as VLDL or LDL. The transport properties of a second protein, identified as selenoprotein P, have been met with opposing viewpoints. The protein is found in the plasma and is believed to be a carrier by some. Others believe that the presence of selenocysteine within the structure inhibits the transport abilities of the protein.

Storage

Selenium that is absorbed becomes a part of both transport and storage proteins. Selenium is believed to influence the formation of the proteins. The uptake of selenium is a complex process that involves numerous factors. The heart, kidney, lung, liver, pancreas, and muscle contain very high levels of selenium as a component of glutathione. In addition, type I (slow twitch) muscle likely contains greater amounts of reduced glutathione than type IIb (fast twitch) because of their oxidative capacity. The liver is a major supplier of circulating reduced glutathione, which is reflected in the amount of its reserves. The volume of glutathione in the liver is from 5-7 mM; that in the heart ranges between 2-3 mM. With the exception of the lens of the eye, the levels found in the liver are the highest within the body. Noteworthy is the fact that red blood cells contain four times more GSH than the plasma (2.0 mM vs. .5 mM).

Excretion

Selenium homeostasis is regulated primarily through excretion via two main paths: urinary (50 to 67 %) and fecal (40 to 50 %). Extremely high intakes of selenium can lead to ventilatory elimination of the mineral in the form of dimethylselenide. Excretion via the lungs is characterized by a garlic smell odor of the volatile selenium compound. Urinary excretion is the primary route of regulation under normal physiological conditions.

Physiological Role

Currently, eleven different selenium-containing proteins (seleno-proteins) are identified in animals. Most of these proteins have enzymatic functions that have been characterized. Some hypothesized functions of selenium include: maintenance of the cytochrome P450 system, DNA repair, enzyme activation, and immune system function. Better understood roles of selenium are: selenium is best known for the role it plays in the glutathione peroxidase (GSH-Px) enzyme system (Fig. 17.1).

Four separate glutathione peroxidases have been identified. Within the cell total (GSH-Px) is distributed ~2:1 between the cytosol and the mitochondrial matrix. The distribution of the enzyme allows for increased efficiency of free radicals by the GSH-Px system. These enzyme systems are well established as being the major antioxidant defense systems within the body. Reduced glutathione is the first line of defense against free radicals. The glutathione system is key in the coordination of the water and lipid soluble antioxidant defense systems. The peroxidases use reduced glutathione to stop peroxidation of cells by breaking down hydrogen peroxide (H_2O_2) and lipid peroxides. The majority of research involving the glutathione system has addressed GSH-Px, the enzyme responsible for the breakdown of hydrogen peroxide to water. Adequate levels of the intracellular substrate, reduced glutathione, are required in order for GSH-Px to exhibit antioxidant properties. As reduced glutathione is utilized to remove H_2O_2 from the body oxidized glutathione is formed.

An equally important selenium-containing enzyme that converts oxidized glutathione back to reduced glutathione for use by the antioxidant defense systems is glutathione reductase. Iodine metabolism also relies heavily on selenium availability. More specifically the enzyme involved in the conversion of thyroxine (T4) to tri-iodothyronine (T3) appears to be selenium dependent. Both of these enzymes play a very important role during metabolic activities, which in turn demonstrates the importance of selenium in the system.

Recommended Daily Allowance (RDA)

After some corrections for body weight and subject variability the RDA was set at 70 ug for men and 55 ug for women.

Enzymes: Basic Concepts and Kinetics

18

The enzymes support almost all of the chemical reactions that maintain animal homeostasis. Because of their role in maintaining life processes, the assay and pharmacological regulation of enzymes have become key elements in clinical diagnosis and therapeutics. Almost all enzymes are proteins, with the exception of ribozymes, which are molecules of ribonucleic acid that catalyze reactions on the phosphodiester bond of other RNAs.

Enzymes are Found in all Tissues and the Body Fluids

1. *Intracellular enzymes* catalyze the reactions of metabolic pathways.
2. *Plasma membrane enzymes* regulate catalysis within cells in response to extracellular signals, and
3. *Enzymes of the circulatory system* are responsible for regulating the clotting of blood. Almost every significant life process is dependent on enzyme activity.

Enzymes Transform Different Forms of Energy

Most biochemical reactions in the living system use enzymes to convert energy from one form to another usable form, e.g. 1) Photosynthesis converts light energy to chemical energy, 2) Respiration converts chemical energy into ATP.

Number	Classification	Action
1	Oxidoreductases	Act on many chemical groupings to add or remove hydrogen atoms.
2	Transferases	Transfer functional groups between donor and acceptor molecules. Kinases are specialized transferases that regulate metabolism by transferring phosphate from ATP to other molecules.
3	Hydrolases	Add water across a bond, hydrolyzing it.
4	Lyases	Add water, ammonia or carbon dioxide across double bonds, or remove these elements to produce double bonds.
5	Isomerases	Carry out many kinds of isomerization: L to D isomerization, mutase reaction (shifts of chemical groups) and others.
6	Ligases	Catalyze reactions in which two chemical groups are joined (or ligated) with the use of energy from ATP.

Enzyme Classifications

According to the International Union of Biochemists (IUB) enzymes are grouped into six functional classes, each with 4-13 subclasses. The IUB system while complex is precise, descriptive, and informative. The enzyme name has two parts, the first part names the substrate or substrates; the second ending with -ase indicates the type of reaction catalyzed. Further each enzyme has a four-digit systemic code number assigned by enzyme commission (EC). The first digit characterizes the reaction type as to class, the second and third digit specifies the sub class, and sub-sub class, the fourth digit specifies the specific enzyme, e.g. E.C.2.7.1.1 denotes: a transferase, transfer of phosphate, an alcohol functions as the phosphate acceptor, the final digit denotes the enzyme Hexokinase (ATP: D-hexose-6-phosphotransferase) an enzyme catalyzing the transfer of phosphate from ATP to the hydroxyl group on carbon 6 of glucose. The six major classes of enzymes with their actions are shown below.

Enzymes are also Classified Based on Their Composition

Enzymes composed of only protein are known as **simple enzymes** in contrast to **complex enzymes**, which are composed of protein plus a relatively small organic molecule. Complex enzymes are also known as holoenzymes. In this terminology, the **protein component** is known as the **apoenzyme**. When the **non-protein component** is bound to apoenzyme by non-covalent interactions it is known as **coenzyme**, when it is bound covalently we call it a **prosthetic group**. Many prosthetic groups and coenzymes are water-soluble derivatives of vitamins. It should be remembered that the main clinical symptoms of dietary vitamin insufficiency generally arise from the malfunction of enzymes, which lack sufficient cofactors derived from vitamins to maintain homeostasis.

Enzymes that require a metal in their composition are known as **metalloenzymes**. Their metal atom(s) is bound under all conditions. Those enzymes, which have a lower affinity for metal ion, but still require them for activity, are known as **metal-activated enzymes**.

Functional Role of Coenzymes

Coenzymes act to carry chemical groups from one reactant to another. The chemical groups carried can be as simple as the hydride ion (H^+ + $2e^-$) carried by NAD or hydrogen carried by FAD, or they can be even more complex such as an amine ($-NH_2$) carried by pyridoxal phosphate.

Since coenzymes are chemically changed as a consequence of enzyme action, they are often considered as special class of substrates, or **second substrates**. In all cases, the coenzymes donate the chemical group they carried, to an acceptor molecule and are thus regenerated to their original form. This regeneration of coenzyme and holoenzyme fulfills the definition of an enzyme as a chemical catalyst.

Enzyme Reaction Relative to Substrate Type

Although the type of reaction catalyzed by a given enzyme is highly specific, the same is not always true of substrates they act on. For example, succinic dehydrogenase (SDH) always catalyzes an oxidation-reduction **reaction** and its substrate is invariably succinic acid. Whereas the enzyme **alcohol dehydrogenase** (ADH) that catalyzes **oxidation-reduction reactions** can act on a number of **different substrates**, ranging from methanol to butanol, but is most active against ethanol.

Enzymes are generally specific for a particular steric configuration (optical isomer) of a substrate. Enzymes that attack D-sugars will not attack the corresponding L-isomer. Enzymes that act on L-amino acids will not act on the corresponding D-optical isomer. The striking exception to these generalities is racemases, whose function is to convert D-isomers to L-isomers and vice versa.

As enzymes have a more or less broad range of substrate specificity, it follows that a given substrate may be acted on by a number of different enzymes, each of which uses the same substrate(s) and produces the same product(s). The individual members of a set of enzymes sharing such characteristics are known as **isozymes**. These are the products of genes that differ only slightly; often, various isozymes of a group are expressed in different tissues of the body. The best-studied set of isozymes is the lactate dehydrogenase (LDH) system. LDH is a tetrameric enzyme composed of all possible arrangements of two different protein subunits; the subunits are known as H (for heart) and M (for skeletal muscle). These subunits combine in various combinations leading to 5 distinct isozymes. The all H (H4) isozymes are typically found in heart muscle, and the all-M (M4) isozymes are typically found in skeletal muscle and liver. Both these isozymes catalyze the same chemical reaction, but they exhibit differing degrees of efficiency. The detection of specific LDH isozymes in the blood is highly diagnostic of tissue damage such as the one that occurs during cardiac infarct.

RATE OF CHEMICAL REACTIONS

The rate of a chemical reaction is described by the number of molecules of reactant(s) that are converted into product(s) in a specified period of time. Reaction rate is always dependent on the enzyme and substrate concentrations involved in the process, and on rate constants that are characteristic of the reaction. For example, the reaction in which A is converted to B is written as follows:

A ⟶ B   **Eqn. 1**

The rate of this reaction is expressed algebraically as either a decrease in the concentration of reactant A: $-[A] = k[B]$ **Eqn. 2**

Or an increase in the concentration of product B: $[B] = k[A]$
Eqn. 3

In the second equation (of the three above), the negative sign signifies a decrease in concentration of A as the reaction progresses, brackets define molar concentration, and the k is known as a rate constant.

Rate constants are simply proportionality constants that provide a quantitative relationship between chemical concentrations and reaction rates. Each chemical reaction has characteristic values for its rate constants; this in turn is directly related to the **equilibrium constant** for that reaction. Thus, reaction can be rewritten as an equilibrium expression in order to show the relationship between reaction rates, rate constants and the equilibrium constant for this simple case.

The rate constant for the forward reaction is defined as k_{+1} and the reverse as k_{-1}.

At equilibrium the rate/velocity (v) of the forward reaction $(A \rightarrow B)$ is by definition equal to that of the reverse or back reaction $(B \rightarrow A)$, a relationship which is algebraically symbolized as: $v_{forward} = v_{reverse}$

Where, for the forward reaction: $v_{forward} = k_{+1}[A]$

and for the reverse reaction: $v_{reverse} = k_{-1}[B]$

In the above equations, k_{+1} and k_{-1} represent rate constants for the forward and reverse reactions, respectively. The negative subscript refers only to a reverse reaction, not to an actual negative value for the constant. To put the relationships of the two equations into words, we state that the rate of the forward reaction $[v_{forward}]$ is equal to the product of the forward rate constant k_{+1} and the molar concentration of A. The rate of the reverse reaction is equal to the product of the reverse rate constant k_{-1} and the molar concentration of B.

At equilibrium, the rate of the forward reaction is equal to the rate of the reverse reaction leading to the **equilibrium constant** of the reaction and is expressed by:

$[B]/[A] = k_{+1}/k_{-1} = K_{eq}$

This equation demonstrates that the equilibrium constant for a chemical reaction is not only equal to the equilibrium ratio of product and reactant concentrations, but is also equal to the ratio of the characteristic rate constants of the reaction.

CHEMICAL REACTION ORDER

Reaction order refers to the number of molecules involved in forming a reaction complex that can proceed to product(s). Empirically, order is easily determined by summing the exponents of each concentration term in the rate equation for a reaction. A reaction characterized by the conversion of one molecule of **A** to one molecule of **B** with no influence from any other reactant or solvent is a *first-order* reaction. The exponent on the substrate concentration in the rate equation for this type of reaction is **1**. A reaction with two substrates forming two products would be a **second-order** reaction. However, the reactants in second- and higher- order reactions need not be different chemical species. An example of a second order reaction is the formation of ATP through the condensation of ADP with orthophosphate:

$$ADP + H_2PO_4 \leftrightarrow ATP + H_2O$$

For this reaction the forward reaction rate would be written as:

$$v_{forward} = k_1[ADP][H_2PO_4]$$

EXPRESSION OF ENZYME KINETIC

In typical enzyme-catalyzed reactions, reactant and product concentrations are usually hundreds or thousands of times greater than the enzyme concentration. Consequently, each enzyme molecule catalyzes the conversion of many reactant molecules to product. In biochemical reactions, reactants are commonly known as substrates. The catalytic event that converts substrate to product involves the formation of a transition state, and it occurs most easily at a specific binding site on the enzyme. This site on the enzyme is called the **catalytic site**, which is evolutionarily structured to provide specific high-affinity binding of substrate (S), and to provide an environment that favors the catalytic events. The complex, that forms when substrate (S) and enzyme combine is called the **enzyme-substrate (ES) complex**. When the **ES** complex breaks down, the products and enzyme are released. Between the binding of substrate to enzyme, and the reappearance of free enzyme and product, a series of complex events must take place. These events are: an **ES** complex is formed; the complex passes through a transition state (**ES***), and the transition state complex advance to an enzyme product complex (**EP**), which finally dissociated to product and free enzyme.

The rate or velocity (v) of enzyme-catalyzed reaction depends on both enzyme concentration **[E]** and substrate concentration **[S]**.

The reaction rate plot versus substrate concentration of a typical enzyme-catalyzed reaction is usually hyperbolic (Fig. 18.1).

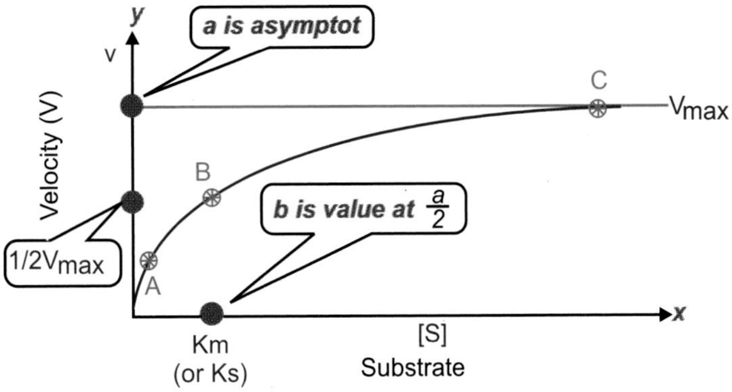

This plot is known as a ***saturation plot***, it means that when the enzyme becomes "saturated" with substrate (i.e. each active-site of enzyme molecule is associated with substrate molecule), the rate becomes independent of substrate concentration. The simplest scheme for an enzyme-catalyzed reaction is given in the following equation:

Fig. 18.1: Michaelis-Menten plot (saturation plot of enzyme catalyzed reaction)

$$E + S \underset{K1}{\overset{K1}{\rightleftharpoons}} ES \xrightarrow{K2} E + P$$

Where k1 and k-1 are the rates of association and disassociation of ES (enzyme substrate complex), and K2 is the turnover number or catalytic constant.

Usually an enzyme's velocity is measured under initial conditions of [S] and [P].

These same reactions can be described graphically:

At low [S], velocity (V) increases as [S] increases.

At high [S], enzymes become saturated with substrates, and the reaction is independent of [S]

Elevated [S] displays saturation kinetics. $\mathbf{V_{max} = k_2[ES]}$
Since [S] is irrelevant at high [S] the above equation can be rewritten as $\mathbf{V_{max} = K_2[E]}$
The above saturation plot is a graph of a hyperbola, and the equation for a hyperbola is

$$Y = \frac{ax}{b+x}$$ Where a is the asymptote and b is value $\frac{a}{2}$

Substituting our equation parameters,

$$V = \frac{Vmax\,[S]}{Km + [S]}$$ Is transformed to Michaells-Menten equation

Different enzymes reach V_{max} at different [S] because enzymes differ in their affinity for the substrate or K_m.
1. If the tendency for a pair of enzyme and substrate to form an ES complex is greater, the enzyme's affinity for the substrate is greater or the K_m is low.
2. An enzyme with a higher affinity form more ES at a given substrate concentration [S], i.e. the greater the affinity, the lower the [S] needed to saturate the enzyme or to reach maximal velocity (V_{max}).
Enzyme-substrate affinity and reaction kinetics are closely associated:

[S] at which V $=1/2V_{max} = K_m$

Michaelis-Menten constant (K_m) is the substrate concentration [S] at which the reaction rate (V) is half the maximal ($1/2\,V_{max}$).
K_m is a measure of enzyme affinity, meaning that the lower the K_m, the less substrate is needed to saturate the enzyme.

$$K_m = \frac{K_{-1}}{K_1}$$ reflection of association and dissociation of ES

a small K_m (high affinity) favors $E + S \longrightarrow ES$
a large K_m (low affinity) favors $ES \longrightarrow E + S$

We would like numerical values of V_{max} and K_m for a means of comparison among enzymes.
It is difficult to estimate V_{max} and K_m from a typical hyperbolic graph of [substrate] vs. velocity.
These two parameters are used to describe the efficiency of enzymes but there must be an easier method for estimating these parameters.
The Michaelis-Menten equation is a quantitative description of the relationship among the rate of an enzyme-catalyzed reaction [v], the concentration of substrate [S] and two constants, V_{max} and K_m (which are set by the particular equation). The symbols used in the Michaelis-Menton equation refer to the reaction rate [v], maximum reaction rate (V_{max}), substrate concentration [S] and the Michaelis-Menten constant (K_m). This equation demonstrates that the substrate concentration, which produces exactly half of the maximum reaction rate (**$1/2\,V_{max}$**) is numerically equal to K_m. This fact provides a simple yet powerful bioanalytical tool that has been used to characterize both normal and altered enzymes, such as those that produce the symptoms of genetic diseases.

Rearranging the Michaelis-Menten equation leads to: $[S]\{V_{max}/[v-1]\} = K_m$

From this equation it is clear that when the substrate concentration is half that required to support the maximum rate of reaction, the observed rate **v** will be equal to V_{max} divided by 2; in other words, **v** = $[V_{max}/2]$. At this substrate concentration V_{max}/v_1 will be exactly equal to 2, with the result that $[S](1) = K_m$

The latter is an algebraic statement of the fact that, for enzymes of the Michaelis-Menten type, when the observed reaction rate is half of the maximum possible reaction rate, the substrate concentration is numerically equal to the Michaelis-Menten constant. In this derivation, the units of K_m are those used to specify the substrate concentration, usually molarity. The Michaelis-Menten equation has the same form as the equation for a rectangular hyperbola; graphical analysis of reaction rate (v) versus substrate concentration [S] produces a hyperbolic rate plot.

The key features of Michaelis-Menten plot are marked by points **A, B** and **C** (Fig. 18.1). At high substrate concentrations the rate represented by point **C** is almost equal to V_{max}, and the difference in rate at nearby concentrations of substrate is almost negligible. If the Michaelis-Menten plot is extrapolated to infinitely high substrate concentrations, the extrapolated rate is equal to V_{max}. When the reaction rate becomes independent of substrate concentration, the rate is said to be zero order. If the reaction has two substrates, it may or may not be zero order with respect to the second substrate. The very small differences in reaction velocity at substrate concentrations around point **C** (near V_{max}) reflect that at these concentrations almost all of the enzyme molecules are bound to substrate and the rate is virtually independent of substrate, hence it is zero order. At lower substrate concentrations, such as at points **A** and **B**, indicate that at any moment only a portion of the enzyme molecules are bound to the substrate. In fact, at the substrate concentration denoted by point **B**, exactly half the enzyme molecules are in an ES complex at any instant and the rate is exactly one half of V_{max}. At substrate concentrations near point **A** the rate appears to be directly proportional to substrate concentration, and the reaction rate is said to be first order.

INHIBITION OF ENZYME CATALYZED REACTION

To avoid dealing with Michaelis-Menten curvilinear plots of enzyme catalyzed reactions, Lineweaver and Burk introduced an analysis of enzyme kinetics based on the following rearrangement of the Michaelis-Menten equation: done by transformation of the data by taking the reciprocal of both sides of the equation, popularly known as double reciprocal plot or Lineweaver-Burk plot (Fig. 18.2).

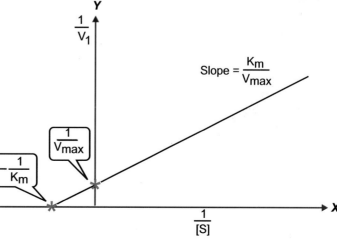

Fig. 18.2: Lineweaver-Burk plot

$$v = \frac{V_{max}\,[S]}{K_m + [S]} \quad OR \quad \frac{1}{V} = \left[\frac{K_m}{V_{max}}\right]\frac{1}{[S]} + \frac{1}{V_{max}}$$

Plots of $1/v$ versus $1/[S]$ yield straight lines having a slope of K_m/V_{max} and an intercept on the ordinate at $1/V_{max}$.

An alternative linear transformation of the Michaelis-Menten equation is the Eadie-Hofstee transformation (Fig.18. 3). When $v/[S]$ is plotted on the x-axis versus v on the y-axis, the result is a linear plot with a slope of $-1/K_m$ and the value V_{max}/K_m as the intercept on the y-axis (Fig. 18.3).

$$\frac{V}{[S]} = -V\left[\frac{1}{K_m}\right] + \left[\frac{V_{max}}{K_m}\right]$$

Both the Lineweaver-Burk and Eadie-Hofstee transformations of the Michaelis-Menten equation are useful in the analysis of enzyme inhibition. Since most clinical drug therapy is based on enzyme inhibition, analysis of enzyme reactions using the tools described is useful to the modern design of pharmaceuticals. Well known examples of such therapy include the use of methotrexate in cancer chemotherapy to semi-selectively inhibit DNA synthesis of malignant cells, the use of aspirin to inhibit the synthesis of prostaglandins which are at least partly responsible for the aches and pains of arthritis, the use of sulfa drugs to inhibit the folic acid synthesis that is essential for the metabolism and growth of disease-causing bacteria, and the use of trimethoprim that inhibit folate reductase and so the formation of tetrahydrofolate essential for growth and metabolism of pathogenic bacteria. In addition, many poisons such as cyanide, carbon monoxide and polychlorinated biphenols (PCBs) produce their life-threatening effects by enzyme inhibition.

Enzyme inhibitors fall into two broad classes: those causing irreversible inactivation of enzymes and those whose inhibitory effects can be reversed.

Irreversible inhibitors usually cause enzyme inactivation by covalent modification of enzyme structure. Cyanide is a classic example of an irreversible enzyme inhibitor, which covalently binds to Fe^{2+} of mitochondrial cytochrome oxidase and inhibits all the reactions associated with electron transport. The kinetic effect of irreversible inhibitors is to decrease the concentration of active enzyme, thus decreasing the maximum possible concentration of ES complex. Since the limiting enzyme reaction rate is often k_2 [ES], under these circumstances the reduction in enzyme concentration will lead to *decreased reaction rates* (V_{max}), but the turnover number and the K_m are not altered. **Turnover number,** related to V_{max}, is defined as the maximum number of moles of substrate that are converted to product per mole of catalytic site per second. Irreversible inhibitors are usually poisons and are unsuitable for therapeutic purposes.

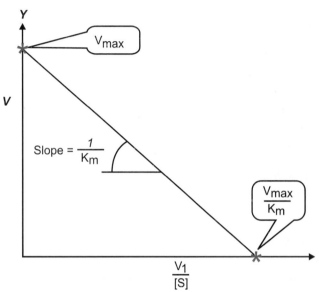

Fig. 18.3: Eadie-Hofstee plot

Reversible inhibitors can be divided into two main categories, **competitive inhibitors** and **noncompetitive inhibitors**, with a third category, **uncompetitive inhibitors**, rarely encountered.

Inhibitor type	Binding site on enzyme	Kinetic effect
Competitive Inhibitor	Normally at the catalytic site of E, where it competes with substrate for binding in a dynamic equilibrium-like process. Inhibition is reversible by substrate.	V_{max} is unchanged; K_m is increased.
Noncompetitive Inhibitor	Binds E or ES complex other than at the catalytic site. Substrate binding is unaltered, but ESI complex cannot form products. Inhibition cannot be reversed by substrate. K_m appears unaltered; V_{max} is decreased proportionately to inhibitor concentration.	K_m appears unaltered; V_{max} is decreased proportionately to inhibitor concentration
Uncompetitive Inhibitor	Uncompetitive inhibitor binds only to ES complexes at locations other than the catalytic site. Substrate binding modifies enzyme structure, making inhibitor-binding site available. Inhibition cannot be reversed by substrate.	Apparent V_{max} decreased; K_m is decreased.

The characteristic feature of all the reversible inhibitors is that when the inhibitor concentration drops, enzyme activity is regenerated. Usually these inhibitors bind to enzymes by non-covalent forces and the inhibitor maintains a reversible equilibrium with the enzyme. The equilibrium constant for the dissociation of enzyme inhibitor complexes is known as K_I: $K_I = [E][I]/[EI]$.

The importance of K_I is that in all enzyme reactions where substrate, inhibitor and enzyme interact, the normal K_m and/or V_{max} for substrate enzyme interaction appear to be altered. These changes are a consequence of the influence of K_I on the overall rate equation for the reaction.

Competitive Inhibition

The best-known reversible inhibitors are competitive inhibitors, which bind at the catalytic or active site of the enzyme. Majority of drugs that alter enzyme activity belong to this type. Competitive inhibitors are the best clinical modulators of enzyme activity, since they offer two routes for the reversal of enzyme inhibition. *First,* a decreasing concentration of the inhibitor reverses the equilibrium and regenerates the active free enzyme. *Second,* since both substrates and competitive inhibitors compete with each other for the same binding site, raising the concentration of substrate (S), while holding the concentration of inhibitor constant, reverses competitive inhibition.

The greater the proportion of substrate, the greater is the proportion of enzyme present in ES complexes. High concentrations

$$E + S \underset{}{\overset{K_s}{\rightleftharpoons}} ES \xrightarrow{K2} E + P$$
$$+$$
$$I$$
$$\downarrow K_1$$
$$EI$$

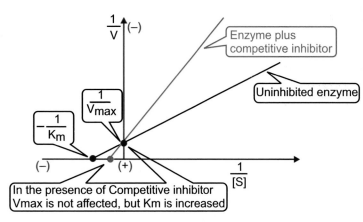

Fig. 18.4: Features of competitive inhibition

of substrate virtually displace all competitive inhibitor bound to active sites. Thus, V_{max} is *unchanged* by competitive inhibitors, but *increases the apparent* K_m *value.*

The effects of the inhibitor are best observed in Lineweaver-Burk plots (Fig. 18.4).

This characteristic of competitive inhibitors is reflected in the identical vertical-axis intercepts of Lineweaver-Burk plots, with and without inhibitor. Since attaining V_{max} requires appreciably higher substrate concentrations in the presence of competitive inhibitor, K_m (the substrate concentration at half maximal velocity) is also higher, as demonstrated by the differing negative intercepts on the horizontal axis (Fig. 18.4).

Noncompetitive Inhibition

From the definition of noncompetitive inhibitor the following equilibria can be written:

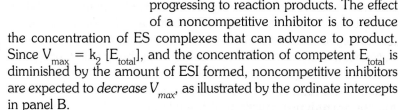

Analogously, the Fig. 18.5 illustrates that noncompetitive inhibitors appear to have no effect on the intercept of the negative abscissa implying that noncompetitive inhibitors have *no effect on* K_m *of the enzymes they inhibit.* Since noncompetitive inhibitors do not interfere in the binding of the substrate (the dissociation constant of ES and ESI have the same value Ks) the K_m's of Michaelis-Menten type enzymes are not expected to be affected by noncompetitive inhibitors, as demonstrated by the abscissa intercepts. However, increasing substrate concentration cannot abolish the inhibition, because more complexes that contain inhibitor (ESI) are formed and these are incapable of progressing to reaction products. The effect of a noncompetitive inhibitor is to reduce the concentration of ES complexes that can advance to product. Since $V_{max} = k_2 [E_{total}]$, and the concentration of competent E_{total} is diminished by the amount of ESI formed, noncompetitive inhibitors are expected to *decrease* V_{max}, as illustrated by the ordinate intercepts in panel B.

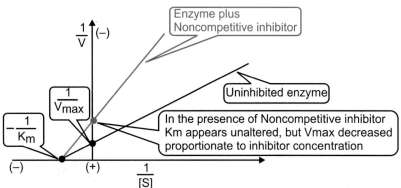

Fig. 18.5: Features of noncompetitive inhibition

Uncompetitive Inhibition

From the definition of uncompetitive inhibitor (an inhibitor which binds only to ES complexes) the following equilibria can be written:

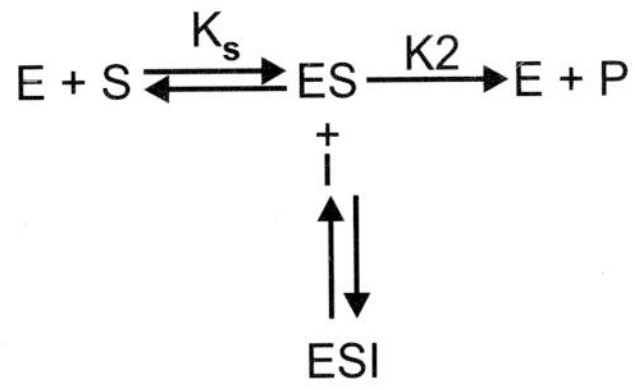

$$E + S \underset{}{\overset{K_s}{\rightleftharpoons}} ES \xrightarrow{K2} E + P$$

ESI

Uncompetitive Inhibition

From the definition of uncompetitive inhibitor (an inhibitor which binds only to ES complexes) the following equilibria can be written:

The ES complex dissociates the substrate with a dissociation constant equal to Ks, whereas the ESI complex does not dissociate it (i.e. it has a Ks value equal to zero). The K_m's of Michaelis Menten type enzymes, are expectedly reduced.

Increasing substrate concentration leads to increasing ESI concentration (a complex incapable of progressing to reaction products); therefore the inhibition cannot be removed. *Changing both* K_m *and* V_{max} leads to double reciprocal plots, in which intercepts on the vertical and horizontal axis are proportionately changed; this leads to the production of parallel lines in inhibited and uninhibited reactions (Fig. 18.6).

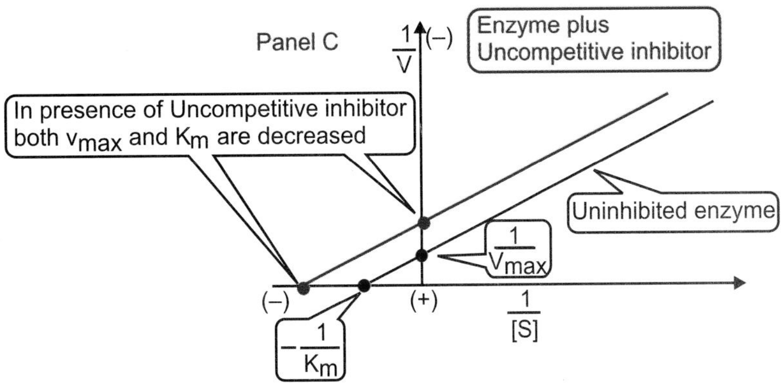

Panel C

In presence of Uncompetitive inhibitor both v_{max} and K_m are decreased

Enzyme plus Uncompetitive inhibitor

Uninhibited enzyme

$\frac{1}{V_{max}}$

$-\frac{1}{K_m}$

$\frac{1}{[S]}$

Fig. 18.6: Features of uncompetitive inhibition

ENZYMES ARE BIOLOGICAL CATALYSTS

Within cells, enzymes catalyze most reactions. Enzymes are regenerated during the course of a reaction. These enzymes are physiologically important because they speed up the rates of reactions that would otherwise be too slow to support life. Enzymes increase reaction rates by about one thousand folds, sometimes by as much as one million fold. Any catalyst speeds up the forward and reverse reactions proportionately so that, although the magnitude of the rate constants of the forward and reverse reactions are increased, the ratio of the rate constants remains the same in the presence or absence of enzyme.

Enzymes increase reaction rates by decreasing the amount of energy required (activation energy) to form a complex of reactants that is able to produce reaction products. This complex is known as the activated state or **transition state complex** for the reaction. Enzymes and other catalysts accelerate reactions by lowering the energy of the transition state. The free energy required to form an activated complex is much lower in the catalyzed reaction (Fig. 18.7). The amount of energy required to

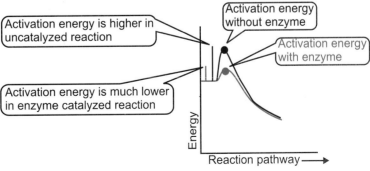

Fig. 18.7: Activation energy and catalyzed reaction

The favored model of enzyme-substrate interaction is known as the **induced fit model.** This model proposes that the initial interaction between enzyme and substrate is relatively weak, but these weak interactions rapidly induce conformational changes in the enzyme that strengthen binding and bring catalytic sites close to substrate bonds, to be altered. After binding takes place, one or more of the following mechanisms of catalysis generates transition—state complexes and reaction proceeds to form products.

COMMON FEATURES OF ENZYME ACTIVE SITES (CATALYTIC SITES)

Even though enzymes differ widely in structure, specificity, and mode of catalysis, their active sites share common features.

1. Active site takes up a relatively small part of the total volume of an enzyme.
2. Active site is a three-dimensional entity formed by specific amino acid residues.
3. Substrates are bound to enzymes by multiple weak interactions mediated by electrostatic bonds, hydrogen bonds, van der Waals forces, and hydrophobic interactions.
4. Active sites are mainly nonpolar clefts or crevices, from where water is excluded as a reactant. Some polar residues present at active site create a microenvironment, with special properties necessary for catalysis.
5. Specificity of binding depends on precisely defined arrangement of atoms at the active site as defined by:
   a. Emil Fischer's idea of lock-and-key (rigid model), and
   b. Induced fit model (flexible), which proposes that active sites assume shapes complementary to substrate only after substrate is bound.

FOUR POSSIBLE MECHANISMS OF ENZYME CATALYSIS

Catalysis by Bond Strain

The binding of substrate at the active site induces structural rearrangements and ultimately produces strained substrate bonds, which more easily attain the transition state. The new confirmation often forces substrate atoms and bulky catalytic groups, such as 'R' groups of aspartate and glutamate residues into conformations that strain existing substrate bonds.

Catalysis by Proximity and Orientation

Interactions between enzyme and substrate orient reactive groups and bring them into proximity with one another. In addition to inducing strain, chemically reactive groups such as 'R' groups of aspartate, and their proximity and orientation toward the substrate favors their participation in catalysis.

Other mechanisms such as general acid-base catalysis also contribute significantly to the completion of catalytic events initiated by strained substrate bonds, e.g. glutamate act as a general acid catalyst (proton donor).

Covalent Catalysis

The substrate is oriented to active sites on the enzymes in such a way that a covalent intermediate forms between the enzyme or coenzyme and the substrate. One of the best-known examples of this mechanism is that involving proteolysis by serine proteases, which include digestive enzymes (trypsin, chymotrypsin, and elastase) and several enzymes of the blood-clotting cascade. These proteases contain serine at active site whose 'R' group hydroxyl forms a covalent bond with a carbonyl carbon of a peptide bond, thereby causing hydrolytic cleavage of the peptide bond.

INFLUENCE OF pH AND TEMPERATURE ON ENZYME ACTIVITY

Enzymes are very sensitive to changes in temperature and pH. Enzyme activity increases with temperature up to about 45 degrees Centigrade. Enzyme activity falls rapidly above a critical temperature because the enzyme denatures (unfolds). Heat sterilization is based on this principle of denaturing bacteria enzymes.

Effect of pH

Enzymes have a pH optimum; if the pH is too low or too high the activity will fall, pH sensitivity is due to acidic and basic side groups of amino acids present at active site, which undergo protonation and deprotonation with change in pH. When enzyme activity is measured at several pH values, optimal activity is generally observed between pH values of 5.0 and 9.0. However, certain enzymes (e.g. pepsin) are active at pH values well outside this range. The shape of pH-activity curves is determined by the following factors:
1. Denaturation of enzymes at extremely high or low pH.
2. Effects on the charged state of the substrate or enzyme. The charge changes in the surrounding may affect enzyme activity either by changing structure or by changing the charge on a functional residue involved in substrate binding or catalysis. A change in pH can change the ionic state of the substrate as well. Optimal activity is possible, only when maximum number of substrates and enzymes are in the correctly charged state.

Enzymes are adapted to their pH environment and have optimal activity at certain pH. Cells, blood and saliva have pH close to 7, stomach has a pH of 1 to 2 during digestion, and lysosomes (cell organelles) have pH about 4.5. The hydrolytic enzymes are adapted to the pH of their environment (Fig. 18.8).

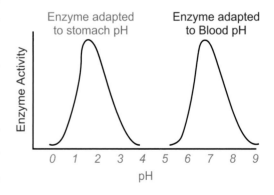

Fig. 18.8: Enzyme adapted to different pH

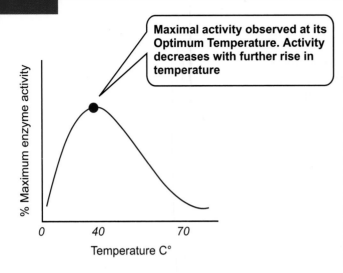

Fig. 18.9: Effect of temperature on enzyme activity

The graph (Fig. 18.8) shows the activities of two different enzymes, one adapted to work in the stomach and the other adapted to work in the blood.

Effect of Temperature

As temperature rises, the velocity of enzyme-catalyzed reactions increases over a limited range of temperature (Fig. 18.9). The velocity of many biological reactions roughly doubles with a 10°C rise in temperature, and is halved if temperature is decreased by 10°C. When enzyme-catalyzed reactions are measured at several temperatures, there is an optimal temperature at which the reaction is maximal. Above this, the reaction drops sharply, mainly due to denaturation of protein enzyme by heat. Changes in temperature also affect the state of ionization of both enzyme and substrate.

ENZYME ACTIVITY IS ALSO INFLUENCED BY THE CONCENTRATION OF ENZYME, SUBSTRATE AND PRODUCT

When velocity of enzyme-catalyzed reaction is assayed with increasing concentration of substrate (holding the temperature and pH constant), the velocity increases in the initial phase; but the curve flattens latter. This phenomenon is explained by the fact; in the initial stage by increasing the amount of substrate, more and more catalytic sites on the enzyme are occupied and the velocity increases. But once all the catalytic sites are saturated with substrate, there is no further rise in velocity with an increase in substrate concentration.

Velocity of enzyme-catalyzed reaction increases proportional to enzyme concentration, provided the substrate concentration is unlimited. This property of enzyme kinetics is made use of in quantitating enzymes in biological samples. A known volume of biological sample is incubated with substrate for a fixed time, then reaction is stopped and product is quantitated. The product formed is proportional to enzyme concentration when all other parameters are held constant.

When enzyme catalyzed reactions are allowed to continue, a point is reached where the concentration of product equals concentration of substrate-equilibrium is reached. At a state of equilibrium, the reaction slows down, stops, or even reversed as per law of mass reaction. In inborn errors of metabolism, the deficiency or absence of one enzyme of a metabolic pathway can block the whole pathway, because of the accumulation of an intermediate of the pathway.

REGULATION OF ENZYME ACTIVITY

Enzymatic activity is regulated in three principal ways:
1. Allosteric control (stimulation and inhibition by control proteins)
2. Reversible covalent modification and
3. Proteolytic activation.

Allosteric Control

The enzyme *aspartate transcarbamolyase* involved in pyrimidine (thymine and cytosine) biosynthesis catalyzes the synthesis of N-carbamoylaspartate. It is feedback inhibited by cytidine triphosphate (CTP), which is the final product of the pathway. CTP works by decreasing ATCase affinity for substrates without affecting V_{max}. Extent of inhibition is substrate-dependent. ATP is an activator of ATCase, which enhances ATCase affinity for substrate, but leaves V_{max} unaffected. ATP and CTP compete with each other for binding to allosteric site on ATCase.

High levels of ATP prevent CTP from inhibiting enzyme. The purpose of this regulation is two fold:
1. Activation by ATP signals that energy is available for DNA replication and synthesis of needed pyrimidine nucleotides
2. Feedback inhibition by CTP assures that N-carbamoylaspartate and intermediates are not needlessly formed when pyrimidines are abundant.

$$A+B \rightarrow C \overset{E1}{\rightarrow} D \rightarrow E \rightarrow F \rightarrow P \quad \text{Feedback inhibition}$$
$$\searrow$$
$$G \rightarrow H$$

ATCase consists of six subunits, three catalytic and three regulatory subunits. Regulatory subunit can bind CTP or ATP; catalytic subunits bind substrate. Enzyme has one of catalytic trimers lying above and the other two subunits lying below an equatorial belt of three regulatory subunits. Enzyme contains a large central cavity, which displays a threefold axis of symmetry. When ATCase binds the substrate, the enzyme expands in size, due to changes in the quaternary structure of the enzyme. The active site of the enzyme is at the interface among catalytic subunits.

Reversible Covalent Modification

Phosphorylation of enzymes catalyzed by *protein kinases* is the most common reversible covalent modification. Substrates include other enzymes, membrane channels, and other target proteins. Transfer of terminal phosphate of ATP to serine or threonine residues of enzymes is carried out by one type of protein kinase and transfer to tyrosine residues is carried out by another type of protein kinase. The effects are reversed by *protein phosphatases*, which hydrolyze phosphoryl group attached to target protein. Because hydrolysis of ATP to ADP and Pi has such a large -G, this is essentially irreversible under physiological conditions. The target proteins cycle between phosphorylated and unphosphorylated forms depending upon activities of protein kinases and protein phosphatases. Phosphorylation is an effective means for regulating protein activity because:
1. A phosphoryl group adds two negative charges to modified protein and allows for disruption of electrostatic interactions in unphosphorylated protein so that new ones can be formed.
2. A phosphoryl group can form three hydrogen bonds.
3. Can change equilibrium between different functional states of a protein.

4. Phosphorylation and dephosphorylation can occur in less than one second or over several hours, which can be adjusted to meet physiological needs in the cell.

5. Phosphorylation evokes highly amplified effects; a single activated protein kinase can result in phosphorylation of several hundred target-proteins in a short time period.

Proteolytic Cleavage

Many enzymes are synthesized as zymogens and are subsequently cleaved to form active molecule. Proteolytic cleavage can only occur once in the "life" of a protein, not repeatedly as is the case for allosteric control and reversible covalent modification. Activation of enymes by proteolysis occurs in the following cases:

1. Digestive enzymes—synthesized as zymogens in stomach and pancreas cells
2. Blood clotting—mediated by cascade of proteolytic activations
3. Some protein hormones are synthesized as inactive precursors
4. Collagen is derived for procollagen
5. Developmental processes are controlled by activation of zymogens. Chymotrypsin is a digestive enzyme that hydrolyzes proteins in the small intestine; its inactive precursor is called chymotrypsinogen, synthesized in acinar cells of pancreas and stored inside membrane-bounded vesicles. When a hormonal signal or nerve impulse reaches acinar cell, contents of vesicles are released into duct leading into duodenum. Chymotrypsinogen consists of 245 amino acids; cleaved into active enzyme when peptide bond between Arg-15 and Ile-16 is cleaved by trypsin to form α-chymotrypsin. Two dipeptides are removed from α-chymotrypsin (a. a. 14 and 15 and a. a. 147 and 148) to produce α-chymotrypsin. α-chymotrypsin is composed of three subunits (A,B,C) held together by disulfide bonds between A and B and between B and C.

How does Cleavage of a Single Peptide Bond Activate the Zymogen?

1. Newly formed amino-terminal group of isoleucine 16 turns inward and interacts with aspartate 194 in interior of molecule; protonation of amino group stabilizes active site of chymotrypsin.
2. Methionine 192 moves from being deeply buried to the surface and residues 187 and 193 are more extended, the formation of substrate specificity site for aromatic and bulky nonpolar groups; one side of site is formed by a. a. 189-192, which is not fully formed in zymogen.
3. Tetrahedral transition state normally stabilized in active molecule cannot be formed because NH group is not located in right place in zymogen.

Pancreatic Trypsin Inhibitor (PTI)

Pancreatic trypsin inhibitor stops proteolysis because cleavage of peptide bond permanently activates enzyme. There are specific protease inhibitors that stop proteolysis. PTI inhibits trypsin by binding very tightly to active site (binding of Lys 15 of inhibitor to Asp 189 at specificity pocket of enzyme and hydrogen bonds between inhibitor and enzyme). PTI has very high affinity for trypsin because its structure is almost perfectly complementary to that of active site of trypsin.

α1-antitrypsin is a protein that protects tissues from digestion by the enzyme elastase, which is secreted by neutrophils; it works by binding nearly irreversibly to active site of elastase. In individuals with genetic disorder of antitrypsin deficiency, excess elastase destroys alveolar walls of lungs by digesting elastic fibre and other connective tissue proteins, resulting in emphysema (destructive lung disease). Cigarette smoking increases likelihood that a heterozygote will develop emphysema, since smoke oxidizes methionine 358 in α1-antitrypsin leading to unchecked activity of elastase.

PLASMA ENZYMES IN CLINICAL PRACTICE

Certain enzymes occur predominantly in cells of certain tissues, where they may be located in different cell organelles. Normal levels of plasma enzymes reflect the balance between the rate of synthesis and release into plasma during cell turnover, and the rate of clearance from the circulation. Elevated levels of enzymes in plasma is a reflection of its reduced clearance or increased proliferation of cells, increased rate of cell turnover, increased cell damage or increased rate of enzyme synthesis (induction of microsomal enzymes by certain drugs). Decreased levels of enzymes activity in plasma is very rare, it could be either due to reduced synthesis, or to congenital deficiency or due to presence of inherited variants of relatively low biological activity, e.g. cholinesterase variants.

Transaminases

Transaminases are widely distributed in the body, which need pyridoxal phosphate as cofactor, and are involved in transfer of an amino group from an α-amino to an α-keto acid.

Aspartate transaminase (AST)/glutamate oxaloacetate transaminase (GOT) is found in high concentration in heart, liver, skeletal muscle, kidneys and erythrocytes. Damage to any of these tissues results in elevated level of plasma AST.

Normal range of plasma AST is 8-20 IU/L.

Causes of elevated plasma AST are: *in vitro* hemolysis, neonatal period (about 1.5 times more than adult values), hypoxia, myocardial infarction, and viral or toxic hepatitis (about 10 to 100 times the upper limit of adult values). Moderately elevated in skeletal muscle diseases, severe hemolytic anemia, cholestatic jaundice, and malignant infiltration.

Alanine transaminase (ALT)/glutamate pyruvate transaminase (GPT) is present in high concentration in liver, and to a lesser extent in skeletal muscle, kidney and heart.

Normal range of plasma ALT is 10-40 IU/L.

Causes of elevated plasma ALT are: *in vitro* hemolysis or delayed separation of plasma from whole blood. Moderately elevated in viral hepatitis, pulmonary embolism, and malignancy. Grossly elevated in shock and circulatory failure, myocardial infarction, muscular dystrophies, and skeletal muscle damage.

Lactate dehydrogenase (LDH) catalyses reversible interconversion of lactate and pyruvate. The enzyme is widely distributed in the body, with high concentrations found in heart, skeletal muscle, liver, kidney, brain and erythrocytes, therefore measurement of plasma LDH as a specific-marker of cardiac muscle damage is not advisable.

The normal range of total LDH in plasma is 100-200 IU/L.

LDH is composed of four protein subunits (H and M types); hence it can exist in five isoenzyme forms. LDH1 (4H), LDH2 (3H and 1M), LDH3 (2H and 2M), LDH4 (1H and 3M), and LDH5 (4M).

Causes of LDH elevation in plasma are: in myocardial infarction LDH1 and LDH2 are predominantly elevated, in malignancy and acute leukemia LDH2 and LDH3 are predominantly elevated, in skeletal muscle and liver damage LDH5 is predominantly elevated.

Creatine phosphokinase (CK/CPK) activity in plasma is elevated in all types of muscular dystrophy (usually with the exception of neurogenic muscle diseases), and myocardial infarction.

Normal range of plasma total CK is 10-100 U/L.

CK is composed of two protein subunits, M and B that combine to form three isoenzymes, BB (CK-1), MB (CK-2), and MM (CK-3). The predominant isoenzyme in skeletal muscle and heart is CK-MM and is detectable in plasma of normal individuals. In the heart muscles, about 35 percent of total CK is CK-MB and about 5 percent is CK-MM. Brain and smooth muscles have high concentration of CK-BB fraction.

CK-MB fraction is elevated in myocardial infarctions, whereas CK-MM is elevated in muscular dystrophies.

α-amylase is the enzyme that breaks down starch and glycogen to maltose. This enzyme is found in high concentrations in pancreas and salivary glands, other tissues having appreciable quantities of amylase are, fallopian tubes, gonads and skeletal muscles. Most of the amylase found in plasma is contributed from pancreas and salivary glands, since they are of low molecular weight they are excreted in the urine.

The normal range of amylase in plasma is 80-180 somogyi U/dl (50-20 IU/L).

Causes of elevated plasma amylase activity are: acute pancreatitis, parotitis, severe diabetes ketoacidosis, perforated pancreatic ulcer, severe glomerular impairment, and macroamylasemia.

Alkaline phosphatases (ALP) are a group of enzymes that hydrolyze phosphates at alkaline pH. They are found in high concentrations in osteoblasts of bone, hepatobiliary tract, intestinal wall, placenta and renal tubules. Most of the plasma ALP is derived from bone and liver. The normal range of plasma ALP is 40-125 IU/L.

Causes of elevated plasma ALP are: increased osteoblastic activity, preterm infants (upto five times the adult value), pubertal growth, pregnancy (last trimester), osteomalacia and rickets, secondary deposits of malignancy in bone, cholestasis in the liver diseases.

Acid phosphatase is found in prostate, liver, erythrocytes, bone and placenta. Indications for estimation of acid phosphatase are in the diagnosis of prostatic cancer and monitoring the treatment. It has two important isoenzymes tartarate labile and tartarate resistant.

Normal range of plasma acid phosphatase is less than 1 IU/L.

Causes of elevated plasma acid phosphatase are: tartarate labile isoenzyme in plasma is elevated in prostatic cancer, acute retention of urine and following rectal examination. Total acid phosphatase in plasma is elevated in hemolysed specimens, Paget's disease, and metastatic bone diseases.

γ-glutamyltransferase (GGT) occurs mainly in the liver, kidney, prostate and pancreas. Plasma GGT values are higher in men than women.

Normal range of plasma GGT value is 10-30 IU/L.

Causes of raised plasma GGT activity are: induction of enzymes by drugs such as phenytoin, phenobarbitone and alcohol, hepatocellular damage, and cholestatic liver disease.

Hormones and Receptors

19

Hormones are Blood Borne Chemical Messengers Secreted by Endocrine Glands

Hormones by definition are chemical agents produced by ductless organs, and transported to all parts of the body through blood. Only those organs having specific receptors respond to the hormone, and their secretion is controlled by feedback loops. They are involved in homeostasis and adaptation, and are rapidly destroyed so that new message can be sent.

Cytokines are Hormone-like Proteins that Act Locally

Cytokines are small proteins that act on same cell that produces them (autocrine) or on nearby cells (paracrine), rarely do they enter the blood or transported to distant parts of the body. They are mainly involved in defense of the body (many are produced by white blood cells). Examples are nerve growth factor, tumor necrosis factor, vascular endothelial growth factor (VEGF) involved in angiogenesis (production of new capillaries), and interleukins. Insulin-like growth factor-I (IGF-I), prolactin, and growth hormone behaves both as endocrine, and cytokine (paracrine, and autocrine).

Many Hormones Control the Activity of Other Endocrine Glands

Tropic hormones of the anterior pituitary (ACTH, TSH, FSH. LH) control many endocrine glands. There are many other interactions between endocrine glands such as epinephrine increases the secretion of glucagons.

Several Hormones are Involved in Control of Water, Salt, and Osmotic Pressure

Blood pressure, activity of nerves and muscles, and other physiological functions depend upon close regulation of salt and water in the body.

ADH (antidiuretic hormone) causes water retention by inserting water pores (aquaporines) in the collecting duct of the kidney. ADH secretion is increased in response to elevated blood osmotic pressure.

Aldosterone increases sodium reabsorption in the renal tubules. Aldosterone secretion is increased (this involves two more hormones, renin and angiotensin) when the blood volume falls.

Many Hormones Regulate Reproductive Functions

Growth of the ovaries and testes and secretion of sex hormones is controlled by FSH and LH. Oxytocin causes contraction of uterine muscles, aiding in delivery, milk ejection when the baby suckles is also caused by oxytocin. Milk production involves many hormones, including prolactin.

Hormones Control Metabolism and Growth

Thyroid hormone is extremely important in growth and increases the metabolic rate of many tissues. Growth hormone is the major hormone, which supports body growth. Some of its effects are due to secondary hormones, called somatomedins produced in the liver. Deficiency of either growth hormone or thyroid hormone during development will produce dwarfism. Gigantism in children and acromegaly in adults are the result of elevated production of growth hormone. Several hormones such as glucagon, epinephrine, cortisol, and growth hormone aid metabolism by raising blood glucose, whereas insulin lowers blood glucose. Erythropoietin supports metabolism by regulating the number of red cells in the blood.

Hormones Help the Body Respond to Stress

The immediate response to stress is the fight or flight reaction, which has both nervous and hormonal components, the hormonal component is the release of large amounts of epinephrine by the adrenal medulla; this hormone stimulates the heart, lungs and other organs involved in the emergency response. Long-term stress will cause release of large amounts of cortisol from the adrenal cortex that elevates blood glucose level. *Deleterious effects of prolonged stress are increased blood pressure and inhibition of the immune system.*

STRUCTURE AND FUNCTION OF HORMONES

Hormones secreted by endocrine tissues generally bind to a specific carrier protein in the blood, and is transported to distant tissues. Carrier proteins for peptide hormones prevent hormone destruction by plasma proteases. Carriers for steroid and thyroid hormones allow transportation of these hydrophobic substances in the aqueous plasma. Carriers for small hydrophilic *amino acid-derived hormones*, prevent their filtration through the renal glomeruli.

Tissues capable of responding to endocrines have two properties in common: they posses' receptors that have high affinity for hormone, and the receptor is coupled to intracellular events that regulates metabolism of the target cells. Receptors for most amino acid-derived hormones and all peptide hormones are located on the plasma membrane. Activation of these receptors by hormones leads to the intracellular production of a **second messenger**, such as cAMP, which is responsible for initiating a sequence of intracellular biochemical events. Steroid and thyroid hormones being hydrophobic diffuse across the plasma membrane and bind to intracellular receptors. The resultant complex of steroid and receptor is translocated into the nucleus, where it binds to a *hormone response elements* on nuclear DNA, and regulates the production of mRNA for specific proteins.

Metabolic Responses to a Rise in cAMP

Tissue	Inducing hormone	Metabolic response
Adipose	Epinephrine; ACTH; Glucagon	Increase in triglyceride hydrolysis decrease in amino acid uptake
Liver	Epinephrine; Norepinephrine; Glucagon	Increase in conversion of glycogen to glucose inhibition of synthesis of glycogen increase in amino acid uptake increase in gluconeogenesis
Follicle	FSH; LH	Increase in synthesis of estrogen, progesterone
Adrenal cortex	ACTH	Increase in synthesis of aldosterone, cortisol
Cardiac muscle	Epinephrine	Increase in contraction rate
Thyroid	TSH	Secretion of thyroxin
Bone cells	Parathyroid hormone	Increase in resorption of calcium from bone
Skeletal muscle	Epinephrine	Conversion of glycogen to glucose
Intestine	Epinephrine	**Fluid secretion**
Kidney	Vasopressin	Reabsorption of water
Blood platelets	Prostaglandin I	inhibition of aggregation and secretion

Common Vertebrate Hormones

Pituitary Hormones

Hormone	Structure	Functions
Oxytocin	polypeptide of 9 amino acids **CYIQNCPLG** (C's are disulfide bonded)	Uterine contraction, causes milk ejection in lactating females, responds to suckling reflex and estradiol, lowers steroid synthesis in testes
Vasopressin (antidiuretic hormone, ADH)	Polypeptide of 9 amino acids **CYFQNCPRG** (C's are disulfide bonded)	Responds to osmoreceptor which senses extracellular [Na$^+$], blood pressure regulation, increases H$_2$O reabsorption from distal tubules in kidney

Melanocyte-stimulating hormones (MSH)	α polypeptide = 13 amino acids β polypeptide = 18 amino acids γ polypeptide = 12 amino acids	Pigmentation
Corticotropin (adrenocorticotropin, ACTH)	Polypeptide = 39 amino acids	Stimulates cells of adrenal gland to increase steroid synthesis and secretion
Lipotropin (LPH)	β polypeptide = 93 amino acids γ polypeptide = 60 amino acids	Increases fatty acid release from adipocytes
Thyrotropin (thyroid-stimulating hormone, TSH)	2 proteins: α is 96 amino acids; β is 112	Acts on thyroid follicle cells to stimulate thyroid hormone synthesis
Growth hormone (GH, or somatotropin)	Protein of 191 amino acids	General anabolic stimulant, increases release of insulin-like growth factor-I (IGF-I), cell growth and bone sulfation
Prolactin (PRL)	Protein of 197 amino acids	Stimulates differentiation of secretory cells of mammary gland and stimulates milk synthesis
Luteinizing hormone (LH); human chorionic gonadotropin (hCG) is similar and produced in placenta	2 proteins: α is 96 amino acids; β is 121	Increases ovarian progesterone synthesis, luteinization; acts on Leydig cells of testes to increase testosterone synthesis and release and increase interstitial cell development
Follicle-stimulating hormone (FSH)	2 proteins: α is 96 amino acids; β is 120	Ovarian follicle development and ovulation, increases estrogen production; acts on Sertoli cells of semeniferous tubule to increase spermatogenesis

Hypothalamic Hormones

Hormone	Structure	Functions
Corticotropin-releasing factor (CRF or CRH)	Protein of 41 amino acids	Acts on corticotrope to release ACTH and β-endorphin (lipotropin)
Gonadotropin-releasing factor (GnRF or GnRH)	Polypeptide of 10 amino acids	Acts on gonadotrope to release LH and FSH
Prolactin-releasing factor (PRF)	This may be TRH	Acts on lactotrope to release prolactin
Prolactin-release inhibiting factor (PIF)	May be derived from GnRH precursor, 56 amino acids	Acts on lactotrope to inhibit prolactin release
Growth hormone-releasing factor (GRF or GRH)	Protein of 40 and 44 amino acids	Stimulates GH secretion
Somatostatin (SIF, also called growth hormone-release inhibiting factor, GIF)	Polypeptide of 14 and 28 amino acids	Inhibits GH and TSH secretion
Thyrotropin-releasing factor (TRH or TRF)	Polypeptide of 3 amino acids: Glutamyl-Histidyl-Proline	Stimulates TSH and prolactin secretion

Thyroid Hormones

Hormone	Structure	Functions
Thyroxin and triiodothyronine	Iodinated di-tyrosin derivatives	Responds to TSH and stimulates oxidations in many cells
Calcitonin	Protein of 32 amino acids	Produced in parafollicular C cells of the thyroid, regulation of Ca^{2+} and P_i metabolism
Calcitonin gene-related peptide (CGRP)	Protein of 37 amino acids, product of the calcitonin gene derived by alternative splicing of the precursor mRNA in the brain	Acts as a vasodilator

Parathyroid Hormone

Hormone	Structure	Functions
Parathyroid hormone (PTH)	Protein of 84 amino acids	Regulation of Ca^{2+} and P_i metabolism, stimulates bone resorption thus increasing serum $[Ca^{2+}]$, stimulates P_i secretion by kidneys

Gastrointestinal Hormones

Hormone	Structure	Functions
Gastrin	Polypeptide of 17 amino acids	Produced by stomach antrum, stimulates acid and pepsin secretion, also stimulates pancreatic secretions
Secretin	Polypeptide of 27 amino acids	Secreted from duodenum at pH values below 4.5, stimulates pancreatic acinar cells to release bicarbonate and H_2O
Cholecystokinin (CCK)	Polypeptide of 33 amino acids	Stimulates gallbladder contraction and bile flow, increases secretion of digestive enzymes from pancreas
Motilin	Polypeptide of 22 amino acids	Controls gastrointestinal muscles
Vasoactive intestinal peptide (VIP)	Polypeptide of 28 residues	Produced by hypothalamus and GI tract, relaxes the GI, inhibits acid and pepsin secretion, acts as a neurotransmitter in peripheral autonomic nervous system, increases secretion of H_2O and electrolytes from pancreas and gut
Gastric inhibitory peptide (GIP)	Polypeptide of 43 amino acids	Inhibits secretion of gastrin
Somatostain	14 amino acid version	Inhibits gastrin secretion from stomach and glucagon secretion from pancreas

Pancreatic Hormones

Hormone	Structure	Functions
Insulin	Disulfide bonded dipeptide of 21 and 30 amino acids	Produced by β-cells of the pancreas, increases glucose uptake and utilization, increases lipogenesis, general anabolic effects
Glucagon	Polypeptide of 29 amino acids	Produced by α-cells of the pancreas, increases lipid mobilization and glycogenolysis in order to increase blood glucose levels
Pancreatic polypeptide	Polypeptide of 36 amino acids	Increases glycogenolysis, regulation of gastrointestinal activity
Somatostatin	14 amino acid version	Inhibition of glucagon and somatotropin release

Placental Hormones

Hormone	Structure	Functions
Estrogens	Steroids	Maintenance of pregnancy
Progestins	Steroids	Mimic action of progesterone
Chorionic gonadotropin	2 proteins: α is 96 amino acids; β is 147	Activity similar to LH
Placental lactogen	Protein of 191 amino acids	Acts like prolactin and GH
Relaxin	2 proteins of 22 and 32 amino acids	Produced in ovarian corpus luteum, inhibits myometrial contractions, secretion increases during gestation

Gonadal Hormones

Hormone	Structure	Functions
Estrogens (ovarian)	Steroids; estradiol and estrone	Maturation and function of female secondary sex organs
Progestins (ovarian)	Steroid; progesterone	Implantation of ovum and maintenance of pregnancy
Androgens (testicular)	Steroid; testosterone	Maturation and function of male secondary sex organs
Inhibins A and B	1 protein (α is 134 amino acids; β is 115 and 116 amino acids	Inhibition of FSH secretion

Adrenocortical Hormones

Hormone	Structure	Functions
Glucocorticoids	Steroids; cortisol and corticosterone	Diverse effects on inflammation and protein synthesis
Mineralocorticoids	Steroids; aldosterone	Maintenance of salt balance

Adrenomedullary Hormones

Hormone	Structure	Functions
Epinephrine (adrenalin)	Derived from tyrosine	Glycogenolysis, lipid mobilization, smooth muscle contraction, cardiac function
Norepinephrine (noradrenalin)	Tyrosine derivative	Lipid mobilization, arteriole contraction

Liver Hormones

Hormone	Structure	Functions
Angiotensin	Polypeptide of 8 amino acids derived from α_2-globin which is cleaved by the kidney enzyme **renin** to give the decapeptide, pro-angiotensin, the C-terminal 2 amino acids are then released to yield angiotensin	Responsible for essential hypertension through stimulated synthesis and release of aldosterone from adrenal cells

Kidney Hormone

Hormone	Structure	Functions
Calcitriol [1,25-$(OH)_2$-vitamin D_3]	Derived from 7-dehydrocholesterol	Responsible for maintenance of calcium and phosphorus homeostasis, increases intestinal Ca^{2+} uptake, regulates bone mineralization

Cardiac Hormone

Hormone	Structure	Functions
Atrial natriuretic	Several active peptides cleaved from a 126 amino acid precursor	Released from heart atria in response to hypovolemia, acts on outer adrenal cells to decrease aldosterone production; smooth muscle relaxation peptide (ANP)

Pineal Hormone

Hormone	Structure	Functions
Melatonin	N-acetyl-5-methoxytryptamine	Regulation of cardiac rhythms

RECEPTORS FOR PEPTIDE HORMONES

The receptors for amino acid-derived, and peptide hormones (with the exception of the thyroid hormone receptor), are located in the plasma membrane. Structure of receptors is varied:

i. Some receptors consist of a single polypeptide chain with a domain on either side of the membrane connected by a membrane-spanning domain.

ii. Some receptors are comprised of a single polypeptide chain that is passed back and forth in serpentine fashion across the membrane giving multiple intracellular, transmembrane, and extracellular domains.

iii. Other receptors are composed of multiple polypeptides. For example, the insulin receptor is a disulfide-linked tetramer with the β-subunits spanning the membrane and the α-subunits located on the exterior surface.

When the hormone molecule binds to the receptor on the outside of the cell, a signal is transduced to the interior of the cell, where second messengers and phosphorylated proteins generate appropriate metabolic responses. The main second messengers are **cAMP, Ca^{2+}, inositol-1,4,5-triphosphate (IP_3), and diacylglycerol (DAG)**. Serine and threonine residues of proteins are phosphorylated by **cAMP-dependent protein kinase (PKA)** and **DAG-activated protein kinase C (PKC)**. Additionally, specific tyrosine residues on target enzymes and other regulatory proteins are phosphorylated by membrane-associated and intracellular *tyrosine kinases*.

Binding of hormone to (most but not all) plasma membrane receptor is transduced to the interior of cells, by the binding of *receptor-ligand complexes* to a series of membrane-localized GDP/GTP binding proteins called **G-proteins**.

The classical interactions between receptors, G-protein transducer, and membrane-localized *adenylate cyclase* are illustrated using the pancreatic hormone **glucagon** as an example (Fig. 19.1). When glucagon binds to its receptor, GTP exchanges with GDP bound to the α subunit of the G-protein that is in association with receptor. The Gα-GTP complex then dissociates leaving behind the β and α subunits of G-protein. In the next step, Gα-GTP complex binds to membrane bound *adenylate cyclase* and activates it. The activation of *adenylate cyclase* leads to cAMP production in the cytosol and to the activation of PKA, followed by regulatory phosphorylation of numerous enzymes. Stimulatory G-proteins are designated G_s inhibitory G-proteins are designated G_i.

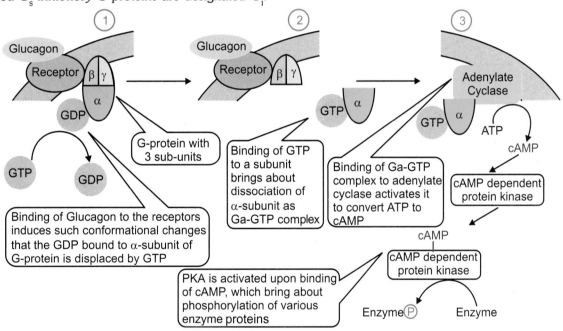

Fig. 19.1: Interaction between receptor and G-protein

A second class of peptide hormones induces the transduction of two, second messengers, DAG and IP_3 (Fig. 19.2). Hormone binding is followed by interaction with a stimulatory G-protein that is followed in turn by G-protein activation of membrane-localized *phospholipase C-γ, (PLC-γ)*. PLC-γ hydrolyzes phosphatidylinositol bisphosphate to produce two messengers: IP_3, which is soluble in the cytosol, and DAG that remains in the membrane phase.

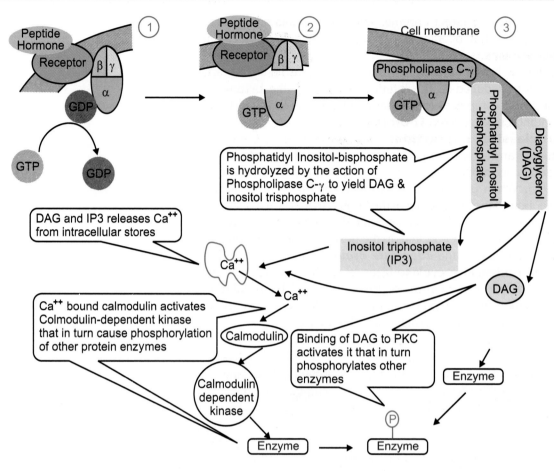

Fig. 19.2: Transduction of second messengers DAG and IP3 by peptide hormone

Cytosolic IP_3 binds to sites on the endoplasmic reticulum that opens Ca^{2+} channels and allow stored Ca^{2+} to flood the cytosol. Calcium activates numerous enzymes by activating their calmodulin or calmodulin-like subunits.

DAG has two roles: it binds and activates PKC, and it opens Ca^{2+} channels in the endoplasmic reticulum that reinforce the effect of IP_3.

Like PKA, PKC phosphorylates serine and threonine residues of many proteins, thus modulating their catalytic activity.

Only one class of receptor, that for the **atrial natriuretic factor (ANF)** is coupled to the production of intracellular cGMP. The receptors for the natriuretic factors are integral plasma membrane proteins, whose intracellular domains catalyze the formation of cGMP following natriuretic factor binding. Intracellular cGMP activates a protein kinase G (PKG), which phosphorylates and modulates enzyme activity, leading to the biological effects of the natriuretic factors.

Basics of Peptide Hormones

Releasing hormones belong to the class of peptide hormones that are synthesized in neural cell bodies of the hypothalamus and secreted at the axon terminals into the portal hypophyseal circulation, which bathes the anterior pituitary. These peptide hormones initiate a series of biochemical reactions that culminate in hormone-regulated, whole-body biological end points. Cells of the anterior pituitary, with specific receptors for individual releasing hormones, generally respond through a Ca^{2+}, IP_3, PKC-linked pathway that stimulates exocytosis of vesicles containing the various anterior pituitary hormones. The pituitary hormones are carried via the systemic circulation to target tissues throughout the body. At the target tissues they generate unique biological activities.

The secretion of hypothalamic, pituitary, and target tissue hormones is under tight regulatory control by a series of feedback and feed-forward loops. This complexity can be demonstrated using the growth hormone (GH) regulatory system as an example. Both, *growth hormone releasing hormone* (stimulatory substance) and *somatostatin* (inhibitory substance) are products of the hypothalamus, which control pituitary GH secretion. Under the influence of GRH, growth hormone is released into the systemic circulation, causing the target tissue to secrete IGF-1. The principal source of systemic IGF-1 is the liver, although most other tissues secrete and contribute to systemic IGF-1. Liver IGF-1 is considered to be the principal regulator of tissue growth. In particular, the IGF-1 secreted by the liver is believed to synchronize growth throughout the body, resulting in a homeostatic balance of tissue size and mass. IGF-1 secreted by peripheral tissues is generally considered to be autocrine or paracrine in its biological action.

Systemic IGF-1 also has hypothalamic and pituitary regulatory targets. The negative feedback loops cause down-regulation of GH secretion directly at the pituitary. The longer positive feedback loop, involving IGF-1 regulation at the hypothalamus, stimulates the secretion of somatostatin, which in turn inhibits the secretion of growth hormone by the pituitary. The latter is a relatively unusual negative feed-forward regulatory process. Similar feedback loops exist for all the major endocrine hormones, and many subtle nuances modulate each regulatory loop.

STEROID HORMONES

All steroid hormones are derived from cholesterol. With the exception of vitamin D, all steroid hormones contain the same cyclopentano-phenanthrene ring as cholesterol. The important steroid hormones are shown along with the structure (Fig. 19.3).

Pregnenolone: synthesized directly from cholesterol, the precursor molecule for all C-18, C-19 and C-21 steroids.

Progesterone: a progestin, synthesized directly from pregnenolone and secreted from the *corpus luteum*, responsible for changes associated with luteal phase of the menstrual cycle, and differentiation factor for mammary glands.

Aldosterone: the principal mineralocorticoid, synthesized from progesterone in the *zona glomerulosa* of adrenal cortex, raises blood pressure and fluid volume, increases sodium uptake.

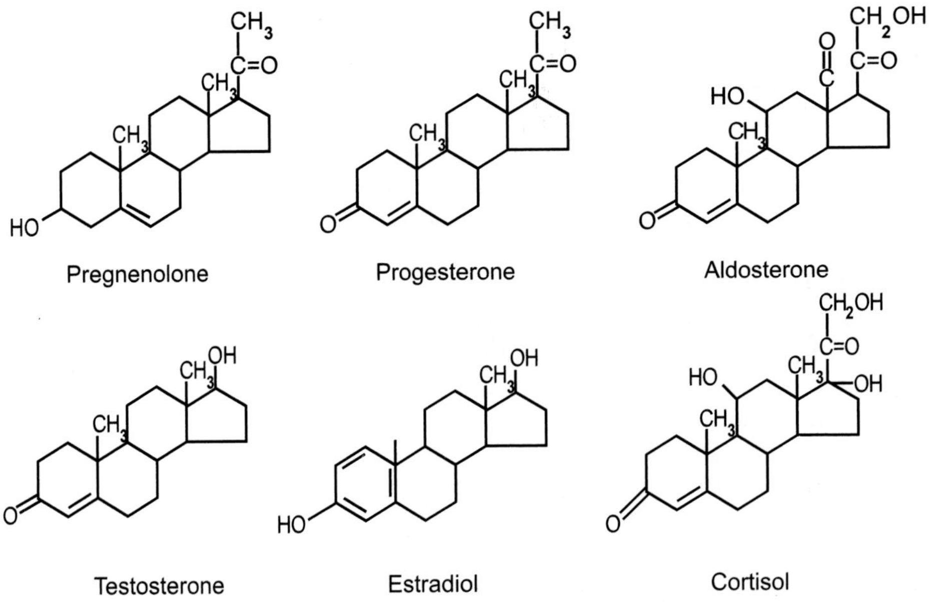

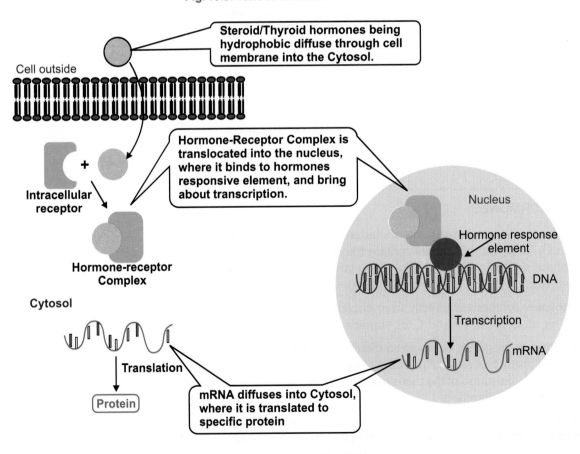

Fig. 19.3: Various steroidal hormones

Fig. 19.4: Mechanism of action of steroid hormone

Testosterone: an androgen, male sex hormone synthesized from progesterone in the testes, responsible for secondary male sex characteristics.

Estradiol: an estrogen, principal female sex hormone, synthesized in the ovary is responsible for secondary female sex characteristics.

Cortisol: dominant glucocorticoid in humans, synthesized from progesterone in the *zona fasciculata* of the adrenal cortex is involved in stress adaptation, elevation of blood pressure and sodium uptake; it also has numerous effects on the immune system.

MECHANISM OF ACTION OF STEROID HORMONES

All the steroid hormones and thyroid hormones exert their action by passing through the plasma membrane and binding to intracellular receptors (Fig. 19.4). Both the steroid and thyroid hormone-receptor complexes exert their action by binding to specific nucleotide sequences in the DNA of responsive genes. These DNA sequences are identified as **hormone response elements (HREs)**. The interaction of steroid-receptor complexes with DNA leads to altered rates of transcription of the associated genes.

Nutritional Needs

20

BALANCED DIET

Balanced diet should include adequate quantities of fats, proteins, carbohydrates, water, vitamins and minerals.

Food choices that promote health and prevent diseases should include a variety of foods

a. Low in saturated fat, and cholesterol.
b. Moderate amounts of sugar, salt, and alcohol
c. Plenty of fruits, vegetable, and grain products

Amount of energy provided by food is measured in *kilocalories*, which is the amount of heat required to raise the temperature of 1Kg of water by 1 degree Celsius. The caloric value provided by major foods are: 1 gram of carbohydrate provides 4 kilocalories, 1 gram of protein provides 4 kilocalories, and 1 gram of fat provides 9 kilocalories.

Ideal body weight (IBW) calculations is done as follows:

Women; for 5 feet height the reasonable weight is 100 pounds, for each inch over 5 feet add 5 pounds or for each inch under 5 feet subtract 5 pounds. For a large-framed individual add 10 pounds and for a small-framed individual subtract 10 pounds.

Men; for 5 feet height the reasonable weight is 106 pounds, for each inch over 5 feet add 6 pounds or for each inch under 5 feet subtract 6 pounds. For a large-framed individual add 10 pounds and for a small-framed individual subtract 10 pounds.

Daily energy needs are calculated based on individual's basal metabolic rate (BMR), thermal effect of food (TEF), physical activity energy cost (PAEC), and individual's total energy out-put (TEO).

a. **Basal metabolic rate (BMR)** is the energy required to carry out involuntary activities of the body at rest and in a fasting state. Calculation of BMR for women: 0.9 kilocalories **X** Weight (Kg) **X** 24 (hours in a day).

Calculation of BMR for men: 1.0 kilocalories **X** Weight (Kg) **X** 24 (hours in a day).

Factors that increase BMR are lean body tissue, childhood growth periods, exercise, sympathetic stimulation, shivering, fever (7% for every degree above 98.6^{0}F), hyperthyroidism, pregnancy, stress and male sex hormones.

Factors that decrease BMR are fat tissue, aging process, end-stage illness, dieting starvation, hypothyroidism and sleep.

b. **Specific dynamic action (SDA)/thermal effect of food (TEF)** is the energy the body uses in the process of digestion and absorption, which is approximately 10 percent of the total kilocalories in food consumed. BMR should be measured 12 hours after eating because of the immediate postabsorptive thermogenic effect of food.

c. **Physical activity energy cost** is the energy the body uses in the process of physical activity PAEC for both men and women:

Sedentary lifestyle (Typing, writing and playing cards) is 20 percent of the BMR.

Very light active lifestyle (walking on level surface at 2 - 3 mph, making beds and painting) is 40 percent of BMR.

Moderately active lifestyle (walking on level surface at 3.5 – 4 mph, pulling weeds and golfing without carting) is 40 percent of BMR.

Heavy active lifestyle (shoveling, cross-country running and jogging 5mph) is 50 percent of BMR.

d. **Total energy output** is the sum of the body's three uses of energy BMR, TEF and PAEC.

Illustration I: *Calculate the TEO for a woman weighing 130 lbs (59Kg), who eats 1800 kilocalories a day and maintain a regular exercise program.*

Calculation:

i.   BMR = 0.9 × 59 × 24 = 1274 kilocalories

ii. TEF = 1800 × 10% = 180 kilocalories

iii. PAEC = BMR × 40% = 510 kilocalories

iv. TEO = 1274 + 180 + 510 = 1964 kilocalories

Illustration II: Estimate the daily kilocalorie adjustment necessary for weight loss of one pound of body fat per week.

i.   Calculate the amount kilocalories in 1 gram of pure fat and body fat

1 gram of pure fat = 9 kilocalories

1 gram of body fat = 7.7 kilocalories (some water is present in fat cells)

ii. Calculate the amount of kilocalories in 1 pound of pure fat and body fat

1 pound of pure fat = 454 grams × 9 kilocalories/gram = 4086 kilocalories

1 pound of body fat = 454 grams × 7.7 kilocalories/gram = 3500 kilocalories

iii. Calculate the amount of kilocalorie adjustment necessary for 1 pound (3500 kilocalories) of body fat per week

3500 kilocalories, 7 days (1 week) = 500 kilocalories/day

CARBOHYDRATES

Carbohydrates are organic compounds composed of carbon, hydrogen and oxygen. They provide an immediate and reserve source of energy at 4 kcal/gm, spare protein from being used as a source of energy so that it can be used for other functions, and prevent ketosis as a result of inefficient fat metabolism for energy. A normal diet should compose 55 to 60 percent carbohydrate of the total kilocalories.

Dietary simple sugars include monosaccharide such as glucose (corn syrup), fructose (fruits and honey), and galactose (milk). Disaccharides include maltose (sweetners in food products, intermediates of starch digestion), sucrose (table sugars, sugar cane, sugar beets and molasses), and lactose (milk).

Complex sugars include starch and fibers. Starch (grains and grain products, legumes and potatoes) is polysaccharide made of hundreds of sugars linked together by glycosidic bonds that human digestive enzymes can break. Fibers include cellulose, hemicellulose, gums and mucilage found in stems and leaves of vegetables, covering of seeds and grains, algae and seaweed. They are found in plant cell walls composed of hundreds of sugars linked together by bonds that human digestive enzymes cannot break.

The indigestible fibers add to the bulk of diet, absorb water in the intestinal lumen to produce larger, softer feces that are easier to eliminate, alter the composition of intestinal bacteria, reduce enterohepatic circulation of cholesterol, delay intestinal sugar absorption and reduce the absorption of certain minerals.

Carbohydrate Metabolism

a. Storage and Conversion

Carbohydrates are stored primarily in the liver and skeletal muscle as glycogen (a large polymer of glucose) through the process of glycogenesis (formation of new glycogen) to remove excess glucose out of the bloodstream while maintaining a blood glucose level of 70 - 120 mg/dl. When the blood glucose level drops below 70 -120 mg/dl, glycogen stores in the liver and skeletal muscle are converted back to glucose through the process of glycogenolysis (breakdown of glycogen into glucose). If glycogen stores are depleted, proteins and fats are converted in the liver to glucose through the process of gluconeogenesis (creation of a new glucose). Each glucose molecule is broken down into two molecules of pyruvic acid (glycolysis), which is then converted into two molecules of acetyl coenzyme A (acetyl - CoA). Each acetyl - CoA molecule is completely oxidized in the citric acid cycle (Krebs cycle) and its energy is donated to energy storage compounds (adenosine triphosphate - ATP).

b. Digestion

Simple sugars (monosaccharides) require no digestion; quickly absorbed from the intestine and transported to the liver.

Disaccharides require digestion; quickly absorbed from the intestine and transported to the liver only after being digested by a series of enzymes to monosaccharides.

The enzymes involved are
- Ptyalin (saliva): Starch → dextrins → maltose
- Pancreatic amylase: Starch → dextrins → maltose
- Sucrase (intestine): Sucrose → glucose + fructose
- Lactase (intestine): Lactose → glucose + galactose
- Maltase (intestine): Maltose → glucose + glucose
- Fibers (cellulose, hemicellulose, gums, mucilages) are never digested.

PROTEINS

Proteins are polymers of amino acids linked together by peptide bonds, these are organic substances composed of four elements: carbon (C), hydrogen (H), oxygen (O), nitrogen (N). They are essential for tissue growth and repair, component of the body framework and fluids, help regulate fluid and acid-base balance, form antibodies, and provide a source of energy when carbohydrate intake is low at 4 kcal/gm. Protein in the diet should compose about 15 percent of the total kilocalories.

Amino acids are classified as ***essential and nonessential amino acids***.

Essential Amino Acids

The essential amino acids are those that the body cannot manufacture and, therefore, must be supplied for the body as part of the diet. The ten essential amino acids are: threonine, leucine, isoleucine, valine, lysine, methionine, phenylalanine, tryptophan, arginine and histidine.

Nonessential amino acids

The nonessential amino acids are those that the body can manufacture and, therefore, do not need to be supplied as part of the diet. The ten nonessential amino acids are: glycine, alanine, aspargine, aspartic acid, glutamic acid, glutamine, proline, cysteine, tyrosine, and serine.

From dietary point of view, proteins are classified as complete proteins, incomplete proteins and complementary proteins.
  i. Complete proteins contain all the essential amino acids and many nonessential ones, e.g. meats, poultry, fish, dairy products, and eggs.
  ii. Incomplete proteins lack one or more of the essential amino acids, e.g. grains, legumes, and vegetables
  iii. Complementary proteins are two or more proteins whose amino acid assortments complement each other in such a way that the essential amino acids missing from each is supplied by the other. A person should select from two or more of the following groupings to create complementary amino acid combinations:

- Grains: e.g. oats, rice, whole grain breads, and pasta.
- Legumes: e.g. peanuts, soy products, pinto beans, black beans
- Seeds and nuts: e.g. cashews, nut butters, sesame seeds
- Vegetables: e.g. broccoli, cabbage, peppers, squash, spinach.

Metabolism

a. Storage and Catabolism

Proteins are synthesized from amino acids and stored as body tissue and plasma proteins, e.g. tissue proteins, albumin, globulin, and fibrinogen. Proteins are catabolized by breakdown of the body's tissue proteins to amino acids in the liver in the following way; a) Removing the nitrogen-containing amino part of the amino acid through the process of deamination and either: converting it to ammonia to be excreted as urea in the urine, or using it to make another compound, such as a nonessential amino acid. b) Converting the remaining non-nitrogen containing part of the amino acid to either: pyruvic acid, which can be converted to glucose, or acetyl Co A, which can enter the citric acid cycle (Krebs cycle).

Positive nitrogen balance exists when the body takes in more nitrogen than it excretes, usually occurs during periods of rapid growth such as childhood and adolescence, pregnancy, and phases of physical exercise when muscle mass increases.

Negative nitrogen balance exists when the body takes in less nitrogen than it excretes, usually occurs during periods of convalescence from a protein-depleting illness or after fasting or inadequate intake of protein and calories.

b. Digestion

Proteins are broken down by a series of enzymes to small peptide and amino acids that are absorbed from the intestine and transported to the liver. The enzymes involved are:
- Pepsin (stomach); protein → polypeptides
- Trypsin (pancreas); protein, polypeptides → polypeptides, dipeptides
- Chymotrypsin (pancreas); protein, polypeptides → polypeptides, dipeptides
- Carboxypeptidases (pancreas); polypeptides → simpler peptides, dipeptides, amino acids
- Aminopeptidase (small intestine); polypeptides → peptides, dipeptides, amino acids
- Dipeptidase (small intestine); dipeptides → amino acids

LIPIDS

Lipids are organic compounds composed of three elements: carbon (C), hydrogen (H), and oxygen (O).

Functions of lipids Lipids are structural components, insulate the body, cushion the internal organs, help absorption of fat-soluble vitamins, and provide a source of energy when carbohydrate intake is low at 9 kcal/gram. Normal diet should compose 25-30 percent of the total kilocalories

Classification of Lipids

i. **Fatty acids** (saturated fatty acids, unsaturated fatty acids, and essential fatty acids).

    Saturated fatty acids are composed of a chain of carbon atoms and hydrogen atoms in which all carbon atoms are filled (saturated) with hydrogen. The sources are bacon, meat fat, lean red meat, poultry, seafood, egg yolk, and dairy fat.

    Unsaturated fatty acids composed of a chain of carbon atoms and hydrogen atoms in which there is at least one double bond between two carbon atoms so all carbon atoms are not filled (saturated) with hydrogen. The two types of unsaturated fatty acids are: monounsaturated fatty acids, which have one double bond between two carbon atoms, and polyunsaturated fatty acids, which have double bonds between four or more carbon atoms. The sources are olives, olive oil, and vegetable oils.

    Essential fatty acids are those that the body cannot manufacture and, therefore, must be supplied for the body as part of the diet. The two essential fatty acids are: linoleic (Omega 6) and linolenic (Omega 3). The sources are; (a) linoleic (Omega 6) from seeds of plants, and oils harvested from seeds (b) linolenic (Omega 3) from fish oils.

ii. **Glycerides** are composed of one glycerol molecule and one, two, or three fatty acids. The three types of gylcerides are: monoglycerides, which have one glycerol molecule and one fatty acid, diglycerides, which have one glycerol molecule and two fatty acids, and triglycerides, which have one glycerol molecule and three fatty acids. Almost 90 percent of all lipids are triglycerides.

iii. **Phospholipids** are composed of one glycerol molecule, two fatty acids, and choline or some other compound instead of a third fatty acid, e.g. lecithin.

iv. **Sterols** are composed of interconnected rings of carbon, e.g. cholesterol, vitamin D, sex hormones.

v. **Lipoproteins** are composed of an interior of triglycerides and cholesterol (both water insoluble) surrounded by phospholipids and protein (water-soluble) to provide a means to transport water insoluble triglycerides and cholesterol in the bloodstream. Lipoproteins are classified as:

    a. *Very low-density lipoproteins (VLDL)* have 50% triglyceride, 20% phospholipid, 20% cholesterol, and 10% protein.

    b. *Low-density lipoproteins (LDL)* are larger, lighter, and more lipids filled composed of 10% triglyceride, 20% phospholipid, 50% cholesterol, and 20% protein. They are known as "bad" cholesterol because LDL's transport cholesterol to all the body tissues.

    c. *High-density lipoproteins (HDL)* are smaller, denser, and packaged with more protein composed of 10% triglyceride,

20% phospholipid, 20% cholesterol, and 50% protein. They are known as "good" cholesterol because HDL's transport cholesterol back to the liver to be broken down and excreted.

Metabolism

Triglycerides are broken down to glycerol and fatty acids, glycerol is converted to pyruvic acid, which can be converted to glucose, and fatty acids are converted to acetyl CoA that can enter the citric acid cycle (Krebs cycle).

Digestion

Lipids are absorbed from the intestine and transported throughout the body only after being emulsified by bile salts from gallbladder and digested by a series of enzymes:

Lingual lipase (mouth); some initial fat breakdown
Steapsin (pancreas);
Triglycerides → diglycerides
Diglycerides → monoglycerides
Monoglycerides → fatty acids and glycerol

PROTEIN-ENERGY MALNUTRITION

Protein-energy malnutrition is a condition that is specifically severe in growing children of particularly underdeveloped or developing countries that leads to wide range of clinical symptoms of starvation. This can also be seen in adults as a consequence of malabsorption, gastrointestinal surgery or severe illness.

Kwashiorkor (protein malnutrition) is seen in children who consume adequate energy but limited protein, leading to generalized edema.

Marasmus (protein-calories deficiency) occurs with deficient intake of both calories and protein.

VITAMINS

Vitamins are organic compounds that are non-caloric, essential nutrients necessary in very small amounts for specific metabolic control and disease prevention that cannot be manufactured by the body.
Vitamins are classified as follows:
Water-soluble vitamins are those that the body cannot store and, therefore, must be supplied daily in the diet. They are: C (ascorbic acid), thiamin (B_1), riboflavin (B_2), niacin (B_3), pyridoxine (B_6), folic acid (B_9), cobalamin (B_{12}), pantothenic acid, and biotin.
Sources:
C (ascorbic acid); citrus fruits, green peppers, tomatoes, white potatoes, cabbage, broccoli, chard, kale, turnip greens, asparagus, berries, melons, pineapples, and guavas.
Thiamin (B_1); pork, beef, liver, whole or enriched grains, and legumes.

Riboflavin (B_2); milk, meats, enriched cereals, and green vegetables.

Niacin (B_3); meats, peanuts, legumes, and enriched grains.

Pyridoxine (B_6); grains, seeds, liver and kidney, meats, milk, eggs, and vegetables.

Pantothenic acid: meats, cereals, legumes, milk, vegetables, and fruits.

Biotin: liver, egg yolk, soy flour, tomatoes, and yeast.

Fat-soluble vitamins are those that the body can store to a certain extent and, therefore, do not need to be supplied daily in the diet. They are: Vitamin A (retinol), D (cholecalciferol), E (tocopherol), and K.

Sources:

A (retinol); fish liver oils, liver, egg yolk, butter, and cream

D (cholecalciferol); yeast, fish liver oils, and enriched milk

E (tocopherol); vegetable oils

K; green leafy vegetables

MINERALS

Minerals are inorganic elements, widely distributed in nature, required by the human body in different amounts to do numerous metabolic tasks.

Minerals are classified as:

a. **Macrominerals** Those are required by the body in amounts more than 100 milligrams a day. They are calcium, phosphorus, sodium, potassium, magnesium, chloride, and sulfur.

Sources:

Calcium; milk, cheese, whole grains, egg yolk, legumes, nuts, and green leafy vegetables

Phosphorus; milk, cheese, meat, egg yolk, whole grains, legumes, and nuts

Sodium; table salt, milk, meat, egg, baking soda, baking powder, carrots, beets, spinach, celery

Potassium; fruits, vegetables, meats, whole grains, and legumes

Magnesium; whole grains, nuts, legumes, and green vegetables

Chloride; table salt

Sulfur; meat, egg, cheese, milk, nuts, and legumes

b. **Microminerals** are those required by the body in amounts less than 100 milligrams a day. They include; iron, iodine, zinc, copper, manganese, chromium, cobalt, selenium, molybdenum, and fluorine

Sources:

Iron; liver, meats, egg yolk, whole grains, enriched bread and cereal, dark green vegetables, legumes, nuts

Iodine; iodized salt, seafood

Zinc; meat, seafood, eggs, milk, whole grains, legumes

Copper; liver, seafood, whole grains, legumes, nuts

Manganese; cereals, whole grain, soybeans, legumes, nuts, tea, vegetables, fruits

Chromium; whole grains, cereal products
Cobalt; preformed vitamin B_{12}
Selenium; seafoods, kidney, liver, meats, whole grains
Molybdenum; organ meats, milk, whole grains, leafy vegetables, legumes
Fluorine; fluoridated water

FOOD GUIDE PYRAMID

Bread, cereal, rice, pasta; 6-11 servings a day.

Vegetable group; 3 to 5 servings a day, 1 or 2 of them should be good sources of vitamin C, one of them should be a good source of vitamin A every other day.

Fruit group; 2 to 4 servings a day, 1 to 2 of them should be good sources of vitamin C, one of them should be a good source of vitamin A every other day.

Meat, poultry, fish, bacon, eggs, nuts; 2 to 3 servings a day.
Milk, yogurt, cheese:
Children less than 9: 2 to 3 servings a day
Children 9 to 12: 3 or more servings a day
Teenager: 4 or more servings a day
Adult: 2 or more servings a day
Pregnant: 3 or more servings a day
Lactating: 4 or more servings a day
Fat, oils, sweets; use sparingly

FACTORS INFLUENCING DIET

Ethnicity and culture, age, religion, economic status, peer groups, personal preference and uniqueness.

Life-style, beliefs about health effects of food, alcohol abuse, advertising, psychological factors, health status, therapy, and medications.

METHODS TO STIMULATE THE APPETITE

Relieve illness symptoms that depress the appetite, e.g.: analgesic for pain, and antipyretic for fever.

Provide familiar food the client likes
Select small portions
Avoid unpleasant, uncomfortable treatments immediately before or after meals
Provide tidy, clean, pleasant, odor-free environment around meals
Encourage/provide oral hygiene before meals
Reduce psychological stress around meals.

DIAGNOSTIC STUDIES

1. Blood Tests

a. Hemoglobin and hematocrit; collection of a specimen of blood to measure the amount of hemoglobin and hematocrit in the blood to ascertain state of hydration and protein and iron deficiencies.

b. Serum albumin; collection of a specimen of blood to measure the amount of serum albumin in the blood to ascertain state of hydration and protein and iron deficiencies.

c. Transferrin; collection of a specimen of blood to measure the amount of transferrin in the blood to ascertain protein and iron deficiencies.

d. Total iron-binding capacity (TIBC); a collection of specimen of blood to measure the iron-binding capacity of a red blood cell and ascertain iron deficiencies.

e. Total lymphocyte count; collection of a specimen of blood to measure the amount of lymphocytes in the blood to ascertain immune function and presence of infection.

f. Blood urea nitrogen; collection of a specimen of blood to measure the amount of urea nitrogen in the blood to ascertain protein status.

g. Mean corpuscular volume (MCV); collection of a specimen of blood to measure the average size of an RBC to ascertain the presence and type of anemia.

h. Mean corpuscular hemoglobin (MCH); collection of a specimen of blood to measure the average weight of hemoglobin in an RBC to ascertain the presence and type of anemia.

i. Mean corpuscular hemoglobin concentration (MCHC); collection of a specimen of blood to measure the average concentration of hemoglobin in an RBC to ascertain the presence and type of anemia.

2. Urine Tests

a. Urine urea nitrogen; collection of a 24-hour composite specimen of urine to measure the amount of urea nitrogen to ascertain protein balance.

b. Urinary creatinine; collection of a 24-hour composite specimen of urine to measure the amount of creatinine to ascertain protein balance.

3. Anthropometric Measurements

a. Height

b. Weight

c. Triceps skin-fold (TSF); measurement of the skin-fold in the midpoint of the back of the upper arm with calipers to determine the amount of leanness and fatness.

d. Subscapular skin-fold (SSF); measurement of the skin-fold of the skin just below the scapula with calipers to determine the amount of leanness and fatness.

e. Mid-upper arm circumference (MAC); measurement of the midpoint of the upper arm, halfway between the acromion process and the olecranon process, with a tape measure to determine skeletal muscle mass.

ALTERNATIVE FEEDING METHODS

I. Enteral

a. Nasogastric; instillation of specially prepared nutrients through a tube that is inserted through one of the nostrils, down the nasopharynx, and into the stomach.

b. Nastrostomy; instillation of specially prepared nutrients through a tube that is surgically placed through the abdominal wall into the stomach.

c. Percutaneous endoscopic gastrostomy (PEG) tube; instillation of specially prepared nutrients through a tube that is placed through the abdominal wall into the stomach under the guidance of an endoscope.

d. Jejunostomy; instillation of specially prepared nutrients through a tube that is surgically placed through the abdominal wall into the jejunum.

II. Parenteral

a. Peripheral parenteral nutrition (PPN); instillation of specially prepared nutrients through a tube that is inserted into a peripheral vein.

b. Total parenteral nutrition (TPN); instillation of specially prepared nutrients through a tube that is inserted into a large central vein (usually subclavian).

Biochemistry of Nerve Impulse Transmission

21

The propagation of nerve impulses from one nerve cell to another is called synaptic transmission. Such transmission occurs at specialized cellular structures known as **synapse**. Synapse is a junction at which the axon of the presynaptic neuron terminates upon the postsynaptic neuron. The end of a presynaptic axon, where it is juxtaposed to the postsynaptic neuron, is enlarged and forms a structure known as the **terminal button**. The presynaptic axon can make contact anywhere along the second neuron. The presynaptic axon forms three types of synapses.

i. When it makes contact with the dendrites of postsynaptic neuron it is called an **axodendritic synapse**

ii. The contact with the cell body of postsynaptic neuron is called an **axosomatic synapse**, and

iii. The contact with the axons of postsynaptic neuron is called an **axo-axonal synapse**.

Nerve impulses are transmitted at synapses by the release of chemicals called **neurotransmitters**. As a nerve impulse or **action potential** reaches the end of a presynaptic axon, molecules of neurotransmitter are released into the synaptic space (Fig. 21.1). The neurotransmitters are a diverse group of chemical compounds such as dopamine (simple amine, GABA (amino acid), and enkephalins (polypeptide).

Neuromuscular Transmission

A different type of nerve transmission occurs when an axon terminates on a skeletal muscle fiber, which is a specialized structure called the **neuromuscular junction** (Fig. 21.2). The action potential occurring at this site is known as **neuromuscular transmission**. At neuromuscular junction, the axon subdivides into numerous terminal buttons that reside within depressions formed in the **motor end plate**. The transmitter at the neuromuscular junction is **acetylcholine.**

The receptors for chemical transmitters are destroyed in myasthenia gravis (an autoimmune disease that causes muscular weakness). Drugs used to relax skeletal muscle, competitively block these receptors

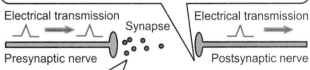

Electrical transmission   Synapse   Electrical transmission

Presynaptic nerve   Postsynaptic nerve

Chemical transmitters made and stored at presynaptic nerve endings are released on arrival of nerve impulse. postsynaptic nerve endings senses the chemical transmitter and generate action potential.

Fig. 21.1: Chemical transmission of nerve impulse

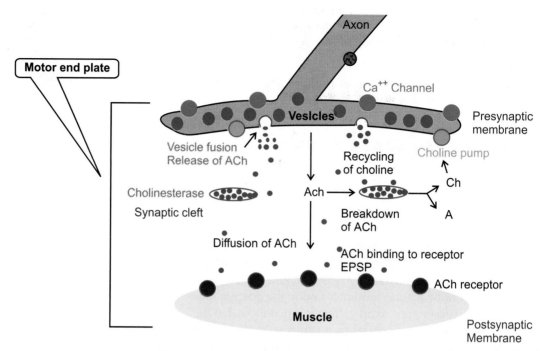

Fig. 21.2: Neuromuscular junction

Neurotransmitter Receptors

Upon firing of an action potential, the neurotransmitter molecules are released from the presynaptic nerve endings, which bind to specific receptors on the surface of the postsynaptic neuron. There are numerous subtypes of receptor for any given neurotransmitter. Neurotransmitter receptors are found on both postsynaptic and presynaptic neurons. In general, presynaptic neuron receptors act to inhibit further release of neurotransmitter. The vast majority of neurotransmitter receptors belong to a class of proteins known as the **serpentine receptors** that spans the cell membrane seven times. The link between neurotransmitters and intracellular signaling is carried out in association either with G-proteins, protein kinases, or by the receptor itself in the form of a ligand-gated ion channel (e.g, the acetylcholine receptor). One additional characteristic of neurotransmitter receptors is that they are subject to **ligand-induced desensitization**: i.e. they can become unresponsive upon prolonged exposure to their neurotransmitter.

ACETYLCHOLINE

Neurons that synthesize and release ACh are termed **cholinergic neurons**. When an action potential reaches the terminal button of a presynaptic neuron a voltage-gated calcium channel is opened. The influx of calcium ions (Ca^{++}) stimulates the exocytosis of presynaptic vesicles containing ACh, there by ACh is released into the synaptic cleft. Once released, ACh must be removed rapidly by the action of acetylcholine esterase, in order to allow repolarization to take place (Fig. 21.3).

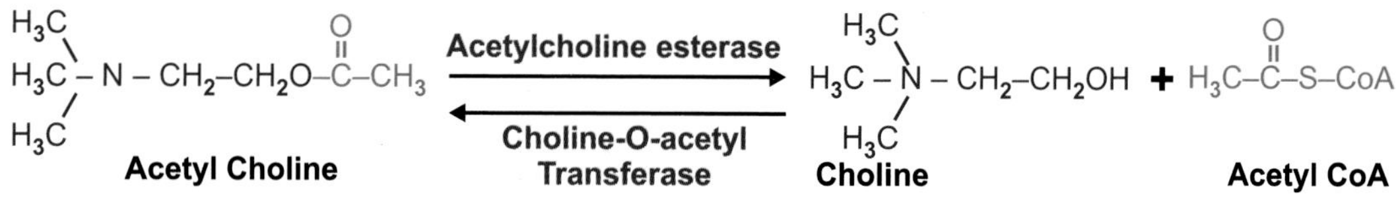

$$H_3C-N-CH_2-CH_2O-\overset{O}{\overset{\|}{C}}-CH_3 \quad \underset{\text{Choline-O-acetyl Transferase}}{\overset{\text{Acetylcholine esterase}}{\rightleftharpoons}} \quad H_3C-N-CH_2-CH_2OH + H_3C-\overset{O}{\overset{\|}{C}}-S-CoA$$

Acetyl Choline   **Choline**   **Acetyl CoA**

Fig. 21.3: Action of acetylcholine esterase

Acetylcholine receptors are ligand-gated cation channels. Two main classes of ACh receptors have been identified on the basis of their responsiveness to muscarine (toadstool alkaloid) or to nicotine, designated respectively as **muscarinic receptors** and the **nicotinic receptors**. Both receptor classes are abundant in the human brain. Nicotinic receptors are further subdivided into those found at neuromuscular junctions and those found at neuronal synapses. The activation of ACh receptors by ACh binding, leads to an influx of Na^+ into the cell and an efflux of K^+ out of the cell that results in a depolarization of the postsynaptic neuron and the initiation of a new action potential.

CHOLINERGIC AGONISTS AND ANTAGONISTS

Numerous compounds have been identified that act as either agonists or antagonists of cholinergic neurons. The principal action of cholinergic agonists is the excitation or inhibition of autonomic effector cells that are innervated by *postganglionic parasympathetic neurons* and as such are referred to as *parasympathomimetic agents*. The cholinergic agonists include choline esters (such as ACh itself) as well as protein-based or alkaloid-based compounds. Several naturally occurring compounds have been shown to affect cholinergic neurons, either positively or negatively.

The responses of cholinergic neurons can also be enhanced by administration of cholinesterase (ChE) inhibitors. ChE inhibitors have been used as components of nerve gases but also have significant medical application in the treatment of disorders such as glaucoma and myasthenia gravis (an autoimmune disease, where the ACh receptors are destroyed) as well as in terminating the effects of neuromuscular blocking agents such as atropine.

Cholinergic agonists	Source of compound	Mode of action
Nicotine	Alkaloid prevalent in the tobacco plant	Activates nicotinic class of ACh receptors, locks the channel open
Muscarine	Alkaloid produced by *Amanita muscaria* mushrooms	Activates muscarinic class of ACh receptors
α-Latrotoxin	Protein produced by the black widow spider	Induces massive ACh release, possibly by acting as a Ca^{2+} ionophore

Cholinergic antagonists

Atropine (and related compound scopolamine)	Alkaloid produced by the deadly nightshade, *Atropa belladonna*	Blocks ACh actions only at muscarinic receptors
Botulinus toxin	Eight proteins produced by *Clostridium botulinum*	Inhibits the release of ACh
α-bungarotoxin	Protein produced by *Bungarus* genus of snakes	Prevents ACh receptor channel opening
δ-tubocurarine	Active ingredient of curare	Prevents ACh receptor channel opening at motor end-plate

CATECHOLAMINES

The principal catecholamines are **epinephrine, norepinephrine**, and **dopamine**. These compounds are synthesized from phenylalanine and tyrosine. In the catecholamine-secreting neurons, tyrosine undergoes a series of reactions to form dopamine, norepinephrine and finally to epinephrine.

Catecholamines exhibit both excitatory and inhibitory effects on peripheral nervous system, as well as the CNS, such as respiratory stimulation and increased psychomotor activity. The excitatory effects are exerted upon smooth muscle cells of the blood vessels in the skin and mucous membranes. Cardiac function is also subject to excitatory effects, which lead to an increased heart rate and forced contraction. Inhibitory effects, by contrast, are exerted upon smooth muscle cells in the wall of the gut, the bronchial tree of the lungs, and the vessels that supply blood to skeletal muscle.

In addition to the neurotransmitter effects, norepinephrine and epinephrine can influence the metabolic rates, both by modulating endocrine function such as insulin secretion and by increasing the rate of glycogenolysis and fatty acid mobilization.

Catecholamines bind to two different classes of receptors termed the α- and β-adrenergic receptors. The catecholamines therefore are also known as **adrenergic neurotransmitters**; neurons that secrete epinephrine are **adrenergic neurons**, and the neurons that secrete norepinephrine are **noradrenergic neurons**. Some of the norepinephrine released from presynaptic noradrenergic neurons is recycled in the presynaptic neuron by a reuptake mechanism.

CATECHOLAMINE CATABOLISM

Epinephrine and norepinephrine are catabolized to inactive compounds through the sequential actions of **catecholamine-O-methyltransferase (COMT)** and **monoamine oxidase (MAO)**. Compounds that inhibit the action of MAO have been shown to have beneficial effects in the treatment of clinical depression, even when tricyclic antidepressants are ineffective. The utility of MAO inhibitors was discovered unexpectedly when patients treated for tuberculosis with isoniazid showed signs of an improvement in mood.

SEROTONIN

Hydroxylation and decarboxylation of tryptophan yields serotonin (5-hydroxytryptamine/ 5-HT). The greatest concentration of 5-HT (about 90%) is found in the enterochromaffin cells of the gastrointestinal tract and the remainder of the body's 5-HT is found in platelets and the CNS. The effects of 5-HT are felt most prominently in the cardiovascular system, with additional effects in the respiratory system and the intestines. Vasoconstriction is the classic response to 5-HT administration. Neurons that secrete 5-HT are termed **serotonergic**. A portion of 5-HT that is released is taken up by the presynaptic serotonergic neuron, in a manner similar to that of the reuptake of norepinephrine. The actions of 5-HT follow binding to specific cell surface receptors. At least seven distinct subtypes of 5-HT receptors have been identified (5-HT$_{1A}$, 5-HT$_{1B}$, 5-HT$_{1C}$, 5-HT$_{1D}$, 5-HT$_2$, 5-HT$_3$ and 5-HT$_4$). The whole family of 5-HT receptors is serpentine receptors coupled to activation of adenylate cyclase by G-protein; the only exception is 5-HT$_3$ receptors that are ion channels.

GABA

Several amino acids have distinct excitatory or inhibitory effects upon the nervous system. The amino acid derivative, **γ-amino butyrate (GABA)** is a well-known inhibitor of presynaptic transmission in the CNS, and in the retina.

GABA is formed by the decarboxylation of glutamate catalyzed by **glutamate decarboxylase (GAD).** GAD is present in many nerve endings of the brain as well as in the β-cells of the pancreas. Neurons that secrete GABA are termed **GABAergic**.

GABA exerts its effects by binding to two distinct receptors, GABA-A and GABA-B. The GABA-A receptors form a Cl⁻ channel. The binding of GABA to GABA-A receptors increases the Cl⁻ conductance of presynaptic neurons. The benzodiazepine family of anxiolytic drugs exerts their soothing effects by potentiating the responses of GABA-A receptors to GABA binding. The GABA-B receptors are coupled to an intracellular G-protein and act by increasing conductance of an associated K^+ channel.

Contractile Proteins (Muscle) the Sarcomere

22

There are 3 Basic Types of Muscle in the Body

Skeletal muscle attached to bones form levers, which help bodily movement.

Cardiac muscle forms the heart that pumps blood through circulatory system.

Smooth muscle lines blood vessels and gut that controls diameter of these tubular structures that helps to propel blood in vessels and the digested food in gut.

To perform these different operations each muscle type has different properties

Comparison of Different Types of Muscle

Property	Skeletal muscle	Cardiac muscle	Smooth muscle
Striations	Yes	Yes	No
Speed of contraction	Fast	Intermediate	Slow
Voluntary control	Yes	No	No
Refractory period	Short	Long	
Nuclei per cell	Many	Single	Single
Control of contraction	Nerves	Beats spontaneously but modulated by nerves	Nerve and hormones
Cells connected by discs or gap junctions	No	Yes	Yes

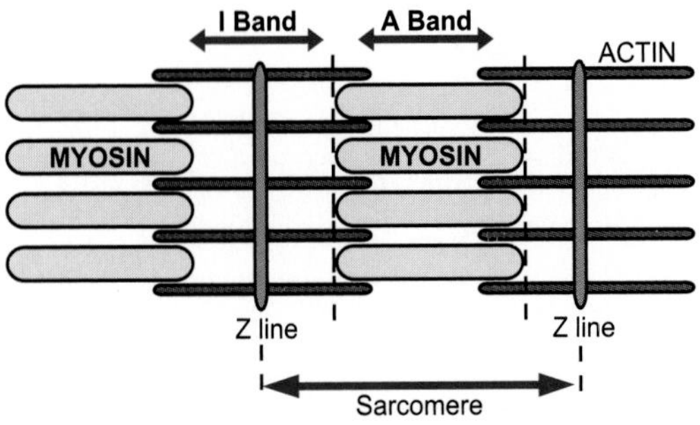

Fig. 22.1: Structure of sarcomere

Basic Unit of Muscle Contraction is Sarcomere

Skeletal and cardiac muscles are striated but smooth muscle does not show striations. The striations are caused by alignment of bands: the most prominent are the A bands, I bands, and the Z line. Sarcomere is the basic unit of contraction between two Z lines (Fig. 22.1).

The major proteins of these bands are actin and myosin. In the 'A' band, the two proteins overlap but the 'I' band has only actin.

When muscle contracts the sarcomere shortens and the 'Z' lines move closer to each other.

"Sliding Filament" Model

Muscle is composed of two contractile proteins:
a. Thin filaments: actin attached to 'Z' line is found in both 'A' and 'I' bands
b. Thick filaments: myosin is found only in 'A' band
    When muscle contracts the actin filaments slide into the 'A' band, overlapping with myosin (Fig. 22.2):
a. The 'Z' lines move closer to each other
b. The 'I' band becomes shorter
c. But the length of 'A' band remains the same.
    This is called the "sliding filament" model of muscle contraction. Sarcomere can contract to a maximum of 30 percent.

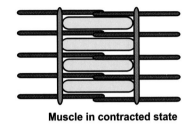

Fig. 22.2 Relaxed and contracted state of muscle

ACTIN

The globular actin (G-actin) with bound ATP polymerizes to form filamentous actin (F-actin) that spiral around the axis of the filament. The G-actin monomer has a deep cleft where ATP binds along with magnesium ion (Fig. 22.3).

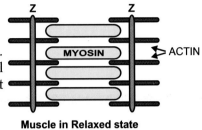

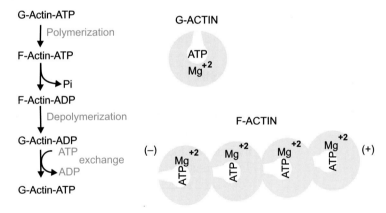

Fig. 22.3: Polymerization actin units

The conformation of actin, depend on whether there is ATP or ADP in the nucleotide-binding site.

The G-actin-ATP polymerizes to F-actin-ATP, whereas the F-actin-ADP depolymerizes to G-actin-ADP.

The F-actin may hydrolyze its bound ATP to ADP and phosphate, but ADP release from the filament does not occur since the cleft opening is blocked. G-actin-ADP can release ADP and bind ATP, which is usually present in the cytosol at higher concentration than ADP.

Actin filaments have polarity. The actin monomers all orient with their cleft toward the same end of the filament (designated the minus end). Filament growth at the end designated plus (+), exceeded that at the other end designated minus (–).

Myosin Cross-bridging with Actin Causes Muscle Contraction

The filaments slide together because myosin attaches to actin and pulls on it (Fig. 22.4). Myosin head attaches to actin filament, forming a cross-bridge, then the myosin head bends, pulling on the actin filaments and causing them to slide. The cross-bridge cycle is: grab → pull → release, repeated over and over.

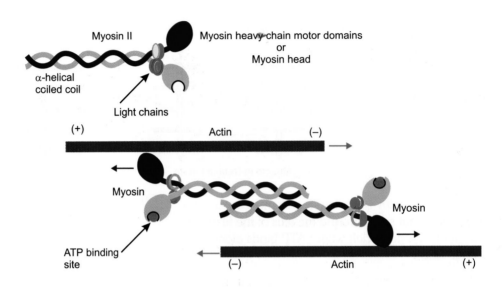

Fig. 22.4: Actin and myosin interaction

MYOSIN

The myosins are a family of motor proteins that move along actin filaments. Myosin II (Fig. 22.4), the form found in skeletal muscle includes two heavy chains, each with a globular motor domain that includes a binding site for ATP and a domain that interacts with actin. Tail domains of the heavy chains are associated in a rod-like α-helical coiled coil structure. Two light chains associate with each heavy chain in the neck region. Light chains of different myosin types are calmodulin or calmodulin-like regulatory proteins. They may provide stiffening in neck domains.

The coiled coil tail domains of myosin II molecules interact to form antiparallel bipolar complexes that contain many myosin molecules.

The movement of myosin heads along actin filaments is accompanied by ATP hydrolysis.

Actin filaments may move relative to one another, as heads at the opposite ends of bipolar myosin complexes move toward the plus ends of adjacent antiparallel actin.

Both Contraction and Relaxation of Muscle Need ATP

ATP is required for sliding of the filaments that are accomplished by a bending movement of the myosin heads during contraction, and separation of actin and myosin, which relaxes the muscle.

Heads of myosin II interact with actin filaments in a reaction cycle that may be summarized as follows (Fig. 22.5).

ATP binding to myosin causes a conformational change that makes it to let go of actin. The active site closes and ATP is hydrolyzed, the conformational change that follows makes myosin bind to actin weakly, at a different place on the filament. Phosphate release results in further conformational change that lead to stronger myosin

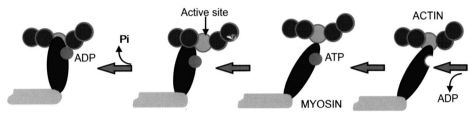

Fig. 22.5: Interaction between myosin head and action filament

binding, and the power stroke. ADP release leaves the myosin head tightly bound to actin. In the absence of ATP, this state continues and results in muscle rigidity called rigor.

Muscle Contraction is Triggered by Calcium Ions

The complex of tropomyosin and troponin that includes a calmodulin-like protein regulates actin-myosin interaction in skeletal muscle. Actin-myosin interactions are regulated by calcium in differing ways in different tissues.

In the resting state, the protein tropomyosin winds around actin and covers the myosin binding sites. One of the troponin subunits, **troponin-C (Tn-C)**, is a calmodulin-like calcium-binding protein. When Tn-C binds calcium, the whole troponin molecule undergoes the conformational change that moves the attached tropomyosin away from the myosin binding sites on actin with the sites exposed. This event permits nearby myosin heads to interact with myosin binding sites, and contractile activity ensues.

Some myosins are regulated by Ca^{++} binding to calmodulin-like light chains, in the neck region.

Some myosins are regulated by phosphorylation of myosin light chains, catalyzed by a calcium-dependent kinase or by a kinase that is activated by a small GTP-binding protein.

A protein called caldesmon that is regulated by phosphorylation and calcium ions controls actin-myosin interaction in smooth muscle.

Sarcoplasmic Reticulum is the Storehouse of Calcium in Muscles

Calcium that causes muscle contraction is stored in the sarcoplasmic reticulum (SR). Skeletal muscle is stimulated by nerves, which contact muscle through a neuromuscular junction. The nerve releases acetylcholine and generates a muscle action potential. The action potential travels down the T-tubule and causes the SR to release calcium. After the contraction calcium is rapidly pumped back into the SR so that muscle can again contract.

Special Junctions help Spread the Excitation from One Cell to Another in Cardiac and Smooth Muscles

In skeletal musclse, each fiber (cell) can contract independently but in cardiac and smooth muscles, the cells are interconnected by special junctions: *intercalated disks* in cardiac and *gap junctions* in smooth muscles. They help spread the excitation from one cell to another and causes cardiac and most smooth muscle to contract as a unit.

Cardiac muscle beats spontaneously, even if all nerves to the heart are cut. The nerves do speed up or slow down the heartbeat; however, cutting the nerve to skeletal muscle will cause it to degenerate.

MUSCLE RELAXATION

Cessation of electrical impulse at myoneural junction relaxes muscle, and sarcoplasmic membrane returns to its resting electrical potential, as does the entire T tubule system and the SR membrane. Subsequently, sarcoplasmic calcium is pumped back into the SR by an extremely active ATP- driven calcium pump, an integral protein of SR membrane. For each ATP hydrolyzed, two calcium ions are moved out of the sarcoplasm, into the SR. The cisternal surface of the SR membrane contains large quantities of a glycoprotein known as **calsequestrin**. Calsequestrin avidly binds calcium, decreasing its concentration in the cisternae, and thus favoring calcium accumulation.

TETANY AND RIGOR MORTIS

Tetany is a condition of hypercontracted muscle that follows a prolonged period of repetitive muscle stimulation. It is caused by the depletion of ATP and other high-energy phosphates that help maintain normal ATP levels.

The high-energy phosphates include other nucleoside triphosphates (NTPs), creatine phosphate (CP), and ADP. The three reactions are carried out by *nucleoside diphosphokinase*, *creatine kinase* and *adenylate kinase*, respectively.

NTP + ADP → NDP + ATP
CP + ADP → Creatine +ATP
ADP + ADP → AMP + ATP

Tetanic stimulation raises sarcoplasmic calcium and ATP depletion, which ends up in a highly contracted muscle with calcium bound to Tn-C and no ATP available to resequester calcium into the cisternae of the SR, nor to break actomyosin cross-bridges. Under these conditions, mitochondria will preferentially pump calcium into the mitochondrial matrix, ultimately removing calcium bound to Tn-C, obscuring myosin binding sites on thin filaments, and, allowing the muscle to assume a flaccid state. Muscles in this physiological state are said to be fatigued. In death, all reactions tend toward equilibrium. Among the first of these processes is that of ion equilibration across all compartments as ion pumps loose their energy supplies. In muscle cells, both cisternal and extracellular calcium leak into the sarcoplasm.

The high levels of calcium induce conformational changes in the troponin-tropomyosin complex, and exposes myosin-binding sites on thin filaments. This uncontrolled contractile activity leads to total exhaustion of ATP supplies and ends with all myosin molecules in cross-linked actomyosin complexes. The rigid state of muscles that develops shortly after death is known as **rigor mortis**.

Blood Coagulation

23

The body's ability to control bleeding following vascular injury is important for survival. Blood clotting is a good example of a clinically relevant process that is controlled by sequential enzymatic reactions. The events of blood clotting and the subsequent dissolution that follow tissue repair, involves a **cascade of zymogen activations**, what is termed as **hemostasis.** Hemostasis includes four major sequential events that follow vascular injury:

1. The **vascular constriction** that decreases blood flow to the injured area is the first phase.
2. The formation of loose **platelet plug** at the site of injury by platelets activated by thrombin is the second phase. Collagen is the primary stimulus for platelet clumping. Platelets are activated on binding to collagen, which is exposed following damage to the endothelial lining of vessels. Activation of platelets changes their shape to accommodate the formation of plug and induces release of its contents: **adenosine-5'-diphosphate, ADP** and **TXA$_2$, serotonin, phospholipids, lipoproteins**, and **other proteins** important for the coagulation cascade.
3. *Stabilization of loose* **platelet plug** by a *fibrin mesh* (also called the clot) is the third phase. If the plug contains only platelets it is termed a *white thrombus*; if it also includes red blood cells it is called a *red thrombus*.
4. *Dissolution of clot* to restore blood flow following tissue damage repair is the fourth phase. The dissolution of the clot occurs through the action of **plasmin**.

Fibrin mesh formation occurs by two pathways—one intrinsic and the other extrinsic. The two pathways are initiated by different mechanism, but converge on a common pathway that leads to clot formation. The formation of a **red thrombus** or a clot in response to an **abnormal vessel wall** without tissue injury is the result of the **intrinsic pathway**. The formation of **fibrin clot** following **tissue injury** is the result of the **extrinsic pathway**. Both pathways are complex and involve numerous different proteins termed clotting factors.

Von Willebrand Factor (vWF) is a Platelet Adherence Factor that Activates Platelets

The von Willebrand factor (vWF) mediates adhesion and aggregation of platelets to the exposed collagen on endothelial cell surfaces and the release of platelet contents. Von Willebrand disease is an inherited deficiency of vWF, which acts as a bridge between a specific glycoprotein on the platelets surface and collagen fibrils, in addition factor VIII binding by vWF is required for normal survival of factor VIII in the circulation.

Von Willebrand factor is a complex multimeric glycoprotein that is produced by and stored in the α-granules of platelets. It is also synthesized by megakaryocytes and found associated with subendothelial connective tissue.

The initial activation of platelets that initiate a signal transduction cascade is the result of thrombin binding to specific receptors on the platelet surface, which is coupled to a G-protein. Such binding activates phospholipase C-γ (PLC-γ) that hydrolyzes phosphatidylinositol-4, 5-biphosphate (PIP_2) leading to the formation of inositol-3, 4, 5- triphosphate (IP_3) and diacylglycerol (DAG). In turn stored intracellular Ca^{2+} is released by IP_3, and *protein kinase* C (PKC) is activated by DAG.

Platelets adhesion to collagen and release of intracellular Ca^{2+} leads to the activation of $4(PLA_2)$, which then hydrolyzes membrane phospholipids, leading to liberation of arachidonic acid. The arachidonic acid release leads to the production and subsequent release of thromboxane A_2 (TXA_2). This is another platelet activator that functions through the PLC-γ pathway. The released Ca^{2+} from intracellular stores also activates *myosin light chain kinase* (MLCK) that phosphorylates the light chain of myosin, which then interacts with actin, resulting in altered platelet morphology and motility.

One of the many effects of PKC is the phosphorylation and activation of a specific 47,000-Dalton platelet protein. This activated protein induces the release of platelet granule contents; one of which is ADP. ADP further stimulates platelets increasing the overall activation cascade; it also modifies the platelet membrane in such a way to allow fibrinogen to adhere to two platelet surface glycoproteins, GPIIb and GPIIIa, leading to fibrinogen-induced platelet aggregation.

Activation of platelets is required for aggregation into a platelet plug. However, equally significant is the activation of platelet surface phospholipids in the activation of the coagulation cascade.

PRIMARY FACTORS OF BLOOD COAGULATION

Factor	Trivial Name	Pathway	Characteristic
Prekallikrein	Fletcher factor	Intrinsic	——
High-molecular-weight kininogen (HMWK)	Contact activation cofactor; Fitzgerald, Flaujeac William's factor	Intrinsic	——
I	Fibrinogen	Both	——
II	Prothrombin	Both	Contains N-term *gla* segment
III	Tissue factor	Extrinsic	——
IV	Calcium	Both	——
V	Proaccelerin, labile factor, accelerator (Ac-) globulin	Both	Protein cofactor
VI (Va)	Accelerin	——	This is Va, reduntant to factor V
VII	Proconvertin, serum prothrombin conversion accelerator (SPCA), cothromboplastin	Extrinsic	Endopeptidase with *gla* residues
VIII	Antihemophilic factor A, antihemophilic globulin (AHG)	Intrinsic	Protein cofactor
IX	Christmas factor, antihemophilic factor B, plasma thromboplastin component (PTC)	Intrinsic	Endopeptidase with *gla* residues
X	Stuart-Prower factor	Both	Endopeptidase with *gla* residues
XI	Plasma thromboplastin antecedent (PTA)	Intrinsic	Endopeptidase
XII	Hageman's factor	Intrinsic	Endopeptidase
XIII	Protransglutaminase, fibrin stabilizing factor (FSF) fibrinoligase	Both	Transpeptidase

FUNCTIONAL CLASSIFICATION OF CLOTTING FACTORS

Functional class	Activity
Fibrinogen	
Factor I	Cleaved by thrombin to form fibrin clot
Transglutaminase	
Factor XIII	Activated by thrombin in presence of Ca^{2+}; stabilizes fibrin clot by covalent cross-linking
Cofactors	
Factor VIII	Activated by thrombin; Factor VIIIa is a cofactor in the activation of factor X by factor IXa
Factor V	Activated by thrombin; Factor Va is a cofactor in the activation of prothrombin by factor Xa
Factor III (tissue factor)	A subendothelial cell-surface glycoprotein that acts as a cofactor for Factor VII
Zymogene of serine proteases	
Factor XII	Binds to exposed collagen at site of vessel wall injury, activated by high-MW kininogen and Kallikrein
Factor XI	Activated by factor XIIa
Factor IX	Activated by factor XIa in presence of Ca^{2+}
Factor VII	Activated by thrombin in presence of Ca^{2+}
FactorX	Activated on surface of activated platelets by tenase complex and by factor VIIa in presence of tissue factor and Ca^{2+}
Factor II	Activated on surface of activated platelets by prothrombinase complex
Regulatory and other proteins	
Von Willebrand factor	Associated with subendothelial connective tissue; serves as a bridge between platelet and glycoprotein GPIb/ IX and collagen
Protein C	Activated to protein Ca by thrombin bound to thrombomodulin; then degrades factors VIIIa and Va.
Protein S	Acts as a cofactor of protein C; both proteins contain gla (γ-carboxyglutamyl) residues
Thrombomodulin	Protein on the surface of endothelial cells; binds thrombin, which then activates protein C
Antithrombin III	Most important coagulation inhibitor, controls activities of thrombin, and factors IXa, Xa, XIa and XIIa.

THE CLOTTING CASCADES

Intrinsic Clotting Cascade Functions in the Absence of Tissue Injury

Intrinsic pathway commences with the exposure of prekalikrein, high molecular weight kininogen, factors XII and XI to an activating surface (perhaps collagen exposed at vessel surface *in vivo*), which is called "contact phase". The intrinsic pathway also requires factors VIII, IX, calcium ions and phospholipids of platelet membrane.

The assemblage of contact phase components results in conversion of prekallikrein to kallikrein, which in turn activates factor XII to factor XIIa. Factor XIIa can then hydrolyze more prekallikrein to kallikrein, establishing a reciprocal activation cascade (water fall effect). Factor

XIIa also activates factor XI to factor XIa and leads to the release of bradykinin, a potent vasodilator, from high-molecular-weight kininogen (Fig. 23.1).

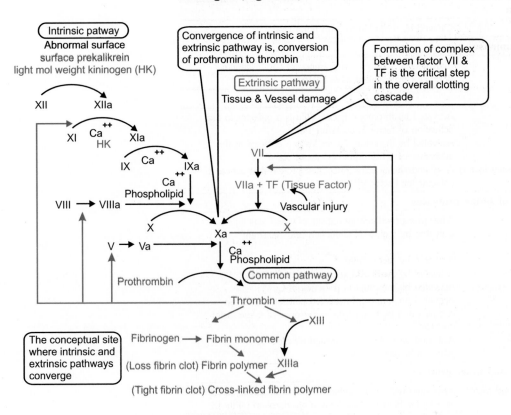

Fig. 23.1: Blood clotting cascade

In the presence of Ca^{2+}, factor XIa activates factor IX to factor IXa. Factor IX is a proenzyme that contains γ-carboxyglutamate (*gla*) residues, whose serine protease activity is activated following Ca^{2+} binding to these gla residues. Several of the serine proteases of the cascade (II, VII, IX, and X) are also gla-containing proenzymes. Active factor IXa cleaves factor X at an internal arginine-isoleucine bond leading to its activation to factor Xa.

The activation of factor X to Xa requires assemblage of *tenase complex* (Ca^{2+} and factors VIIIa, IXa and X) on the surface of activated platelets. One of the responses of platelets to activation is the presentation of phosphatidylserine and phosphatidylinositol on their surfaces. The exposure of these phospholipids allows the tenase complex to form. The role of factor VIIIa in this process is to act as a receptor for factor IXa as it cleaves the Arg-Ile bond of factorX. The activation of factor VIII to factor VIIIa (the actual receptor) occurs in the presence of minute quantities of thrombin. As the concentration of thrombin increases, factor VIIIa is ultimately cleaved by thrombin and inactivated. This dual action of thrombin, upon factor VIII, acts to limit the extent of tenase complex formation and thus the extent of the coagulation cascade.

Extrinsic Clotting Cascade is in Response to Tissue Injury

The extrinsic pathway is initiated at the site of injury in response to the release of tissue factor (factor III), which is a cofactor in the factor VIIa-catalyzed activation of factor X. Factor VIIa, a *gla* residue containing serine protease, cleaves factor X to factor Xa in a manner identical to that of factor IXa of the intrinsic pathway. The activation of factor VII occurs through the action of thrombin or factor Xa.

The ability of factor Xa to activate factor VII creates a link between the intrinsic and extrinsic pathways. An additional link between the two pathways exists through the ability of tissue factor and factor VIIa to activate factor IX.

The formation of complex between factor VIIa and tissue factor is believed to be a principal step in the overall clotting cascade. Evidence for these stems from the fact, that persons with hereditary deficiencies in the components of the contact phase of the intrinsic pathway do not exhibit clotting problems.

A major mechanism for the inhibition of the extrinsic pathway occurs at the complex formed by tissue factor, factor VIIa, Ca^{2+} and factor Xa. The lipoprotein-associated coagulation inhibitor (LACI, formerly named anticonvertin) specifically binds to this complex. LACI is composed of three tandem protease inhibitor domains. Domain 1 binding to factor Xa and domain 2 binding to factor VIIa occurs only in the presence of factor Xa.

Activation of Prothrombin to Thrombin Occurs on the Platelet

The actual convergence point of intrinsic and extrinsic pathways is the conversion of prothrombin to thrombin by factor Xa, which occurs on the platelet. Thrombin in turn, converts fibrinogen to fibrin. The activation of prothrombin (factor II) to thrombin (factor IIa) that occurs on the surface of activated platelets requires formation of a **prothrombinase complex**. This complex is composed of the platelet phospholipids; phosphatidylinositol and phosphatidylserine (exposed by platelet disruption and degranulation), Ca^{2+}, factors Va from platelet which acts as a receptor for factor Xa, which in turn binds prothrombin.

Factor V is a cofactor in the formation of the prothrombinase complex, similar to the role of factor VIII in **tenase complex** formation.

Like factor VIII activation, factor V is activated to factor Va by means of minute amounts and is inactivated by increased levels of thrombin. Factor Va binds to specific receptors on the surfaces of activated platelets and forms a complex with prothrombin and factor Xa.

Prothrombin is a 72,000-Dalton, single-chain protein containing ten gla residues in its N-terminal region. Within the prothrombinase complex, prothrombin is cleaved at two sites by factor Xa. This cleavage generates a two-chain active thrombin molecule containing an A and a B chain, which are held together by a single disulfide bond.

Thrombin in addition to activation of fibrin clot formation plays an important regulatory role in coagulation. The complex formation between thrombin and thrombomodulin present on endothelial cell surfaces converts protein C to protein Ca. Protein Ca and protein S degrade factors Va and VIIIa, thereby their activity in coagulation cascade is regulated.

Antithrombin-III (AT-III) is an Important Regulator of Thrombin Activation

Uncontrolled activity of circulating levels of active form of thrombin would lead to serious consequences, which is regulated by two principal mechanisms. The predominant form of thrombin in the circulation is the inactive prothrombin, whose activation requires the pathways of proenzyme activation described earlier for the clotting cascade. At each step in the cascade, feedback mechanisms regulate the balance between active and inactive forms of enzymes.

Four specific thrombin inhibitors regulate thrombin activation of which ***antithrombin-III*** is the most important since it can also inhibit the activities of factors IXa, Xa, XIa and XIIa. The basis for clinical use of heparin as an anticoagulant is its ability to bind to specific site on antithrombin-III, thereby inducing a conformational change in the antithrombin-III molecule (Fig. 23.2). Antithrombin-III with the new conformation has higher affinity for binding and inactivating thrombin as well as its other substrates. The naturally occurring activator of antithrombin-III is present as heparan and heparan sulfate on the surface of vessel endothelial cells. It is the feature that controls the activation of the intrinsic coagulation cascade.

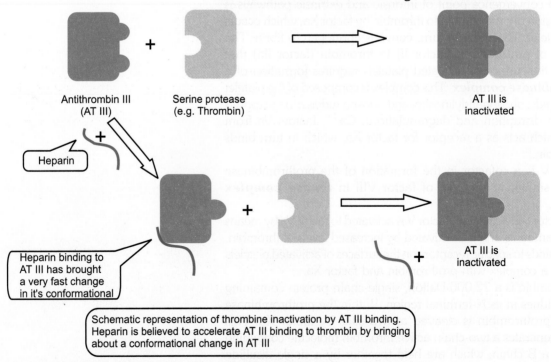

Antithrombin III (AT III) Serine protease (e.g. Thrombin) AT III is inactivated

Heparin

Heparin binding to AT III has brought a very fast change in it's conformational

AT III is inactivated

Schematic representation of thrombine inactivation by AT III binding. Heparin is believed to accelerate AT III binding to thrombin by bringing about a conformational change in AT III

Fig. 23.2: Schematic representation of thrombine inactivation by AT III binding. Heparin is believed to accelerated AT III binding to thrombin by bringing about a conformational change in AT III

However, thrombin activity is also inhibited by α_2-**macroglobulin**, **heparin cofactor II** and α_1-**antitrypsin**. Although α_1-antitrypsin is a minor player in thrombin regulation, it is the primary serine protease inhibitor of human plasma. Its physiological significance is demonstrated by the fact that lack of this protein plays a causative role in the development of emphysema particularly in tobacco smokers.

Activation of Fibrinogen to Fibrin is by Proteolysis between Fibrinopeptides

Fibrinogen (factor I) consists of three pairs of polypeptides ([A-α], [B-β], and [γ])$_2$, which are covalently linked near their N-terminals through disulfide bonds. The A and B portions of the A-α and B-β chains comprise the fibrinopeptides, A and B, respectively. The fibrinopeptide regions of fibrinogen contain several glutamate and aspartate residues imparting a high negative charge to this region and aid in the solubility of fibrinogen in plasma. Active thrombin is a serine protease that hydrolyses fibrinogen at four arg-gly bonds between the fibrinopeptides and the α and β portions of the protein (Fig. 23.3).

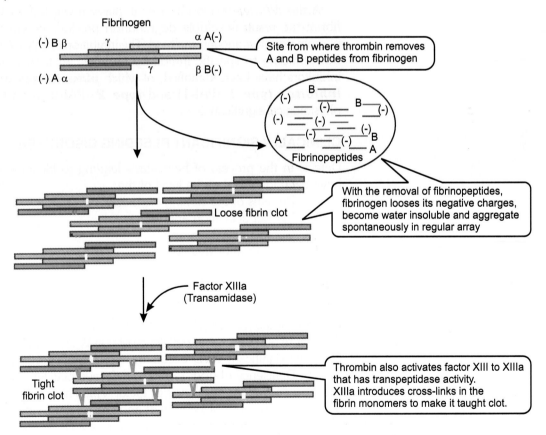

Fig. 23.3: Fibrin clot formation

Thrombin-mediated release of the fibrinopeptides generates fibrin monomers with a subunit structure (α–β-and $\gamma)_2$. These monomers spontaneously aggregate in a regular array, forming a somewhat weak fibrin clot. In addition to fibrin activation, thrombin converts factor XIII to factor XIIIa, a highly specific transglutaminase that introduces cross-links composed of covalent bonds between the amide nitrogen of glutamines and ϵ-amino group of lysines in the fibrin monomers.

Function of Plasmin is Dissolution of Fibrin Clots

Fibrin clots are degraded by plasmin, a serine protease that circulates as plasminogen (the inactive proenzyme). Any free circulating plasmin is rapidly inhibited by α_2-antiplasmin. Plasminogen binds to both fibrinogen and fibrin, thereby being incorporated into a clot as it is formed. **Tissue plasminogen activator** (tPA) and **urokinase** are serine proteases, which convert plasminogen to plasmin. Inactive tPA is released from vascular endothelial cells following injury; it binds to fibrin and is consequently activated. Urokinase is produced as the precursor, **prourokinase** by epithelial cells lining excretory ducts. The role of urokinase is to activate the dissolution of fibrin clots that may be deposited in these ducts.

Active tPA cleaves plasminogen to plasmin which then digests the fibrin; the result is soluble degradation product to which neither plasmin nor plasminogen can bind. The inhibition of tPA activity results from binding to specific inhibitory proteins. At least four distinct inhibitors have been identified, of which **plasminogen activator-inhibitor type 1** (PAI-1) and **type 2** (PAI-2) are of greatest physiological significance.

CLINICALLY SIGNIFICANT BLEEDING DISORDERS

Defects in the process of hemostasis leading to bleeding disorders have been identified at the level of the:

- a. Proteins of the clotting cascades,
- b. Platelet activation and function,
- c. Contact activation and
- d. Antithrombin function.

Von Willebrand Disease Leads to Defective Platelet Adhesion

Von Willebrand disease (vWD) is the most common inherited bleeding disorder of humans due to deficiency of von Willebrand factor (vWF). Clinically significant vWD occurs in approximatley 125 people per million. Deficiency of vWF results in defective platelet adhesion and causes a secondary deficiency of factor VIII. The result is that vWF deficiency can cause bleeding that appears similar to that caused by platelet dysfunction or hemophilia. vWD is an extremely heterogeneous disorder that has been classified into several major subtypes. Type I vWD is the most common and is inherited as an autosomal dominant trait. This variant is due to simple quantitative deficiency of all vWF multimers. Type 2 vWD is subdivided further dependent upon whether the dysfunctional protein has decreased or paradoxically increased function in certain laboratory tests of binding to platelets. Type 3 vWD is clinically severe and is characterized by recessive inheritence and total absence of vWF.

Factor XI Deficiency Affect Contact Activation

Factor XI deficiency is an autosomal disorder with either homozygosity or compound heterozygosity, which is very common in Ashkenazic Jews. Three independent point mutations in factor XI have been identified. This deficiency was originally termed hemophilia C. When blood makes contact with negatively charged surfaces it triggers a series of interactions that involve factor XI, prekallikrein and high molecular weight kininogen leading to blood coagulation. This process is referred to as contact activation. Deficiency in factor XI leads to an injury-related bleeding tendency.

Hemophilia A (Inability to Clot Blood) is due to Deficiency of Factor VIII

It is an X-linked disorder resulting from a deficiency in factor VIII, which is a key component of the coagulation cascade. The level of active factor VIII in the plasma is reflected as severe, moderate and mild forms of hemophilia A.

Variety of different point mutations have been characterized in the factor VIII gene in hemophilia A. Frequency of inheritance of the disorder is about 1:10,000 males. Factor VIII is a cofactor in the activation of factor X to factor Xa in a reaction catalyzed by factor Xa. Activation of factor VIII occurs via proteolytic cleavage by thrombin and factor Xa. Inactivation of factor VIIIa occurs by limited proteolysis by factor Xa or activated protein C.

Individuals with factor VIII deficiencies suffer hemorrhage in joint and muscle, easy bruising and prolonged bleeding from wounds. Treatment of hemophilia A is by infusion of factor VIII concentrates prepared from either human plasma or by recombinant DNA technology.

Hemophilia B is the Result of Factor IX Deficiency

The prevalence of hemophilia B is approximately 1:100,000. All patients with hemophilia B have prolonged coagulation time and decreased factor IX clotting activity. Like hemophilia A, there are severe, moderate and mild forms of hemophilia B and reflect the factor IX activity in plasma.

More than 300 unique factor IX mutations have been identified, 85 percent are point mutations, 3 percent are short nucleotide deletions or insertions and 12 percent are gross gene alterations.

Disorders of Fibrinogen is Linked to Several Diseases

An elevated plasma fibrinogen levels have been observed in patients with coronary artery disease, diabetes, hypertension, peripheral artery disease, hyperlipoproteinemia and hypertriglyceridemia. In addition, pregnancy, menopause, hypercholesterolemia, use of oral contraceptives and smoking lead to increased plasma fibrinogen levels.

Inherited disorders in fibrinogen are rare. These disorders include *afibrinogenemia* (a complete lack of fibrinogen), *hypofibrinogenemia* (reduced levels of fibrinogen) and *dysfibrinogenemia* (presence of dysfunctional fibrinogen). Afibrinogenemia is an inherited autosomal recessive disorder characterized by neonatal umbilical cord hemorrhage, ecchymoses, mucosal hemorrhage, internal hemorrhage, and recurrent abortion. Hypofibrinogenemia is either acquired or inherited condition characterized by fibrinogen levels below 100 mg/dL (normal is 250-350 mg/dL). Symptoms of hypofibrinogememia are less severe than afibrinogenemia. Dysfibrinogenemias are extremely heterogeneous affecting any of the functional properties of fibrinogen. Clinical consequences of dysfibrinogenemias include hemorrhage, spontaneous abortion and thromboembolism.

Factor XIII Deficiency is Characterized by Delayed Bleeding

Factor XIII is the proenzyme form of plasma *transglutaminase* and is activated by thrombin in the presence of calcium ions. Active factor XIII catalyzes the cross-linking of fibrin monomers. Factor XIII is a tetramer of two different peptides, α and β (forming $\alpha_2\beta_2$). It is an autosomal recessive inherited disorder resulting in the absence of either subunit. Factor XIII deficiency is characterized by normal primary hemostasis but delayed bleeding. Deficiency leads to neonatal umbilical cord bleeding, intracranial hemorrhage and soft tissue hematomas.

Antithrombin Deficiency Manifests as Venous Thromboembolic Disorders

Several activated coagulation factors including thrombin, factor IXa and factor Xa, are inhibited by antithrombin forming a stable complex. Antithrombin activity is enhanced at least 1000 fold by heparan and heparan sulfate.

It is inherited as autosomal dominant trait. Approximately 2 percent of venous thromboembolic diseases are due to deficiency of antithrombin. Deficiencies are the result of mutations that affect synthesis or stability of antithrombin or from mutations that affect the protease and/or heparin binding sites of antithrombin.

Common clinical manifestations of antithrombin deficiency are deep vein thrombosis and pulmonary embolism. Arterial thrombosis is rare in antithrombin deficiency. Thrombosis may occur spontaneously or in association with surgery, trauma or pregnancy. Acute episodes of thrombosis are treated with heparin infusion (for 5 to 7 days) followed by oral anticoagulant therapy.

PHARMACOLOGICAL INTERVENTIONS IN BLEEDING

Useful anticoagulants in treating bleeding disorders include coumarin drugs, such as warfarin as well as the glycosaminoglycans, heparin and heparan sulfate.

a. *Heparin* is useful as an anticoagulant because it binds to, and activates, antithrombin-III, which then inhibits the serine proteases of the coagulation cascade.

b. *Coumarin drugs* inhibit coagulation by inhibiting the vitamin K-dependent γ-carboxylation reactions necessary to the function of thrombin, factors VII, IX, and X as well as proteins C and S. These drugs act by inhibiting the reduction of the quinone derivatives of vitamin K to their active hydroquinone forms. Because of the mode of action of coumarin drugs, it takes several days for their maximum effect to be realized. For this reason, heparin is normally administered first followed by warfarin or warfarin-related drugs.

c. *Plasminogen activators* (Streptokinase) also are useful for controlling coagulation. Because tPA is highly selective for the degradation of fibrin in clots, it is extremely useful in restoring the patency of the coronary arteries following thrombosis, in particular during the short period following myocardial infarct. *Streptokinase* (an enzyme from the *streptococci* bacterium) is a plasminogen activator useful from a therapeutic standpoint. However, it is less selective than tPA, being able to activate circulating plasminogen as well as that bound to a fibrin clot.

d. *Aspirin* is an important inhibitor of platelet activation. By virtue of inhibiting the activity of *cyclooxygenase*, aspirin reduces the production of TXA_2. Aspirin also reduces the endothelial cells' production of prostacyclin (PGI_2), an inhibitor of platelet aggregation and a vasodilator. Since endothelial cells regenerate active *cyclooxygenase* faster than platelets, the net effect of aspirin is more in favor of endothelial cell-mediated inhibition of the coagulation cascade.

UNIT-II
Metabolism and Biochemical Genetics

Signal Transduction Cascades

24

The overall cellular metabolism is regulated by three principal ways:

1. **Amount of enzymes available** depends upon rate of synthesis and degradation. Altering the rate of transcription mostly brings about changes in enzyme concentration.

2. **Catalytic activities of enzymes** are altered by allosteric modulation (e.g. feedback inhibition) and reversible covalent modification

3. **Flux of substrates**: Transfer of substrates from one compartment to another (e.g. pyruvate from cytosol to mitochondria), compartmentalization of biosynthetic and degradative pathways, and the energy status of the cell.

    Ribonucleotides play an important role in overall control of cellular metabolism. Activated carrier molecules such as ATP, NADH, $FADH_2$, and coenzyme A all contain adenine phosphate units. Earliest catalysts were RNA molecules called ribozymes. Non-RNA units were accommodated later in evolution to serve as efficient carriers of activated electrons and chemical units, a function that RNA cannot do. Even when proteins replaced RNA as catalysts, ribonucleotide coenzymes remained the same.

    Signal transduction cascades direct the overall control of cellular metabolism.

Signal Transduction Cascades

At a cellular level *signal transduction* refers to movement of signals from outside of the cell to inside of the cell. Such movement of signals can be simple, like that associated with receptor molecules of the acetylcholine class involved in propagation of nerve impulse. These receptors constitute channels, which upon ligand interaction allow signals to be passed in the form of small ion movement, either into or out of the cell. Such ion movements result in changes in the electrical potential of the cells that in turn propagates the signal along the cell. More complex signal transduction involves the coupling of ligand-receptor interactions to many intracellular events. These events include phosphorylation of enzyme proteins by serine/threonine kinases and tyrosine kinases, or the phosphorylation and dephosphorylation of protein enzyme by kinases and phosphatases, which change their conformation and activities. The final outcome is an alteration in cellular activity and expression of the program of genes within the responding cells.

CLASSIFICATION OF SIGNAL TRANSDUCING RECEPTORS

Receptors of signal transduction broadly fall under three classes:

1. **Transmembrane receptors with intrinsic enzyme activity,** which includes *Tyrosine kinases* (e.g. PDGF, insulin, EGF and FGF receptors), *Tyrosine phosphatases* (e.g. CD45 [*cluster determinant-45*] and protein of T cells and macrophages) *Guanylate cyclases* (e.g. natriuretic peptide receptors), and *serine/ threonine kinases* (e.g. activin and TGF-β receptors).

   Receptors with intrinsic tyrosine kinase activity are capable of autophosphorylation as well as phosphorylation of other substrates. Additionally, several families of receptors lack intrinsic enzyme activity yet are coupled to intracellular tyrosine kinases by direct protein-protein interactions.

2. **G-protein coupled receptors** that are coupled inside the cell to GTP-binding and hydrolyzing proteins. These receptors are called serpentine receptors, since they have seven transmembrane spanning domains. Examples of this class are the adrenergic receptors, odorant receptors, and certain hormone receptors (e.g. glucagon, angiotensin, vasopressin and bradykinin).

3. **Intracellular receptors** that upon ligand binding is translocated into the nucleus, where the *ligand-receptor complex* binds to specific sequences on the DNA and affects the gene transcription. Many enzymes are regulated by covalent modifications, wherein a phosphate group is attached to the hydroxyl group of one or more of its aminoacyl residues such as serine, threonine, or tyrosine. Such phosphorylation reactions are catalyzed by **protein kinases**, which transfer the terminal phosphate group of ATP to a hydroxyl group on a protein (Fig. 24.1). **Protein phosphatase** is another enzyme that catalyzes the hydrolytic removal of these phosphate groups. These two enzymes together regulate the activity of other enzymes by phosphorylating and dephosphorylating them.

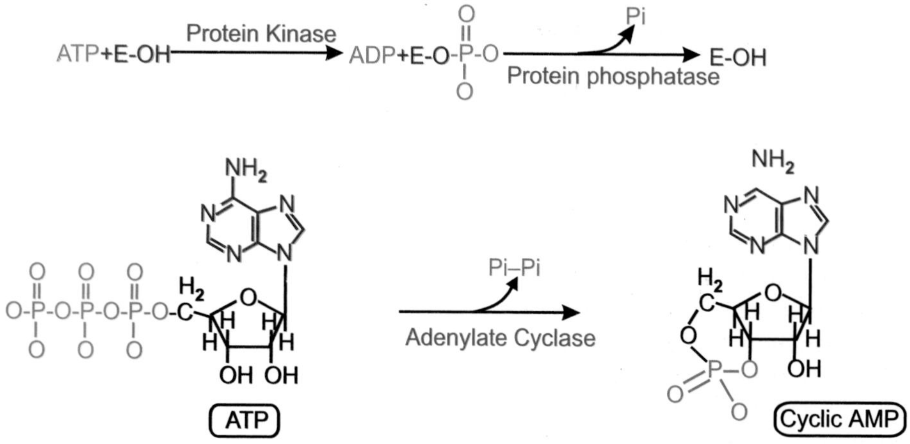

Fig. 24.1: Cyclic AMP formation

Protein kinases and phosphatases themselves are under complex regulatory signal cascades that are often initiated by binding of a hormone to a membrane receptor on the outer surface of a cell. One such kinase that regulates enzymes of metabolism is **cyclic AMP-dependent protein kinase** (Protein kinase A).

Cyclic-AMP (**cAMP**) is suited to function as a transient signal since it hydrolyzes spontaneous, but is kinetically stable in the absence of an enzyme that catalyzes its hydrolysis. Enzymes that synthesize and degrade cAMP are tightly regulated.

Adenylate cyclase catalyzes (Fig. 24.1): $ATP \rightarrow cAMP + PP_i$

Pyrophosphatase drives the reaction forward by hydrolyzing: $PP_i \rightarrow 2 P_i$

Phosphodiesterase catalyzes: $cAMP \rightarrow AMP$

Cyclic AMP is called a "**second messenger**" since binding of certain hormones (e.g., epinephrine) to specific receptors on the outer surface of a cell, activates *adenylate cyclase* that catalyzes formation of cAMP within the cell. Binding of cAMP activates *cAMP-dependent protein kinase*, which in turn bring about phosphorylation of the hydroxyl group of a serine or threonine that is part of a particular 5-amino acid sequence.

cAMP-dependent protein kinase (PKA) is a tetramer consisting of two regulatory subunits -'**R**' and two catalytic subunits -'**C**'. Each regulatory subunit contains a **pseudosubstrate** sequence comparable to the substrate domain of a target protein for protein kinase A, but with alanine substituting for the serine or threonine thus lack hydroxyl groups that can be phosphorylated. When PKA is inactive the pseudosubstrate domain of the regulatory subunit, binds to the active site of the catalytic subunit, blocking its activity. When cAMP molecules bind to each of the regulatory subunits, a conformational change makes the regulatory subunits to get separated from catalytic subunits. Each catalytic subunit '**C**' can then catalyze phosphorylation of serine or threonine residues on target proteins.

$$R_2C_2 + 4\ cAMP \rightarrow R_2\ 4cAMP + 2C$$

G-PROTEIN SIGNAL CASCADE

Binding of hormone (epinephrine or glucagons) to a 7-helix receptor (Rhodopsin) also called **G-protein coupled receptor (GPCR)** at the outer surface of cell membrane bring about the activation of **G-protein** that is in contact with the GPCR on the inner surface of the membrane. The *G-protein* has 3 subunits: α, β, and γ. The α subunit binds **GTP**, and can hydrolyze it to GDP. If part of a stimulatory pathway, G-protein may be called G_s, and subunits $G_{s\,\alpha}$, etc.

The complex of β and γ subunits inhibits G_α. The α and γ subunits have covalently attached lipid tails that is embedded in the plasma membrane that bind the G-protein to the cytosolic surface of the plasma membrane. Adenylate cyclase (AC) is a transmembrane protein, with cytosolic domains forming the catalytic site.

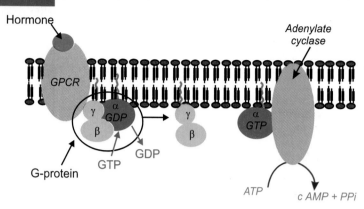

Hormone

GPCR

G-protein

Adenylate cyclase

GTP

GDP

ATP

c AMP + PPi

Fig. 24.2: cAMP dependent protein kinase activation

The Sequence of Eevents in the Signal Cascade

Initially the α, β, and γ subunits of G-protein are complexed together and GDP is bound to the α-subunit. Hormone binding to GPCR causes a conformational change in the receptor that is transmitted to the G-protein. The nucleotide-binding site on G_α becomes more accessible to the cytosol, where GTP concentration is usually higher than GDP. The G_α releases GDP and binds GTP (GDP-GTP exchange). Substitution of GTP for GDP causes another conformational change in G_α. Now the G_α-GTP subunit dissociates from the inhibitory β–γ subunit complex, and can now bind to and activate adenylate cyclase. The *adenylate cyclase*, activated by G_α-GTP, catalyzes synthesis of cAMP. Binding of cAMP, to cAMP *dependent protein kinase* catalyzes phosphorylation of various cellular proteins, and alters their activity (Fig. 24.2).

Turning Off of the Signal

GTPase activity of G_α hydrolyzes bound GTP to GDP + P_i. The presence of GDP on G_α causes it to re-associate with the inhibitory β–γ complex and there are no more stimuli for *adenylate cyclase* to synthesize cAMP. Whatever quantity of cAMP that has already been formed is hydrolyzed to AMP by the activity of *phosphodiesterase*.

Desensitization of hormone receptors occurs by a complex process, which varies with the hormone. Protein phosphatase catalyzes hydrolytic removal of phosphates that were attached to proteins by protein kinase A.

Signal Amplification is an Important Feature of Signal Cascades

One hormone molecule can lead to formation of many cAMP molecules. Each catalytic subunit of cAMP dependent protein kinase catalyzes phosphorylation of many proteins during the lifetime of the cAMP.

Some species of $\mathbf{G_\alpha}$ are inhibitory rather than stimulatory. Different effectors and their receptors induce $\mathbf{G_{i\alpha}}$ to exchange GDP for GTP than those that activate $\mathbf{G_{s\alpha}}$. In some cells $\mathbf{G_{\beta\gamma}}$, which is released when G_α binds GTP is itself an effector that binds to and activates other proteins.

Some clinically important compounds that affect these signal cascades include:

Cholera toxin that catalyzes covalent modification of $\mathbf{G_{s\alpha}}$. ADP-ribose is transferred from NAD^+ to $G_{s\alpha}$. ADP-ribosylated $G_{s\alpha}$ cannot hydrolyze GTP. Thus $\mathbf{G_{s\alpha}}$ becomes permanently activated.

Pertussis toxin (whooping cough disease) catalyzes ADP-ribosylation of $\mathbf{G_{i\alpha}}$, making it incapable of exchanging GDP for GTP. Thus the inhibitory pathway is blocked.

The family of *heterotrimeric G-proteins* includes:

Transducin present in rods and cones of retina is involved in perception of light.

A G-protein present in olfactory neurons is involved in **odorant sensing**.

There is a larger family of small GTP-binding switch-proteins related to G_α

They include:

Initiation and elongation factors (protein synthesis)

Ras (growth factor signal cascades)

Rab (membrane vesicle targeting and fusion)

ARF (formation of vesicle coatomer coats)

Ran (transport of proteins into and out of the nucleus)

Rho (regulation of actin cytoskeleton)

All GTP-binding proteins undergo conformational change depending on whether GTP or GDP is present at their nucleotide-binding site. In general, GTP-binding proteins are in the active state when GTP is bound.

Most enzymes have evolved to maximize catalytic efficiency. G-proteins and the small GTP-binding proteins are relatively inefficient at hydrolyzing GTP. This results in a relatively long-lived activated state, and provides opportunities for regulation.

Many GTP-binding proteins depend on helper proteins. GTPase activating proteins (GAPs) promote GTP hydrolysis.

Guanine nucleotide exchange factors (GEFs) promote GDP/GTP exchange.

One of the GAPs provides an essential active site residue, while promoting a conformation that favors catalysis. GAPs and GEFs are themselves regulated. The activated receptor (GPCR) serves as GEF for a heterotrimeric G-protein.

The *nucleotide-binding site* in each GTP-binding switch-protein consists of loops that extend out from the edge of a β-sheet, which is usually 6-stranded. The P-loop that connects one of the β-strands with an α-helix makes contact with the terminal phosphates of GTP.

Three switch domains have been identified, that change position when GTP substitutes for GDP on G_α. These domains include residues adjacent to the terminal phosphate of GTP and/or the Mg^{++} associated with the two terminal phosphates.

The β subunit of the inhibitory G-protein has a β-propeller structure, formed from multiple repeats of a sequence called the WD-repeat. The β-propeller acts as a scaffold for the binding site for G_α.

PHOSPHATIDYLINOSITOL CASCADE

The membrane lipid **phosphatidylinositol** (Fig. 24.3) activates the signal cascade of some hormones.

The sequences of events are:

1. The inosital part of phosphatidylinositol found in plasma membrane is sequentially phosphorylated (ATP is the phosphate

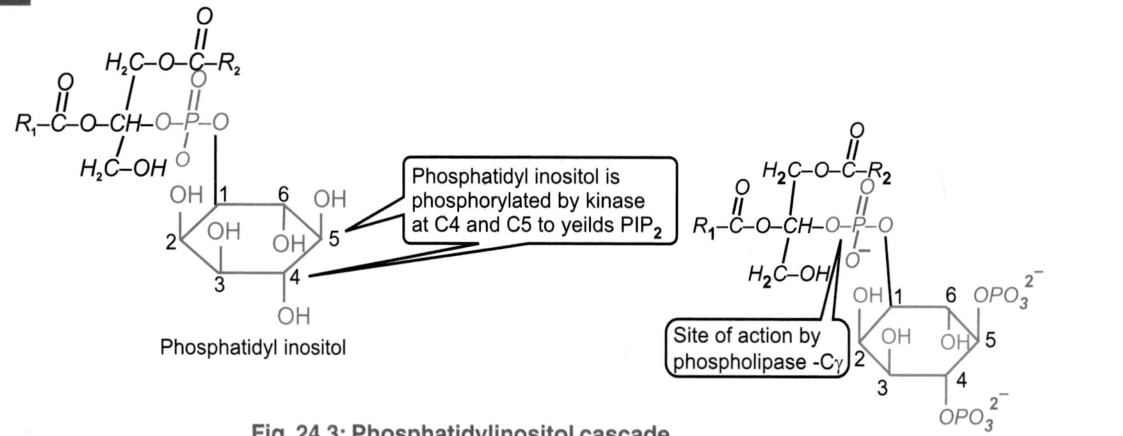

Phosphatidyl inositol

Phosphatidylinositol 4,5-bisphosphate (PIP_2)

Fig. 24.3: Phosphatidylinositol cascade

donor) by a *kinase* to yield phosphatidylinositol-4, 5-bisphosphate (**PIP_2**).

2. Phosphatidylinositol-4,5-bisphosphate is cleaved by *phospholipase C-γ (PLC-γ)* an enzyme that has active site domain, a domain that anchors it to the plasma membrane, and a Ca^{++}-binding domain. Binding of a hormone or other extracellular agonist activates GPCR by GTP exchange for GDP. Then G_{α}-GTP activates phospholipase C-γ.
3. Cleavage of PIP_2 by phospholipase C yields two second-messengers, inositol trisphosphate (**IP_3**), and diacylglycerol (**DG**) (Fig. 24.4).

Diacylglycerol, with Ca^{++}, activates *protein kinase C (PKC),* which catalyzes phosphorylation of several cellular proteins and alter their activity. Inositol-1, 3,4-trisphosphate (IP_3) activates Ca^{++} channels in endoplasmic reticulum (ER) membranes. Ca^{++} stored in the ER is released to the cytosol, where it may bind to calmodulin, or may

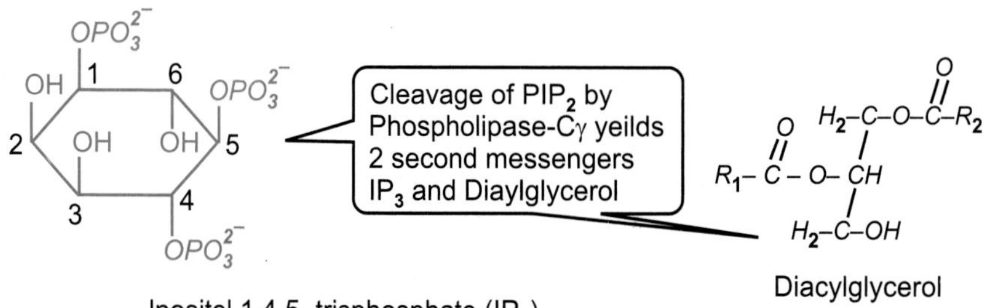

Inositol 1,4,5. trisphosphate (IP_3)

Diacylglycerol

Fig. 24.4: Calcium-ATPase pump activation

help to activate PKC (Fig. 24.5).

Signal turn-off includes removal of Ca^{++} from the cytosol, by action of Ca^{++}-ATPase pumps, dephosphorylation of IP_3, and regeneration of phosphatidylinositol (Fig.24.5).

Sequential dephosphorylation of IP_3 (by hydrolysis) yields **inositol**. Inositol may then be used for synthesis of phosphatidylinositol. Phosphatidylinositol (PI) is then phosphorylated at 4 and 5 hydroxyl

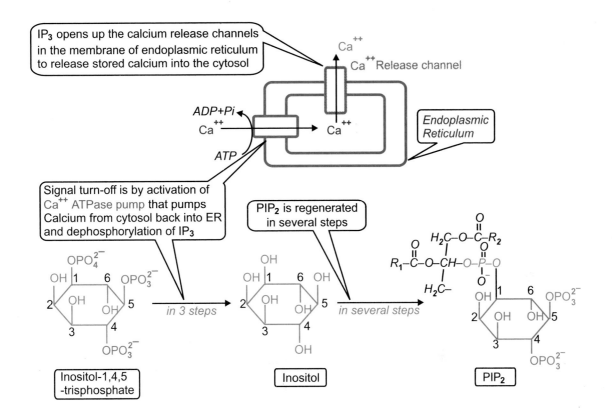

IP$_3$ opens up the calcium release channels in the membrane of endoplasmic reticulum to release stored calcium into the cytosol

Ca^{++}

Ca^{++} Release channel

ADP+Pi

Ca^{++}

Ca^{++}

ATP

Endoplasmic Reticulum

Signal turn-off is by activation of Ca^{++} ATPase pump that pumps Calcium from cytosol back into ER and dephosphorylation of IP$_3$

PIP$_2$ is regenerated in several steps

in 3 steps

in several steps

Inositol-1,4,5 -trisphosphate

Inositol

PIP$_2$

Fig. 24.5: Calcium release from endoplasmic reticulum

groups of inositol ring catalyzed by ATP dependent kinase to yield PIP$_2$ (PI-4, 5-P$_2$). **PI 3-kinases** catalyze phosphorylation at the 3-position of the inositol ring of PI.

The PI-3-P, PI-3, 4-P$_2$ PI-3, 4, 5-P$_3$, and PI-4, 5-P$_2$ have signaling roles. They are ligands for particular protein domains rich in Phe-Tyr-Val-Glutamate residues that bind proteins to membrane surfaces.

Signal cascades often involve complexes of proteins that assemble at the cytosolic surface of the plasma membrane. Signal proteins having pleckstrin homology domains may be recruited into such complexes when PI derivatives recognized by those domains are transiently formed in the cytosolic leaflet of the plasma membrane.

RECEPTOR TYROSINE KINASES CASCADE

These proteins have four major domains: An extracellular *ligand binding domain*, an intracellular *tyrosine kinase domain*, a *regulatory domain*, and a *transmembrane domain*.

The amino acid sequences of the tyrosine kinase domains are highly conserved with those of *cAMP-dependent protein kinase* (PKA) within the ATP binding and substrate binding regions.

Some receptor tyrosine kinases (RTKs) have an insertion of non-kinase domain amino acids into the kinase domain termed the kinase insert. Receptor tyrosine kinases are classified into at least 14 different families based on the structural features in their extracellular portions (as well as the presence or absence of a kinase insert) which include the cysteine rich domains, immunoglobulin-like domains, leucine-rich domains, Kringle domains, cadherin domains, fibronectin type III repeats, discoidin I-like domains, acidic domains, and EGF-like domains.

Receptors that have intrinsic tyrosine kinase activity, as well as those tyrosine kinases that are associated with cell surface receptors contain tyrosine residues, which upon phosphorylation, interact with other proteins of the signaling cascade (Fig. 24.6). These other proteins contain a domain of amino acid sequences that are homologous to a domain first identified in the c-Src proto-oncogene (*c*-designates the cellular form of proto-oncogenes that were first identified in transforming retrovirus). These domains are termed SH2 domains (Src homology domain 2). Another conserved protein-protein interaction domain identified in many signal transduction proteins is related to a third domain in c-Src identified as the SH3 domain.

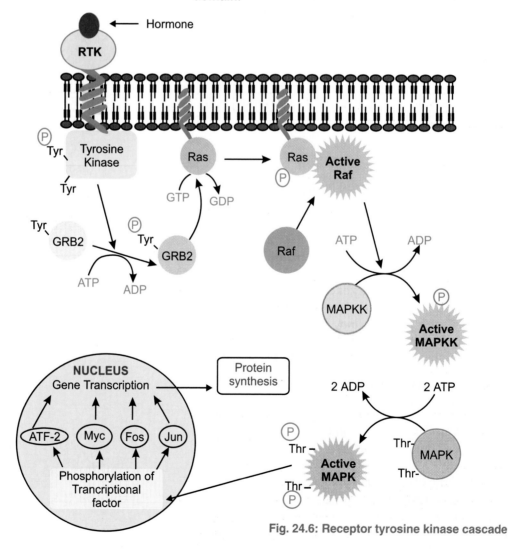

Fig. 24.6: Receptor tyrosine kinase cascade

The interactions of SH2 domain containing proteins with RTKs or receptor associated tyrosine kinases leads to tyrosine phosphorylation of the SH2 containing proteins. The result of the phosphorylation of SH2 containing proteins that have enzymatic activity is an alteration (either positively or negatively) in that activity. Several SH2 containing proteins that have intrinsic enzymatic activity include phospholipase C-γ (PLC-γ), the proto-oncogene c-Ras associated GTPase activating protein (rasGAP), phosphatidylinositol-3-kinase (PI-3K), protein phosphatase-1C (PTP1C), as well as members of the Src family of protein tyrosine kinases (PTKs).

There are numerous intracellular PTKs that are responsible for phosphorylating tyrosine residues of a variety of intracellular proteins following activation of cellular growth and proliferation signals. There are now two recognized distinct families of non-receptor PTKs.

One such intracellular PTK is the Src protein is a tyrosine kinase first identified as the transforming protein in Rous sarcoma virus. Subsequently, a cellular homolog was identifed as c-Src. Numerous proto-oncogenes were identified as the transforming proteins carried by retroviruses. The second family is related to the Janus kinase (Jak).

OTHER SIGNAL CASCADES

Nitric oxide (NO), a free radical species, is a membrane-permeable signal synthesized from arginine (Fig.24.7). It acts only locally, and for a brief time, because it quickly degrades.

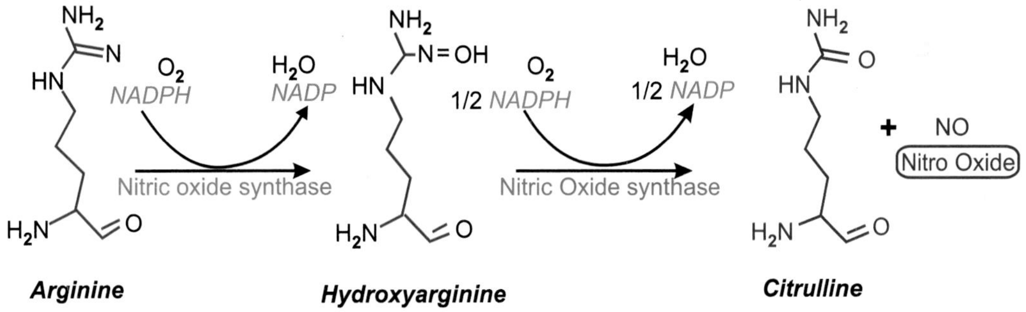

Fig. 24.7: Nitric oxide synthesis

Nitric oxide, produced in endothelial cells lining the lumen of small arterial blood vessels, diffuses into smooth muscle cells in the blood vessel wall to activate *Guanylate cyclase* that catalyzes production of cGMP (analogous in structure to cyclic-AMP). The cGMP-dependent protein kinase then phosphorylates various other proteins, including Ca^{++} channels and Ca^{++}-ATPase pumps, which may result in decreased Ca^{++} within smooth muscle cells. Ultimately smooth muscles relax and arterioles dilate.

Nitroglycerin, used clinically to dilate blood vessels in ischemic heart diseases, acts by releasing NO as it breaks down.

Sildenafil citrate (Viagra), used for the treatment of male impotency is a specific inhibitor of phosphodiesterase 5 (PDE5). Phosphodiesterase 5 cleaves the ring form of cyclic GMP (**cGMP**) a cellular second messenger similar to cAMP. The inhibition of the phosphodiesterase allows for the persistence of *cGMP*, which promotes the effects of cGMP production. In this case, it allows for increased blood flow into the penis, which may result in an erection.

Normally, sexual stimulation in the male is followed by release of nitric oxide (NO) in the corpus cavernosum of the penis. NO activates the enzyme guanylate cyclase in the smooth muscle cells that allows for the relaxation of the penile arteries and an increase flow of blood into the penile cavity. The effect of Sildenafil citrate (Viagra) is to allow the accumulation of cGMP by inhibiting the phosphodiesterase action that tends to magnify the effect of NO release.

Clearly, the mechanism of penile erection is a case of when NO means yes.

One of the curious side effects of Viagra is an effect on the visual discrimination of certain colors. This appears to be due to the reduced affinity of the drug for the phosphodiesterase enzyme found in the retina (PDE6). Viagra has an even more reduced affinity for PDE3 that is critical since PDE3 is active in heart muscle cells.

Insulin and various *growth factors* (proteins that regulate cell growth and division) act via *receptor tyrosine kinases*. The insulin-activated signal cascade can lead to stimulation of a *protein phosphatase* that "turns off" effects of the glucagon-activated cAMP cascade.

Prostaglandins are local hormones formed from the fatty acid arachidonate, which is one of the fatty acids in PIP_2. Arachidonate may be released from diacylglycerol as part of the phosphoinositide cascade.

INTRACELLULAR HORMONE RECEPTORS

Hormone receptors are proteins that bypass all of the signal transduction pathways described above by residing within the cytoplasm. All the hormone receptors are bi-functional. They are capable of binding hormone as well as directly activating gene transcription.

The steroid/thyroid hormone receptor superfamily (e.g. glucocorticoid, vitamin D, retinoic acid and thyroid hormone receptors) is a class of proteins that reside in the cytoplasm and bind the hydrophobic hormones. Upon binding ligand the hormone-receptor complex translocates to the nucleus and bind to specific DNA sequences termed **hormone response elements (HREs)**. The binding of the complex to an HRE results in altered transcription rates of the associated gene.

Amino Acid Metabolism

25

The liver is the major site of nitrogen metabolism in the body. However, all tissues have the ability to synthesize nonessential amino acids, remodeling of amino acids, and conversion of carbon skeletons of nonessential amino acids into amino acids and other nitrogen containing derivatives.

When supplies of dietary amino acids are in surplus, the potentially toxic nitrogen of amino acids is eliminated by reactions of *transaminations, deamination*, and *urea formation*. However, the carbon skeletons of amino acids are generally converted to carbohydrates (by gluconeogenesis), and to fatty acid (by fatty acid synthesis pathways).

Amino acids are categorized based on the metabolic fate of their carbon skeletons as: *glucogenic, ketogenic*, or *glucogenic and ketogenic amino acids*. Glucogenic amino acids are those that give rise to a net production of pyruvate or TCA cycle intermediates, which are precursors for the synthesis of glucose by gluconeogenesis. *Lysine and leucine are solely ketogenic amino acids*, since their carbon skeleton yields only acetyl-CoA or acetoacetyl-CoA, which are precursors for the synthesis of ketone bodies and fatty acids. A small group of amino acids comprised of *isoleucine, phenylalanine, tyrosine, tryptophan* and *threonine*, yield precursors of both glucose and fatty acid and are hence *categorized as both glucogenic and ketogenic*. The *remaining amino acids are purely glucogenic*. During times of starvation the reduced carbon skeleton of amino acid is oxidized to CO_2 and H_2O to meet energy requirement.

BIOSYNTHESIS OF NONESSENTIAL AMINO ACIDS

Those amino acids that are synthesized in the body by transamination reactions are termed nonessential amino acids, which include glycine, alanine, serine, cysteine, tyrosine, proline, aspartate, asparagine, glutamate and glutamine.

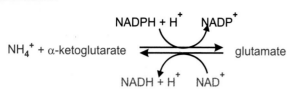

$$NH_4^+ + \alpha\text{-ketoglutarate} \rightleftharpoons \text{glutamate}$$

with $NADPH + H^+ \rightarrow NADP^+$ and $NADH + H^+ \rightarrow NAD^+$

Fig. 25.1: Reactions of glutamate dehydrogenase

Glutamate and Aspartate Biosynthesis

Glutamate and aspartate are synthesized from their widely distributed α-keto acids by simple one-step transamination reactions. The former catalyzed by **glutamate dehydrogenase** (Fig. 25.1) and the latter by **aspartate aminotransferase**. Aspartate is also derived from asparagine through the action of **asparaginase**.

Alanine and the Glucose-Alanine Cycle

Alanine plays a unique role in carrying the nitrogen from peripheral tissue to the liver. Many tissues (mainly muscle) transfer alanine that is formed by transamination of pyruvate at a rate proportional to intracellular pyruvate production into the circulation.

Liver accumulates plasma alanine and reverses the transamination that occurred in muscle, and proportionately increases urea production. The pyruvate is either oxidized or converted to glucose via gluconeogenesis. *Alanine transfer from muscle to liver coupled with glucose transport from liver back to muscle is known as the glucose-alanine cycle* (Fig. 25.2). The key feature of the cycle is that the peripheral tissue exports pyruvate and ammonia (which are potentially rate-limiting for metabolism) in the form of alanine to the liver, where the carbon skeleton is recycled and most of the nitrogen eliminated as urea.

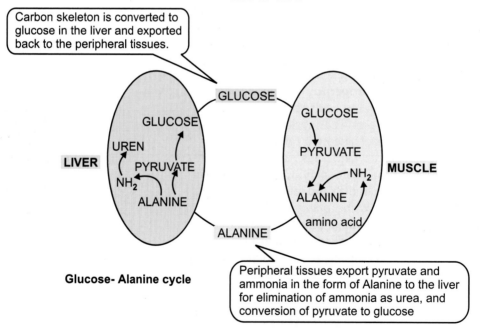

Carbon skeleton is converted to glucose in the liver and exported back to the peripheral tissues.

Glucose- Alanine cycle

Peripheral tissues export pyruvate and ammonia in the form of Alanine to the liver for elimination of ammonia as urea, and conversion of pyruvate to glucose

Fig. 25.2: Glucose-alanine cycle

There are two main sources of muscle alanine: directly from protein degradation, and by transamination of pyruvate by *glutamate-pyruvate aminotransferase* (GOT), which is also called **alanine transaminase** (Fig. 25.3).

Cysteine Biosynthesis

The source of sulfur for cysteine synthesis is the essential amino acid methionine.

Condensation of ATP and methionine catalyzed by *methionine adenosyltransferase* yields S-adenosylmethionine (Fig. 25.4).

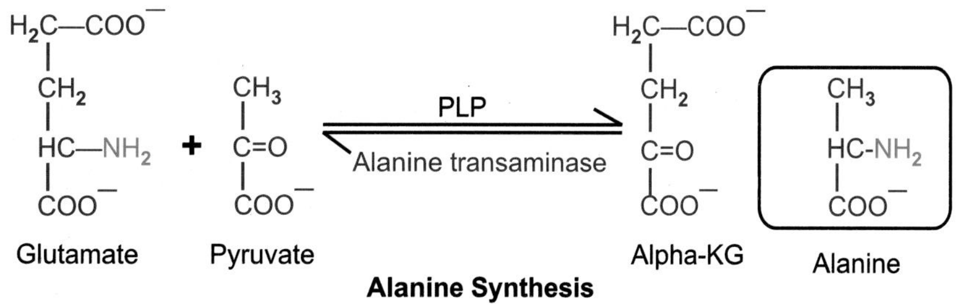

Alanine Synthesis

Fig. 25.3: Alanine synthesis

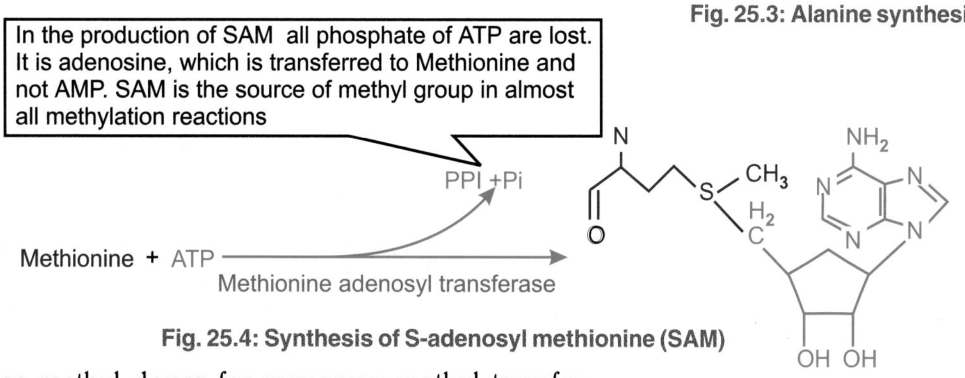

In the production of SAM all phosphate of ATP are lost. It is adenosine, which is transferred to Methionine and not AMP. SAM is the source of methyl group in almost all methylation reactions

Methionine + ATP $\longrightarrow$ Methionine adenosyl transferase

PPI +Pi

Fig. 25.4: Synthesis of S-adenosyl methionine (SAM)

SAM serves as methyl donor for numerous methyl transfer reactions (e.g. the conversion of norepinephrine to epinephrine, and specialized products of amino acids). Upon transfer of methyl group of SAM, it is converted to S-adenosylhomocysteine, which is then cleaved by *adenosylhomocysteinase* to yield homocysteine and adenosine. Homocysteine can be converted back to methionine, by *methionine synthase*, a reaction that occurs under methionine-sparing conditions that requires N^5-methyl-tetrahydrofolate as methyl donor (Fig. 25.5). This reaction is also discussed in the context of vitamin B_{12}-requiring enzymes.

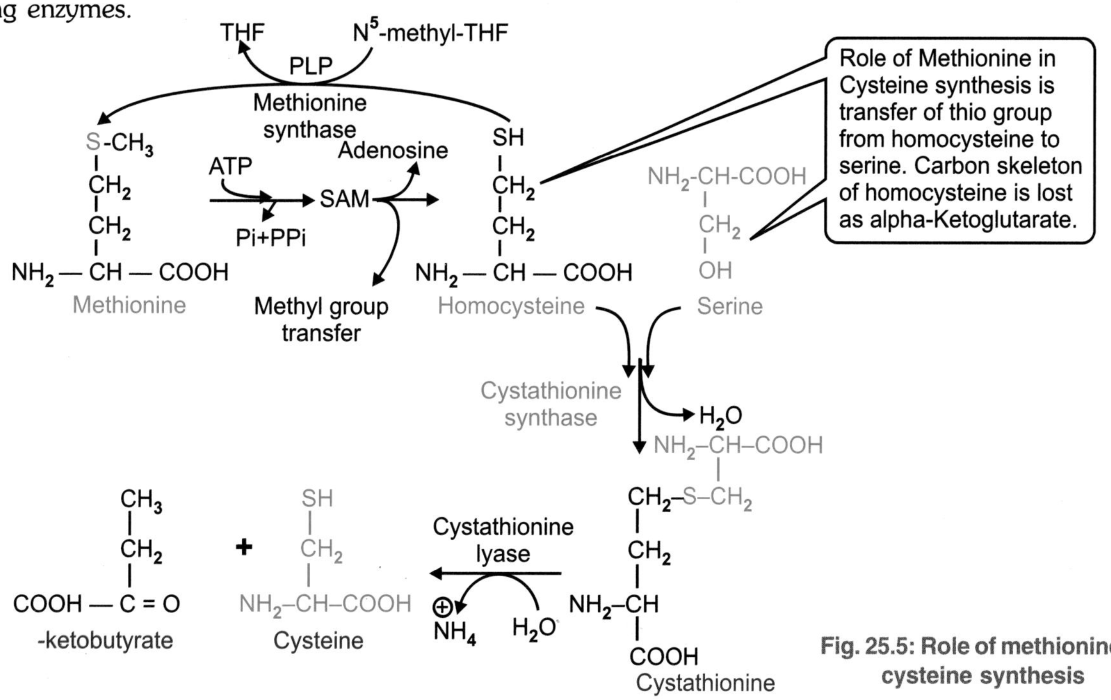

Role of Methionine in Cysteine synthesis is transfer of thio group from homocysteine to serine. Carbon skeleton of homocysteine is lost as alpha-Ketoglutarate.

Fig. 25.5: Role of methionine in cysteine synthesis

Transmethylation reactions employing SAM are extremely important, but in this case the role of S-adenosylmethionine in transmethylation is secondary to the production of homocysteine (essentially a by-product of *transmethylase* activity). In the production of SAM, all phosphates of an ATP are lost: one as P_i and two as PP_i. It is adenosine, which is transferred to methionine and not AMP. In cysteine synthesis, homocysteine condenses with serine to produce cystathionine, which is subsequently cleaved by *cystathionine lyase* to produce cysteine and α-ketobutyrate (Fig. 25.5). The sum of the latter two reactions is known as trans-sulfuration.

Cysteine is used for protein synthesis and other body needs, while the α-ketobutyrate is decarboxylated and converted to propionyl-CoA. While two cysteine molecules readily oxidizes in air to form the disulfide cystine, the ubiquitous reducing agent, glutathione effectively reverses the formation of cystine by a nonenzymatic reduction reaction.

The two key enzymes of this pathway, *cystathionine synthase* and *cystathionine lyase (cystathionase)*, require pyridoxal phosphate as a cofactor, and both are under regulatory control. *Cystathionase* is under negative allosteric control by cysteine, as well cysteine inhibits the expression of the *cystathionine synthase* gene.

Genetic defects associated with both *cystathionine synthase* and the cystathionine lyase enzymes are known. Absence or impaired cystathionine synthase activity leads to **homocystinuria** and is often associated with mental retardation, although the complete syndrome is multifaceted and many individuals with this disease are mentally normal. Some instances of genetic homocystinuria respond favorably to pyridoxine therapy, suggesting that in these cases the enzyme *cystathionine synthase* has decreased affinity for the cofactor. Absence or altered activity of *cystathionine lyase* leads to excretion of cystathionine in the urine without any other untoward effects. Rare cases in which *cystathionine lyase* are defective and their activity low, will lead to methioninuria with no other ill effects.

Tyrosine Biosynthesis

Tyrosine is synthesized in cells by hydroxylation of phenylalanine. Half the dietary phenylalanine is converted to tyrosine under normal conditions. If the diet is rich in tyrosine, the requirement for phenylalanine is reduced by about 50 percent.

Phenylalanine hydroxylase is a mixed-function oxygenase: one atom of oxygen is incorporated into water and the other into phenylalanine, which becomes the hydroxyl of tyrosine. The reducing equivalents are provided by the cofactor tetrahydrobiopterin, which is maintained in the reduced state by the NADH-dependent enzyme *dihydropteridine reductase* (Fig. 25.6).

Absence or deficient *phenylalanine hydroxylase* leads to the genetic disease known as **phenylketonuria (PKU)**, which if untreated leads to severe mental retardation. The mental retardation is caused by the accumulation of phenylalanine, which becomes a major amino groups donor in aminotransferase activity and depletes

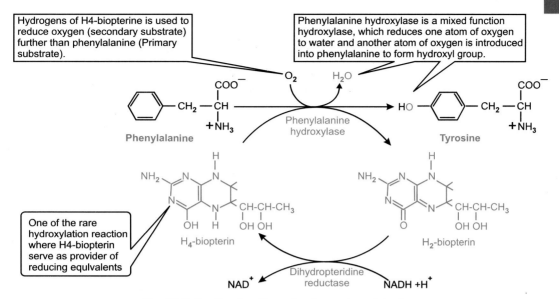

Fig. 25.6: Synthesis of tyrosine from phenylalanine

α-ketoglutarate in neural tissue. The depletion of α-ketoglutarate shuts down the TCA cycle and the associated production of aerobic energy (a mechanism similar to that is caused by hyperammonemia), which is essential for normal brain development (Fig. 25.7).

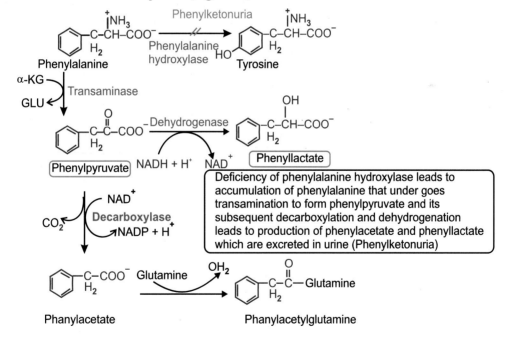

Fig. 25.7: Phenylalanine metabolism

Transamination of phenylalanine yields phenylpyruvic acid, which is reduced to phenylacetate and phenyllactate, and all three compounds appear in the urine. The presence of phenylacetate in the urine imparts a "mousy" odor. If the problem is diagnosed early, the addition of tyrosine and restriction of phenylalanine in the diet can minimize the extent of mental retardation.

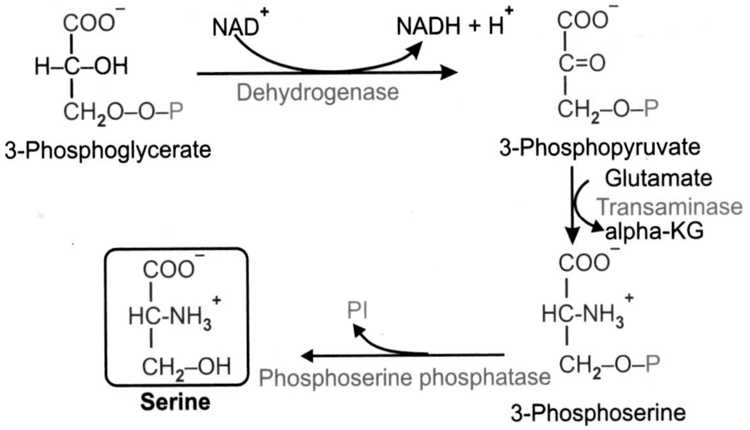

Fig. 25.8: Serine synthesis

The absence or impaired dihydropteridine reductase for which tetrahydrobiopterin is a cofactor cause even more severe neurological deficits than those usually associated with PKU caused by deficient hydroxylase activity.

Serine Biosynthesis

The major pathway of serine biosynthesis starts with the glycolytic intermediate 3-phosphoglycerate. The 3-phosphoglycerate is converted to 3-phosphopyruvate, by an NADH linked dehydrogenase. Subsequently in a coupled transamination reaction with glutamate, the 3-phosphoserine is formed, which is converted to serine by *phosphoserine phosphatase* (Fig. 25.8).

Ornithine and Proline Biosynthesis

Glutamate is the precursor molecule for the biosynthesis of both proline and ornithine. Glutamate semialdehyde is the branch point intermediate leading to one or the other of these two products. Ornithine is not one of the amino acids of protein, but it plays important role as an acceptor of carbamoyl phosphate in the urea cycle, and is also the precursor for synthesis of polyamines. When dietary arginine is limited, the production of ornithine from glutamate assumes importance.

The metabolic fate of glutamate semialdehyde depends on prevailing cellular conditions. Ornithine production occurs from the glutamate semialdehyde via a simple glutamate-dependent transamination, producing ornithine. When arginine concentrations become elevated, the ornithine contributed from the urea cycle and that formed from glutamate semialdehyde inhibit the amino transferase reaction, with accumulation of the semialdehyde, as a result the semialdehyde cyclizes spontaneously to form d^1pyrroline-5-carboxylate which is then reduced by an NADPH-dependent reductase to yield proline (Fig. 25.9).

Glycine Biosynthesis

The major pathway of glycine synthesis is a one-step reaction catalyzed by *serine hydroxymethyltransferase* (Fig. 25.10). This reaction involves the transfer of the hydroxymethyl group from serine to the cofactor tetrahydrofolate (THF), producing glycine and N^5, N^{10}-methylene-THF.

Glycine is involved in many anabolic reactions other than protein synthesis including the synthesis of purine nucleotides, heme, glutathione, creatine and serine.

Glutamate/Glutamine and Aspartate/Asparagine Biosynthesis

Glutamate is synthesized by the reductive amination of α-ketoglutarate catalyzed by *glutamate dehydrogenase*; it is thus a

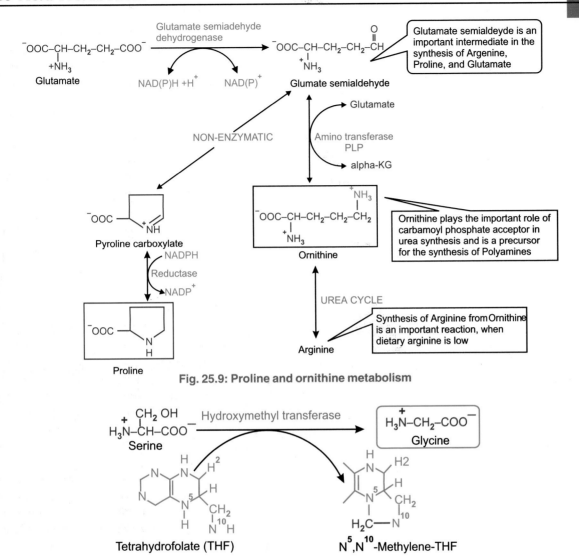

Fig. 25.9: Proline and ornithine metabolism

Fig. 25.10: Glycine synthesis

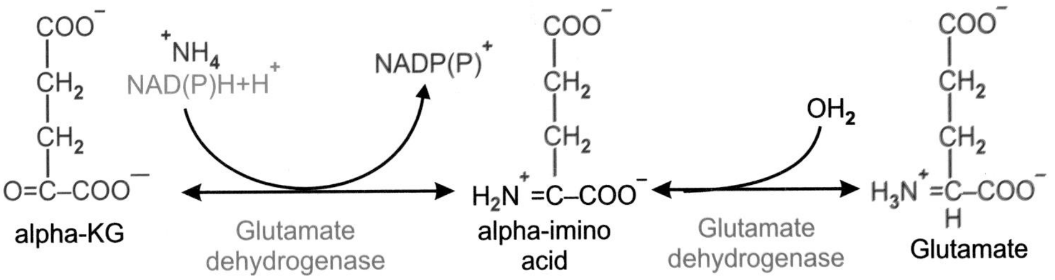

nitrogen-fixing reaction (Fig. 25.11). In addition, glutamate is formed by transamination reactions, in which α-ketoglutarate accepts the amino nitrogen from a number of different amino acids. Thus, glutamate is a general collector of amino nitrogen.

Fig. 25.11: Reductive amination

Aspartate is formed by coupled transamination reaction catalyzed by *aspartate transaminase* (AST), where glutamate is amino donor and oxaloacetate is the amino group acceptor. Aspartate is also formed by deamination of asparagine catalyzed by *asparaginase* (Fig. 25.12).

Asparagine synthetase and *glutamine synthetase* catalyze the production of asparagine and glutamine from their respective α-amino acids (Fig. 25.13). Glutamine is produced from glutamate by

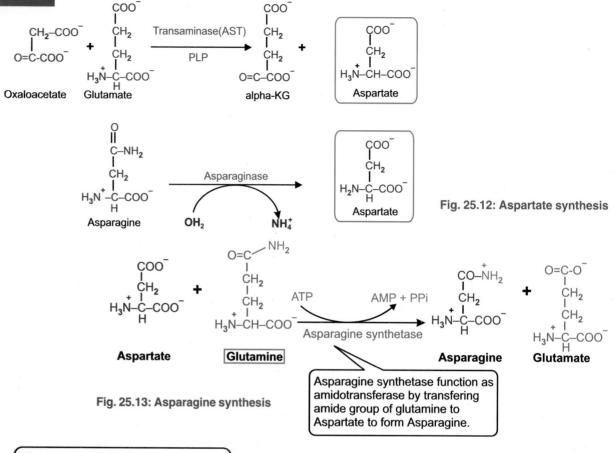

Fig. 25.12: Aspartate synthesis

Fig. 25.13: Asparagine synthesis

Asparagine synthetase function as amidotransferase by transfering amide group of glutamine to Aspartate to form Asparagine.

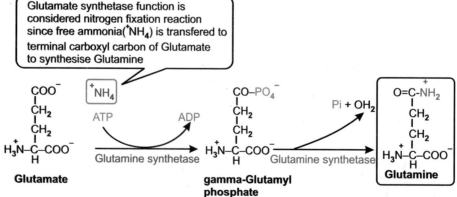

Glutamate synthetase function is considered nitrogen fixation reaction since free ammonia($^+NH_4$) is transferred to terminal carboxyl carbon of Glutamate to synthesise Glutamine

Fig. 25.14: Glutamine synthesis

the direct incorporation of ammonia (Fig. 25.14); and this can be considered another nitrogen fixing reaction. Asparagine, however, is formed by an amidotransferase reaction.

Transaminase reactions are readily reversible. The direction of any individual transamination depends mainly on the concentration ratio of reactants and products. In contrast, transamidation reactions, which are dependent on ATP, are considered irreversible.

As a consequence, the degradation of asparagine and glutamine takes place by a hydrolytic pathway rather than by a reversal of the pathway by which they are formed. As indicated in Figure 25.13, asparagine can be degraded to aspartate.

CATABOLISM OF AMINO ACIDS

Glutamine/Glutamate and Asparagine/Aspartate Catabolism

Glutaminase is an important enzyme in kidney tubule, which is involved in converting glutamine (from liver and other tissues) to

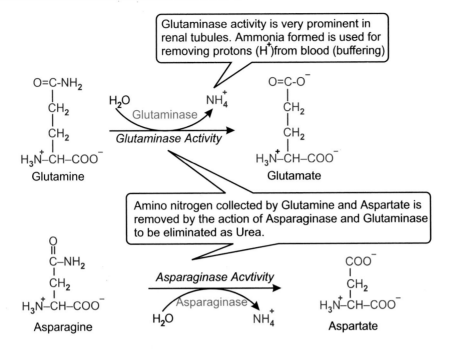

Fig. 25.15: Synthesis of aspartate and glutamate

glutamate with the releases of ammonia (NH_3), which is excreted as ammonium ion (NH_4^+) in the urine (Fig. 25.15).

Glutaminase activity is present in many other tissues as well, although its activity is not nearly as prominent as in the kidney. The glutamate produced from glutamine is converted to α-ketoglutarate; hence glutamine is a glucogenic amino acid.

Asparaginase is also widely distributed within the body, where it converts asparagine into ammonia and aspartate (Fig. 25.14). Aspartate then undergoes transamination to yield oxaloacetate, which enters gluconeogenic pathway to yield glucose.

Glutamate and aspartate are important in collecting and eliminating amino nitrogen via *glutamine synthetase* and the urea cycle, respectively. The catabolic path of the carbon skeletons involves simple one-step transamination reactions that directly produce TCA cycle intermediates. The *glutamate dehydrogenase* reaction operating in the direction of α-ketoglutarate production provides a second avenue leading from glutamate to gluconeogenesis.

Alpha-decarboxylation of glutamate yields α-amino butyric acid (GABA), which is a neurotransmitter.

Alanine Catabolism

Alanine is also important in inter-tissue nitrogen transport as part of the glucose-alanine cycle. Alanine catabolic pathway involves a simple amino transferase reaction that directly produces pyruvate (Fig. 25.16). Generally pyruvate produced by this pathway will result in the formation of oxaloacetate, but when the energy charge of a cell is low the pyruvate will be oxidized to CO_2 and H_2O via the PDH complex and the TCA cycle. This makes alanine a glucogenic amino acid.

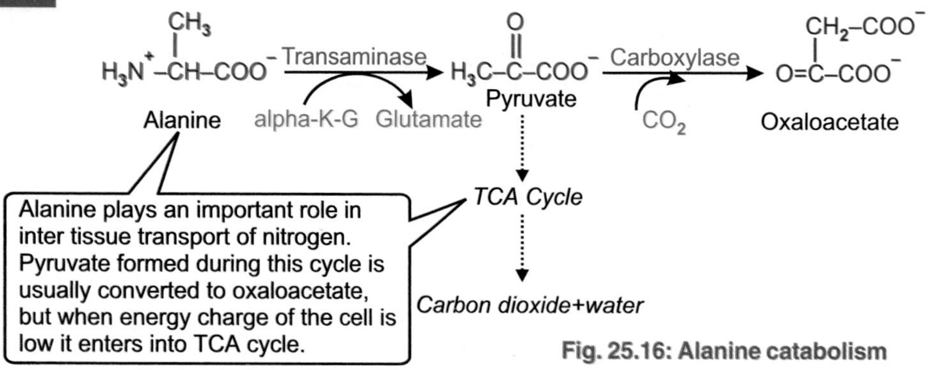
Transaminase
Alanine
alpha-K-G
Glutamate
Pyruvate
Carboxylase
CO2
Oxaloacetate
TCA Cycle
Carbon dioxide+water
Alanine plays an important role in inter tissue transport of nitrogen. Pyruvate formed during this cycle is usually converted to oxaloacetate, but when energy charge of the cell is low it enters into TCA cycle.

Fig. 25.16: Alanine catabolism

Arginine, Ornithine and Proline Catabolism

The catabolism of arginine begins within the urea cycle where it is hydrolyzed to urea and ornithine by the enzyme *arginase*.

Ornithine in excess of urea cycle requirements is transaminated to form glutamate semialdehyde, which serves as the precursor for proline biosynthesis as described earlier or it can be converted to glutamate (Fig. 25.9).

Proline catabolism is a reversal of its synthesis process. The glutamate semialdehyde generated from ornithine and proline catabolism is oxidized to glutamate by an ATP-independent *glutamate semialdehyde dehydrogenase*. The glutamate is then converted to α-ketoglutarate in a transamination reaction. Thus arginine, ornithine and proline are glucogenic.

Serine Catabolism

Conversion of serine to glycine and its oxidation to CO_2 and NH_3, with the production of two equivalents of N^5, N^{10}-methylene THF is described earlier. Serine can also be catabolized to the glycolytic intermediate, 3-phosphoglycerate, by a pathway that is essentially a reversal of serine biosynthesis (Fig. 25.17). However, the enzymes are different. Serine can also be converted to pyruvate through a deamination reaction catalyzed by *serine/threonine dehydratase*.

Threonine Catabolism

Threonine is catabolized by at least three different pathways (Fig.25.18). The first pathway is catalyzed by *threonine aldolase*. The products of this reaction are acetaldehyde and glycine. The second pathway is catalyzed by *threonine dehydrogenase* yielding α-amino-β-ketobutyrate, which is either converted to acetyl-CoA and glycine or spontaneously decarboxylates to form aminoacetone, which is converted to pyruvate. The third pathway involves *serine/threonine dehydratase* yielding α-ketobutyrate which is further catabolized to propionyl-CoA and finally the TCA cycle intermediate, succinyl-CoA.

Glycine Catabolism

Glycine is classified as a glucogenic amino acid, since it can be converted to serine, by *serine hydroxymethyltransferase*, and serine

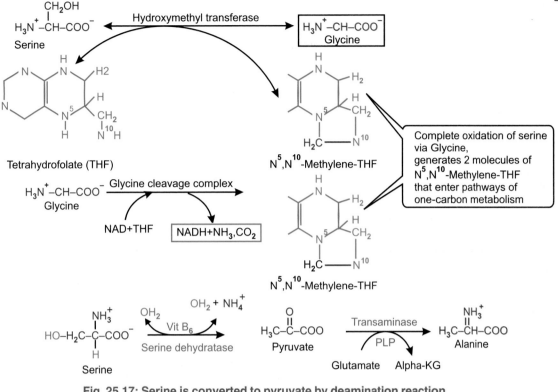

Fig. 25.17: Serine is converted to pyruvate by deamination reaction

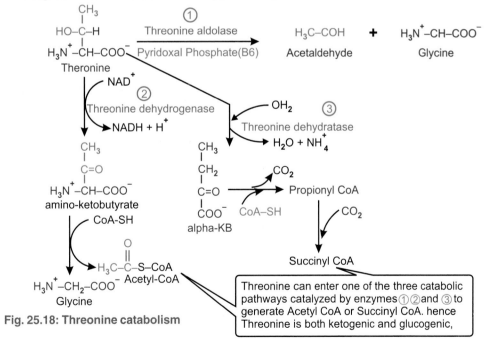

Fig. 25.18: Threonine catabolism

can be converted back to the glycolytic intermediate, 3-phosphoglycerate or to pyruvate by *serine/threonine dehydratase*. However, the main glycine catabolic pathway in mitochondria leads to the production of CO_2, ammonia, and one equivalent of N^5, N^{10}-methylene THF by *glycine cleavage complex* (Fig. 25.19).

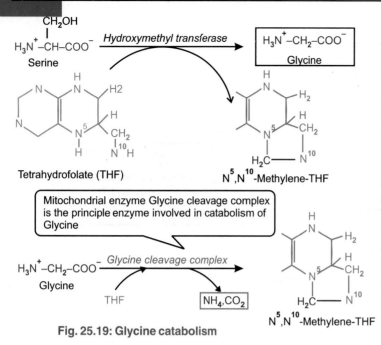

Fig. 25.19: Glycine catabolism

Cysteine Catabolism

Different pathways catabolize cysteine. The simplest, but least important pathway is catalyzed by a liver desulfurase that produces hydrogen sulfide, (H_2S) and pyruvate. The more important catabolic pathway is via a cytochrome-P_{450} coupled enzyme, *cysteine dioxygenase* that oxidizes the cysteine sulfhydryl to sulfinate, producing the intermediate cysteinesulfinate (Fig. 25.20). Cysteinesulfinate serves as a biosynthetic intermediate for taurine, which is used to form the bile acid conjugates, taurocholate and taurochenodeoxycholate. Catabolism of cysteinesulfinate proceeds through transamination to β-sulfinylpyruvate, which undergoes desulfuration yielding bisulfite, (HSO_3^-) and pyruvate. The enzyme *sulfite oxidase* uses O_2 and H_2O to convert HSO_3^- to sulfate, (SO_4^-) and H_2O_2. The resultant sulfate is used as a precursor for the formation of 3'-phosphoadenosine-5'-phosphosulfate (PAPS), which function as sulfate donor to biological molecules such as the sugars of the glycosphingolipids.

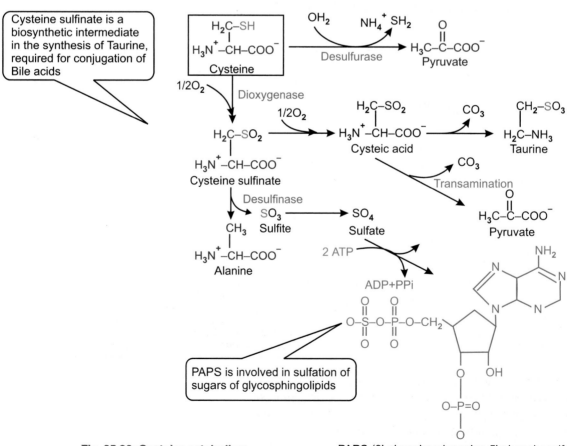

Fig. 25.20: Cysteine catabolism

PAPS (3'-phosphoadenosine 5'-phosphosulfate)

The enzyme *cystathionase* catalyzes the transfer of the sulfur from one cysteine to another, generating thiocysteine and pyruvate. Transamination of cysteine yields mercaptopyruvate, which reacts with sulfite (SO_3^{2-}), to produce thiosulfate ($S_2O_3^{2-}$) and pyruvate. Both thiocysteine and thiosulfate are used by the enzyme *rhodanase* to incorporate sulfur into cyanide (CN^-) that detoxifies cyanide to thiocyanate.

Methionine Catabolism

The principal fates of the essential amino acid methionine are incorporation into polypeptide chains, and use in the production of α-ketobutyrate and cysteine via SAM as described earlier. The transulfuration reactions that produce cysteine from homocysteine and serine also produce α-ketobutyrate, the latter being converted to succinyl-CoA.

Regulation of the methionine metabolic pathway is based on the availability of methionine and cysteine. If both amino acids are present in adequate quantities, SAM accumulates and acts as positive effector on *cystathionine synthase*, encouraging the production of cysteine and α-ketobutyrate (both of which are glucogenic). However, if methionine is scarce, SAM is formed in small quantities, thus limiting *cystathionine synthase* activity. Under these conditions accumulated homocysteine is remethylated to methionine, using N^5-methyl THF and other compounds as methyl donors.

Valine, Leucine and Isoleucine Catabolism

This group of essential amino acids is identified as the branched-chain amino acids (BCAAs). Since humans cannot make the carbon skeletal of these amino acids, these amino acids are an essential element in the diet. The catabolism of all three amino acids is initiated in muscle and yields NADH and $FADH_2$, which is utilized for ATP generation (Fig. 25.21). The first two steps of catabolism of all three amino acids use the same enzymes. The first step is α-ketoglutarate coupled transamination reaction catalyzed by *BCAA aminotransferase*. As a result, three different α-keto acids are produced and are oxidized using a common *branched-chain α-keto acid dehydrogenase*, which yields three different CoA derivatives. Subsequently the metabolic pathways diverge to produce many intermediates.

The principal product from valine is propionyl-CoA, the glucogenic precursor of succinyl-CoA. Leucine gives rise to acetyl-CoA and acetoacetyl-CoA, which are strictly ketogenic. Isoleucine catabolism terminates with production of acetyl-CoA and propionyl-CoA, which are both glucogenic and ketogenic.

There are number of genetic diseases associated with faulty catabolism of the BCAAs. The most common defect is in the *branched-chain α-keto acid dehydrogenase*. Since there is only one dehydrogenase enzyme for all three amino acids, all three α-keto acids accumulate and are excreted in the urine (Fig. 25.20). The

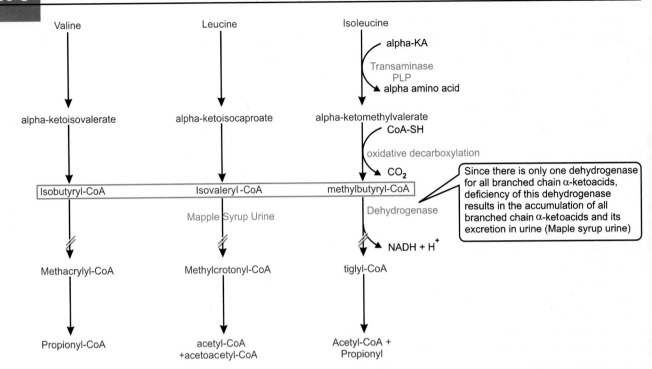

Fig. 25.21: Branched chain amino acid catabolism

disease is known as maple syrup urine disease because of the characteristic odor of the urine in afflicted individuals. Mental retardation in these cases is extensive. Unfortunately, since these are essential amino acids, they cannot be heavily restricted in the diet; ultimately, the life of afflicted individuals is short and development is abnormal. The neurological problems are due to poor myelin formation in the CNS.

Phenylalanine and Tyrosine Catabolism

Phenylalanine normally has two fates: one is protein biosynthesis and the other the synthesis of tyrosine by tetrahydrobiopterin-dependant enzyme *phenylalanine hydroxylase*. Thus the catabolism of phenylalanine always follows the pathway of tyrosine catabolism. The main pathway of tyrosine degradation involves its conversion to fumarate and acetoacetate; hence both phenylalanine and tyrosine are classified as both glucogenic and ketogenic (Fig. 25.22).

Tyrosine is equally important for protein biosynthesis as well as an intermediate in the biosynthesis of several physiologically important metabolites, e.g. dopamine, norepinephrine and epinephrine (discussed later in the chapter 27: Specialized Products of Amino Acids).

As in phenylketonuria (deficiency of *phenylalanine hydroxylase*), deficiency of *tyrosine transaminase* leads to urinary excretion of tyrosine and the intermediates between phenylalanine and tyrosine. The adverse neurological symptoms are the same for the two diseases.

Genetic diseases such as various tyrosinemias and alkaptonuria are also associated with other defective enzymes of the tyrosine catabolic pathway (Fig. 25.22). The first genetic disease ever recognized, alkaptonuria, is caused by defective *homogentisic acid oxidase*. Homogentisic acid accumulation is relatively innocuous, causing urine to darken on exposure to air, but no life-threatening effects accompany the disease. The other genetic deficiencies lead to more severe symptoms, most of which are associated with abnormal neural development, mental retardation, and shortened life-span.

Lysine Catabolism

Lysine catabolism is unusual in the way that the α-amino group is transferred to α-ketoglutarate and that enter the general nitrogen pool. The reaction is a transamination in which the α-amino group is transferred to the α-keto carbon of α-ketoglutarate forming the metabolite, saccharopine (Fig. 25.23).

Unlike the majority of transamination reactions, this one does not employ pyridoxal phosphate as a cofactor. Saccharopine is immediately hydrolyzed by the enzyme *α-aminoadipic semialdehyde synthase* (this enzyme has both transaminase and dehydrogenase activity) in such a way that the amino nitrogen remains with the α-carbon of α-ketoglutarate, producing glutamate and α-amino adipic semialdehyde. Because this transamination reaction is not reversible, lysine is an essential amino acid. The ultimate end product of lysine catabolism is acetoacetyl-CoA

Genetic deficiencies in the enzyme *α-aminoadipic semialdehyde synthase* have been observed in individuals who excrete large quantities of lysine and some saccharopine in urine, which is a benign condition. Other serious disorders associated with lysine metabolism are due to failure of the transport system for lysine and the other dibasic amino acids across the intestinal wall. Lysine is essential for protein synthesis; a deficiency of its transport into the body can cause seriously diminished levels of protein synthesis. Probably more significant, however, is the fact that arginine is transported on the same dibasic amino acid carrier, and resulting arginine deficiencies limit the quantity of ornithine available for the urea cycle. The result is severe hyperammonemia after a meal rich in protein. The addition of citrulline to the diet prevents the hyperammonemia.

Lysine is also important as a precursor for the synthesis of carnitine, which transports fatty acids into the mitochondria. Some proteins modify lysine to trimethyllysine using SAM as the methyl donor to transfer methyl groups to the α-amino of the lysine side chain. Hydrolysis of proteins containing trimethyllysine provides the substrate for the subsequent conversion to carnitine.

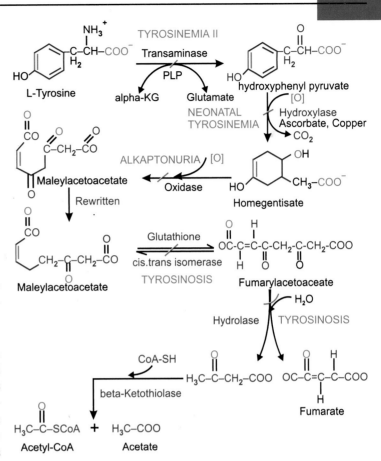

Fig. 25.22: Tyrosine catabolism

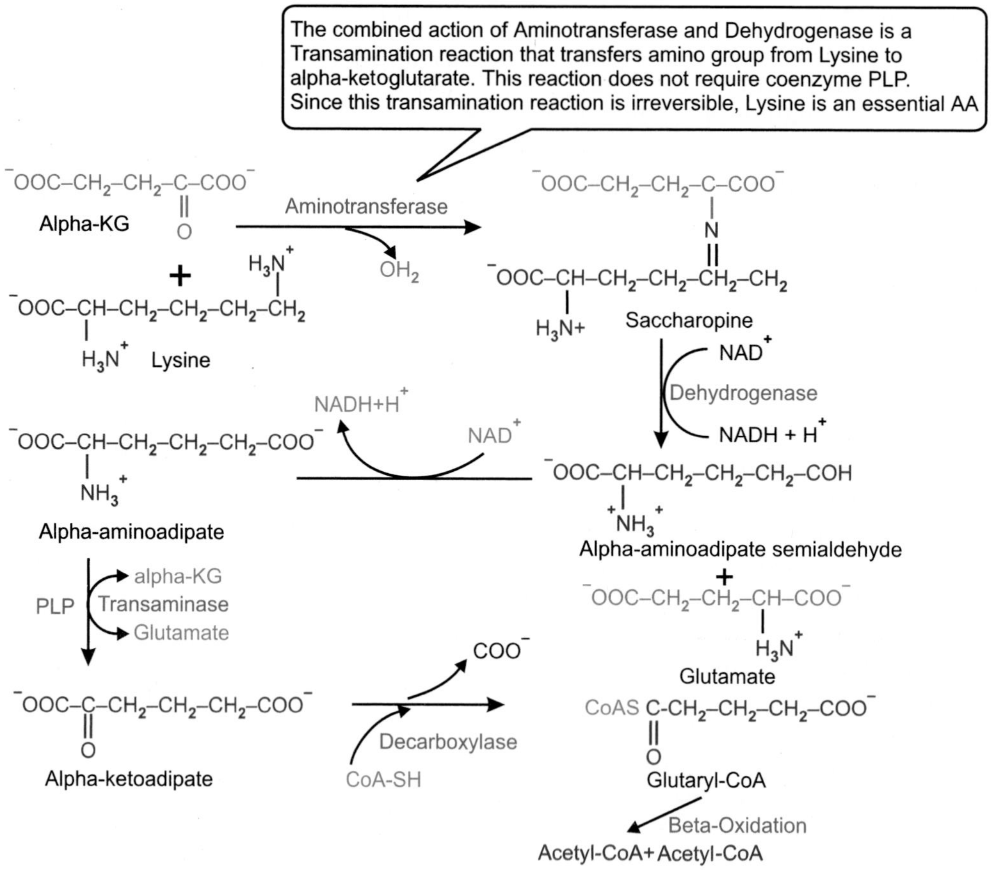

The combined action of Aminotransferase and Dehydrogenase is a Transamination reaction that transfers amino group from Lysine to alpha-ketoglutarate. This reaction does not require coenzyme PLP. Since this transamination reaction is irreversible, Lysine is an essential AA

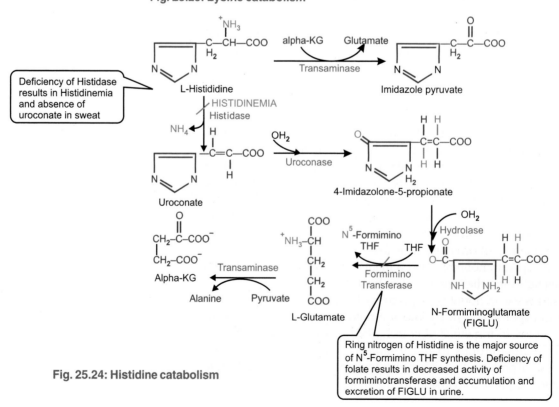

Fig. 25.23: Lysine catabolism

Deficiency of Histidase results in Histidinemia and absence of uroconate in sweat

Fig. 25.24: Histidine catabolism

Ring nitrogen of Histidine is the major source of N^5-Formimino THF synthesis. Deficiency of folate results in decreased activity of formiminotransferase and accumulation and excretion of FIGLU in urine.

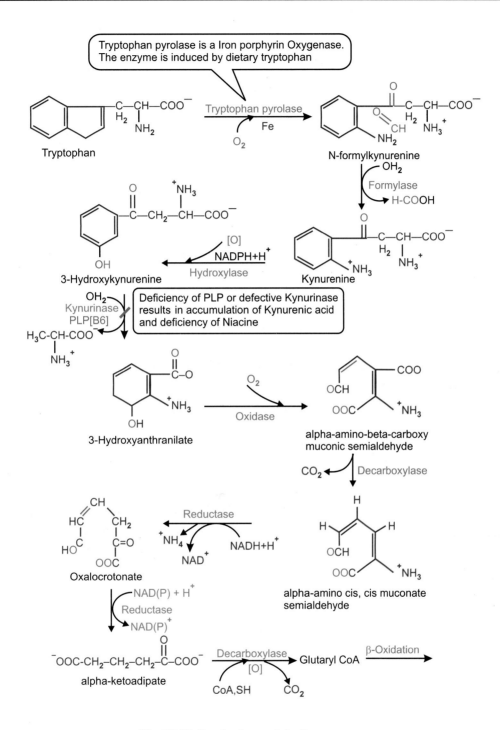

Fig. 25.25: Tryptophan catabolism

Histidine Catabolism

The first reaction of histidine catabolism is the release of the α-amino group catalyzed by *histidase* (Fig. 25.24). As a result, the deaminated product urocanate is not the usual α-keto acid associated with loss of α-amino nitrogens. The end product of histidine catabolism is glutamate, which is glucogenic amino acid. Another key feature of histidine catabolism is that it serves as a source of ring nitrogen to combine with tetrahydrofolate (THF), producing the one-carbon THF intermediate known as N^5-formiminoTHF (FIGLU).

The important genetic deficiency associated with histidine metabolism is absence or deficiency *histidase*. The resultant histidinemia is relatively benign but has relatively high incidence. Decarboxylation of histidine in the intestine by bacteria gives rise to histamine. Similarly, histamine arises in many tissues by the decarboxylation of histidine, which in excess causes constriction or dilation of various blood vessels. The general symptoms are those of asthma and various allergic manifestations.

Tryptophan Catabolism

The first enzyme of the catabolic pathway is tryptophan pyrolase (an iron porphyrin oxygenase) that opens the indole ring. This enzyme is highly inducible and its concentration rising almost ten-fold on a diet high in tryptophan. A number of other important side reactions occur during the catabolism of tryptophan on the pathway to acetoacetate (Fig. 25.25).

Kynurenine is the first key branch point intermediate in the pathway. Kynurenine undergoes deamination in a standard transamination reaction yielding kynurenic acid. Kynurenic acid and metabolites have been shown to act as anti-excitotoxics and anti-convulsives.

A second side branch reaction produces anthranilic acid and alanine. Another equivalent of alanine is produced further along the main catabolic pathway, and it is the production of these alanine residues that allows tryptophan to be classified among the glucogenic and ketogenic amino acids.

The second important branch point converts kynurenine to *2-amino-3-carboxymuconic semialdehyde*, which has two metabolic fates. The main flow of carbon elements from this intermediate is to glutarate. An important side reaction in liver is a transamination and several rearrangements to produce limited amounts of nicotinic acid, which leads to production of a small amount of NAD^+ and $NADP^+$

Beside its role as an amino acid in protein biosynthesis, tryptophan also serves as a precursor for the synthesis of serotonin and melatonin.

Nitrogen Metabolism

26

Humans are entirely dependent on other organisms for converting atmospheric nitrogen to forms available to the body. Nitrogen fixation is carried out by bacterial **nitrogenases** that form reduced nitrogen (NH_4^+), which is then utilized by all other forms of living organisms to synthesize amino acids. The sources of reduced nitrogen to human body are dietary protein, free amino acids, and the ammonia produced by bacteria harboring intestinal tract.

The two principal enzymes found in all organisms that utilize ammonia for the synthesis of amino acids *glutamate* and *glutamine* are **Glutamate dehydrogenase** and **glutamine synthetase** respectively. Amino and amide groups of these two amino acids are freely transferred to other carbon skeletons by *transamination* and *transamidation* reactions.

Aminotransferases exist for each of the amino acids except threonine and lysine. The most common compounds involved as a donor/ acceptor pair in transamination reactions are glutamate and α-ketoglutarate (α-KG), which participate in reactions with many different aminotransferases (Fig. 26.1). Serum aminotransferases such as **serum glutamate-oxaloacetate aminotransferase/aspartate transaminase** (SGOT/AST) and **serum glutamate-pyruvate aminotransferase/alanine transaminase** (SGPT/ALT) are used as clinical markers of tissue damage. **Alanine transaminase** plays an important role in the transfer of carbon and nitrogen formed in skeletal muscle to the liver, in the form of alanine. In skeletal muscle, pyruvate is

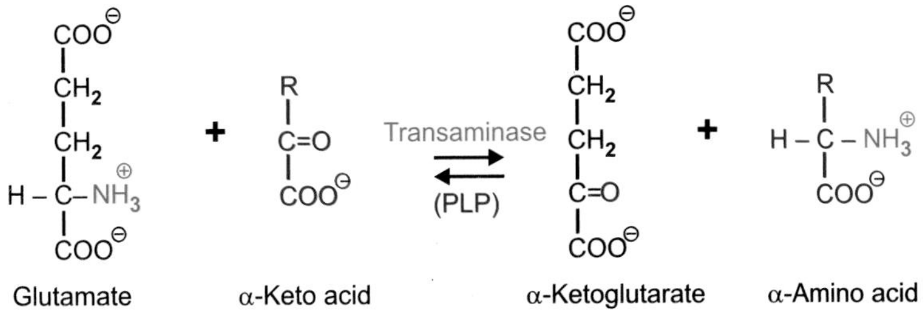

Fig. 26.1: Representative aminotransferase catalyzed reaction

transaminated to form alanine, which provides an additional route for transport of nitrogen from muscle to liver. In liver, ***alanine transaminase*** facilitates transfer of ammonia from alanine to α-KG; thereby pyruvate is regenerated that is then diverted to gluconeogenesis. This process is referred to as the glucose-alanine cycle.

Glutamate Dehydrogenase Reaction

The *glutamate dehydrogenase* utilizes both NAD^+ and NADPH as cofactors. The NAD^+ is utilized in the direction of nitrogen liberation and NADPH for nitrogen incorporation.

In the forward reaction, *glutamate dehydrogenase* incorporates free ammonia into α-ketoglutarate (α-KG) to form glutamate (Fig. 26.2). However, the reverse reaction is a key anaplerotic process linking amino acid metabolism with TCA cycle activity. This reaction provides an oxidizable carbon source used for the production of energy as well as a reduced electron carrier NADH. Glutamate dehydrogenase being a branch point enzyme linking energy metabolism is regulated by energy charge of the cell. The ATP and GTP are positive allosteric effectors of the formation of glutamate, whereas ADP and GDP are positive allosteric effectors of the reverse reaction. Thus, when the level of cellular ATP is high, conversion of glutamate to α-KG and other TCA cycle intermediates is limited; when the cellular energy charge is low, glutamate is converted to ammonia and oxidizable intermediates of TCA cycle. Glutamate is also a principal amino donor to other amino acids in transamination reactions. The multiple roles of glutamate in nitrogen balance make it an important link between free ammonia and the amino groups of most amino acids.

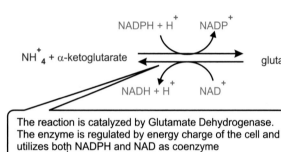

The reaction is catalyzed by Glutamate Dehydrogenase. The enzyme is regulated by energy charge of the cell and utilizes both NADPH and NAD as coenzyme

Fig. 26.2: Glutamate dehydrogenase catalyzed reaction

Glutamine Synthetase Reaction

The reaction catalyzed by *glutamine synthetase* is:

Glutamate + NH_4^+ + ATP $\rightarrow$ glutamine + ADP + P_i + H^+ —— **Reaction 1**

The *glutamine synthetase* reaction is important in several respects. First it produces glutamine, one of the 20 major amino acids. Second, in animals, glutamine is the major amino acid found in the circulatory system. Its role in the circulatory system is to carry ammonia from peripheral tissues to the kidney, where the amide nitrogen is hydrolyzed by the enzyme *glutaminase*, this process regenerates glutamate and free ammonia, which is excreted in the urine as ammonium ion (NH_4^+).

Glutamine + H_2O $\rightarrow$ glutamate + NH_3 —— **Reaction 2**

In reaction 1, ammonia arising in peripheral tissue is carried in a nonionizable form, which has none of the neurotoxic or alkalosis-generating properties of free ammonia.

Liver contains both *glutamine synthetase* and *glutaminase* but the enzymes are localized in different cellular segments. This ensures that the liver is neither a net producer nor consumer of glutamine. The differences in cellular location of these two enzymes allow the liver to scavenge ammonia that has not been incorporated into urea. The enzymes of the urea cycle are located in the same cells as those that contain *glutaminase*. The result of the differential distribution of these two hepatic enzymes makes it possible to control ammonia incorporation into urea or glutamine, the latter leads to excretion of ammonia by the kidney.

In acidosis, more glutamine is diverted from the liver to the kidney. This allows for the conservation of bicarbonate ion since the incorporation of ammonia into urea requires bicarbonate. When glutamine reaches the kidney, *glutaminase* releases the amide nitrogen of glutamine as ammonia to from glutamate and then *glutamate dehydrogenase* releases α-amino nitrogen of glutamate as another mole of ammonia to generate α-ketoglutarate. The ammonia formed in these two reactions undergoes protonation to form ammonium ion (NH_4^+) that is excreted in the urine, where it helps maintain urine pH in the normal range of pH 4 to pH 8.

Digestive Tract Nitrogen

Most of the amino acids found in human tissues necessarily come from dietary sources. Protein digestion begins in the stomach, where a proenzyme called *pepsinogen* is secreted, which is autocatalytically converted to *Pepsin A* that bring about the first step of proteolysis. However, most proteolysis takes place in the duodenum where pancreatic enzymes are secreted into the duodenum. Serine proteases and the zinc peptidases of pancreatic secretions are in the form of their respective proenzymes. These proteases are both endopeptidase and exopeptidase, their combined action on dietary proteins in the intestine leads to the production of *amino acids, dipeptides, and tripeptides*, all of which are taken up by enterocytes of the mucosal wall.

Presence of food in the intestinal lumen triggers secretion of proenzymes into the intestine. Special mucosal endocrine cells secret the peptide hormones *cholecystokinin (CCK)* and *secretin* into the circulatory system, which cause contraction of the gallbladder and the exocrine secretion of a bicarbonate-rich alkaline fluid containing protease proenzymes from the pancreas into the intestine. A second, paracrine role of CCK is to stimulate adjacent intestinal cells to secrete *enteropeptidase*, a protease that cleaves *trypsinogen* to produce *trypsin*. *Trypsin* in turn activates *trypsinogen* and all the other proenzymes in the pancreatic secretion, producing the active proteases and peptidases that hydrolyze dietary polypeptides.

Small peptides and amino acids are transferred through enterocytes into the portal circulation by **diffusion, facilitated diffusion,** or **active transport**. A number of Na^+-dependent amino acid transport systems with overlapping amino acid specificity have been described. In these transport systems, Na^+ and amino acids at high luminal concentrations are co-transported down their concentration gradient to the interior of the enterocytes. The ATP-dependent Na^+/K^+ pump exchanges the accumulated Na^+ for extracellular K^+, thereby reducing intracellular Na^+ levels and maintaining the high extracellular Na^+ concentration required to drive this transport process.

Small peptides accumulated in the enterocytes by a proton (H^+) driven transport process are hydrolyzed by intracellular peptidases. Amino acids in the circulatory system and in extracellular fluids are transported into cells of the body by different ATP-requiring active transport systems with overlapping amino acid specificities.

Hartnup disease is an autosomal recessive impairment of neutral amino acid transport, affecting the kidney tubules and small intestine. It is believed that the defect lies in a specific system responsible for neutral amino acid transport across the brush-border membrane of renal and intestinal epithelium. The characteristic diagnostic feature of Hartnup disease is a dramatic neutral hyperaminoaciduria. Additionally, individuals excrete indolic compounds that originate from the bacterial degradation of unabsorbed tryptophan. The reduced intestinal absorption and increased renal loss of tryptophan lead to a reduced availability of tryptophan for biosynthesis of niacin and nicotinamide nucleotide. As a consequence affected individuals frequently exhibit pellagra-like rashes.

Some of the products of protein digestion by intestinal bacteria have powerful vasopressor effects. *E. coli* present in intestine can make the carbon skeletons of all 20 amino acids and transaminate those carbon skeletons with nitrogen from glutamine or glutamate to complete the amino acid structures.

Products of intestinal bacterial activity

Substrate	Vasopressor aminase	Other
Lysine	Cadaverene	
Arginine	Agmatine	
Tyrosine	Tyramine	
Ornithine	Putrescine	
Histidine	Histamine	
Tryptophan		Indole and skatole
All amino acids		NH_4^+

Human cells cannot synthesize the branched carbon chains of branched chain amino acids or the ring systems of aromatic amino acids such as phenylalanine, nor can incorporate sulfur into covalently bonded structures. Therefore, the so-called essential amino acids must be supplied from the diet. Nevertheless, it should be recognized that, depending on the composition of the diet and physiological state of the individual, one or another of the non-essential amino acids might also become a required dietary component. For example, arginine is considered as an essential amino acid only during early childhood development because enough of adult needs are made by the urea cycle.

To take a different type of example, cysteine and tyrosine that are considered nonessential are formed from the essential amino acids methionine and phenylalanine respectively. If sufficient cysteine and tyrosine are present in the diet, the requirements for methionine and phenylalanine are markedly reduced; conversely, if dietary supply of methionine and phenylalanine is in limited quantities, cysteine and tyrosine will become essential dietary components.

It should be recognized that if the α-keto acids corresponding to the carbon skeletons of the essential amino acids are supplied in the diet, aminotransferases in the body could convert the keto acids to their respective amino acids that will largely supply the basic needs.

Unlike fats and carbohydrates, nitrogen has no designated storage depots in the body. Since the half-life of many proteins is short (on the order of hours), insufficient dietary quantities of even one amino acid can quickly limit the synthesis of many essential proteins. The limited synthesis of protein and normal rates of its degradation result in significant imbalance of nitrogen intake and its excretion. Healthy adults are generally in nitrogen balance, with intake and excretion being very well matched. Young growing children, adults recovering from major illness, and pregnant women are often in ***positive nitrogen balance***. Their uptake of nitrogen exceeds their loss, as net protein synthesis proceeds. An individual is said to be in ***negative nitrogen balance*** when more nitrogen is excreted than is incorporated into the body. Insufficient supply of even one essential amino acid is enough to turn an otherwise normal individual into one with a negative nitrogen balance.

The term, ***biological value of dietary proteins*** is related to the extent to which they provide all the necessary amino acids. Proteins of animal origin generally have a high biological value; plant proteins have a wide range of values from almost none to quite high. In general, plant proteins are deficient in lysine, methionine, and tryptophan and are much less concentrated and less digestible than animal proteins. The absence of lysine in low-grade cereal proteins, used as staple food in many underdeveloped countries, leads to an inability to synthesize protein and ultimately to a syndrome known as ***kwashiorkor.***

Essential vs. Nonessential Amino Acids

The amino acids arginine, methionine and phenylalanine are considered essential for reasons not directly related to lack of synthesis. Arginine is synthesized by mammalian cells but at a rate that is insufficient to meet the growth needs of the body and the majority that is synthesized is cleaved to form urea.

Nonessential amino acids	*Essential amino acids*
Alanine, asparagine, aspartate, cysteine, glutamate, glutamine, glycine, Proline, serine, tyrosine	Arginine*, histidine, isoleucine Leucine, lysine, methionine* Phenylalanine, threonine, Tryptophan, valine

Methionine is required in large amounts to produce cysteine if the latter amino acid is not adequately supplied in the diet. Similarly, large amounts of phenylalanine are needed to form tyrosine if the latter is not adequately supplied in the diet.

Removal of Nitrogen from Amino Acids

The predominant reactions that remove nitrogen of amino acid in the body are transamination reactions. This class of reactions is involved in funneling nitrogen from all free amino acids into a small number of compounds; then, either they are oxidatively deaminated to release ammonia, or their amine groups are converted to urea in the urea cycle. Transamination reactions involve transfer of α-amino group from a donor α-amino acid to the keto carbon of an acceptor α-keto acid. These reversible reactions are catalyzed by a group of intracellular enzymes known as aminotransferases, which generally employ covalently bound pyridoxal phosphate as a cofactor. However, *some aminotransferases employ pyruvate as a cofactor.*

Therapeutic Use of Asparaginase

Most cells have an active pathway to synthesize asparagine they need.
Aspartate + glutamine + ATP → glutamate + asparagine + AMP + PP$_i$
However, some leukemia cells require exogenous asparagine, which they obtain from the plasma. Chemotherapy using the *enzyme asparaginase* takes advantage of this property of leukemic cells by hydrolyzing serum asparagine to ammonia and aspartic acid, thus depriving the neoplastic cells of the asparagine that is essential for their characteristic rapid growth.

In the peroxisomes of mammalian hepatic tissues, there exist a minor enzymatic pathway for the removal of amino groups from amino acids by an FMN-linked *L-amino acid oxidase* that has broad specificity for the L-amino acids. A number of substances including oxygen act as electron acceptors from reduced flavoproteins. If oxygen is the acceptor the product is hydrogen peroxide, which is then rapidly degraded by the *catalases* found in liver and other tissues. Absence or defective peroxisomes or *L-amino acid oxidase* causes generalized hyperaminoacidemia and hyperaminoaciduria, generally leading to neurotoxicity and early death.

UREA CYCLE

About 80 percent of nitrogen excreted from the human body are in the form of urea that is largely made in the liver. A series of reactions that are distributed between the mitochondrial matrix and the cytosol are responsible for synthesis of urea. The series of reactions that lead to urea formation is known as *urea cycle* or Krebs-Henseleit cycle (Fig. 26.3).

The essential features of the urea cycle reactions and their metabolic regulation are as follows:

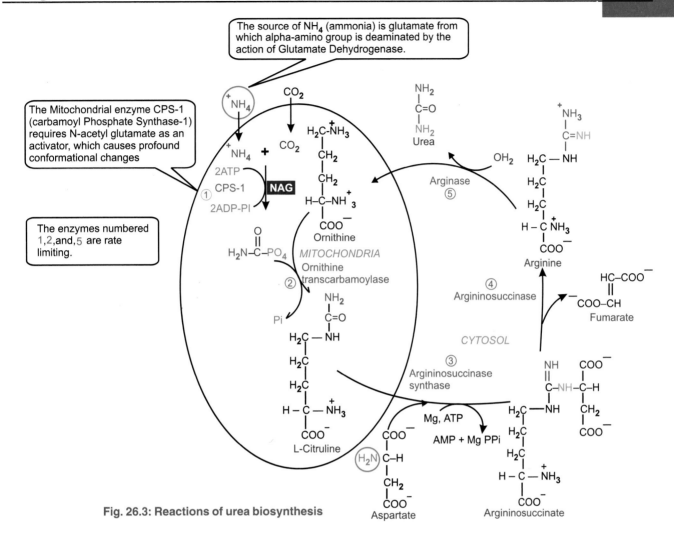

Fig. 26.3: Reactions of urea biosynthesis

a. Arginine from the diet or from protein breakdown is cleaved by the cytosolic enzyme *arginase*, generating urea and ornithine.

b. In subsequent reactions of the urea cycle, a new urea residue is built on the ornithine, regenerating arginine and perpetuating the cycle.

c. Ornithine arising in the cytosol is transported to the mitochondrial matrix, where it condenses with carbamoyl phosphate catalyzed by *ornithine transcarbamoylase* to produce citrulline. The energy for the reaction is provided by the high-energy anhydride of carbamoyl phosphate. The citrulline is then transported to the cytosol, where the remaining reactions of the cycle take place. The synthesis of citrulline requires a prior activation of carbon and nitrogen as carbamoyl phosphate (CP). This activation step requires two equivalents of ATP and the mitochondrial matrix enzyme *carbamoyl phosphate synthetase-I* (CPS-I). There are two CP synthetases: a mitochondrial CPS-I, which forms CP destined for inclusion in the urea cycle, and another is a cytosolic CP synthetase (CPS-II), which is involved in pyrimidine nucleotide biosynthesis.

d. The allosteric effector N-acetyl-glutamate positively regulates CPS-I, while the cytosolic enzyme is acetylglutamate independent.

e. In a 2-step reaction, catalyzed by cytosolic *argininosuccinate synthetase*, citrulline and aspartate are condensed to form argininosuccinate. The reaction involves the addition of AMP (from ATP) to the amido carbonyl of citrulline, forming an activated intermediate on the enzyme surface (AMP-citrulline), and the subsequent addition of aspartate to form argininosuccinate.

f. In the next step catalyzed by a cytosolic enzyme *argininosuccinate lyase* (also called *argininosuccinase*), argininosuccinate is cleaved to yield arginine and fumarate.

g. In the final step of the cycle arginase cleaves urea from arginine, regenerating cytosolic ornithine, which is transported to the mitochondrial matrix for another round of urea synthesis. The fumarate generated via the action of *argininosuccinate lyase* is reconverted to aspartate for use in the *argininosuccinate synthetase* reaction. This occurs through the actions of cytosolic versions of the TCA cycle enzymes, *fumarase* (that yields malate) and *malate dehydrogenase* (that yields oxaloacetate). The oxaloacetate is then transaminated to aspartate by AST.

Energetic of Urea Cycle

The reactions of the cycle consume three equivalents of ATP and a total of four high-energy nucleotide phosphates. Urea is the only new compound generated by the cycle; all other intermediates and reactants are recycled. The energy consumed in the production of urea is more than recovered by the release of energy formed during the synthesis of the urea cycle intermediates. Ammonia released during the *glutamate dehydrogenase* reaction is coupled to the formation of NADH. In addition, when fumarate is converted back to aspartate, the *malate dehydrogenase* reaction used to convert malate to oxaloacetate generates a mole of NADH. These two moles of NADH, thus, are oxidized in the mitochondria yielding six moles of ATP.

Regulation of the Urea Cycle

The urea cycle operates only to eliminate excess nitrogen On high-protein diets the carbon skeletons of the amino acids are oxidized for energy or stored as fat and glycogen, but the amino nitrogen must be excreted. To facilitate this process, enzymes of the urea cycle are controlled at the gene level:

The long-term changes A significant increase in dietary proteins raises the enzyme concentrations of urea cycle up to twenty-fold. On return to a balanced diet, enzyme levels decline. Under conditions of starvation, enzyme levels are elevated as more proteins are degraded and carbon skeletons of amino acids are used to provide energy, thus increasing the quantity of nitrogen that must be excreted.

The short-term regulations Occurs principally at *CPS-I*, which is relatively inactive in the absence of its allosteric activator

N-acetylglutamate. The steady-state concentration of N-acetylglutamate is set by the concentration of its components acetyl-CoA and glutamate, and by arginine, which is a positive allosteric effector of **N-acetyl glutamate synthetase.**

Acetyl-CoA + glutamate $\rightarrow$ N-acetyl glutamate + CoA

Genetic Defects of Urea Cycle

A complete lack of any one of the enzymes of the urea cycle will result in death shortly after birth. However, deficiencies in each of the enzymes of the urea cycle, including *N-acetyl glutamate synthase*, have been identified. These disorders are referred to as urea cycle disorders or UCDs. A common finding in most UCDs is hyperammonemia leading to ammonia intoxication with the consequences described hereunder.

The clinical symptoms of UCDs are most severe with *carbamoyl phosphate synthetase-I* deficiency and the least manifested with *arginase deficiency*. Symptoms of UCDs usually manifest at birth, which include ataxia, convulsions, lethargy, poor feeding and eventually coma and death if not recognized and treated properly. In fact, the mortality rate is 100 percent for UCDs that are left undiagnosed. Several UCDs manifest with late-onset such as in adulthood. In these cases, the symptoms are hyperactivity, hepatomegaly and avoidance of protein-rich foods.

Treatment of UCDs

The mainstay of treatment includes a reduction in dietary protein, removal of excess ammonia and replacement of intermediates missing from the urea cycle. ***Administration of levulose reduces ammonia through its action of acidifying the colon***. Bacteria metabolize levulose to acidic by-products, which then promotes excretion of ammonia in the feces as ammonium ions (NH_4^+). Antibiotics can be administered to destroy intestinal bacteria that produce ammonia. Sodium benzoate and sodium phenylbutyrate can be administered, which covalently bind glycine (forming hippurate) and glutamine (forming phenylacetylglutamine) respectively. These latter compounds, which contain the ammonia nitrogen, are excreted in the feces. Dietary supplementation with arginine or citrulline can increase the rate of urea production in certain UCDs.

Type-I Hyperammonemia (Carbamoylphosphate Synthetase I Deficiency)

Within 24 to 72 hours after birth infant becomes lethargic and needs stimulation to feed. The infant starts vomiting, respiratory rate increases and becomes hypothermic; without measurement of serum ammonia levels and appropriate intervention infant will die. Treatment with arginine activates N-acetyl glutamate synthetase.

N-acetyl Glutamate Synthetase Deficiency (N-acetyl Glutamate Synthetase Deficiency)

Clinical symptoms include mild to severe hyperammonemia associated with deep coma, acidosis, recurrent diarrhea, ataxia, hypoglycemia, and hyperornithinemia. Treatment includes administration of carbamoyl glutamate to activate CPS I.

Type-2 Hyperammonemia (Ornithine Transcarbamoylase Deficiency)

It is the only X-linked and most commonly occurring UCD. Ammonia, amino acids and orotic acid are elevated in the serum, increased serum orotic acid due to mitochondrial carbamoylphosphate entering cytosol and getting incorporated into pyrimidine nucleotides, which leads to excess production and consequently excess catabolic products (orotic acid). Treatment includes high carbohydrate low protein diet, and ammonia detoxification with sodium phenylacetate or sodium benzoate.

Classic Citrullinemia (Argininosuccinate Synthetase Deficiency)

Clinical signs and symptoms include episodic hyperammonemia, vomiting, lethargy, ataxia, seizures, and eventual coma. Treat with arginine administration to enhance citrulline excretion, and also with sodium benzoate for ammonia detoxification.

Argininosuccinic Aciduria (Argininosuccinase Deficiency)

The symptoms are similar to classic citrullinemia with elevated plasma and cerebral spinal fluid argininosuccinate. Treat with arginine and sodium benzoate.

Hyperargininemia (Arginase Deficiency)

It is a rare UCD characterized by progressive spastic quadriplegia and mental retardation. The serum and CSF levels of ammonia and arginine are elevated. Urinary excretion of arginine, lysine and ornithine are high. Treatment includes low protein diet that includes essential amino acids but exclude arginine.

Ammonia is Neurotoxic

Ammonia is neurotoxic and cause marked brain damage if not treated early. Aside from its effect on blood pH (depletes bicarbonate), ammonia readily traverses the blood-brain barrier where it gets converted to glutamate via *glutamate dehydrogenase*, and depletes the α-ketoglutarate in the brain. As the α-ketoglutarate is depleted, oxaloacetate levels fall correspondingly and ultimately TCA cycle activity comes to a halt. In the absence of aerobic oxidative phosphorylation and TCA cycle activity, irreparable cell damage and neural cell death ensue. In addition, the elevated ammonia levels lead to glutamine formation that depletes glutamate stores in neural tissue. Since glutamate is both a neurotransmitter and a precursor for the synthesis of another neurotransmitter γ-aminobutyrate (GABA), glutamate depletion affects the CNS function. Therefore, reductions in brain glutamate affect both energy production as well as neurotransmission.

Specialized Products of Amino Acids

27

Tyrosine-derived Neurotransmitters

Most of tyrosine that is not incorporated into proteins is catabolized for energy production. The other important fate of tyrosine is its conversion to **catecholamines**, which include *epinephrine*, *norepinephrine* and *dopamine* (Fig. 27.1).

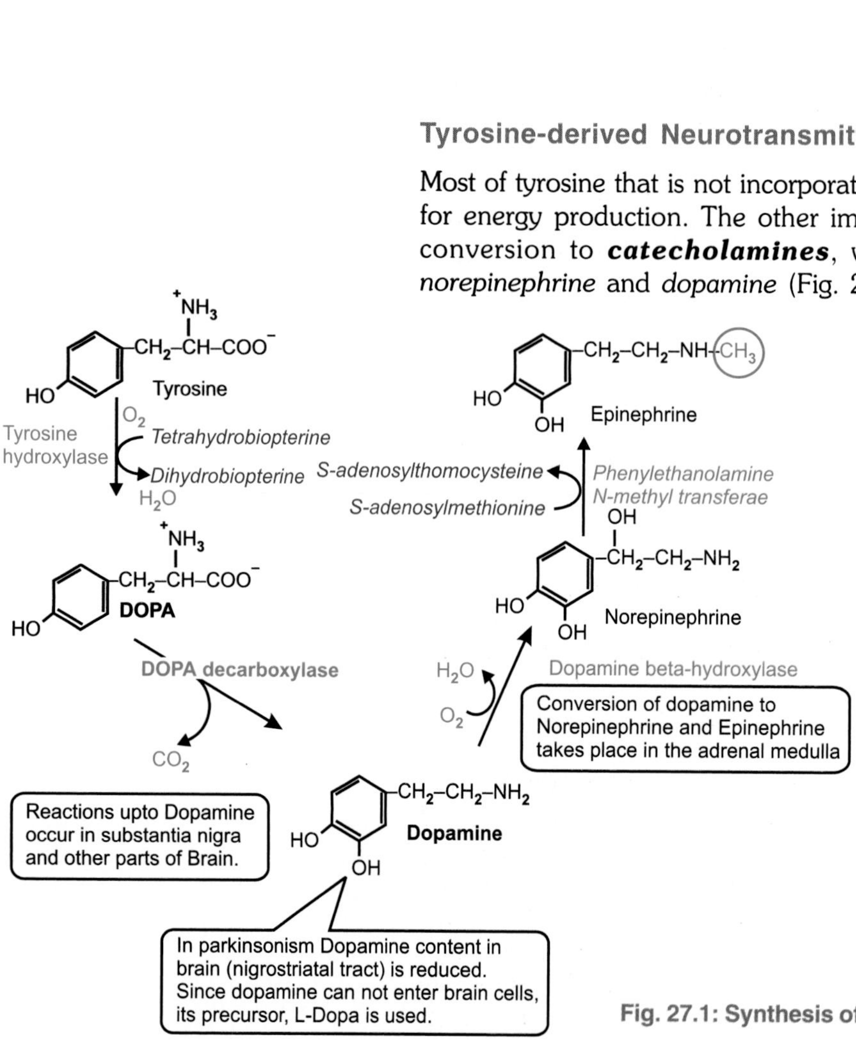

Fig. 27.1: Synthesis of catecholamines

Norepinephrine is the principal neurotransmitter of sympathetic postganglionic endings. Both norepinephrine and its methylated derivative epinephrine are stored in synaptic knobs of neurons that secrete it. However, epinephrine is not a mediator at postganglionic sympathetic endings.

Tyrosine is transported into catecholamine-secreting neurons and adrenal medullary cells where catecholamine synthesis takes place. The first step in the process is catalyzed *tyrosine hydroxylase*, which like *phenylalanine hydroxylase* requires tetrahydrobiopterin as cofactor. The hydroxylation reaction generates DOPA (3,4-dihydrophenylalanine), which is converted to dopamine by DOPA *decarboxylase*. Dopamine is converted to norepinephrine and by *dopamine β-hydroxylase*. Norepinephrine is then methylated to form epinephrine by *N-methyltransferase*. This latter reaction is one of the several in the body that uses SAM as a methyl donor generating S-adenosylhomocysteine.

Within the substantia nigra and some other regions of the brain, synthesis proceeds only up to dopamine. Within the adrenal medulla dopamine is converted to norepinephrine and epinephrine

Once synthesized, dopamine, norepinephrine and epinephrine are packaged in granulated vesicles. Within these vesicles, norepinephrine and epinephrine are stored bound to ATP and a protein called *chromogranin A*.

Metabolism of the catecholamines occurs through the actions of *catecholamine-O-methyltransferase* (COMT) and *monoamine oxidase* (MAO). Both of these enzymes are widely distributed throughout the body. However, COMT and MAO are not found in nerve endings.

Tryptophan-derived Neurotransmitters

Tryptophan is the precursor for the synthesis of *serotonin* (5-hydroxy-tryptamine, 5-HT), and *melatonin* (N-acetyl-5-methoxytryptamine).

Serotonin

Synthesis of serotonin is a two-step process involving tetrahydro-biopterin-dependent hydroxylation catalyzed by tryptophan-5-monooxygenase and then decarboxylation catalyzed by **aromatic L-amino acid decarboxylase** (Fig. 27.2). Since the hydroxylase system is not saturated under normal conditions, an *increased dietary tryptophan will lead to increased brain serotonin content.*

Highest concentrations of serotonin are found in platelets and the gastrointestinal tract. Lesser amounts are found in the retina and brain, where it is involved with alertness. Serotonin containing neurons have their cell bodies in the *midline raphe nuclei* of the brainstem and project to portions of the hypothalamus, the limbic system, the neocortex and the spinal cord. Most of the serotonin released from serotonergic neurons is recaptured by an active reuptake mechanism. Mental depression correlates with low levels of serotonin. **Prozac,** used in treating depressive disorder is a selective serotonin reuptake inhibitor (SSRIs). It inhibits serotonin reuptake process, thereby prolongs the presence of serotonin at the synaptic cleft. Serotonin exerts its functions through interaction with specific receptors. Several serotonin receptors have been cloned and are identified. Most of these receptors are coupled to G-proteins that

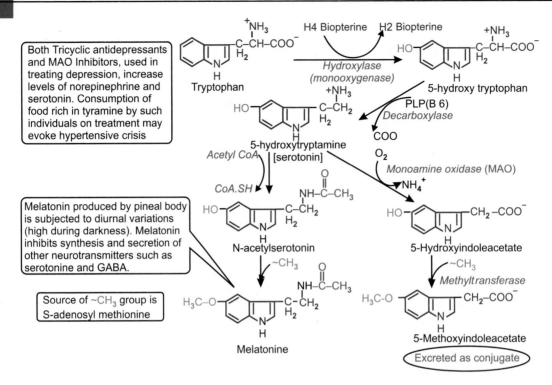

Fig. 27.2: Serotonine and melatonine synthesis

affect the activities of either *adenylate cyclase* or *phospholipase C-γ (PLC-γ)*. The $5HT_3$ class of receptors present in the gastrointestinal tract (related to vomiting) is ion channels. Some serotonin receptors are presynaptic and others postsynaptic. The $5HT_{2A}$ receptors mediate platelet aggregation and smooth muscle contraction. The $5HT_{2C}$ receptors are suspected in control of food intake. The $5HT_4$ receptors present in the gastrointestinal tract are involved in secretion and peristalsis. The $5HT_6$ and $5HT_7$ receptors are distributed throughout the limbic system of the brain and the $5HT_6$ receptors have high affinity for antidepressant drugs.

Melatonin

Melatonin is derived from serotonin within the pineal gland and the retina, where the necessary *N*-acetyltransferase enzyme is found. The pineal parenchymal cells secrete melatonin into the blood and cerebrospinal fluid. Synthesis and secretion of melatonin increase during the dark period of the day and are maintained at a low level during daylight hours. This diurnal variation in melatonin synthesis is regulated by norepinephrine secreted by the postganglionic sympathetic nerves that innervate the pineal gland. The effects of norepinephrine are exerted through its interaction with β-adrenergic receptors. This leads to increased levels of cAMP, which in turn activate the N-acetyltransferase required for melatonin synthesis. Melatonin functions by inhibiting the synthesis and secretion of other neurotransmitters such as dopamine and GABA.

Creatine Biosynthesis

Creatine is synthesized in the liver by methylation of guanidoacetate by SAM (the methyl donor). Guanidoacetate itself is formed in the kidney from the amino acids arginine and glycine (Fig. 27.3).

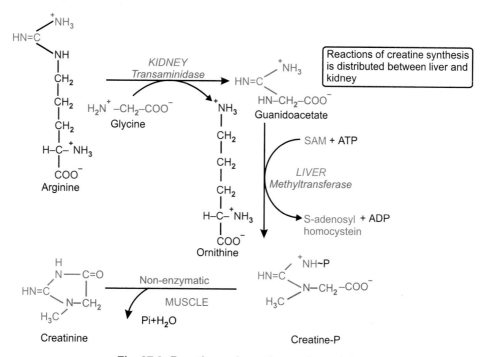

Fig. 27.3: Reactions of creatine and creatinine

Creatine phosphate, which is used as storage form of high-energy phosphate, is formed by phosphorylation of creatine, catalyzed by **creatine phosphokinase**. The reaction is reversible such that when energy demand is high (e.g. during muscle exertion) creatine phosphate donates its phosphate to ADP to yield ATP.

Both creatine and creatine phosphate are found in muscle, brain and blood. Creatinine is formed in muscle from creatine by nonenzymatic dehydration. The amount of creatinine formed is proportional to muscle mass and remains remarkably constant from day to day. Creatinine excreted by the kidneys and the level of excretion (creatinine clearance rate) is a measure of renal function.

Glutathione Functions

Glutathione (abbreviated as GSH) is a tripeptide composed of glutamate, cysteine and glycine (Fig. 27.4). Glutathione has many important functions within cells. It serves as a reductant, gets conjugated to drugs to make them more water-soluble, is

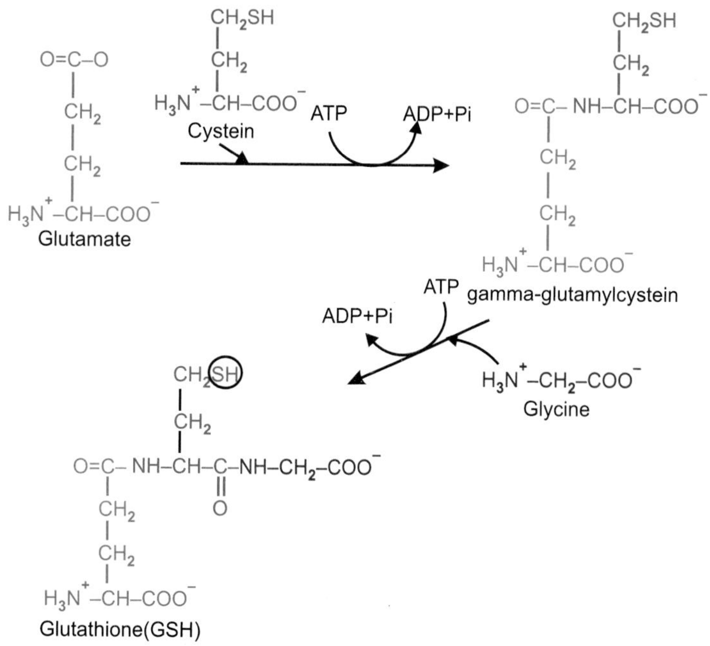

Fig. 27.4: Glutathione sythesis

involved in amino acid transport across cell membranes (the γ-**glutamyl cycle**), is a part of the peptidoleukotrienes, serves as a cofactor for some enzymatic reactions and helps in the rearrangement of protein disulfide bonds.

The role of GSH as a reductant is extremely important particularly in the highly oxidizing environment of the erythrocyte. The sulfhydryl of GSH can be used to reduce peroxides formed during oxygen transport. The resulting oxidized form of GSH consists of two molecules disulfide bonded together (abbreviated GS-SG). The enzyme **glutathione reductase** utilizes NADPH as a cofactor to reduce GS-SG back to two moles of GSH. Hence, the pentose phosphate pathway is an extremely important pathway of erythrocytes for the continuing production of the NADPH needed by **glutathione reductase**. Erythrocytes consume as much as 10 percent of its total glucose consumption for pentose phosphate pathway.

Several mechanisms exist for the transport of amino acids across cell membranes. Many are symport or antiport mechanisms that couple amino acid transport to sodium transport. The γ-glutamyl cycle is an example of a group transfer mechanism of amino acid transport. Although this mechanism requires more energy input, it is rapid and has a high capacity. The cycle functions primarily in the kidney, particularly renal epithelial cells. The enzyme **γ-glutamyl transpeptidase** is located in the cell membrane and shuttles GSH to the cell surface to interact with an amino acid. Reaction with an amino acid liberates cysteinylglycine and generates a γ-glutamyl-amino acid, which is transported into the cell and hydrolyzed to release the amino acid. Glutamate is released as 5-oxoproline and the cysteinylglycine is cleaved to its component amino acids. Regeneration of GSH requires an ATP-dependent conversion of 5-oxoproline to glutamate and then the 2 additional moles of ATP that are required during the normal generation of GSH.

Polyamine Biosynthesis

One of the earliest signals for the cells to enter their replication cycle is the appearance of elevated levels of mRNA for *ornithine decarboxylase* (ODC). The ODC is the first enzyme in the pathway of polyamine synthesis (Fig. 27.5). Since polyamines are highly cationic and tend to bind nucleic acids with high affinity, it is believed that the polyamines are important participants in DNA synthesis and its regulation.

The key features of the pathway are that it involves **putrescine** an ornithine catabolite, and S-adenosylmethionine (SAM) as a donor of two propylamine residues. The first propylamine conjugation yields **spermidine** and addition of another to spermidine yields **spermine**. The function of ODC is to produce the 4-carbon saturated diamine, putrescine. At the same time, *SAM decarboxylase* cleaves the SAM carboxyl residue, producing decarboxylated SAM (S-adenosylmethylthiopropylamine), which retains the methyl group usually involved in **SAM** *methyltransferase* activity. The *SAM decarboxylase*

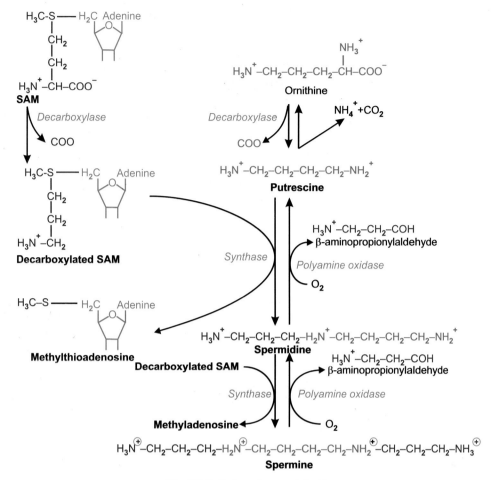

Fig. 27.5: Polyamine metabolism

activity is regulated by product inhibition and allosterically stimulated by putrescine. The *spermidine synthase* catalyzes the condensation reaction, producing spermidine and 5'-methylthioadenosine. A second propylamine residue is added to spermidine producing spermine.

The signal for regulating ODC activity is unknown, but since the product of its activity, putrescine regulates *SAM decarboxylase* activity, it appears that polyamine production is principally regulated by ODC concentration.

The butylamino group of spermidine is used in a post-translational modification reaction important to the process of translation. A specific lysine residue in the translational initiation factor **eIF-4D** is modified. Following the modification the residue is hydroxylated yielding a residue in the protein termed **hypusine**.

Nitric Oxide: Synthesis and Function

Vasodilators, such as acetylcholine, do not exert their effects upon the vascular smooth muscle cell in the absence of the overlying endothelium. When acetylcholine binds its receptor on the surface of endothelial cells, a signal cascade coupled to the activation *phospholipase* C-γ (PLC-γ) is initiated. The PLC-γ-mediated release of inositol trisphosphate, IP$_3$ (from membrane associated phosphatidylinositol-4, 5-bisphosphate, PIP$_2$), leads to the release of intracellular stores of Ca^{2+}. In turn, the elevation in Ca^{2+} leads to the liberation of *endothelium-derive relaxing factor (EDRF)* which then diffuses into the adjacent smooth muscle. Within smooth muscle cells, EDRF reacts with the heme moiety of a soluble **guanylyl cyclase,** resulting in its activation and a consequent elevation of intracellular levels of cGMP that causes calcium ions to enter storage areas of the cell. The lowered concentrations of calcium ions (Ca^{++}) set off a cascade of cellular reactions that cause the smooth muscle cell's contractile filaments (myosin and actin) to slide apart and relax, the net effect is dilatation of blood vessels.

The widely used nitroglycerine a coronary artery vasodilator, acts to increase intracellular release of EDRF and thus of cGMP. The EDRF is the free radical diatomic gas, nitric oxide (NO) that is formed by the action of *nitric oxide synthase* (NOS) on the amino acid arginine.

Arginine → citrulline + NO

NOS is a very complex enzyme, employing five redox cofactors: NADPH, FAD, FMN, heme and tetrahydrobiopterin. NO can also be formed from nitrite, derived from vasodilators such as glycerin trinitrate during their metabolism. The half-life of NO is extremely short, lasting only 2 to 4 seconds. This is because it is a highly reactive free radical and interacts with oxygen and superoxide. NO is inhibited by hemoglobin and other heme proteins which bind it tightly.

Chemical inhibitors of NOS are available and can markedly decrease production of NO. The effect is a dramatic increase in blood pressure due to vasoconstriction. Another important cardiovascular effect of NO is exerted through the production of cGMP, which acts to inhibit platelet aggregation.

Sildenafil citrate (Viagra) used for the treatment of male impotency is a specific inhibitor of phosphodiesterase 5. Phosphodiesterase 5 (PDE5) cleaves the ring form of cyclic GMP (**cGMP**) a cellular second messenger similar to cAMP. The inhibition of the phosphodiesterase allows for the persistence of **cGMP**, which promotes the effects of cGMP production. In this case, it allows for increased blood flow into the penis, which may result in an erection.

Normally, sexual stimulation in the male is followed by release of nitric oxide (NO) in the corpus cavernosum of the penis. NO activates the enzyme guanylate cyclase in the smooth muscle cells, which allows for the relaxation of the penile arteries and an increased blood flow into the penile cavity. The effect of Viagra is to allow the accumulation of **cGMP** by inhibiting the phosphodiesterase action, which tends to magnify the effect of NO release. Clearly, the mechanism of penile erection is a case of when NO means yes. One of the curious side effects of Viagra is an effect on the visual discrimination of certain colors. This appears to be due to the reduced affinity of the drug for the phosphodiesterase enzyme found in the retina (PDE6). Viagra has an even more reduced affinity for PDE3, which is critical since PDE3 is active in heart muscle cells.

Intestinal Uptake and Transport of Lipids

28

Intestinal Uptake of Lipids

The ingested dietary lipids are emulsified in the aqueous environment of the intestine, with the help of bile salts. Bile salts are catabolites of cholesterol formed in the liver and then stored in the gallbladder; they are secreted following the ingestion of fat.

Emulsification of dietary fats is essential to make them accessible to pancreatic lipases (primarily *lipase* and phospholipase-A_2) that are secreted into the intestine from the pancreas. These enzymes are essentially esterases that hydrolyze the dietary triacylglycerol to generate free fatty acids and mixtures of mono- and diacylglycerols. Pancreatic lipase degrades triacylglycerols at the 3 and 1 positions sequentially to generate 1,2-diacylglycerols and 2-acylglycerols. The phospholipids are hydrolyzed at the 2 positions by the pancreatic phospholipase-A_2 releasing free fatty acid and lysophospholipid. The products of hydrolysis by the action of pancreatic lipases then diffuse into the intestinal epithelial cells, where triacylglycerols are re-synthesized.

Triacylglycerols and cholesterol of dietary origin, as well as those synthesized by the liver are secreted in the form of water-soluble lipid-protein complexes called *lipoproteins*. The *lipoproteins are water-soluble transport form of particulate lipid-protein complexes, secreted by small intestine and liver into the circulating blood.* They are composed of triacylglycerol and cholesteryl esters surrounded by polar phospholipids and apolipoproteins. These lipid-protein complexes differing in their content of lipid and protein are classified based on their density and the net charge they carry. Since lipid is less dense than protein, the lipoproteins with low protein content have lower density. On electrophoresis lipoproteins separate into four bands as α, pre-β, β, and chylomicrons depending on the net charge they carry.

Composition of the Major Lipoprotein Complexes

Complex	Source	Density (g/ml)	%Protein	%TG[a]	%PL[b]	%CE[c]	%C[d]	%FFA[e]
Chylomicron	Intestine	<0.95	1-2	85-88	8	3	1	0
VLDL	Liver	0.95-1.006	7-10	50-55	18-20	12-15	8-10	1
IDL	VLDL	1.006-1.019	10-12	25-30	25-27	32-35	8-10	1
LDL	VLDL	1.019-1.063	20-22	10-15	20-28	37-48	8-10	1
*HDL$_2$	Intestine, liver (chylomicrons and VLDLs)	1.063-1.125	33-35	5-15	32-43	20-30	5-10	0
*HDL$_3$	Intestine, liver (chylomicrons and VLDLs)	1.125-1.21	55-57	3-13	26-46	15-30	2-6	6
Albumin-FFA	Adipose tissue	>1.281	99	0	0	0	0	100

[a]Triacylglycerols, [b]Phospholipids, [c]Cholesteryl esters, [d]Free cholesterol, [e]Free fatty acids
*HDL2 and HDL3 derived from nascent HDL as a result of the acquisition of cholesterylesters

Functions and Classification of Apolipoproteins

Apoprotein MW(Da)	Lipoprotein Association	Function and Comments
apo-A-I - 29,016	Chylomicrons, HDL	Major protein of HDL, activates LCAT
apo-A-II - 17,400	Chylomicrons, HDL	Primarily in HDL, enhances hepatic lipase activity
apo-A-IV - 46,000	Chylomicrons and HDL	Present in triacylglycerol rich lipoproteins
apo-B-48 - 241,000	Chylomicrons	Exclusively found in chylomicrons, derived from apo-B-100 gene by RNA editing in intestinal epithelium; lacks the LDL receptor-binding domain of apo-B-100
apo-B-100 - 513,000	VLDL, IDL and LDL	Major protein of LDL, binds to LDL receptor; one of the longest known proteins in humans
apo-C-I - 7,600	Chylomicrons, VLDL, IDL and HDL	May also activate LCAT
apo-C-II - 8,916	Chylomicrons, VLDL, IDL and HDL	Activates lipoprotein lipase
apo-C-III - 8,750	Chylomicrons, VLDL, IDL and HDL	Inhibits lipoprotein lipase
apo-D - 20,000; also called cholesterol ester transfer protein, CETP	HDL	Exclusively associated with HDL, cholesteryl ester transfer
apo-E - 34,000 (at least 3 alleles [E$_2$, E$_3$, E$_4$] each of which have multiple isoforms)	Chylomicron remnants, VLDL, IDL and HDL	Binds to LDL receptor, apo-E$_{e4}$ allele amplification associated with late-onset Alzheimer's disease

Contd...

Contd...

apo-H - 50,000 (also known as β-2-glycoprotein I)	Chylomicrons	Triacylglycerol metabolism
apo (a)-at least 19 different alleles; protein ranges in size from 300,000 - 800,000	LDL	Disulfide bonded to apo-B-100, forms a complex with LDL identified as lipoprotein (a), Lp (a); strongly resembles plasminogen; may deliver cholesterol to sites of vascular injury, high risk association with premature coronary artery disease and stroke

Chylomicrons

Chylomicrons are formed in the mucosal cells of the intestine to *mobilize dietary lipids* to the rest of the body (Fig. 28.1). The predominant lipids of chylomicrons are triacylglycerols. The predominant apolipoproteins found in chylomicrons before they enter the circulation include apo-B-48 (exclusively found in chylomicrons), apo-A-I, -A-II and IV. The intestine secretes chylomicrons into the lymphatic system that enter the circulation at the left subclavian vein. In the systemic bloodstream, chylomicrons acquire apo-C-II and apo-E from plasma HDLs. The *lipoprotein lipase* (LPL) found on the surface of endothelial cells lining the capillaries in muscle and adipose tissue removes the fatty acids of triacylglycerol in the chylomicrons. The apo-C-II in the chylomicrons

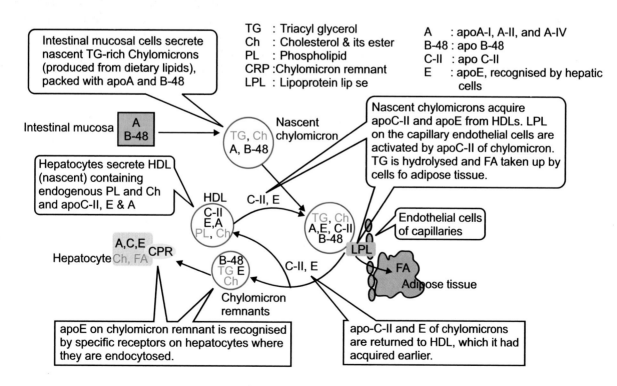

Fig. 28.1: Chylomicron metabolism

activates LPL in the presence of phospholipid. The tissues then absorb the free fatty acids, where as the glycerol backbone of the triacylglycerol is returned via the blood, to the liver and kidneys, where it is converted to the glycolytic intermediate dihydroxyacetone phosphate (DHAP).

Substantial portion of phospholipid, apo-A and apo-C are transferred to HDLs during the process of fatty acid removal from chylomicrons. The loss of apo-C-II prevents LPL from further degrading the chylomicron remnants. Chylomicron remnants, containing primarily cholesterol, apo-E and apo-B-48 are then delivered to, and taken up by, the liver through interaction with the chylomicron remnant receptor. The recognition of chylomicron remnants by the hepatic remnant-receptor requires apo-E. The chylomicrons function to deliver dietary cholesterol to the liver, and triacylglycerols to adipose tissue and muscle.

Very Low-density Lipoproteins (VLDLs)

The dietary intake of both fat and carbohydrates in excess of the body needs are converted to triacylglycerols in the liver. These triacylglycerols are packaged into very low-density lipoproteins (VLDLs) and secreted into the circulation for delivery to the peripheral tissues (primarily muscle and adipose tissue), where they are stored or oxidized to release energy (Fig. 28.2). The VLDLs are therefore, the molecules formed to transport endogenously derived triacylglycerols to extrahepatic tissues. The VLDLs, in addition to triacylglycerols also contain some free cholesterol, cholesteryl esters and the apoproteins apo-B-100, apo-C-I, apo-C-II, apo-C-III and apo-E. Like nascent chylomicrons, newly released VLDLs acquire apo-Cs and apo-E from circulating HDLs.

The fatty acid portion of VLDLs is taken up by adipose tissue and muscle in the same way as for chylomicrons through the action of lipoprotein lipase. The action of lipoprotein lipase coupled to a loss of certain apoproteins (the apo-Cs) converts VLDLs to intermediate density lipoproteins (IDLs), also termed VLDL remnants. The apo-Cs are transferred to HDLs and the predominant remaining proteins are apo-B-100 and apo-E. The further loss of triacylglycerols converts IDLs to LDLs.

Intermediate Density Lipoproteins (IDLs)

The IDLs are formed from VLDLs as its triacylglycerols are removed. The fate of IDLs is either conversion to LDLs or its direct uptake by the liver. IDLs are converted to LDLs as more triacylglycerols are removed. The liver takes up IDLs after they have interacted with the LDL receptor to form a complex, which is endocytosed by the cell. For LDL receptors in the liver to recognize IDLs it requires the presence of both apo-B-100 and apo-E (the LDL receptor is also called the apo-B-100/apo-E receptor).

Low Density Lipoproteins (LDLs)

The cells requirement for cholesterol as a membrane component is satisfied in one of two ways: either it is synthesized *de novo* within

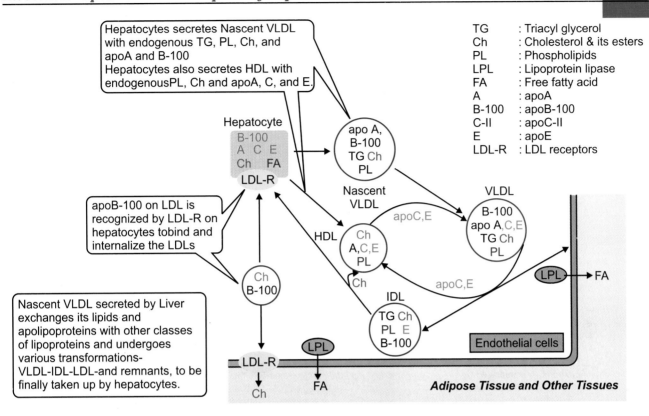

Fig. 28.2: VLDL metabolism

the cell, or it is supplied from extracellular sources, namely, chylomicrons and LDLs. The dietary cholesterol that goes into chylomicrons is delivered to the liver by the interaction of chylomicron remnants with the remnant receptor. In addition, cholesterol synthesized in the liver is transported to extrahepatic tissues, packaged in VLDLs. In the circulation, VLDLs are converted to LDLs through the action of lipoprotein lipase (Fig. 28.2). The LDLs are the primary carriers of cholesterol in the blood for delivery to all peripheral tissues.

Almost 75 percent of LDLs are taken-up by liver, adrenal and adipose tissue cells by LDL receptor-mediated endocytosis. The interaction of LDLs with LDL receptors requires the presence of apo-B-100, which is found exclusively in LDLs. The endocytosed membrane vesicles (endosomes) fuse with lysosomes, in which the apoproteins are degraded and the cholesterol esters are hydrolyzed to yield free cholesterol. The cholesterol is then incorporated into the plasma membranes as necessary and the excess cholesterol is re-esterified by *acyl-CoA-cholesterol acyltransferase* (ACAT) for intracellular storage. The ACAT activity is enhanced by the presence of intracellular cholesterol. The LDL binding to liver cells is enhanced by insulin and tri-iodotyronine (T3), whereas glucocorticoids (e.g., dexamethasone) have the opposite effect. These effects are probably mediated through the regulation of apo-B degradation that explains the hypercholesterolemia and increased risk of atherosclerosis associated with uncontrolled diabetes or hypothyroidism.

An abnormal form of LDL identified as lipoprotein-X (Lp-X), predominates in the circulation of patients suffering from *lecithin-cholesterol acyl transferase* (LCAT) deficiency or cholestatic liver disease. In both cases there is an elevation in the level of circulating free cholesterol and phospholipids.

High Density Lipoproteins (HDLs)

De novo synthesis of HDLs, as protein-rich discoid particles takes place primarily in the liver and small intestine (Fig. 28.3). These newly formed HDLs (nascent HDLs) are almost devoid of any cholesterol. The primary apoproteins of HDLs are apo-A-I, apo-C-I, apo-C-II and apo-E. In fact, *a major function of HDLs is to act as circulating stores of apo-C-I, apo-C-II and apo-E, apart from scavenging cholesterol from peripheral sites.*

Discoid HDLs are converted into spherical lipoprotein particles through the accumulation of cholesteryl esters. This accumulation converts nascent HDLs to spherical HDL_2 and HDL_3 by the action of the HDL-associated enzyme, *lecithin-cholesterol acyl transferase*

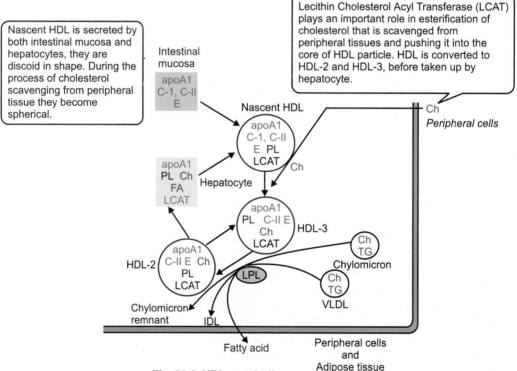

Fig. 28.3: HDL metabolism

(LCAT). Any free cholesterol present in chylomicron remnants and VLDL remnants (IDLs) are also taken up by HDLs and esterified by LCAT, which is synthesized in the liver. The LCAT is so named because it transfers a fatty acid from the C-2 position of lecithin to the C-3 hydroxyl of cholesterol, generating a cholesteryl ester and lysolecithin. The activity of LCAT requires interaction with apo-A-I, which is found on the surface of HDLs.

Cholesterol-rich HDLs are endocytosed by hepatic cells. The hepatic uptake of HDLs or *reverse cholesterol transport* may be mediated through an HDL-specific apo-A-I receptor or through lipid-lipid interactions. Macrophages also take up HDLs through apo-A-I receptor interaction. The HDLs can then acquire cholesterol and apo-E from the macrophages; cholesterol-enriched HDLs are then secreted from the macrophages. The added apo-E in these HDLs leads to an increase in their uptake and catabolism by the liver.

HDLs also acquire cholesterol by extracting it from cell membranes. This process has the effect of lowering the level of intracellular cholesterol, since the cholesterol stored within cells, as cholesteryl esters will be mobilized to replace the cholesterol removed from the plasma membrane. The cholesterol esters of HDLs can also be transferred to VLDLs and LDLs through the action of the HDL-associated enzyme, **cholesterol ester transfer protein (CETP)**, also identified as apo-D. This has the added effect of allowing the excess cellular cholesterol to be returned to the liver through the LDL-receptor pathway as well as the HDL-receptor pathway.

LDL Receptors

The LDLs are the principal carriers of cholesterol in the plasma, which delivers cholesterol from the liver (via hepatic synthesis of VLDLs) to peripheral tissues (primarily the adrenals and adipose tissue). The LDLs also return cholesterol to the liver. The cellular uptake of cholesterol from LDL occurs following the interaction of LDLs with the LDL receptor (also called the apo-B-100/apo-E receptor). The sole apoprotein present in LDLs is apo-B-100 that is required for interaction with the LDL receptor.

The LDL receptor is a polypeptide of 839 amino acids that spans the plasma membrane. An extracellular domain is responsible for apo-B-100/apo-E binding. The intracellular domain is responsible for the clustering of LDL receptors into regions of the plasma membrane termed *coated pits*. When LDL binds to receptor, the complexe is rapidly internalized (endocytosed). The ATP-dependent proton pump lowers the pH in the endosomes, which results in dissociation of the LDL from the receptor. The portion of the endosomal membrane harboring the receptor is then recycled to the plasma membrane and the LDL-containing endosome fuse with the lysosome. Acid hydrolases of the lysosomes degrade the apoproteins and release free fatty acids and cholesterol. As mentioned earlier, the free cholesterol is either incorporated into plasma membrane or esterified (by ACAT) and stored within the cell. The level of intracellular cholesterol is regulated through cholesterol-induced suppression of LDL receptor synthesis and cholesterol-induced inhibition of cholesterol synthesis. The increased level of intracellular cholesterol that results from LDL uptake has the additional effect of activating ACAT, thereby allowing the storage of excess cholesterol within cells.

However, the effect of cholesterol-induced suppression of LDL receptor synthesis is a decrease in the rate at which LDLs and IDLs are removed from the serum. This can lead to excess circulating levels of cholesterol and cholesteryl esters when the dietary intake of fat and cholesterol exceeds the needs of the body. The excess cholesterol tends to be deposited in the skin, tendons and (more gravely) within the arteries, leading to *atherosclerosis*.

LDL Receptor Gene

The LDL receptor gene on chromosome 19 (Fig. 28.4) has 18 exons that define a signal sequence (exon 1 specifying 21 amino acids) and five functional domains. The ligand-binding domain (5 exons from 2 to 6) at the N-terminal end consists of 7 repeated units of 40 amino acids each of which contains 6 cysteines. The next domain (8 exons from 7 to 14) closely resembles the precursor to the epidermal growth factor (EGF). This is followed by a short segment (exon 15) of 58 amino acids including 18 serine or threonines containing O-linked sugars and is followed by a membrane-spanning region involving exons 16 and part of 17. The final domain is coded by exons 17 and 18 and constitutes the cytoplasmic portion of the protein.

Overall, the gene takes up 45 kb of DNA; the mRNA is 5.3 kb of RNA; and the protein consists of 839 amino acids plus a 21 amino acid signal sequence.

Indicated by blue arrows at the bottom of the Figure 28.4 is the effect of mutations in that region on the function of the LDL receptor molecule.

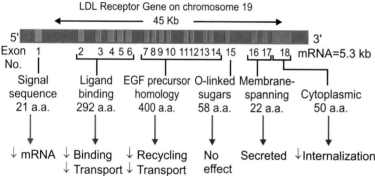

Fig. 28.4: LDL receptor gene

Clinical Significances of Lipoprotein Metabolism

Hyperlipoproteinemias or hypolipoproteinemias due to inherited defects of lipoprotein metabolism are seen in few individuals. Persons suffering from diabetes mellitus, hypothyroidism and kidney disease often exhibit abnormal lipoprotein metabolism as a result of secondary effects of these disorders. For example, since **lipoprotein lipase** (LPL) synthesis is regulated by insulin, LPL deficiencies leading to Type I hyperlipoproteinemia may occur as a secondary outcome of diabetes mellitus. Additionally, insulin and thyroid hormones positively affect hepatic LDL-receptor interactions; therefore, the hyper-cholesterolemia and increased risk of atherosclerosis associated with uncontrolled diabetes or hypothyroidism is likely due to decreased LDL uptake and metabolism by liver.

Familial hypercholesterolemia (FH) may be the most prevalent in the general population. FH is an inherited disorder comprising four different classes of mutation in the LDL receptor gene. The class 1 defect (the most common) results in a complete loss of receptor synthesis. The class 2 defect results in the synthesis of a receptor protein that is not properly processed in the Golgi apparatus and therefore is not transported to the plasma membrane. The class 3 defect results in an LDL receptor that is incapable of binding LDLs. The class 4 defect results in receptors that bind LDLs but do not cluster in coated pits and are, therefore, not internalized.

FH sufferers may be either heterozygous or homologous for a particular mutation in the receptor gene. Homozygotes exhibit grossly elevated serum cholesterol (primarily in LDLs). The elevated levels of LDLs result in their phagocytosis by macrophages. These lipid-laden phagocytic cells tend to deposit within the skin and tendons, leading to xanthomas. A greater complication results from cholesterol deposition within the arteries, leading to atherosclerosis, the major contributing factor of all cardiovascular diseases.

Summary of Lipase

Enzyme	Origin	Site of action	Function	Characteristic features
Gastric Lipase	Stomach	Stomach	Degrade dietary TAG containing short chain FA	Acid stable
Pancreatic Lipase	Pancreas	Lumen of small intestine	Removes FA from carbon 1 and 3, of dietary TAG	Pancreatic co-lipase required for stabilization
Lipoprotein Lipase	Extrahepatic tissue	Endothelial surface of capillaries	Degrades TAG in circulating chylomicrons or VLDL	Released into circulation by heparin; activated by apoC-II
Hormone sensitive Lipase	Adipocytes	Adipocytes	Degrades stored TAG	Activated by cAMP-dependent protein kinase
Acid Lipase	Most tissues	Lysosomes	Removes FA from lipids taken into cells during phagocytosis	Acid pH optimum

Pharmacologic Intervention

Drug treatment to lower plasma lipoproteins and/or cholesterol is primarily aimed at reducing the risk of atherosclerosis and subsequent coronary artery disease. Drug therapy is considered as an option only when non-pharmacologic interventions (altered diet and exercise) fail to lower plasma lipids.

Hypolipoproteinemias

Disorder	Defect	Comments
Abetalipoproteinemia	No chylomicrons, VLDLs or	Rare defect; Intestine and liver
Acanthocytosis and Bassen-Kornweig syndrome	LDLs due to defect in apo-B expression	accumulate lipids Malabsorption of fat, retinitis pigmentosa, atoxic neuropathic disease, erythrocytes have thorny appearance

Contd....

Contd....

Familial hypobetalipo-proteinemia	Apo-B gene mutations, LDL concentrations 10-20% of normal, VLDL slightly lower, HDL normal	Mild or no pathologic changes
Familial alpha-lipoprotein deficiency (Tangier disease, Fish-eye disease. Apo-A-I and –C-III deficiency.	All of these related syndromes have reduced HDL concentrations, no effect on chylomicron or VLDL production	Tendency to hypertriglycerolemia; some elevation in VLDLs; Fish-eye disease characterized by severe corneal opacity

Lovastatin, mevastatin, and mevinolin belong to statin group of drugs that inhibit HMG-CoA reductase. The net result of treatment is an increased cellular uptake of LDLs, since the intracellular synthesis of cholesterol is inhibited and cells are therefore dependent on extracellular sources of cholesterol. However, since mevalonate the product of the HMG-CoA reductase reaction is required for the synthesis of other important isoprenoid compounds besides cholesterol, long-term treatments carry some risk of toxicity.

Nicotinic acid reduces the plasma levels of both VLDLs and LDLs by inhibiting hepatic VLDL secretion, as well as suppressing the flux of free fatty acid release from adipose tissue by inhibiting lipolysis. Because of its ability to cause large reductions in circulating levels of cholesterol, nicotinic acid is used to treat Type II, III, IV and V hyperlipoproteinemias.

Clofibrate, gemfibrozil and fenofibrate are fibric acid derivatives that activate lipoprotein lipase and promote rapid VLDL turnover. They also induce the diversion of hepatic free fatty acids from esterification reactions to those of oxidation, thereby decreasing the secretion of triacylglycerol and cholesterol-rich VLDLs from liver.

Probucol increases the rate of LDL metabolism and may block the intestinal transport of cholesterol. The net result is a significant reduction in plasma cholesterol levels.

Cholestyramine or colestipol (resins) is non-absorbable resins that binds bile acids and prevents its reabsorption. As a result, a greater amount of cholesterol is converted to bile acids to maintain a steady level in circulation. Additionally, the synthesis of LDL receptors increases to allow increased cholesterol uptake for bile acid synthesis, and the overall effect is a reduction in plasma cholesterol. (This treatment is ineffective in homozygous FH patients, since they are completely deficient in LDL receptors.

Hyperlipoproteinemias

Disorder	Defect	Comments
Type I (familial LPL deficiency and hyperchylomicronemia)	(a) Deficiency of LPL; (b) production of abnormal LPL (c) apo-C-II deficiency	Slow chylomicron clearance, reduced LDL and HDL levels; treated by low fat/complex carbohydrate diet; no increased risk of coronary artery disease
Type II (familial hypercholesterolemia, FH)	4 classes of LDL receptor defect	Reduced LDL clearance leads to hypercholesterolemia, resulting in athersclerosis and coronary artery disease
Type III (familial dysbetalipoproteinemia, remnant removal disease, broad beta disease, apolipo-protein E deficiency)	Hepatic remnant clearance impaired due to apo-E abnormality; patients only express the apo-E$_2$ isoform that interacts poorly with the apo-E receptor	Causes xanthomas, hypercholesterolemia and athersclerosis in peripheral and coronary arteries due to elevated levels of chylomicrons and VLDLs
Type IV (familial hypertriacylglycerolemia)	Elevated production of VLDL associated with glucose intolerance and hyperinsulinemia	Frequently associated with type-II non-insulin dependent diabetes mellitus, obesity, alcoholism or administration of progestational hormones; elevated cholesterol as a result of increased VLDLs
Type V familial	Elevated chylomicrons and VLDLs due to unknown cause	Hypertriacylglycerolemia and hypercholesterolemia with decreased LDLs and HDLs
Familial hyperalpha-lipoproteinemia	Increased level of HDLs	Rare condition that is beneficial for health and longevity
Type II Familial hyperbetalipo-proteinemia	Increased LDL production and delayed clearance of triacyl-	Strongly associated with increased risk of coronary artery disease glycerols and fatty acids
Familial ligand-defective apo-B	2 different mutations: Gln for Arg (amino acid 3500) or Cys for Arg (amino acid 3531); both lead to reduced affinity of LDL for LDL receptor	Dramatic increase in LDL levels; no affect on HDL, VLDL or plasma triglyceride levels; significant cause of hypercholesterolemia and premature coronary artery disease
Familial LCAT deficiency	Absence of LCAT leads to inability of HDLs to take up cholesterol (reverse cholesterol transport)	Decreased levels of plasma cholesteryl esters and lysolecithin; abnormal LDLs (Lp-X) and VLDLs; symptoms also found associated with cholestasis
Wolman's disease (cholesteryl ester storage disease)	Defect in lysosomal cholesteryl ester hydrolase; affects metabolism of LDLs	Reduced LDL clearance leads to hypercholesterolemia, resulting in atherosclerosis and coronary artery disease
Hormone-releasable hepatic lipase deficiency	Lipase deficiency leads to accumulation of triacylglycerol-rich HDLs and VLDL remnants	Causes xanthomas and coronary artery disease

Fatty Acid Metabolism

29

FATTY ACID OXIDATION

Mobilization of Fat Stores

Fatty acid oxidation is the major source of cellular ATP in several tissues with the exception of erythrocytes and brain. Liver uses fatty acids for energy when it is carrying out gluconeogenesis. The primary sources of fatty acids for oxidation are dietary fats that are delivered from the gut to cells via transport in the blood as lipoproteins and that mobilized from adipocytes of adipose tissues where it is stored as triacylglycerols. The fatty acids stored as triacylglycerols are mobilized for use by peripheral tissues, when blood insulin level is low and energy demands are more. The release of fatty acids from TAG is controlled by a series of interrelated cascades that result in the activation of *hormone-sensitive lipase*.

The stimulus that activates the cascade in adipocytes could be glucagon, epinephrine or β-corticotropin. Binding of these hormones to cell-surface receptors activate *adenylate cyclase* that are coupled to ligand binding (Fig. 29.1). The resultant increase in cAMP leads to activation of PKA, which in turn phosphorylates and activates hormone-sensitive lipase. This enzyme hydrolyzes fatty acids from carbon atoms 1 or 3 of triacylglycerols. The resulting diacylglycerols are substrates for either *hormone-sensitive lipase* or for the enzyme *diacylglycerolipase*. Finally the monoacylglycerols are substrates for *monoacylglycerol lipase*. The net result of the action of these enzymes is release of three moles of free fatty acid and one mole of glycerol. The free fatty acids diffuse out of adipocytes and transported to other tissues via blood in association with albumin. The glycerol returns to the liver where it is gluconeogenic.

The mobilization of fat from adipose tissue is inhibited by numerous stimuli. The most significant is that exerted by insulin upon *adenylate cyclase*. When an individual is in well-fed state, insulin released from the pancreas diverts the excess fat and carbohydrate to be incorporated into the triacylglycerol pool within adipose tissue and prevent mobilization of stored fat.

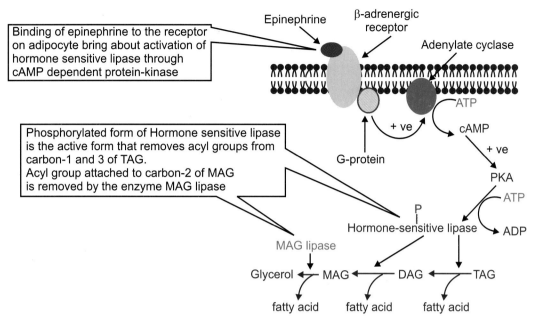

Fig. 29.1: Hormone-induced mobilization of fatty acids from adipocytes

Activation of Fatty Acids

The free fatty acids must be activated (esterified to CoA) in the cytoplasm before being oxidized in the mitochondria. Activation is catalyzed by *acyl-CoA synthetase* that is also called *thiokinase*. This activation process consumes 2 molar equivalents of ATP.

Free fatty acid + ATP + CoA $\rightarrow$ Acyl-CoA + PP$_i$ + AMP.

Oxidation of Fatty Acids Takes Place in the Mitochondrial Matrix

The transport of fatty acyl-CoA into the mitochondrial matrix is achieved via an **acyl-carnitine** intermediate. An enzyme *carnitine acyltransferase I,* that reside on the inner side of the outer mitochondrial membrane catalyze the transfer of acyl group of acyl-CoA to carnitine, forming acyl-carnitine (Fig. 29.2), which is then transported into the mitochondria by an inner mitochondrial membrane transporter *carnitine acyl-carnitine translocase* (Fig. 29.3).

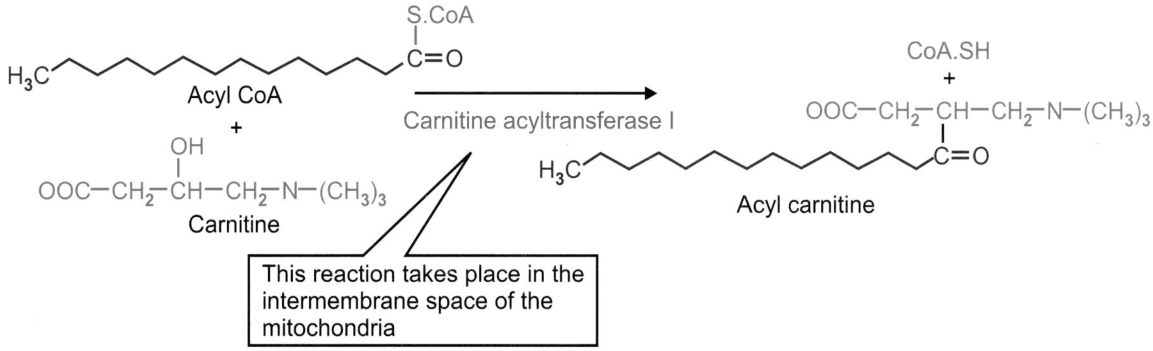

Fig. 29.2: Synthesis of acylcarnitine

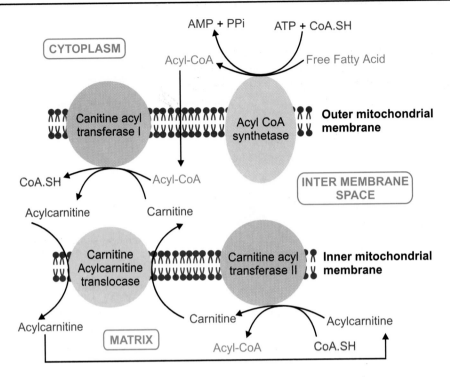

Fig. 29.3: Fatty acid transport into mitochondrial matrix

Fatty acids having less than 12 carbons are carnitine-independent and can cross inner mitochondrial membrane as acyl-CoA.

Within the mitochondrial matrix acyl-carnitine is converted back to acyl-CoA (fatty-CoA), catalysed by an inner mitochondrial membrane enzyme **carnitine acyltransferase II.** Once inside the mitochondrial matrix the fatty-CoA is a substrate for the enzymes of β-oxidation pathway.

Reactions of β-Oxidation

The process of sequential removal of 2-carbon units from the carboxyl end of acyl-CoA by oxidation of the β-carbon of the fatty acyl-CoA is termed β-oxidation. Each successive oxidation step requires a fresh CoA.SH molecule for thiolytic cleavage of β-ketoacyl CoA, to yield acetyl-CoA and acyl-CoA shorter by two carbons. Each round of β–oxidation produces one mole each of NADH, $FADH_2$ and acetyl-CoA. Odd numbered fatty acids are oxidized in the same way except that the last round releases a propionyl-CoA rather than an acetyl-CoA. The acetyl-CoA then enters the TCA cycle, where it is oxidized to CO_2 with the concomitant generation of three moles of NADH, one mole of $FADH_2$ and one mole of GTP. The NADH and $FADH_2$ generated during the β-oxidation of acyl-CoA and oxidation of acetyl-CoA in the TCA cycle, enter the respiratory pathway for the production of ATP.

The oxidation of fatty acids yields significantly more energy per carbon atom than does the oxidation of carbohydrates, since the carbon in fatty acid is more reduced.

β-Oxidation Pathway of Fatty Acids

Step 1. *Acyl-CoA dehydrogenase* catalyzes oxidation of the fatty acid moiety of acyl-CoA, to form a double bond between carbons 2 and 3 (Fig. 29.4). There are different Acyl-CoA dehydrogenases for short-, medium-, and long-chain fatty acids. Hereditary deficiency of medium chain Acyl-CoA dehydrogenase (MCAD) is found in some cases of sudden infant death syndrome (SIDS).

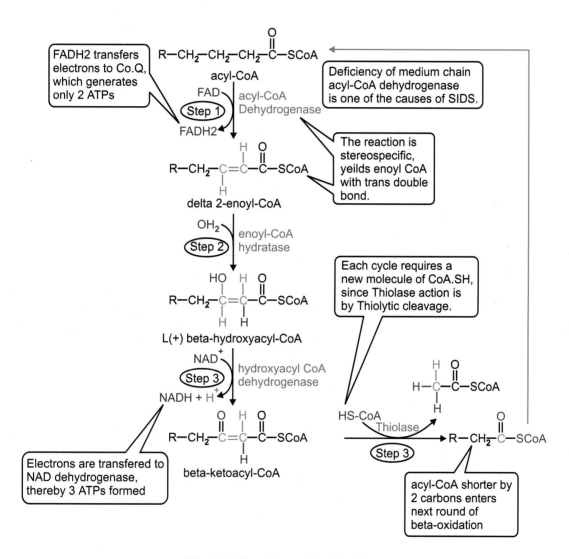

Fig. 29.4: Reactions of β-oxidation

The FAD is the prosthetic group of Acyl-CoA dehydrogenase that functions as electron acceptor. The proposed mechanism is: a glutamyl residue of apoenzyme extracts a proton, facilitating transfer of two e⁻ with H⁺ to FAD. The reduced FAD then accepts a second H⁺ to become $FADH_2$. The reactive glutamyl residues of apoenzyme and FAD are on opposite sides of the substrate at the active site of the enzyme. Thus the reaction is stereospecific, yielding enoyl-CoA with a trans double bond.

The $FADH_2$ of Acyl-CoA dehydrogenase is reoxidized by transfer of two electrons to an electron transfer flavoprotein (ETF), which in turn passes the electrons to coenzyme Q of the respiratory chain.

Step 2. *Enoyl-CoA hydratase* catalyzes stereospecific hydration of the trans double bond produced in the earlier reaction to yield **L-hydroxyacyl-CoA**.

Step 3. *Hydroxyacyl-CoA dehydrogenase* catalyzes the oxidation of hydroxyl group at the β position (C3) to a keto group. The NAD^+ is the electron acceptor in this reaction.

Step 4. *β-ketothiolase* (β-Ketoacyl-CoA thiolase) catalyzes thiolytic cleavage at β-carbon of β-ketoacyl-CoA. Proposed mechanism: The cysteinyl S of incoming CoA.SH attacks the β-keto carbon. Acetyl-CoA is released, leaving the fatty acyl moiety with two carbons less in a thioester linkage to the cysteinyl S of CoA.

The β-oxidation pathway is cyclic. The products are acetyl-CoA and the acyl-CoA shorter by two carbons that become the input to another round of the pathway. If the fatty acid entering the pathway contains an even number of carbon atoms, in the final reaction cycle butyryl-CoA is converted to two molecules of acetyl-CoA. If the fatty acid entering the pathway contains an odd number of carbon atoms, in the final reaction a molecule each of acetyl-CoA and propionyl-CoA are formed. The acetyl-CoA formed enters the Krebs cycle or may contribute to ketone body production, whereas propionyl-CoA can be converted to the Krebs cycle intermediate succinyl-CoA, by a pathway involving vitamin B_{12}.

Summary of one round of the β-oxidation pathway:

Fatty acyl-CoA + FAD + NAD^+ + HS-CoA →

Fatty acyl-CoA (2 C shorter) + $FADH_2$ + NADH + H^+ + acetyl-CoA

Energetics of β-Oxidation (ATP Production)

Reoxidation of $FADH_2$ by transfer of two e^- to coenzyme Q of the respiratory chain is accompanied by H^+ pumping, which leads to production of two ATPs (approximately 1.5 ATPs).

Reoxidation of NADH by transfer of two e^- to the respiratory chain complex I and transfer of two e^- from complex I to oxygen yield three ATPs (approximately 2.5 ATPs).

Oxidation of acetyl-CoA in the Krebs cycle yields 3 NADH, 1 $FADH_2$, and 1 GTP.

Calculate the ATP production when palmitic acid (16 carbon) is completely oxidized.

Oxidation of Unsaturated Fatty Acids

The oxidation of unsaturated fatty acids is essentially the same process as for saturated fats, until either a Δ^3-cis-acyl-CoA compound or a Δ^2-cis-acetyl-CoA compound is formed, depending upon the position of the double bonds (Fig. 29.5). The former compound is isomerized to the corresponding Δ^2-trans-CoA stage, which in turn is hydrated by Δ^2-enoyl hydratase to L(+)-β-hydroxyacyl-CoA. The Δ-cis-acyl-CoA compound first hydrated by Δ-enoyl hydratase to the D(-)-β-hydroxyacyl-CoA derivative. This undergoes epimerization to give the normal L(+)- β-hydroxyaceyl-CoA stage in β-oxidation.

It should be noted that the presence of double bond in the fatty acid spares the action acyl-CoA dehydrogenase thereby $FADH_2$ is not formed. The net result is for each double bond present in the unsaturated fatty acid, the ATP production on oxidation is less by two numbers.

β-oxidation of long-chain fatty acids also occurs within *peroxisomes*. The electron acceptor for peroxisomal acyl-CoA oxidase is FAD, which catalyzes the first oxidative step of the pathway. The resulting $FADH_2$ is reoxidized in the peroxisome producing hydrogen peroxide:

$FADH_2 + O_2 \rightarrow FAD + H_2O_2$

The peroxisomal enzyme catalase degrades H_2O_2 by the reaction: $2\ H_2O_2 \rightarrow 2\ H_2O + O_2$

These reactions produce *no ATP*.

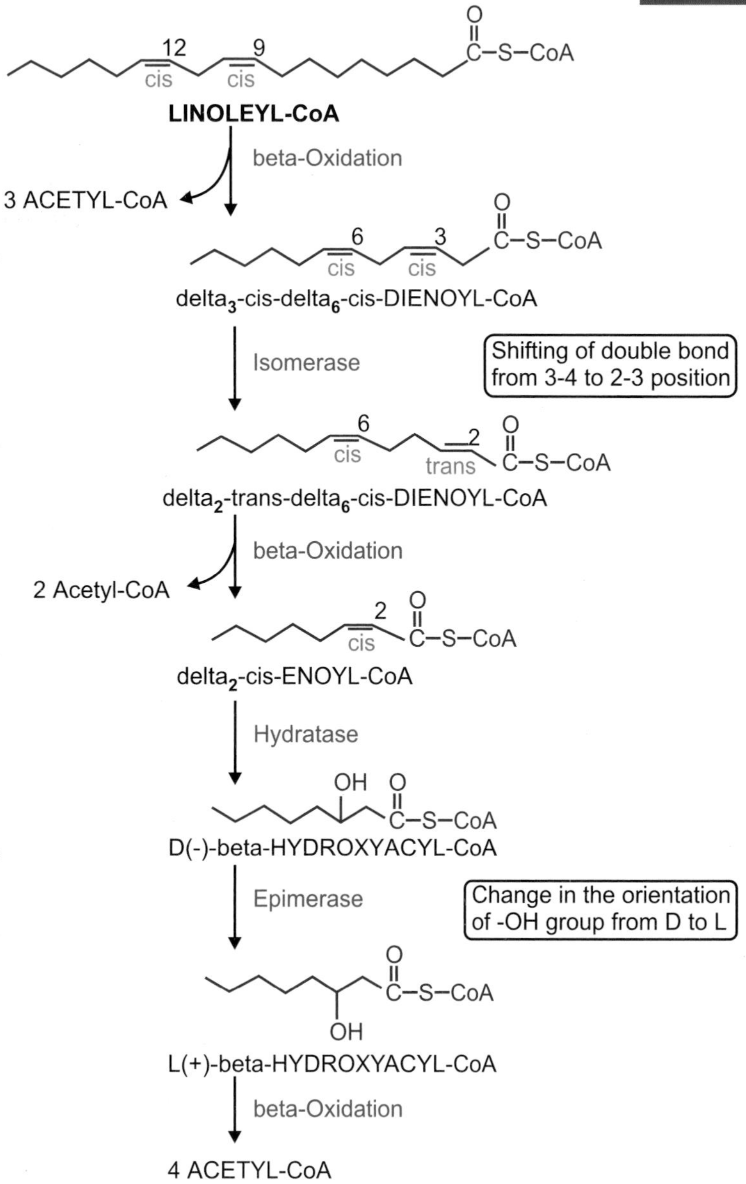

Metabolic Fate of Propionyl-CoA

The majority of natural fatty acids contain an *even* number of carbon atoms. A small proportion of fatty acids that contain odd numbers; upon complete β-oxidation, yield acetyl-CoA units plus a single mole of propionyl-CoA. The propionyl-CoA is converted to succinyl-CoA, in an ATP-dependent pathway that requires biotin and vitamin B_{12}. Succinyl-CoA then enters TCA cycle for further oxidation (Fig. 29.6) or it could be the substrate for heme synthesis.

α- and ω-Oxidation of Fatty Acids

The process of α-oxidation removes one carbon at a time from the carboxyl end of the molecule. This pathway is found active in the brain tissue. It does not require CoA intermediate and does not generate high-energy phosphates. Phytanic acid is a fatty acid present in the tissues of ruminants, dairy products and plant foodstuffs and is therefore an important dietary component. Phytanic acid contains methyl group on the β-carbon that blocks β-oxidation. Hence it

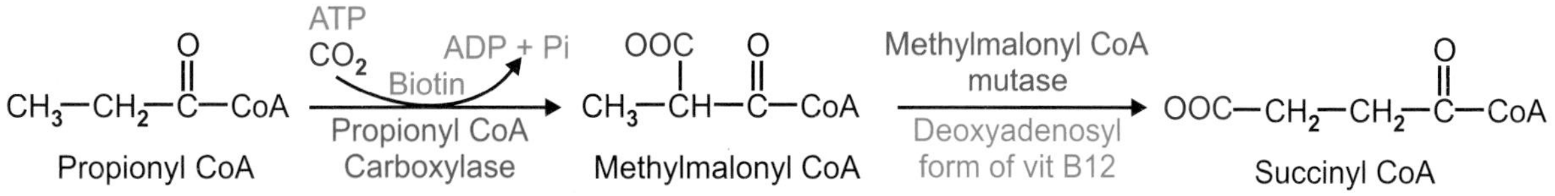

Fig. 29.5: Oxidation of unsaturated fatty acids

Fig. 29.6: Metabolism of propionyl CoA

cannot act as a substrate for the first enzyme of the β-oxidation pathway (acyl-CoA dehydrogenase). An additional mitochondrial enzyme *α-hydroxylase* is required to add a hydroxyl group to the α-carbon of phytanic acid, which then serves as a substrate for the remainder of the normal oxidative enzymes.

ω-oxidation is brought about by a microsomal hydroxylase that involves cytochrome P-450. The methyl group of ω-carbon is converted to $-CH_2OH$ group that is subsequently oxidized to $-COOH$, thus forming a dicarboxylic acid. This is usually β-oxidized to adipic and suberic acid, which are found in the urine of ketotic patients.

FATTY ACID SYNTHESIS

The fatty acid synthesis and its oxidation appears to be reversal of each other, but the distinct regulation of the two pathways and the different cellular compartments in which they occur would not allow the fatty acid synthesis to be a simple reversal of fatty acid oxidation.

The pathway for fatty acid synthesis occurs in the cytoplasm, whereas, oxidation occurs in the mitochondria. The other major differences are: Oxidation of fatty acid involves the reduction of FAD and NAD^+ where as synthesis of fatty acid involves the oxidation of NADPH. Oxidation of fatty acid yields acetyl-CoA, whereas synthesis of fatty acid utilizes an activated acetyl-CoA in the form of malonyl-CoA. However, during fatty acid synthesis the acetyl-CoA exists temporarily bound to the enzyme complex as malonyl-CoA. The malonyl-CoA synthesis is the first committing step in fatty acid synthesis and the enzyme catalyzing this reaction *acetyl-CoA carboxylase* (ACC) is the major site of regulation of fatty acid synthesis. Like other carboxylase, ACC also requires biotin as co-factor.

Acetyl-CoA carboxylase catalyzes a two-step reaction in which acetyl-CoA is carboxylated to form malonyl-CoA (Fig. 29.7). As with pyruvate carboxylase, the prosthetic group is *biotin*.

The mammalian acetyl-CoA carboxylase has two catalytic domains plus a domain, where *biotin* is linked by an amide bond between the terminal carboxyl of the biotin side chain and the ε-amino group of a lysine residue. The combined biotin and lysine side chains act as a long flexible arm that allows the biotin ring to translocate between the two active sites.

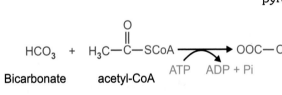

Fig. 29.7: Synthesis of malonyl-CoA

The rate of fatty acid synthesis is controlled by the equilibrium between monomeric ACC and polymeric ACC (Fig. 29.8). It is only the polymeric form of ACC, which is active. Polymerization of ACC is enhanced by citrate and inhibited by long-chain fatty acids (palmitoyl-CoA).

The overall reaction catalyzed by acetyl-CoA carboxylase is *spontaneous*.

ACC, which converts acetyl-CoA to malonyl-CoA, is the *committed step* of fatty acid synthesis.

Mammalian ACC is regulated by *phosphorylation*, and *allosteric* regulation by local metabolites (Fig.29.8).

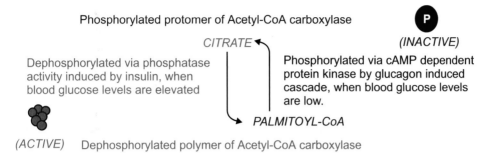

Fig. 29.8: Activation and deactivation of acetyl CoA carboxylase

Regulation acetyl-CoA carboxylase (ACC) is by phosphorylation: A cyclic-AMP cascade is activated by the hormones glucagon and epinephrine when blood glucose is low, which results in phosphorylation of acetyl-CoA carboxylase by cAMP-dependent protein kinase. When phosphorylated, the enzyme filaments dissociate into inactive monomers. Thus acetyl-CoA is kept available for production of ketone bodies, which is the alternative metabolic fuel used when blood glucose is low.

Regulation by local metabolites: Palmitoyl-CoA, the product of fatty acid synthase, promotes the inactive protomer state of ACC (feedback inhibition).

Citrate activates ACC, by promoting enzyme polymerization. Citrate concentration is high when there is adequate acetyl-CoA entering Krebs cycle. Under these conditions, excess acetyl-CoA is converted to fatty acids for storage.

In mammals, fatty acid synthesis starting from acetyl-CoA/propionyl-CoA and malonyl-CoA is carried out by a series of reactions catalyzed by *fatty acid synthase* (FAS) complex. It is a dimer consisting of two polypeptide chains aligned antiparallel to each other. Each chain includes domains corresponding to the several catalytic sites (Fig. 29.9). Its evolution has apparently involved in gene fusion.

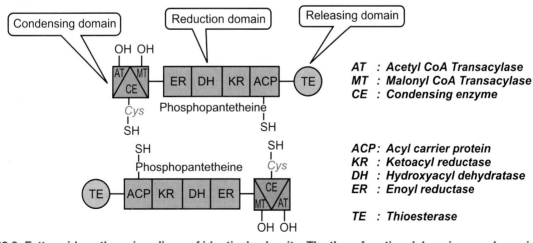

Fig. 29.9: Fatty acid synthase is a dimer of identical subunits. The three functional domains are shown in colour

The **acyl carrier protein (ACP) domain** of the fatty acid synthase enzyme complex has a phosphopantetheine prosthetic group, attached through a serine hydroxyl residue. The thiol of phosphopantetheine forms a *thioester* with carboxyl groups of malonate, and/or the growing fatty acid (Fig. 29.10). The long flexible arm of phosphopantetheine allows its thiol to move from one active site to another within the complex.

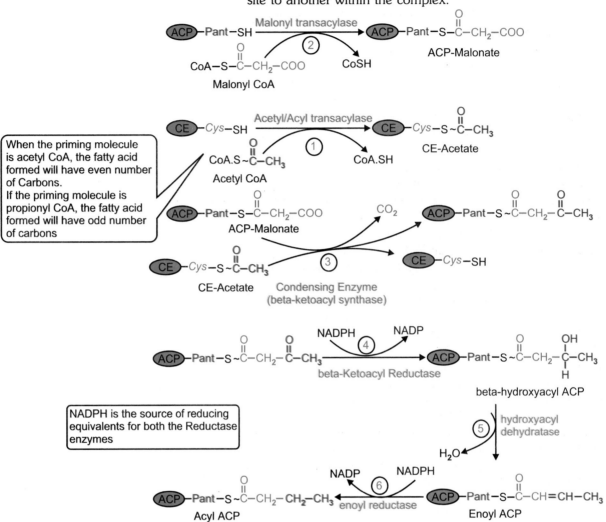

When the priming molecule is acetyl CoA, the fatty acid formed will have even number of Carbons.
If the priming molecule is propionyl CoA, the fatty acid formed will have odd number of carbons

NADPH is the source of reducing equivalents for both the Reductase enzymes

Fig. 29.10: Reactions of fatty acid synthesis

The **condensing enzyme domain (CE)** has a cystinyl thiol group which forms thioester with carboxyl group of acetyl, propionyl or growing acyl molecule (Fig. 29.10).

1. *Acetyl-CoA transacylase* catalyzes transfer of acetyl-CoA or propionyl-CoA to the thiol group of condensing enzyme of one monomer of enzyme complex.
2. *Malonyl-CoA transacylase* catalyzes transfer of malonyl-CoA to the thiol group of ACP domain of another monomer of enzyme complex.
3. In the next step, the *condensing enzyme* catalyzes condensation between the acetyl and malonyl units present on the two monomers of the enzyme complex to form a 4-carbon unit, acetoacetyl ACP. During this reaction one molecule of CO_2 is lost.

4. The acetoacetyl ACP is reduced by NADPH dependent *β-ketoacyl reductase* to form β-hydroxyacyl ACP.

5. The β-hydroxyacyl ACP is then dehydrated to form enoyl ACP, this reaction catalyzed by *hydroxyacyl dehydratase*.

6. The enoyl ACP is again reduced by *enoyl reductase* utilizing a second molecule of NADPH to form butyryl ACP. The butyryl group is now transferred to the thiol group of condensing enzyme on the other monomer of enzyme complex and the second malonyl-CoA molecule binds to the phosphopantothenyl-SH of ACP. The sequence of reactions, namely *condensation, reduction, dehydration* and *reduction* are repeated till the fatty acid of required chain length is formed. Palmitic acid is formed in liver and adipocytes. In lactating mammary gland, capric (10C) and lauric acids (12C) are formed.

7. At the end of the cycle, fatty acid is released by *thioesterase activity*.

All the reactions of fatty acid synthesis are carried out by the multiple enzymatic activities of FAS, which involves four enzymatic activities. These are: *condensing enzyme (β-keto acyl synthase), β-keto acyl reductase, 3-OH acyl dehydratase* and *enoyl reductase*. The two reduction reactions require NADPH as an electron donor. The main pathway of NADPH production is the *pentose phosphate pathway*.

The primary fatty acid synthesized by FAS is palmitate a 16-C saturated fatty acid. Palmitate is then released from the enzyme complex by the action of *thioesterase*. Palmitate can then undergo separate elongation and/or unsaturation reactions to yield other fatty acid molecules.

Summary of palmitate synthesis (ignoring H^+ and water):

acetyl-CoA + 7 malonyl-CoA + 14 NADPH → palmitate + 7 CO_2 + 14 $NADP^+$ + 8 CoA

Summary of palmitate synthesis taking into account ATP-dependent synthesis of malonate:

8 acetyl-CoA + 7 ATP + 14 NADPH → palmitate + 8 CoA + 7 ADP + 7 P_i + 14 $NADP^+$

Origin of Cytoplasmic Acetyl-CoA

Acetyl-CoA is generated in the mitochondria primarily from two sources, one is the pyruvate dehydrogenase (PDH) reaction and other is fatty acid oxidation. In order for these acetyl units to be utilized for fatty acid synthesis they must be present in the cytoplasm. The shift from oxidation of fatty acid and glucose (glycolysis), to synthesis of fatty acids occurs when the need for energy diminishes. This results in reduced oxidation of acetyl-CoA in the TCA cycle. Under these conditions the mitochondrial acetyl-CoA enters the cytoplasm in the form of citrate via the tricarboxylate transport system (Fig. 29.11).

In the cytoplasm, the ***ATP-citrate lyase*** reaction cleaves citrate to oxaloacetate and acetyl-CoA. This reaction is essentially the reverse of that catalyzed by the TCA enzyme *citrate synthase*, except it requires the energy of ATP hydrolysis to drive it forward. The resultant oxaloacetate is converted to malate, by *malate dehydrogenase*

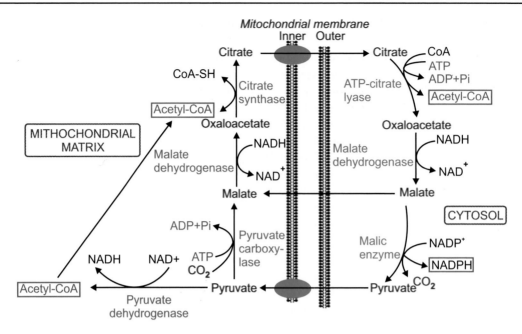

Fig. 29.11: Malate-oxaloacetate shuttle for transfer of mitochondrioal acetyl-CoA to cytoplasm

(MDH). The malate produced by this pathway can undergo oxidative decarboxylation by *malic enzyme*. The coenzyme for this reaction is $NADP^+$ that generate NADPH. The advantage of this series of reactions for converting mitochondrial acetyl-CoA into cytoplasmic acetyl-CoA is that the NADPH produced by the *malic enzyme* reaction can be a major source of reducing co-factor for the *fatty acid synthase* activities.

Fatty Acid Synthase is Transcriptionally Regulated

In **liver cells**, expression of fatty acid synthase is **stimulated by insulin**, which is secreted when blood glucose level is elevated. Thus excess glucose is converted to fatty acids and stored as fat. Transcription factors that mediate the stimulatory effect of insulin includes; upstream stimulatory factors (USFs) and sterol response element binding proteins (SREBP). The SREBPs were first identified for their role in regulating cholesterol synthesis. In **fat cells**, expression of *SREBP-1* and *fatty acid synthase* are inhibited by **leptin** a hormone that regulates food intake and fat metabolism. Leptin is produced by fat cells in response to excess fat storage. Leptin regulates body weight by decreasing food intake, increasing energy expenditure, and inhibiting fatty acid synthesis.

Elongation and Desaturation of Fatty Acids

The predominant fatty acid released from FAS is palmitate (via the action of *palmitoyl thioesterase*), which is a 16:0 fatty acid (16 carbons and no sites of unsaturation). Elongation and unsaturation of fatty acids occur in both the mitochondria and endoplasmic reticulum (microsomal membranes). The predominant site of these processes is in the ER membranes.

Elongation in the ER membrane involves condensation of malonyl-CoA with acyl-CoA, which undergoes reduction, dehydration and reduction to yield a saturated fatty acid that is longer by two carbons (since CO_2 is released from malonyl-CoA as in the FAS reaction). The reduction reactions of elongation require NADPH as cofactor similar to FAS catalyzed reactions.

Mitochondrial elongation involves acetyl-CoA units and is a reversal of oxidation except that the final reduction utilizes NADPH instead of $FADH_2$ as cofactor.

Desaturation of fatty acids takes place in the ER membranes of mammalian cells. It involves four broad-specificity *fatty acyl-CoA desaturases* (non-heme iron containing enzymes). These enzymes introduce unsaturation at C4, C5, C6 or C9 (Fig. 29.12).

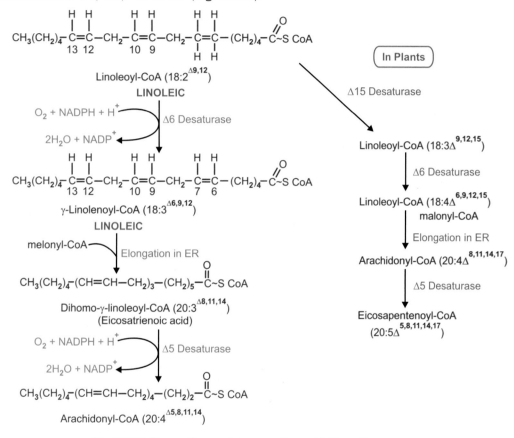

Fig. 29.12: Elongation and desaturation of fatty acids

The electrons from the reduced fatty acid (saturated) and from the desaturase are transferred to molecular oxygen to form water and oxydized fatty acid (unsaturated). NADH is the donor of two electrons, which keep the desaturase in the reduced form through the action of the enzyme *NADH-cytochrome β5 reductase*. These electrons are un-coupled from mitochondrial oxidative phosphorylation and, therefore, do not yield ATP.

Since these enzymes cannot introduce sites of unsaturation beyond C9 they cannot synthesize either *linoleate* ($18:2^{\Delta 9, 12}$) or *linolenate* ($18:3^{\Delta 9, 12, 15}$). These fatty acids must be acquired from the diet and are therefore, referred to as *essential fatty acids*. Linoleic is especially important in that it is required for the synthesis of *arachidonic acid*, which is a precursor for *eicosanoids* (the prostaglandins and *thromboxanes*). It is this role of essential fatty acids in eicosanoid synthesis that leads to poor growth, wound healing and dermatitis in persons on fat free diets. Linoleic acid is also a constituent of sphingolipids in epidermal cell that functions as water permeability barrier.

Comparison of Fatty Acid Synthesis and Degradation

	Beta-oxidation	**Fatty acid synthesis**
Pathway location	Mitochondrial matrix	Cytosol
Acyl carriers (thiols)	Coenzyme-A	Phosphopantetheine (ACP) cysteine
Electron acceptor/ donor	FAD and NAD$^+$	NADPH
Hydroxyl intermediate	L-form	D-form
2-Carbon product/ donor	Acetyl-CoA	Malonyl-CoA & acetyl-CoA

Regulation of Fatty Acid Metabolism

Fat metabolism is regulated by two distinct mechanisms. One is **short-term regulation**, which depends on substrate availability, allosteric effectors and enzyme modification. The other is **long-term regulation** that is achieved by altering the rate of enzyme synthesis and its turnover.

ACC (acetyl-CoA carboxylase) is the rate-limiting (committed) step in fatty acid synthesis. The regulation of ACC by substrate availability (allosteric regulation) and covalent modification by phosphate as discussed earlier is a good example of short-time regulation of metabolic pathways (Fig. 29.13).

Insulin stimulates ACC and FAS synthesis, whereas starvation leads to a decrease in the synthesis of these enzymes. The *lipoprotein lipase* levels in adipose tissue is increased by insulin and decreased by starvation. However, the effects of insulin and starvation on lipoprotein lipase in the heart are just the inverse of those in adipose tissue. This sensitivity allows the heart to absorb any available fatty acids in the blood in order to oxidize them for energy production.

Adipose tissue contains *hormone-sensitive lipase*, which enhance the release of fatty acids into the blood is activated by PKA-dependent phosphorylation. This in turn leads to the increased oxidation of fatty acids in other tissues such as muscle and liver. In the liver, the net result as a result of elevated acetyl-CoA levels is enhanced production of ketone bodies. This would occur under those conditions in which the carbohydrate stores and gluconeogenic precursors available in the liver

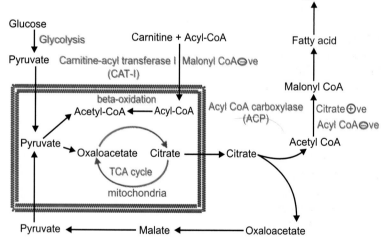

Fig. 29.13: Allosteric regulation of fatty acid metabolism

are not sufficient to allow increased glucose production. The increased levels of fatty acid that become available in response to glucagon or epinephrine are assured of being completely oxidized, because PKA also phosphorylates ACC, which inhibits fatty acid synthesis.

Insulin has the opposite effect of glucagon and epinephrine: it increases the synthesis of triacylglycerols (and glycogen). One of the many effects of insulin is to lower cAMP levels, which leads to increased dephosphorylation through the enhanced activity of protein phosphatases such as PP-1. With respect to fatty acid metabolism, this yields dephosphorylated and inactive hormone-sensitive lipase. Insulin also stimulates certain phosphorylation events through activation of cAMP-independent kinases, one of which phosphorylates and thereby stimulates the activity of ACC.

Since transport of fatty acids into the mitochondria is the rate-limiting step of β-oxidation of fatty acids, the inhibition of CAT I by malonyl-CoA is also an important regulator of β-oxidation (Fig. 29.13). Such regulation serves to prevent *de novo synthesized fatty acids* from entering the mitochondria and getting oxidized.

Genetic Disorders Related to Fatty Acids Metabolism

The majority of genetic disorders related to fatty acid metabolism are associated with fatty acid oxidation. These disorders fall into four main groups:

Carnitine Deficiencies

A deficiency in carnitine leads to an inability to transport fatty acids into the mitochondria for oxidation and accumulation of triacylglycerol deposits in muscle. This can occur in newborns and particularly in pre-term infants. Carnitine deficiencies are also found in patients undergoing hemodialysis or exhibiting organic aciduria. Carnitine deficiencies may manifest systemic symptomology or may be limited to only muscles. Symptoms range from mild, recurrent muscle cramping to severe weakness and death. Treatment is by oral carnitine administration.

Carnitine Acyltransferase-I (CAT I) Deficiency

Deficiencies in this enzyme affect primarily the liver and lead to decreased rate of fatty acid oxidation and ketogenesis. Carnitine acyltransferase II (CAT II) deficiency results in recurrent muscle pain and fatigue and myoglobinuria following strenuous exercise. Sulfonylurea drugs such as tolbutamide and glyburide may also inhibit carnitine acyltransferases.

Deficiencies in Acyl-CoA Dehydrogenases

A group of inherited diseases that impair β-oxidation are the result of deficiencies in acyl-CoA dehydrogenase. The enzymes affected may belong to one of four categories:
   i. Very long-chain acyl-CoA dehydrogenase (VLCAD)
   ii. Long-chain acyl-CoA dehydrogenase (LCAD)
   iii. Medium-chain acyl-CoA dehydrogenase (MCAD)
   iv. Short-chain acyl-CoA dehydrogenase (SCAD).

MCAD deficiency is the most common form of this disease. The deficiency will become apparent within first two years of life following fasting more than 12 hours. Symptoms include hypoglycemia without ketosis, vomiting, lethargy and frequently coma. Excessive urinary excretion of medium-chain dicarboxylic acids as well as their glycine and carnitine esters is diagnostic of this condition. In the case of this enzyme deficiency, taking care to avoid prolonged fasting is sufficient to prevent clinical problems.

Refsum's Disease

Refsum's disease is a rare inherited disorder in which patients lack the mitochondrial α-oxidizing enzyme. As a consequence, they accumulate large quantities of phytanic acid in their tissues and serum. This leads to severe symptoms, including cerebellar ataxia, retinitis pigmentosa, nerve deafness and peripheral neuropathy. As expected, the restriction of dairy products and ruminant meat from the diet can ameliorate the symptoms of this disease.

KETOGENESIS

During carbohydrate starvation, oxaloacetate in liver is depleted because it is used for gluconeogenesis. This slows down the entry of acetyl-CoA into Krebs cycle, which is then converted in liver mitochondria to ketone bodies (*acetoacetate*, *β-hydroxybutyrate*, and *acetone*). Also when the rate of fatty acid oxidation in the liver is high, large amounts of acetyl-CoA generated in excess of the capacity of the TCA cycle is diverted towards ketogenesis. Since ketone bodies are small molecular weight and water-soluble, they are transported in the blood to other tissue cells where they are converted back to acetyl-CoA for catabolism in Krebs cycle.

The formation of acetoacetyl-CoA occurs by condensation of two moles of acetyl-CoA through a reversal of the **thiolase**-catalyzed reaction of fatty acid oxidation (Fig. 29.14). Acetoacetyl-CoA then condenses with an acetyl-CoA molecule to form β-hydroxy-β-methylglutaryl-CoA (HMG-CoA) catalyzed by *HMG-CoA synthase* found in large amounts only in the liver. Some of the HMG-CoA leaves the mitochondria, where it is converted to mevalonate (the precursor for cholesterol synthesis) by *HMG-CoA reductase*. HMG-CoA in the mitochondria is converted to acetoacetate by the action of *HMG-CoA lyase*. Acetoacetate can undergo spontaneous decarboxylation to acetone or be enzymatically converted to β-hydroxybutyrate through the action of NADH dependent *β-hydroxybutyrate dehydrogenase*.

In early stages of starvation when the last remnants of fats are oxidized, heart and skeletal muscle will consume primarily ketone bodies to spare glucose for use by the brain. Acetoacetate and β-hydroxybutyrate in particular, serve as major substrates for the biosynthesis of cerebral lipids in neonates.

Extrahepatic tissues utilize ketone bodies by converting β-hydroxybutyrate to acetoacetate and acetoacetate to acetoacetyl-CoA. The first step involves the reversal of the β-hydroxybutyrate dehydrogenase reaction and the second involves the action of

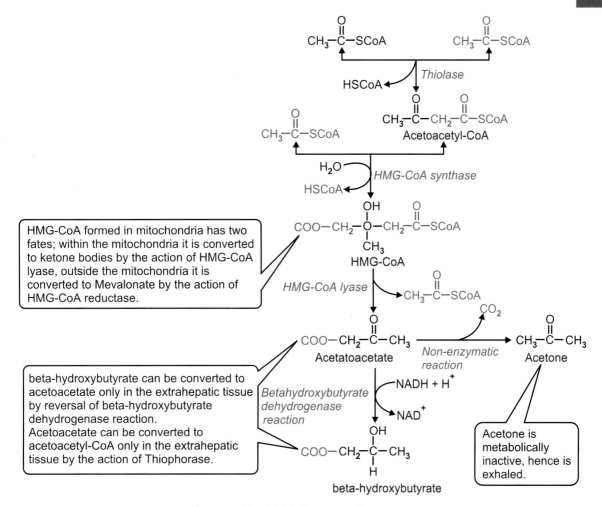

Fig. 29.14: Ketogenesis

acetoacetate: succinyl-CoA transferase (thiophorase) also called *ketoacyl-CoA-transferase.*

Acetoacetate + Succinyl-CoA ↔ Acetoacetyl-CoA + succinate

The latter enzyme is present in all tissues except the liver. The absence of this enzyme in the liver allows the liver to produce ketone bodies but not to utilize them (liver is the net producer of ketone bodies). This ensures that extrahepatic tissues (net utilizers of ketone bodies) have access to ketone bodies as a fuel source during prolonged starvation.

Acetoacetyl-CoA is converted into two molecules of acetyl-CoA by a *thiolase*:

Acetoacetyl-CoA + HS-CoA ↔ 2 Acetyl-CoA

Regulation of Ketogenesis

The fate of the products of fatty acid metabolism is determined by an individual's physiological status. Since ketogenesis takes place primarily in the liver, it may by affected by several factors:

1. Regulation at the level of free fatty acid release from adipose tissue directly affects the level of ketogenesis in the liver. This is an example of substrate-level regulation.
2. Once fatty acids enter the liver they have two distinct fates. They may be activated to acyl-CoAs and oxidized, or esterified with glycerol to form triacylglycerols. If the liver has sufficient supplies of glycerol-3-phosphate, most of the fatty acids will be diverted to the production of triacylglycerols.
3. The acetyl-CoA generated by fatty acid oxidation is completely oxidized in the TCA cycle, when the demand for ATP is high.
4. The rate of fatty acid oxidation is hormonally regulated through phosphorylation of ACC (in response to glucagon) that spares acetyl-CoA for oxidation. The dephosphorylation of ACC (in response to insulin) diverts acetyl-CoA for fatty acid synthesis.

Clinical Significance of Ketogenesis

The ketogenesis occurs at a relatively low rate during normal feeding and physiological status. The normal physiological responses to carbohydrate shortage cause the liver to increase the production of ketone bodies from the acetyl-CoA generated from fatty acid oxidation. This allows the heart and primarily skeletal muscles to use ketone bodies for energy, thereby preserving the limited glucose for use by the brain.

The alterations in the level of ketone bodies, leading to profound clinical manifestations, occur in untreated insulin-dependent diabetes mellitus. The diabetic keto acidosis (DKA) results from a reduced supply of glucose (results in decline in circulating insulin) and a concomitant elevation in fatty acid oxidation (due to a concomitant increase in circulating glucagon). The increased production of acetyl-CoA leads to production ketone bodies in excess of the ability of peripheral tissues to oxidize them. The ketone bodies are relatively strong acids (pK$_a$ around 3.5) and their increase lowers the pH of the blood. This acidification of the blood is dangerous chiefly because it impairs the ability of hemoglobin to bind oxygen.

METABOLISM OF EICOSANOIDS

The eicosanoids are a group of related compounds that includes prostaglandins (PGs), prostacyclines, thromboxanes (TXs) and leukotrienes (LTs). The PGs and TXs are collectively identified as prostanoids. Prostaglandins were originally shown to be synthesized in the prostate gland, thromboxanes from platelets (thrombocytes) and leukotrienes from leukocytes, hence the derivation of their names (Fig. 29.15).

The principal eicosanoids of biological significance to humans are a group of molecules derived from the 20 Carbon (C$_{20}$) fatty acid arachidonic acid. Minor eicosanoids are derived from dihomo-γ-linoleic acid and eicosapentaenoic acid. The major source of arachidonic acid is through its release from membrane phospholipids in cell. Within the cell, it resides predominantly at the C-2 position of membrane phospholipids and is released upon the activation of *phospholipase A$_2$* (Fig. 29.16).

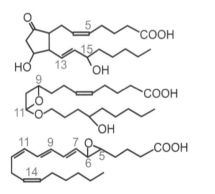

PGE$_2$

TXA$_2$

LTA$_4$

Fig. 29.15: Structures of eicosanoids

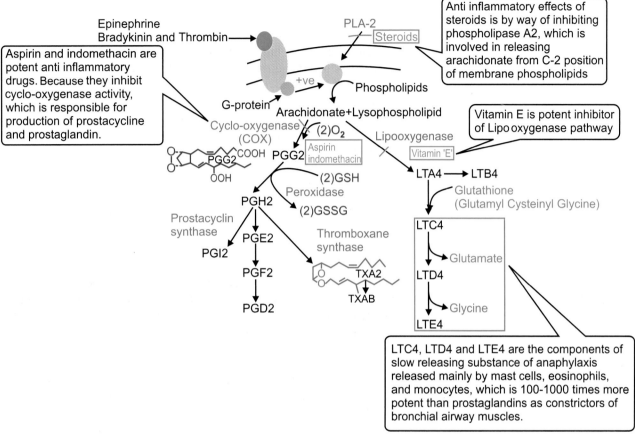

Fig. 29.16: Synthesis of eicosanoids

The immediate dietary precursor of arachidonate is linoleate, which is also the precursor for dihomo-γ-linoleic acid and eicosopentaenoic acid synthesis. Therefore, the absence of linoleic acid from the diet would seriously threaten the body's ability to synthesize eicosanoids.

The eicosanoids produce a wide range of biological effects on inflammatory responses (predominantly those of the joints, skin and eyes), intensity and duration of pain and fever, and on reproductive function (including the induction of labor). They also play important roles in inhibiting gastric acid secretion, regulating blood pressure through vasodilatation or constriction, and inhibiting or activating platelet aggregation and thrombosis.

All mammalian cells except erythrocytes synthesize eicosanoids. These molecules are extremely potent and cause profound physiological effects at very low concentrations. All eicosanoids function locally at the site of synthesis through receptor-mediated G-protein linked signaling pathways leading to an increase in cAMP levels.

Two main pathways are involved in the biosynthesis of eicosanoids. The cyclic pathway synthesizes the prostaglandins and thromboxanes, the linear pathway synthesize leukotrienes (Fig. 29.16).

The cyclic pathway is initiated through the action of **prostaglandin endoperoxide synthetase**. This enzyme possesses two activities, **cyclooxygenase** and **peroxidase**.

The linear pathway is initiated through the action of *lipooxygenases*. It is this enzyme, *5-lipooxygenase* that gives rise to the leukotrienes.

A widely used class of drugs, the non-steroidal anti-inflammatory drugs (NSAIDs) such as ibuprofen, indomethacin, naproxen, phenylbutazone and aspirin, all acts upon the cyclooxygenase activity. Aspirin *acetylates* a serine residue near the cyclooxygenase active site, which prevents binding of arachidonate. The inhibition by aspirin is irreversible. Another class, the corticosteroidal drugs, acts to inhibit phospholipase A_2, thereby inhibiting the release of arachidonate from membrane phospholipids and the subsequent synthesis of eicosanoids. Vitamin E is a potent inhibitor of lipooxygenase.

Functions of Important Eicosanoids

Eicosanoid	Major site(s) of synthesis	Major biological activities
PGD_2	Mast cells	Inhibits platelet and leukocyte aggregation, decreases T cell proliferation and lymphocyte migration and secretion of IL-1α and IL-2; induces vasodilatation and production of cAMP
PGE_2	Kidney, spleen, heart	Increases vasodilatation and cAMP production, enhancement of the effects of bradykinin and histamine, induction of uterine contractions and of platelet aggregation, maintaining the open passageway of the fetal ductus arteriosus; decreases T cell proliferation and lymphocyte migration and secretion of IL-1α and IL-2
$PGF_{2\alpha}$	Kidney, spleen, heart	Increases vasoconstriction, bronchoconstriction and smooth muscle contraction
PGH_2	–	Precursor to thromboxanes A_2 and B_2, induction of platelet aggregation and vasoconstriction
PGI_2	Heart, vascular endothelial cells	Inhibits platelet and leukocyte aggregation, decreases T cell proliferation and lymphocyte migration and secretion of IL-1α and IL-2; induces vasodilatation and production of cAMP
TXA_2	Platelets	Induces platelet aggregation, vasoconstriction, lymphocyte proliferation and bronchoconstriction
TXB_2	Platelets	Induces vasoconstriction
LTB_4	Monocytes, basophils, neutrophils, eosinophils, mast cells, epithelial cells	Induces leukocyte chemotaxis and aggregation, vascular permeability, T cell proliferation and secretion of INF-γ, IL-1 and IL-2
LTC_4	Monocytes and alveolar macrophages, basophils, eosinophils, mast cells, epithelial cells	Component of SRS-A, induces vasodilatation, vascular permeability and bronchoconstriction and secretion of INF-γ
LTD_4	Monocytes and alveolar macrophages, eosinophils, mast cells, epithelial cells	Predominant component of SRS-A, induces vasodilatation, vascular permeability and bronchoconstriction and secretion of INF-γ
LTE_4	Mast cells and basophils	Component of SRS-A, induces vasodilatation and bronchoconstriction

**SRS-A = slow-reactive substance of anaphylaxis

Metabolism of Triglycerides and Phospholipids

30

All cells, but primarily adipocytes store fatty acids for future use in the form of triacylglycerols. Triacylglycerol is composed of a molecule of glycerol, to which three fatty acids are esterified. The fatty acids present in triacylglycerols are predominantly saturated.

Adipocytes cannot use glycerol for triacylglycerol synthesis, because they lack glycerol kinase. Instead they use dihydroxyacetone phosphate (DHAP) produced during glycolysis as the precursor for triacylglycerol synthesis. This means, adipocytes must have adequate supply of glucose in order to store fatty acids in the form of triacylglycerols. Tissues other than adipose tissue also utilize DHAP as a backbone precursor for triacylglycerol synthesis, but to a much lesser extent. In these tissues, the predominant pathway of triacylglycerol synthesis is activation of glycerol to the level of glycerol-3-phosphate by phosphorylation at the C-3 position by *glycerol kinase*. The utilization of DHAP as the backbone is carried out through the action of *glycerol-3-phosphate dehydrogenase*, a reaction that requires NADH (Fig. 30.1). The fatty acids to be incorporated into triacylglycerols are also activated to the level of acyl-CoAs through the action of *acyl-CoA synthetases*. Two molecules of acyl-CoA are esterified to glycerol-3-phosphate at carbon 1 and 2 to yield 1,2-diacylglycerol phosphate (commonly identified as phosphatidic acid). The phosphate group at C3 is then removed by *phosphatidic acid phosphatase*, to yield 1,2-diacylglycerol, which serve as the substrate for addition of the third fatty acid. Intestinal monoacylglycerols, derived from the hydrolysis of dietary fats, can serve as substrates for the synthesis of 1,2-diacylglycerols in the intestinal mucosal cells.

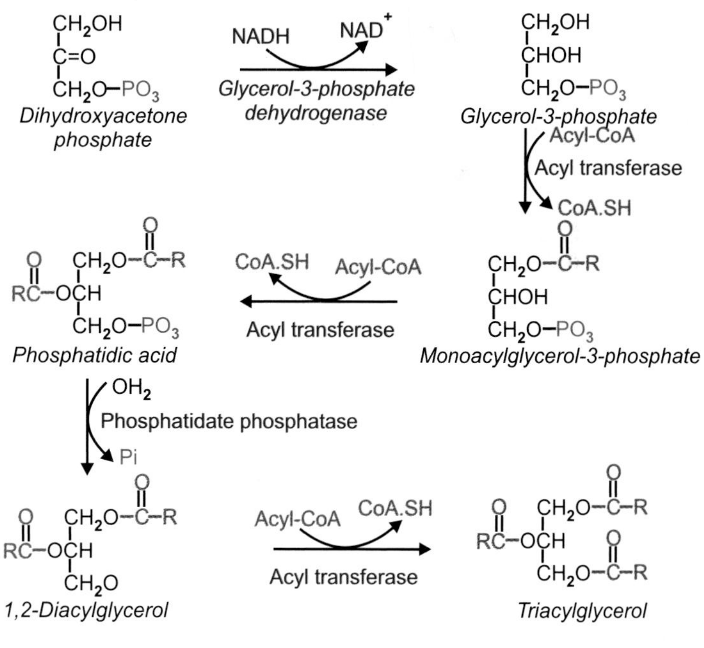

Fig. 30.1: Triacylglycerol synthesis

PHOSPHOLIPID SYNTHESIS

Phospholipids can be synthesized by two mechanisms. One mechanism utilizes a CDP-activated polar head group, which forms phosphodiester bond with C-3 of 1,2-diacylglycerol. The other utilizes CDP-activated 1,2-diacylglycerol (CDP-diacylglycerol) and an inactive polar head group (Fig. 30.2).

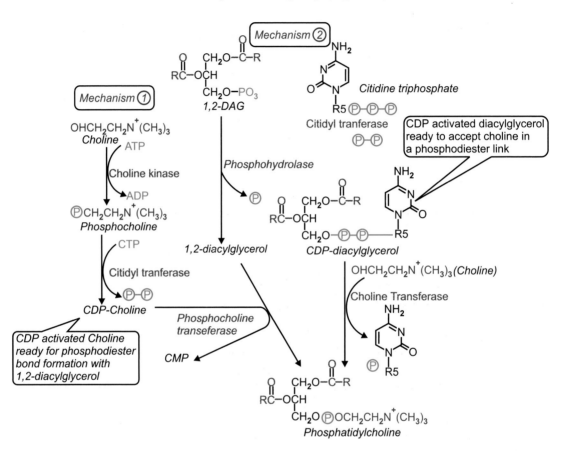

Fig. 30.2: Phosphatidylcholine biosynthesis

Phospholipids are synthesized by the addition of a basic group (predominantly a nitrogenous base) to phosphatidic acid or 1,2-diacylglycerol. Most phospholipids have a saturated fatty acid on C-1 and an unsaturated fatty acid on C-2 of the glycerol backbone.

Major Classes of Phospholipids

The physiologically important phospholipids are phosphatidyl choline, phosphatidyl ethanolamine, phosphatidyl serine, phosphatidyl inositol, phosphatidylglycerol and diphosphatidylglycerol (Fig. 30.3).

Phosphatidyl choline (PC): This class of phospholipids is also known as **lecithins**. At physiological pH, phosphatidylcholines are neutral zwitterions. They contain primarily palmitic or stearic acid at C-1 and oleic, linoleic or linolenic acid at C-2. The lecithin

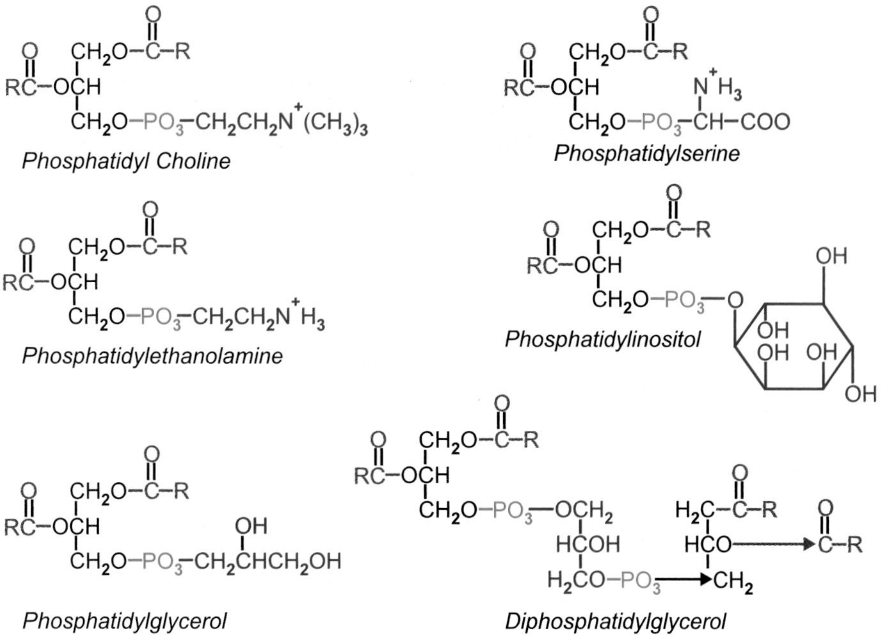

Fig. 30.3: Phospholipid structures

dipalmitoyllecithin is a component of *pulmonary surfactant*. It contains palmitate at both C-1 and C-2 of glycerol and is the major (80%) phospholipid found in the extracellular lipid layer lining the pulmonary alveoli.

Choline is activated first by phosphorylation and then by coupling to CDP prior to attachment to phosphatidic acid (Fig. 30.2). Another pathway to PC synthesis involves the conversion of either phosphatidyl serine (PS) or phosphatidyl ethanolamine (PE) to phosphatidyl choline. The conversion of PS to PC first requires decarboxylation of PS to yield PE, which then undergoes a series of three methylation reactions utilizing S-adenosylmethionine (SAM) as methyl group donor.

Phosphatidyl ethanolamine (PE) is a neutral zwitterion at physiological pH. They contain primarily palmitic or stearic acid on C-1 and a long chain unsaturated fatty acid (e.g. 18:2, 20:4 and 22:6) on C-2. Synthesis of PE can occur by two pathways. The first requires that ethanolamine be activated by phosphorylation and then by coupling to CDP. The ethanolamine is then transferred from CDP-ethanolamine to phosphatidic acid to yield PE. The second involves the decarboxylation of PS.

Phosphatidyl serine (PS) carries a net charge of -1 at physiological pH and is composed of fatty acids similar to the phosphatidyl-ethanolamines. The pathway for PS synthesis involves an exchange reaction of serine for ethanolamine in PE and choline in PC. These exchange occur when PE and PC are in the lipid bilayer of the membrane. As indicated above, PS can serve as a source of PE through a decarboxylation reaction.

Phosphatidyl inositol (PI) contains almost exclusively stearic acid at carbon 1 and arachidonic acid at C-2. Phosphatidylinositols composed exclusively of non-phosphorylated inositol exhibit a net charge of -1 at physiological pH. These molecules exist in membranes with various levels of phosphate esterified to the hydroxyls of the inositol. Molecules with phosphorylated inositol are termed *polyphosphoinositides*. The polyphosphoinositides are important intracellular transducers of signals derived from plasma membrane.

The synthesis of PI involves condensation of CDP-activated 1,2-diacylglycerol with *myo*-inositol. PI subsequently undergoes a series of phosphorylations of the hydroxyls of inositol leading to the production of polyphosphoinositides. One polyphosphoinositide (*phosphatidylinositol 4,5-bisphosphate, PIP$_2$*) is a critically important membrane phospholipid involved in the transmission of signals for cell growth and differentiation from outside the cell to inside.

Phosphatidylglycerol (PG) exhibits a net charge of -1 at physiological pH. These molecules are found in high concentration in mitochondrial membranes and as components of *pulmonary surfactant*. PG is synthesized from CDP-diacylglycerol and glycerol-3-phosphate. The vital role of PG is to serve as the precursor for the synthesis of diphosphatidylglycerols (DPGs).

Diphosphatidylglycerol (DPG) is very acidic, exhibiting a net charge of -2 at physiological pH. They are found primarily in the inner mitochondrial membrane and also as components of *pulmonary surfactant*. Diphosphatidylglycerol is also known as *cardiolipin*, which is synthesized by condensation of CDP-diacylglycerol with PG.

The fatty acids present at the C-1 and C-2 positions of glycerol within phospholipids are continually in flux, owing to phospholipid degradation and the continuous phospholipid remodeling that occurs while these molecules are in membranes. Phospholipid degradation results from the action of **phospholipases**. There are various phospholipases that exhibit substrate specificities for different positions in phospholipids (Fig. 30.4). In many cases, the acyl group, which is initially transferred to glycerol by the action of the acyl transferases, is not the same acyl group present in the phospholipid when it resides in the plasma membrane. The turnover of acyl groups in phospholipids is the result of the action of **phospholipase A$_1$** and **phospholipase A$_2$**. The products of these phospholipids are called lysophospholipids (phospholipids without acyl group at C-2 position), which are substrates for acyl transferases that utilize different acyl-CoA groups. Lysophospholipids can also accept acyl groups from other phospholipids in an exchange reaction catalyzed by *lysolecithin: lecithin acyltransferase* (LLAT). Phospholipase A$_2$ is also an important enzyme, whose activity is responsible for the release of arachidonic acid from the C-2 position of membrane phospholipids. The released arachidonate is then a substrate for the synthesis of the prostaglandins and leukotrienes.

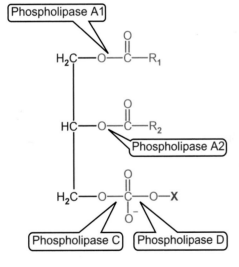

Fig. 30.4: The site of action of various lipases on phospholipids

FATTY LIVER AND LIPOTROPIC FACTORS

Fatty liver or fatty infiltration of liver is a condition where there is excess accumulation of triacylglycerol (TAG) in the liver. Such accumulation over a period of time induces pressure effects on the architecture of liver leading to fibrosis that progress to cirrhosis and impaired liver function.

Some of the etiological factors of fatty liver are uncontrolled diabetes mellitus, toxemia of pregnancy, hepatitis and ethanol abuse.

Causes of Fatty Liver

i. *Increased TAG synthesis in the liver* in excess of its ability to synthesize and secrete it in the form of lipoproteins. Elevated TAG synthesis in the liver could be the result of excessive lipolysis in adipose tissue, increased hydrolysis of chylomicrons or rapid uptake of FFA by the liver.

ii. *Deficiency of lipotropic factors* affects the synthesis of apolipoproteins and phospholipids, which are required for synthesis and secretion of lipoproteins (particularly VLDL) by the liver.

Lipotropic Factors

Lipotropic factors are known to prevent development and progression of fatty liver but are not able to reverse the damage that has already occurred. The examples of lipotropic factors are essential fatty acids, choline, methionine, vitamin E and selenium.

Selenium and vitamin E, being antioxidants prevents lipid peroxidation and fatty liver.

Supply of adequate quantities of essential fatty acids are required for phospholipid synthesis thereby lipoprotein are synthesized and secreted by the liver.

Choline is required for glycation of apolipoproteins, synthesis of lecithin and membrane concerned with lipoprotein assembly and secretion, and carnitine synthesis where choline is the methyl donor. All these processes help TAG removal from liver in the form of lipoproteins.

Causes of choline deficiency are methionine deficiency (SAM is methyl group donor) and diversion of SAM for other process.

Chemicals that cause fatty liver are ethionine, carbon tetrachloride, chloroform, phosphorus, arsenate, lead, puramycin and ethanol.

Ethionine combines with methionine to form SAE (S adenosyl ethionine) thereby ATP is trapped. Ethanol abuse, lead to enhanced fatty acid synthesis. The other chemicals mentioned affect protein synthesis in liver. All these factors can lead to TAG accumulation and development of fatty liver.

PLASMALOGENS

Plasmalogens are glycerol ether phospholipids. They are of two types, alkyl ether and alkenyl ether. Dihydroxyacetone phosphate serves as

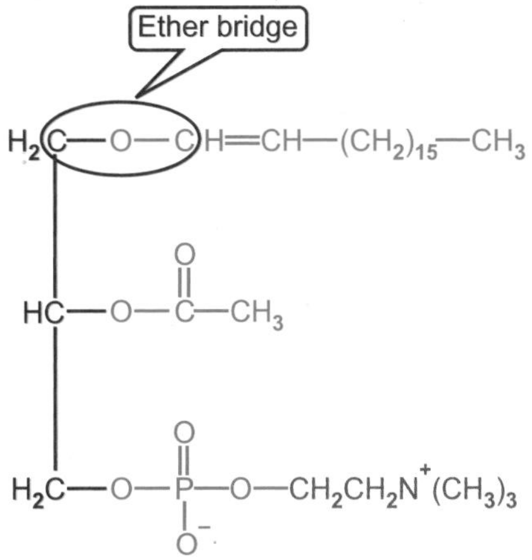

$$H_2C-O-CH=CH-(CH_2)_{15}-CH_3$$

$$HC-O-\overset{\overset{\displaystyle O}{\|}}{C}-CH_3$$

$$H_2C-O-\overset{\overset{\displaystyle O}{\|}}{\underset{\underset{\displaystyle O^-}{|}}{P}}-O-CH_2CH_2\overset{+}{N}(CH_3)_3$$

Ether bridge

Fig. 30.5: Platelet activating factor

the glycerol precursor for the synthesis of glycerol ether phospholipids. Three major classes of plasmalogens have been identified: choline, ethanolamine and serine plasmalogens. Ethanolamine plasmalogen is prevalent in myelin. Choline plasmalogen is abundant in cardiac tissue. One particular choline plasmalogen (1-alkyl, 2-acetyl phosphatidylcholine) has been identified as an extremely powerful biological mediator, capable of inducing cellular responses at concentrations as low as 10^{-11} M. This molecule is called *platelet-activating factor* (Fig. 30.5). The platelet-activating factor (PAF) functions as a mediator of hypersensitivity, acute inflammatory reactions and anaphylactic shock. PAF is synthesized in response to the formation of *antigen-IgE complexes* on the surfaces of basophils, neutrophils, eosinophils, macrophages and monocytes. The synthesis and release of PAF from cells leads to platelet aggregation and the release of serotonin from platelets. PAF also produces responses in liver, heart, smooth muscle, uterus and lung tissues.

METABOLISM OF SPHINGOLIPIDS

The sphingolipids like phospholipids are composed of a polar head group and two nonpolar tails. The core of sphingolipids is the long-chain amino alcohol, sphingosine (Fig. 30.6). The sphingolipids include *sphingomyelins* and *glycosphingolipids* (cerebrosides, sulfatides, globosides and gangliosides). Sphingomyelins are the only sphingolipid that are also phospholipids. Sphingolipids are a component of all membranes but are particularly abundant in the myelin sheath. Ceramide (N-acyl sphingosine) present both in sphingomyelins and glycosphingolipids is derived by N-acylation of amino group of sphingosine with carboxyl carbon of long-chain fatty acid.

Sphingomyelins are important structural lipid components of nerve cell membranes. The predominant sphingomyelins contain palmitic or stearic acid N-acylated at C-2 of sphingosine, and phosphorylcholine is in phosphoester bond with hydroxyl at C-1 of sphingosine in a reaction catalyzed by *sphingomyelin synthase* (Fig. 30.6). Defects in the enzyme *acid sphingomyelinase* result in the lysosomal storage disease known as Niemann-Pick disease. There are at least four related disorders identified as Niemann-Pick disease type A, type B (both of which result from defects in *acid sphingomyelinase*), type C and type D.

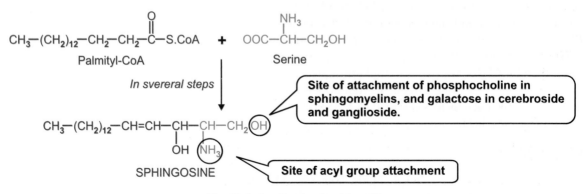

Fig. 30.6: Synthesis of sphingosine

GLYCOSPHINGOLIPIDS

Glycosphingolipids or glycolipids are composed of a ceramide backbone with a wide variety of carbohydrate groups (mono- or oligosaccharides) attached to C-1 of sphingosine. The four principal classes of glycosphingolipids are the cerebrosides, sulfatides, globosides and gangliosides.

Cerebrosides have a single sugar group linked to ceramide. The most common of these is galactose (galactocerebrosides), with a minor level of glucose (glucocerebrosides). Galactocerebrosides are found predominantly in neuronal cell membranes. By contrast glucocerebrosides are not normally found in membranes, especially neuronal membranes; instead, they represent intermediates in the synthesis or degradation of more complex glycosphingolipids.

Galactocerebrosides are synthesized from ceramide and UDP-galactose. Excess accumulation of glucocerebrosides is observed in Gaucher's disease.

Sulfatides are sulfuric acid esters of galactocerebrosides. Sulfatides are synthesized from galactocerebrosides and activated sulfate 3'-phosphoadenosine 5'-phosphosulfate (PAPS). Excess accumulation of sulfatides is observed in sulfatide lipidosis (metachromatic leukodystrophy).

Globosides represent cerebrosides that contain additional carbohydrates, predominantly galactose, glucose or GalNAc. Lactosyl ceramide is a globoside found in plasma membrane of erythrocyte. Globotriosylceramide (also called ceramide trihexoside) contains glucose and two moles of galactose. Accumulation of globosides, primarily in the kidneys is seen in patients suffering from Fabry's disease.

Gangliosides are very similar to globosides except that they also contain NANA in varying amounts. The specific names for gangliosides are a key to their structure. The letter G refers to "ganglioside", and the subscripts M, D, T and Q indicate that the molecule contains mono-, di-, tri and quatra (tetra)-sialic acid. The numerical subscripts 1, 2 and 3 refer to the carbohydrate sequence that is attached to ceramide; 1 stands for Gal-GalNAc-Gal-Glc-ceramide, 2 for GalNAc-Gal-Glc-ceramide and 3 for Gal-Glc-ceramide.

Deficiencies in lysosomal enzymes, which are responsible for the degradation of carbohydrate portions of various gangliosides is responsible for the symptoms observed in rare autosomally inherited diseases termed lipid storage diseases.

Clinical Significances of Sphingolipids

One of the most clinically important classes of sphingolipids confers antigenic determinants on the surfaces of cells, particularly the erythrocytes. The ABO blood group antigens are the carbohydrate moieties of glycolipids that are found on the surface of cells as well as the carbohydrate portion of serum glycoproteins. The ABO

Disorders Associated with Abnormal Sphingolipid Metabolism

Disorder	Enzyme deficiency	Accumulating substance	Symptoms
Tay-Sachs disease	Hexosaminidase A	GM_2 ganglioside	Mental retardation, blindness, early mortality
Gaucher's disease	Glucocerebrosidase	Glucocerebroside	Hepatosplenomegaly, mental retardation in infantile form, long bone degeneration
Fabry's disease	α-Galactosidase A	Globotriaosylceramide; also called ceramide trihexoside (CTH)	Kidney failure, skin rashes
Niemann-Pick disease, more info below Types A and B Type C1 Type C2 Type D	Sphingomyelinase see info below see info below	Sphingomyelin LDL-derived cholesterol LDL-derived cholesterol	All types lead to mental retardation, hepatosplenomegaly, early fatality potential
Krabbe's disease; globoid leukodystrophy	Galactocerebrosidase	Galactocerebroside	Mental retardation, myelin deficiency
Sandhoff-Jatzkewitz disease	Hexosaminidase A and B	Globoside, GM_2 ganglioside	Same symptoms as Tay-Sachs, progresses more rapidly
GM_1 gangliosidosis	GM_1 ganglioside: β-galactosidase	GM_1 ganglioside	Mental retardation, skeletal abnormalities, hepatomegaly
Sulfatide lipodosis; metachromatic leukodystrophy	Arylsulfatase A	Sulfatide	Mental retardation, metachromasia of nerves
Fucosidosis	α-L-Fucosidase	Pentahexosylfucoglycolipid	Cerebral degeneration, thickened skin, muscle spasticity
Farber's lipogranulomatosis	Acid ceramidase	Ceramide	Hepatosplenomegaly, painful swollen joints

carbohydrates present on the surface of cells are linked to membrane sphingolipids and are therefore of the glycosphingolipid class. The ABO carbohydrates associated with serum glycoproteins are referred to as the secreted forms. Some individuals produce the glycoprotein forms of the ABO antigens while others do not. This property distinguishes secretors from non-secretors, a property that has forensic importance such as in cases of rape.

A significant cause of death in infants is respiratory distress syndrome (RDS) or hyaline membrane disease. This condition is caused by an insufficient amount of pulmonary surfactant. Under normal conditions the type II endothelial cells synthesize and secrete the pulmonary surfactants into the alveolar spaces to prevent atelectasis following expiration during breathing. The predominant surfactant is dipalmitoyllecithin; additional lipid components include phosphatidylglycerol and phosphatidylinositol along with proteins termed surfactant proteins. During the third trimester, the type II endothelial cells of fetal lung convert most of its stored glycogen to dipalmitoyllecithin and synthesize sphingomyelin. Determination of fetal lung maturity is done by measuring the ratio of lecithin to sphingomyelin (L/S ratio) in the amniotic fluid. An L/S ratio less than 2.0 indicates a potential risk of RDS. The risk is nearly 75-80 percent when the L/S ratio is 1.5.

The carbohydrate portion of the ganglioside GM_1, found on the surface of intestinal epithelial cells is the site of attachment for cholera toxin (a protein) secreted by. These are just a few examples of how sphingolipids and glycosphingolipids are involved in various recognition functions at the surface of cells. As with the complex glycoproteins, an understanding of all of the functions of the glycolipids is far from complete.

Cholesterol and Bile Acid Metabolism

31

Cholesterol is an extremely important biological molecule unique to animals that has roles in membrane structure as well as being a precursor for steroid hormones, calcitriol and bile acids (Fig. 31.1). Both dietary cholesterol and that synthesized *de novo* are transported as lipoprotein particles in the blood circulation. Cholesterol is stored in cells as cholesteryl esters. The synthesis and utilization of cholesterol must be tightly regulated in order to prevent over-accumulation and abnormal deposition within the body tissues, in particular blood vessels and coronary arteries. Such deposition eventually lead to atherosclerosis, the leading contributory factor in coronary arteries diseases.

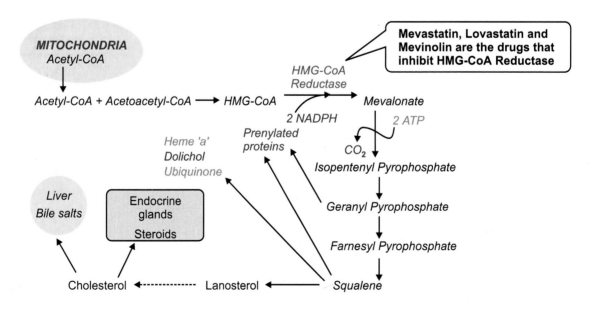

Fig. 31.1: Cholesterol metabolism

BIOSYNTHESIS OF CHOLESTEROL

Almost half the body requirement of cholesterol is met by *de novo synthesis*. The liver accounts for approximately 10 percent, and the intestines 15 percent of cholesterol synthesized each day. The cholesterol synthesis takes place in the cytoplasm and microsomal fraction of all nucleated cells, beginning from two-carbon acetyl-CoA units.

The process of cholesterol synthesis has six major steps, they are:

1. One mole each of acetyl-CoA and acetoacetyl-CoA condenses to form a mole of β-hydroxy-β-methyl glutaryl-CoA (HMG-CoA).
2. HMG-CoA undergoes reduction to form mevalonate.
3. Mevalonate undergoes phosphorylation, decarboxylation and isomerization to form isoprene units: isopentenyl pyrophosphate (IPP), and dimethylallyl pyrophosphate (DAP).
4. Two moles of IPP and one mole of DAP condenses to form farnesyl pyrophosphate
5. Two molecules of farnesyl pyrophosphate condense to form squalene.
6. Squalene is converted to cholesterol by cyclization, demethylation, shift of double bond and reduction.

The acetyl-CoA for cholesterol biosynthesis is derived from oxidation of fatty acids or pyruvate in the mitochondria, which is transported to the cytoplasm by a similar process described earlier for fatty acid synthesis. Acetyl-CoA can also be derived from cytoplasmic oxidation of ethanol by *acetyl-CoA synthetase*. All reduction reactions of cholesterol biosynthesis require NADPH as a cofactor. The isoprene intermediates of cholesterol biosynthesis can be diverted for the synthesis of other molecules such as *dolichol* required in the synthesis of N-linked glycoproteins, *coenzyme Q* of electron transport chain, or the side chains of *heme* a (Fig. 31.1). Additionally, these intermediates are used for the covalent modification of certain proteins.

Acetyl-CoA units are converted to mevalonate by a series of reactions that begins with the formation of HMG-CoA. Unlike the HMG-CoA formed in the mitochondria during ketone body synthesis, the HMG-CoA for cholesterol synthesis is formed in the cytoplasm. However, the substrates and the enzymes involved are the same in both the pathways.

Two moles of acetyl-CoA are condensed in a reversal of the *thiolase* reaction, forming acetoacetyl-CoA. A mole each of acetoacetyl-CoA and acetyl-CoA condenses to form HMG-CoA, catalyzed by *HMG-CoA synthase*. HMG-CoA is converted to mevalonate by *HMG-CoA reductase*. Two moles of NADPH are consumed during the conversion of HMG-CoA to mevalonate catalyzed by *HMG-CoA reductase*, which has absolute requirement for NADPH. The reaction catalyzed by *HMG-CoA reductase* is the rate-limiting step of cholesterol biosynthesis and is regulated by complex mechanisms (Fig. 31.2).

Mevalonate is phosphorylated in three successive steps, by mevalonate kinase to yield 3-P-5-pyrophosphomevalonate (Fig. 31.3). Phosphorylation of mevalonate serves two purposes,

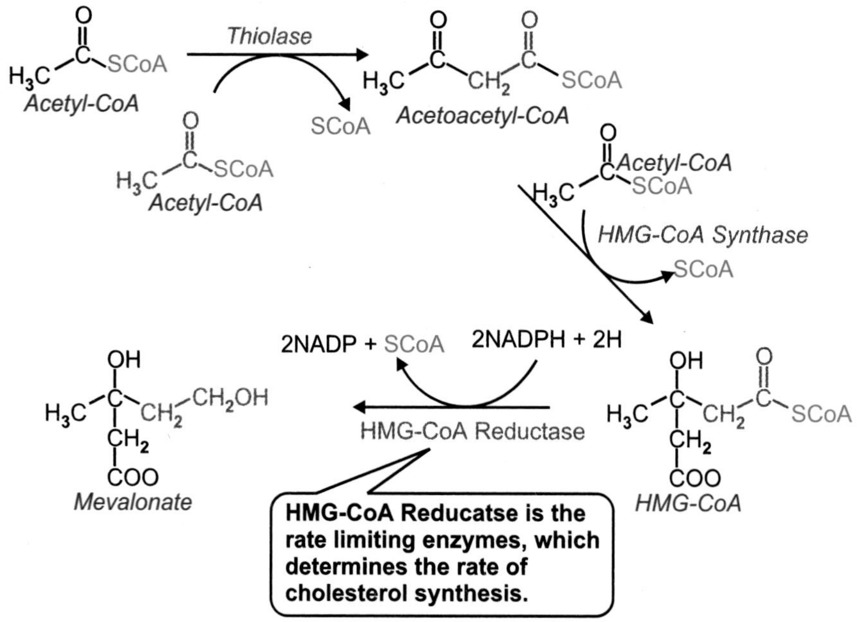

Fig. 31.2: Synthesis of mevalonate

one is to activate it and the other is to maintain its solubility. An ATP dependent decarboxylation of 3-P-5-pyrophosphomevalonate yields isopentenyl pyrophosphate (IPP), which is an activated isoprenoid molecule. Isopentenyl pyrophosphate is in equilibrium with its isomer dimethylallyl pyrophosphate (DMPP), catalyzed by *isomerase*.

Condensation of two molecules of IPP with one molecule of DMPP to generate farnesyl pyrophosphate (FPP) is catalyzed by *isopentenyl transferase*. Finally, the NADPH-requiring enzyme, *squalene synthase* catalyzes the head-to-tail condensation of two molecules of FPP to yield squalene. Squalene undergoes a two-step cyclization to yield lanosterol. The first step is catalyzed by *squalene monooxygenase* that requires NADPH as a cofactor to introduce molecular oxygen as an epoxide at the 2,3 position of squalene. Lanosterol undergoes a series of 19 additional reactions to yield cholesterol.

Regulating Cholesterol Synthesis

Normal healthy adults synthesize cholesterol at a rate of approximately 1g/day and consume approximately 0.3g/day. A relatively constant level of cholesterol in the body (150-200 mg/dL) is maintained primarily by controlling the level of *de novo* synthesis. The level of cholesterol synthesis is regulated in part by the dietary intake of cholesterol. Cholesterol from both diet and *de novo* synthesis is utilized in the formation of membranes, synthesis of the steroid hormones and bile acids. The greatest proportion of cholesterol is diverted to bile acid synthesis.

Steady level of cholesterol supply to cells is maintained by three distinct mechanisms:

1. Regulation of **HMG-CoA reductase** activity and its levels.

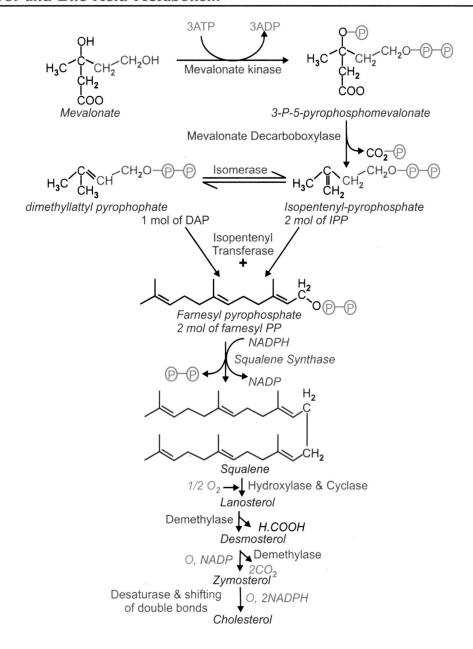

Fig. 31.3: Synthesis of cholesterol

2. Regulation of excess intracellular free cholesterol through the activity of acyl-CoA: cholesterol acyltransferase, ACAT and

3. Regulation of plasma cholesterol levels via LDL receptor-mediated uptake and HDL-mediated reverse transport.

The rate of cholesterol biosynthesis is primarily controlled by the activity of *HMG-CoA reductase* by covalent modification (short-term regulation) and through control of its absolute level (long-term regulation) within cells.

HMG-CoA reductase is a single polypeptide embedded in microsomal membranes; it is most active in its unmodified form and its phosphorylation by *reductase kinase* (RK) decreases the activity.

The RK itself is activated via phosphorylation. The phosphorylation of RK is catalyzed by **reductase** *kinase kinase* (RKK). There are two isoforms of RKK, one independent of cAMP and the other dependent upon cAMP. The cAMP-dependent RKK is activated in the presence of cAMP. Since the intracellular level of cAMP is regulated by hormonal stimuli, regulation of cholesterol biosynthesis also is hormonally controlled. Insulin leads to a decrease in cAMP, which in turn activates cholesterol synthesis. Alternatively, glucagon and epinephrine, which increase the level of cAMP, inhibit cholesterol synthesis.

Long-term control of **HMG-CoA reductase** activity is exerted primarily through control over the synthesis and degradation of the enzyme. When levels of cholesterol are high, the level of expression of the HMG-CoA gene is reduced. Conversely, reduced levels of cholesterol activate expression of the gene. The rate of HMG-CoA reductase synthesis is increased by insulin. The rate of HMG-CoA turnover is also regulated by the supply of cholesterol. The rate of **HMG-CoA reductase** degradation increases, when cholesterol is abundant.

BILE ACID SYNTHESIS AND UTILIZATION

Synthesis of bile acids is the predominant mechanisms by which excess cholesterol is eliminated from the body. However, this mechanism alone is insufficient to compensate for an excess dietary intake of cholesterol and the reminder is excreted as neutral steroids in the bile, but much of it is reabsorbed. The principal sterol in the feces is coprostanol, which is derived from cholesterol formed from bacterial flora inhabiting small intestine.

The end products of cholesterol catabolism in the liver are chenodeoxycholic acid and cholic acid, which are collectively called primary bile acids. The most abundant bile acids in human bile are chenodeoxycholic acid (45 %) and cholic acid (31%).

The committing step in the biosynthesis of bile acids (catabolism of cholesterol) is the 7α-hydroxylation of cholesterol that yields 7α-hydroxycholesterol (Fig. 31.4). This reaction is catalyzed by a microsomal mono-oxygenase system; it requires O_2 and NADPH, and is partially inhibited by carbon dioxide. Vitamin C deficiency appear to interfere with 7α-hydroxylation and leads to cholesterol accumulation and atherosclerosis.

In a sequence of reactions that follow, the terminal three carbons on the side chain of 7α-hydroxycholesterol are removed as propionyl-CoA to yield chenodeoxycholic acid or cholic acid. These two together are called primary bile acids.

The carboxyl group of bile acids is conjugated via an amide bond to either glycine or taurine to yield glycocholic acid and taurocholic acid respectively before their secretion into the bile canaliculi. The bile canaliculi join with the bile ductules, which then form the bile ducts. Bile acids are carried from the liver through these ducts to the gallbladder, where they are stored for future use. The ultimate fate of bile acids is secretion into the intestine, where they aid in the emulsification of dietary lipids.

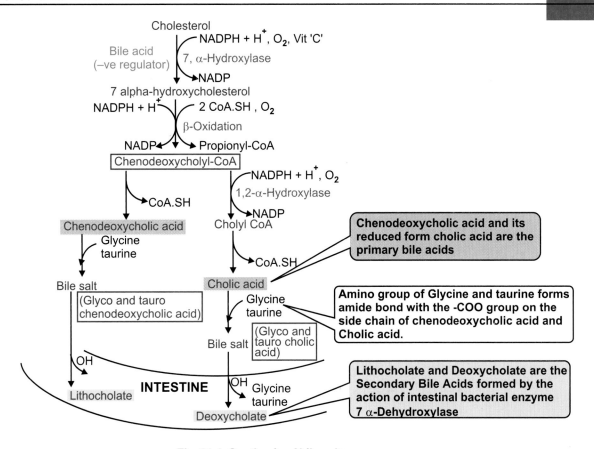

Fig. 31.4: Synthesis of bile salts

In the gut, the glycine and taurine residues of bile salts are removed and the primary bile acid undergoes 7α-dehydroxylation by the action of bacterial enzymes. The products of 7α-dehydroxylation are deoxycholic acid and lithocholic acids, which are collectively called secondary bile acids. The bile acids are either excreted (only to a small extent) or reabsorbed into the portal circulation from the gut and returned to the liver for another round of conjugation and secretion. This process is termed the enterohepatic circulation of bile acids.

Clinical Significance of Bile Acid Synthesis

Bile acids perform four physiologically significant functions, they are:
1. Their synthesis and subsequent excretion in the feces represent the only significant mechanism for the elimination of excess cholesterol.
2. Bile acids and phospholipids help solubilization of cholesterol in the bile, thereby prevent the precipitation of cholesterol in the gallbladder.
3. They facilitate the digestion of dietary triacylglycerols by acting as emulsifying agents that render fats accessible to the action of pancreatic lipases.
4. They facilitate the intestinal absorption of fat-soluble vitamins.

Cholesterol is dissolved in the bile as **'micelles'**, which it forms with **lecithin** and **bile salts**. The normal bile is composed of 5 percent cholesterol, 15 percent lecithin and 80 percent bile salts. Any alterations in the ratio of these three substances in bile can lead to precipitation of cholesterol crystals, which is one of the causes of gallstones formation. Bile composition falling above the green line (Fig. 31.5) would contain excess of cholesterol in either supersaturated or precipitated form, which is the cause of gallstone formation.

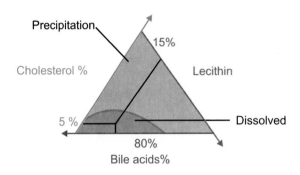

Fig. 31.5: Cholesterol precipitation

The PDH Complex and TCA Cycle

32

Oxidation of pyruvate in mitochondrial matrix generates NADH. The reducing potential of NADH in turn drives oxidative phosphorylation to generate high-energy phosphate in ATP. The metabolic fate of pyruvate depends on energy charge of the cell. When cell energy charge is high pyruvate is directed towards synthesis of fatty acid, but when the energy charge is low pyruvate is completely oxidized to CO_2 and H_2O in the TCA cycle, with generation of 15 equivalents of ATP per pyruvate.

PDH Complex

Oxidative decarboxylation of pyruvate to acetyl-CoA involving coenzyme-A takes place in mitochondrial matrix. The transport of pyruvate from cytosol into the matrix is facilitated by two transporters, one located in the outer mitochondrial membrane called *porin* and the other located in the inner mitochondrial membrane called *pyruvate translocase* (symporter that also moves H^+ into matrix).

All the enzymes of the TCA cycle and of oxidative phosphorylation are located in the mitochondrion. When pyruvate is transported into the mitochondrion, it encounters two principal enzymes: **pyruvate carboxylase** a gluconeogenic enzyme and **pyruvate dehydrogenase (PDH)** the first enzyme of the *PDH complex* (Fig. 32.1). When the cell-energy charge is high all the coenzymeA (CoA) is acylated as acetyl-CoA, which allosterically activates *pyruvate carboxylase* that diverts pyruvate toward gluconeogenesis. When the energy charge is low more of CoA is in free form, pyruvate carboxylase is inactive, and

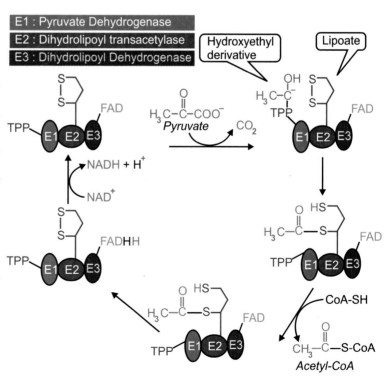

Fig. 32.1: Decarboxylation of pyruvate by PDH complex

pyruvate is diverted towards PDH complex and the enzymes of the TCA cycle for complete oxidation. The NADH and $FADH_2$ generated during the oxidation of pyruvate are used to drive ATP synthesis via oxidative phosphorylation.

The PDH complex has multiple copies of three separate enzymes: **pyruvate dehydrogenase** (20-30 copies), **dihydrolipoyl transacetylase** (60 copies) and **dihydrolipoyl dehydrogenase** (6 copies). The complex also requires 5 different coenzymes: **CoA, NAD$^+$, FAD$^+$, lipoic acid,** and *thiamine pyrophosphate* (TPP). Three of the coenzymes TPP, lipoic acid and FAD$^+$ are tightly bound to enzymes of the complex, and the other two coenzymes CoA and NAD$^+$ are employed as carriers of the products of PDH complex activity (Fig. 32.1).

The first enzyme of the complex is PDH, which oxidatively decarboxylates pyruvate. During the course of the reaction the hydroxyethyl group derived from decarboxylation of pyruvate is bound to TPP. The hydroxyethyl group is oxidized to acetyl group during its transfer to lipoic acid, which is covalently bound to **lipoyl transacetylase**. The transfer of the acetyl group from acyl-lipoamide to CoA results in the formation of two sulfhydryl (SH) groups in lipoate. These sulfhydryl groups should be reoxidized to the disulfide (S-S) form to regenerate lipoate as an acyl acceptor, which is catalyzed by FAD$^+$ dependent **dihydrolipoyl dehydrogenase.** The final activity of the PDH complex is the transfer of reducing equivalents from the $FADH_2$ of dihydrolipoyl dehydrogenase to NAD$^+$. The NADH formed is oxidized via mitochondrial electron transport chain that produces three equivalents of ATP.

The net result of the reactions of PDH complex is:

Pyruvate + CoA + NAD$^+$ $\rightarrow$ CO_2 + acetyl-CoA + NADH + H$^+$

Regulation of the PDH Complex

The reactions of the PDH complex, integrate the pathways of *glycolysis, gluconeogenesis,* and *fatty acid synthesis* with *TCA cycle.* As a consequence, the activity of the PDH complex is highly regulated by a variety of allosteric effectors and by covalent modification.

The diseases associated with deficiencies of the PDH complex have been observed. Affected individuals often do not survive to maturity, since the energy metabolism of highly aerobic tissues such as the brain is dependent on normal conversion of pyruvate to acetyl-CoA and are most sensitive to deficiencies in components of the PDH complex. Genetic diseases associated with PDH complex deficiency are due to mutations in PDH, which are characterized by moderate to severe cerebral lactic acidosis and encephalopathies.

PDH activity is regulated by its' state of phosphorylation, the most active being the dephosphorylated state (Fig. 32.2). Phosphorylation of PDH is catalyzed by a specific *PDH kinase*, whose activity is enhanced by an increase in the cellular level of ATP, NADH and acetyl-CoA. Conversely, an increase in pyruvate strongly inhibits *PDH kinase*. Additional negative effectors of PDH kinase are ADP, NAD$^+$ and CoA.SH, which are elevated when cell energy levels is low. The

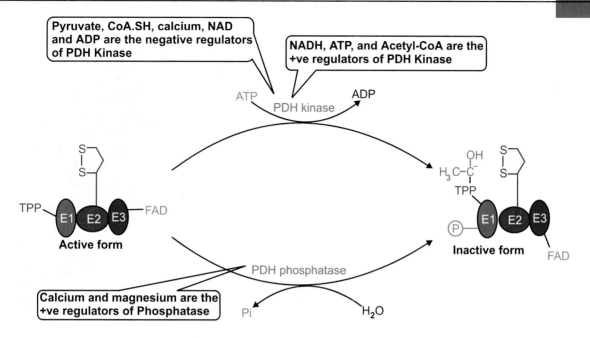

Fig. 32.2: Regulation of PDH activity

regulation of *PDH phosphatase* is not well understood, but Mg^{2+} and Ca^{2+} are known to activate the enzyme. Insulin increases PDH activity in adipose tissue, whereas catecholamines enhance PDH activity in cardiac muscle.

REACTIONS OF TCA CYCLE

Citrate Synthase or Condensing Enzyme

The first reaction of TCA cycle is condensation of the methyl carbon of acetyl-CoA with the keto carbon (C-2) of oxaloacetate (OAA) to form citrate (Fig. 32.4). The standard free energy of the reaction is -8.0 kcal/mol, which drives it strongly in the forward direction. Since the formation of OAA from its precursor is thermodynamically unfavorable, the highly exergonic nature of the *citrate synthase* reaction is of central importance in keeping the entire cycle going in the forward direction, since it *drives* oxaloacetate formation by mass action principles.

When the cellular energy charge increases the rate of flux through the TCA cycle will decline leading to a build-up of citrate. The excess citrate is then used to transport acetyl-CoA carbons out of the mitochondrion into the cytoplasm where they can be used for the biosynthesis of fatty acid or cholesterol. The increased levels of citrate in the cytoplasm activate *acetyl-CoA carboxylase* (ACC) the key regulatory enzyme of fatty acid biosynthesis and inhibit PFK-1. In non-hepatic tissues, citrate can also be used for ketone body synthesis.

Aconitase

The citrate is isomerized to isocitrate by *aconitase*, which is stereospecific. The migration of the -OH group from the central carbon of citrate (formerly the keto carbon of OAA) is always to the

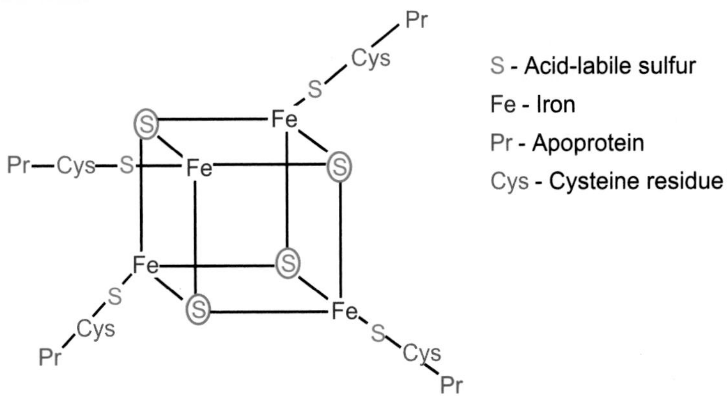

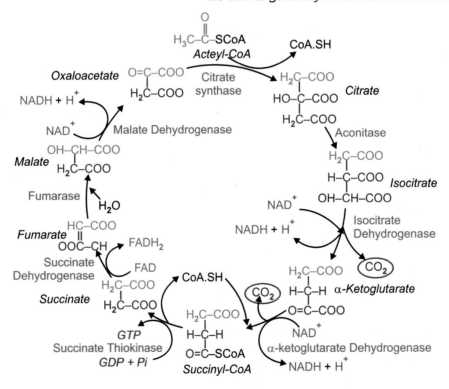

S - Acid-labile sulfur
Fe - Iron
Pr - Apoprotein
Cys - Cysteine residue

Fig. 32.3: Iron-sulfur-protein complex (Fe₄ S₄)

adjacent carbon, which is derived from the methylene (-CH$_2$-) of OAA. The stereospecific nature of the isomerization determines that the CO$_2$ lost during oxidation of isocitrate to succinyl-CoA is the original C-1 of the oxaloacetate used in the citrate synthase reaction. Aconitase is one of several non-heme-iron proteins found in mitochondria. These proteins contain inorganic iron and sulfur known as iron sulfur centers, in a coordination complex with cysteine sulfurs of the protein (Fig. 32.3). There are two prominent classes of non-heme-iron complexes, those containing two equivalents each of inorganic iron and sulfur Fe$_2$S$_2$, and those containing four equivalents of each Fe$_4$S$_4$. Aconitase is a member of the Fe$_4$S$_4$ class. Its iron sulfur centers are often designated as Fe$_4$S$_4$Cys$_4$, indicating that 4 cystine sulfur atoms are involved in the complete structure of the complex. In iron sulfur compounds, the iron is generally involved in oxidation-reduction events.

Fig. 32.4: Reactions of citric acid cycle

Isocitrate Dehydrogenase

Isocitrate is oxidatively decarboxylated to α-ketoglutarate by *isocitrate dehydrogenase* (IDH), which has absolute requirement for NAD$^+$ as a cofactor. The IDH catalyzed reaction is the rate-limiting step, as well as the first NADH-yielding reaction of the TCA cycle.

It is generally considered that control of carbon flow through the cycle is regulated at IDH by its powerful negative allosteric effectors

NADH and ATP, and by the positive effectors; isocitrate, ADP and AMP. It clearly shows that cell energy charge is the key-factor that regulates carbon flow through the TCA cycle.

α-Ketoglutarate Dehydrogenase Complex

α-ketoglutarate is oxidatively decarboxylated to succinyl-CoA catalyzed by *α-ketoglutarate dehydrogenase* (α-KGDH) complex that generates the second TCA cycle equivalent of CO_2 and NADH. This multienzyme complex is very similar to the PDH complex with regard to its protein makeup, cofactors, and its mechanism of action. The reactions of the α-KGDH complex proceed with a large negative standard free energy change. The α-KGDH complex is not subject to covalent modification, but allosteric regulation is quite complex, with activity being regulated by energy charge, the NAD^+/NADH ratio, and effector activity of substrates and products.

Outside the TCA cycle also succinyl-CoA and α-ketoglutarate are important metabolites. α-ketoglutarate represents a key anapleurotic metabolite linking the entry and exit of carbon atoms from the TCA cycle to pathways involved in amino acid metabolism and is also important for driving the malate-aspartate shuttle. Succinyl-CoA along with glycine, contributes all the carbon and nitrogen atoms required for the biosynthesis of protoporphyrin and for ketone body utilization by non-hepatic tissues.

Succinyl-CoA Synthetase or Succinyl Thiokinase

During the *succinyl CoA synthetase* catalyzed conversion of succinyl-CoA to succinate, the high-energy thioester of succinyl-CoA drives the synthesis of a high-energy nucleotide phosphate, by substrate-level phosphorylation. In this process, a high-energy succinyl-phosphate intermediate is formed, with the phosphate subsequently being transferred to GDP. In mitochondrial, the enzyme *nucleoside diphosphokinase* catalyzes a trans-phosphorylation reaction in which the GTP phosphorylates an ADP, producing ATP and regenerating GDP for the continued operation of succinyl-CoA synthetase.

Succinate Dehydrogenase

Succinate dehydrogenase catalyzes oxidation of succinate to fumarate by sequential reduction of enzyme-bound FAD and non-heme-iron. The final electron acceptor is coenzyme Q_{10} (CoQ_{10}), a mobile carrier of reducing equivalents that is restricted to the lipid phase of the mitochondrial membrane.

Fumarase (Fumarate Hydratase)

The fumarase-catalyzed reaction is specific for the *trans* form of fumarate. The result is that the hydration of fumarate precedes stereospecifically with the production of L-malate.

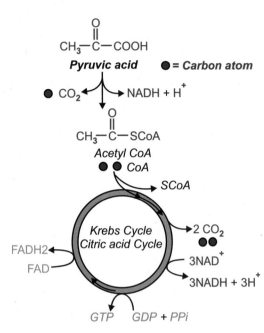

Fig. 32.5: Summary of Krebs cycle

Malate Dehydrogenase (MDH)

The final enzyme of the TCA cycle is MDH that is specific to L-malate. The oxidation of malate yields oxaloacetate (OAA) that has a standard free energy of about +7 kcal/mol, indicating the very unfavorable nature of the forward direction. It should be noted that the citrate synthase reaction has a standard free energy of about -8 kcal/mol and is responsible for pulling the MDH reaction in the forward direction. The overall change in standard free energy change is about -1 kcal/mol for the conversion of malate to oxaloacetate and on to succinate.

Summary of TCA cycle

During each TCA cycle two molecules of CO_2 is released. The GTP generated during the *succinate thiokinase* (succinyl-CoA synthetase) reaction is equivalent to a mole of ATP by virtue of the presence of *nucleoside diphosphokinase*. The 3 moles of NADH and 1 mole of $FADH_2$ generated during each round of the cycle are fed into the oxidative phosphorylation pathway. Each mole of NADH leads to 3 moles of ATP and each mole of $FADH_2$ leads to 2 moles of ATP production. Therefore, for each mole of acetyl-CoA that enters the TCA cycle, 12 moles of ATP can be generated (Fig. 32.5).

The Overall Stoichiometry of the TCA Cycle

$$Acetyl\text{-}CoA + 3NAD^+ + FAD + GDP + P_i + 2H_2O \rightarrow 2CO_2 + 3NADH + FADH_2 + GTP + 2H^+ + CoA.SH$$

Regulation of TCA cycle

The TCA cycle is regulated, both at the level of entry of substrates into the cycle and at the key reactions of the cycle. Fuel for TCA cycle is primarily acetyl-CoA. The generation of acetyl-CoA from carbohydrates is therefore a major control point of the cycle.

The PDH complex is inhibited by acetyl-CoA and NADH and activated by non-acetylated CoA (CoASH) and NAD^+. The *pyruvate dehydrogenase* activities of the PDH complex are regulated by their state of phosphorylation. This modification is carried out by a specific kinase (*PDH kinase*) and the phosphates are removed by a specific phosphatase (*PDH phosphatase*). The phosphorylation of PDH inhibits its activity and, therefore, leads to decreased oxidation of pyruvate. PDH kinase is activated by NADH and acetyl-CoA and inhibited by pyruvate, ADP, CoASH, Ca^{2+} and Mg^{2+}. The *PDH phosphatase*, in contrast, is activated by magnesium and calcium.

Since NAD^+ is required as cofactor for PDH and three reactions of the TCA cycle, it is not difficult to understand why the cellular ratio of $NAD^+/NADH$ has a major impact on the flux of carbon through the TCA cycle.

Substrate availability can also regulate TCA flux. This occurs at the *citrate synthase* reaction as a result of reduced availability of oxaloacetate. Product inhibition also controls the TCA flux, e.g. citrate inhibits *citrate synthase*, and NADH and succinyl-CoA inhibit α-KGDH. Calcium, ATP and ADP also regulate the key enzymes of the TCA cycle allosterically.

Generation of high-energy phosphate bonds when one molecule of pyruvate is completely oxidized to water and carbon dioxide

Reaction catalyzed by	Method of ~P production	No of ~P formed
Pyruvate dehydrogenase	Respiratory chain oxidation of NADH	3
Isocitrate dehydrogenase	Respiratory chain oxidation of NADH	3
α-ketoglutarate dehydrogenase	Respiratory chain oxidation of NADH	3
Succinate thiokinase	Oxidation at substrate level	3
Succinate dehydrogenase	Respiratory chain oxidation of FADH$_2$	3
Malate dehydrogenase	Respiratory chain oxidation of NADH	3
	NET	**15**

Insulin Function and Diabetes

33

The most important function of insulin is to maintain blood glucose levels within a physiological range of 70-140 mg/dl. The other equally important functions of insulin are to maintain and regulate the overall body metabolism. Since there are numerous hyperglycemic hormones in our body at play at any given time, untreated disorders associated with insulin deficiency or dysfunction generally lead to severe hyperglycemia and shortened lifespan.

Insulin is synthesized as a preproinsulin by the β-cells of the islets of Langerhans. Within the cisternae of the endoplasmic reticulum of these cells, the signal peptide of preproinsulin is removed, and the proinsulin is folded to its native structure and locked in this conformation by the formation of two disulfide bonds. In the Golgi apparatus, the center third of proinsulin is cleaved as *C peptide* by a specific protease that generates insulin. The *A* and *B peptides* of insulin held together by two disulfide bonds are packaged into secretory vesicles in the Golgi.

The principal regulator of insulin secretion from the β-cells is the plasma level of glucose, but the precise mechanism by which the glucose signal is transduced is still unclear. One possible explanation is that the increased uptake and metabolism of glucose leads to an elevation in the ATP/ADP ratio in pancreatic β-cells of Langerhans. Elevated level of ATP inhibit ATP-sensitive K^+ channel and depolarize the pancreatic β-cell, leading to Ca^{2+} influx and insulin secretion.

Chronic increases in numerous other hormones such as *growth hormone, placental lactogen, estrogens,* and *progestins*, up-regulate insulin secretion, by increasing the mRNA that codes for preproinsulin and enzymes involved in the preprohormone processing.

In contrast, epinephrine and glucagon diminish insulin secretion by a cAMP-coupled regulatory path as well counters the effect of insulin in liver and peripheral tissue, where it binds to β-adrenergic receptors that induces adenylate cycles activity, increases cAMP, and activates *protein kinase.* The latter events induce glycogenolysis and gluconeogenesis, both of which have hyperglycemic effect and counter insulin's effect on blood glucose levels. In addition, epinephrine influences glucose homeostasis through interaction with α-adrenergic receptors mediated through inosine trisphosphate.

Insulin secreted by the pancreas is directly infused via the portal vein to the liver, where it exerts profound metabolic effects. These insulin effects are receptor mediated, which belongs to the intrinsic tyrosine kinase activity. In liver, the activation of insulin receptor bring about specific phosphorylation events, which lead to an increased glucose storage with a simultaneous decrease in hepatic release of glucose into the circulation.

In most of the tissues, glucose uptake is the result of an increase in the number of plasma membrane glucose transporters in response to insulin, but in liver glucose uptake is increased as a result of increased activity of key glycolytic enzymes (**glucokinase, phosphofructo-kinase-1**, and **pyruvate kinase**) induced by insulin-dependent activation of **phosphodiesterase** (decreased PKA activity, diminished phosphorylation of **pyruvate kinase** and **phosphofructokinase-2**). Dephosphorylation of **pyruvate kinase** and **PFK-2** renders them active. The **PFK-2** converts fructose-6-phosphate into fructose-2,6-biphosphate (F-2,6-BP), which is a potent allosteric activator of the rate limiting enzyme of glycolysis, **PFK-1**, and an inhibitor of the gluconeogenic enzyme, **fructose-1,6-biphosphatase**. In addition, insulin increases the activity of phophatases specific for the phosphorylated forms of the glycolytic enzymes. All these events lead to activation of glycolytic enzymes and a significant increase in glycolysis. In addition, decreased activity of **glucose-6-phosphatase** elevates the phosphorylated derivatives of glucose in hepatocytes, with a consequent fall in blood glucose level.

Insulin generates its intracellular effects in cells by binding to a plasma membrane receptor, which is a disulfide-bonded glycoprotein. One function of insulin (besides its role in signal transduction) is to increase glucose transport into the extrahepatic cells by increasing the number of glucose transport molecules in the plasma membrane. Glucose transporters are in a continuous state of turnover. The plasma membrane content of glucose transporters is increased by enhancing the rate of recruitment of new transporters into the plasma membrane. The transporters are held in a special pool of preformed transporters localized in the cytoplasm.

In addition to its role in regulating glucose metabolism, insulin stimulates lipogenesis, diminishes lipolysis, increases amino acid transport into cells and modulates transcription by altering the cell content of numerous mRNAs. It stimulates the growth, DNA synthesis, and cell replication

DIABETES MELLITUS

Diabetes only means excessive urine excretion. The most common form of diabetes is *diabetes mellitus*, a metabolic disorder in which the ability to oxidize carbohydrate is decreased due to disturbances in insulin function. Diabetes mellitus is characterized by lipemia, elevated glucose in the plasma and episodic ketoacidosis. Additional symptoms of diabetes mellitus include excessive thirst, glucosuria, polyuria and hunger. If left untreated the disease can lead to fatal ketoacidosis. Other forms of diabetes include *diabetes insipidus* and *brittle diabetes*. Diabetes insipidus is the result of a deficiency of *antidiuretic hormone*. The major symptom of diabetes insipidus is excessive urine output as a result of inability of the kidneys to reabsorb water. Brittle diabetes is a form that is very difficult to control. It is characterized by unexplained oscillations between hypoglycemia and acidosis.

Glucose Tolerance Test

Following ingestion of food there is a transient elevation in blood glucose levels, which is in the range of 160 to 180 mg/dl, within 2 to 3 hours time blood glucose levels drop to fasting levels and at times slightly below the fasting values. The effect of ingested carbohydrates can be studied under fairly standard conditions and *the body's ability to assimilate the ingested carbohydrate load* can be studied by glucose tolerance test (GTT)

Method of Carrying Out GTT

The test is carried out best after overnight fasting, but if necessary 4 to 5 hours after the last meal. Any drugs, which affect blood glucose levels, must be withheld at least for three days before the test is performed and the patient should not carry out any physical work or consume any food during the period of test.

Time	Fasting	½ hr	1hr	1½ hr	2hr	2½ hr
Blood glucose mg/dl	75	130	140	100	65	75
Urine glucose	Nil	Nil	Nil	Nil	Nil	Nil

a. The first blood sample is drawn for estimation of fasting blood glucose concentration and a specimen of urine collected simultaneously to check for presence (qualitative test) of glucose in urine.
b. Administer orally 50 gm of glucose dissolved in about 300 ml of water.
c. Thereafter blood is collected at half hourly intervals over next 2½ hours for blood glucose estimations.
d. Two more urine samples are collected at 1 and 2 hour after glucose administration.
e. The glucose concentrations are estimated in all the blood samples collected. Blood glucose concentration in mg/dL is plotted against time on graph paper (Fig. 33.1).

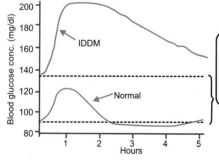

Glucose tolerance curve depicting one for a normal person, and one with Insulin-dependent diabetes mellitus (IDDM, type-1 diabetes). The dotted line indicates the range of glucose concentration expected in a normal individual

Fig. 33.1: Glucose tolerance curve

Criteria to Diagnose Diabetes Mellitus

1. Fasting blood glucose level in excess of 140 mg/dL
2. Or blood glucose levels in excess of 200 mg/dL at two time points during a glucose tolerance test (GTT), one of which must be within 2 hours after ingestion of glucose.

TYPES OF DIABETES MELLITUS

Diabetes mellitus is a heterogeneous clinical disorder of glucose metabolism with varied causes. Two main classifications of diabetes mellitus exist, one is *idiopathic* and the other is *secondary*.

Idiopathic diabetes mellitus is of two main types: insulin dependent (IDD) and non-insulin-dependent (NIDD).

Insulin-dependent diabetes mellitus (IDDM) or Type 1 diabetes, it is defined by the development of ketoacidosis in the absence of insulin therapy. Type-1 diabetes most often manifests in childhood (hence also called juvenile onset diabetes) and is the result of an autoimmune destruction of the β-cells of the pancreas.

Non-insulin-dependent diabetes mellitus (NIDDM) or Type 2 diabetes is characterized by milder hyperglycemia and rarely leads to ketoacidosis, generally manifests after the age of 40 years and is thought to result from genetic defects that cause both insulin resistance and insulin deficiency.

There are three main forms of type-2 diabetes:
1. Late onset associated with obesity.
2. Late onset not associated with obesity.
3. Maturity onset type diabetes of the young (MODY). This form of diabetes mellitus appears to be the result of mutations in the glucokinase gene.

Secondary diabetes mellitus is the esult of:

1. Pancreatic disease: Cystic fibrosis and pancreatitis, which lead to destruction of the pancreas and pancreatectomy.
2. Endocrine disease: Tumors producing counter-regulatory hormones such as glucagon, epinephrine, growth hormone and cortisol.
   a. Glucagonomas are pancreatic cancers that secrete glucagon.
   b. Pheochromocytomas, which secrete epinephrine.
   c. Cushing syndrome results in excess cortisol secretion.
   d. Acromegaly results in excess growth hormone production.
3. Drug-induced diabetes; treatment with glucocorticoids and diuretics can interfere with insulin function.
4. Autoantibodies for insulin receptors (Type B insulin resistance).
5. Mutations in the insulin gene.
6. Mutations in insulin receptor gene, which lead to the syndromes listed below. Two clinical features are common in all syndromes that result from mutations in the insulin receptor gene: acanthosis nigricans and hyperandrogenism (the latter being observed only in females).

a. Leprachaunism
b. Rabson-Mendenhall syndrome
c. Type-A insulin resistance
7. Gestational diabetes; this syndrome sets in during pregnancy and usually resolves itself following childbirth.
8. Many other genetic syndromes have either diabetes or impaired glucose tolerance associated with them; e.g.; lipoatrophic diabetes, Wolfram syndrome, Down syndrome, Klinefelter syndrome (XXY males), Turner syndrome, myotonic dystrophy, muscular dystrophy, Huntington disease, and Friedrich ataxia.

INSULIN-DEPENDENT DIABETES MELLITUS (IDDM)

Etiology of IDDM

Type-1 diabetes is the result of an autoimmune reaction to proteins of the islet cells of the pancreas. There is a strong association between IDDM and other endocrine autoimmunities (e.g. Addison disease). There is an increased incidence of autoimmune disease in family members of IDDM patients.

Types of Autoantibodies

1. *Islet cell cytoplasmic antibodies:* The primary antibodies found in 90 percent of type 1 diabetics are against islet cell cytoplasmic proteins (ICCA). The presence of ICCA is a highly accurate predictor of future development of IDDM.
2. *Islet cell surface antibodies:* Autoantibodies directed against islet cell-surface antigens (ICSA) have also been described in as many as 80 percent of type 1 diabetics. Some patients with type 2 diabetes have been identified that are ICSA positive.
3. *Specific antigenic targets of islet cells:* Antibodies to glutamic acid decarboxylase (GAD) have been identified in over 80 percent of patients newly diagnosed with IDDM. Anti-GAD antibodies decline over time in type-1 diabetics. The presence of anti-GAD antibodies is a strong predictor of the future development of IDDM in high-risk populations. Anti-insulin antibodies (IAAs) have been identified in IDDM patients and in relatives at risk to develop IDDM. These IAAs are detectable even before the onset of insulin therapy in type 1 diabetics. IAA is detectable in around 40 percent of young children with IDDM.

Pathophysiology of IDDM

The autoimmune destruction of pancreatic β-cells leads to a deficiency of insulin secretion. It is this loss of insulin secretion that leads to the metabolic derangements associated with IDDM. In addition to the loss of insulin secretion, the function of pancreatic α-cells is also abnormal. There is excessive secretion of glucagon in IDDM patients. Normally, hyperglycemia leads to reduced glucagon secretion. However, in patients with IDDM, glucagon secretion is not suppressed by hyperglycemia. The resultant inappropriately elevated glucagon levels exacerbate the metabolic defects due to insulin deficiency. The most pronounced example of this metabolic disruption is that patients with IDDM rapidly develop diabetic ketoacidosis in the absence of insulin administration.

Although insulin deficiency is the primary defect in IDDM, there is also a defect in the ability of target tissues to respond to the administration of insulin. There are multiple biochemical mechanisms that account for impairment of tissues to respond to insulin. Deficiency in insulin leads to uncontrolled lipolysis and elevated levels of free fatty acids in the plasma, which suppress glucose metabolism in peripheral tissues such as skeletal muscle. This impairs glucose utilization. Insulin deficiency also decreases the expression of a number of genes necessary for target tissues to respond normally to insulin— such as *glucokinase in liver* and the GLUT 4 class of *glucose transporters in adipose tissue*.

The major metabolic derangements, which result from insulin deficiency in IDDM, are impaired glucose, lipid and protein metabolism.

Glucose metabolism Uncontrolled IDDM leads to increased hepatic glucose output. First, liver glycogen stores are mobilized then hepatic gluconeogenesis is used to produce glucose. Insulin deficiency also impairs non-hepatic tissue utilization of glucose. In particular in adipose tissue and skeletal muscle, insulin stimulates glucose uptake. This is accomplished by insulin-mediated movement of glucose transporter proteins to the plasma membrane of these tissues. Reduced glucose uptake by peripheral tissues in turn leads to a reduced rate of glucose metabolism. In addition, the level of hepatic **glucokinase** is regulated by insulin. Therefore, a reduced rate of glucose phosphorylation in hepatocytes leads to increased delivery to the blood. Other enzymes involved in anabolic metabolism of glucose are affected by insulin (primarily through covalent modifications). The combination of increased hepatic glucose production and reduced peripheral tissues metabolism leads to elevated plasma glucose levels. When the capacity of the kidneys to absorb glucose is surpassed, *glucosuria* ensues. Glucose is an osmotic diuretic and an increase in renal loss of glucose is accompanied by loss of water and electrolytes, termed *polyuria*. The result of the loss of water (and overall volume) leads to the activation of the thirst mechanism (*polydipsia*). The negative caloric balance, which results from the glucosuria and tissue catabolism leads to an increase in appetite and food intake (*polyphagia*).

Lipid metabolism One major role of insulin is to stimulate the storage of food energy in the form of glycogen in hepatocytes and skeletal muscle, following the consumption of a meal. In addition, insulin stimulates hepatocytes to synthesize and store triglycerides in adipose tissue. In uncontrolled IDDM there is a rapid mobilization of triglycerides leading to increased levels of plasma free fatty acids. The free fatty acids are taken up by numerous tissues (except the brain) and metablized to provide energy. In the absence of insulin, malonyl-CoA levels fall and transport of fatty acyl-CoA into the mitochondria increases. Mitochondrial oxidation of fatty acids generates acetyl-CoA that can be further oxidized in the TCA cycle. However, in hepatocytes the majority of the acetyl-CoA is not oxidized by the TCA cycle but is metabolized into the ketone bodies (acetoacetate and β-hydroxybutyrate). These ketone bodies are used for energy production by the brain, heart and skeletal muscle. In IDDM, the increased availability of free fatty acids and ketone bodies exacerbates the reduced utilization of glucose furthering the ensuing hyperglycemia. Production of ketone bodies in excess of the body's ability to utilize them leads to ketoacidosis. A spontaneous breakdown product of acetoacetate is acetone i.e. exhaled by the lungs, which gives a distinctive odor to the breath.

Normally, plasma triglycerides are acted upon by **lipoprotein lipase** (LPL) that requires insulin. LPL is a membrane bound enzyme on the surface of the endothelial cells lining the vessels, which allows fatty acids to be taken from circulating triglycerides for storage in adipocytes. The absence of insulin results in hypertriglyceridemia.

Protein metabolism Insulin regulates the synthesis of many genes, either positively or negatively, which affect overall metabolism. Insulin has an overall effect on protein metabolism, increasing the rate of protein synthesis and decreasing the rate of protein degradation. Thus, insulin deficiency will lead to increased catabolism of protein. The increased rate of proteolysis leads to elevated concentrations of amino acids in plasma, which serve as precursors for hepatic and renal gluconeogenesis that further contributes to the hyperglycemia seen in IDDM.

NON-INSULIN-DEPENDENT DIABETES MELLITUS (NIDDM)

Etiology of NIDDM

NIDDM or type-2 diabetes refers to the common form of idiopathic diabetes is characterized by a lack of the need for insulin to prevent ketoacidosis. It is not an autoimmune disorder; however, there is a strong genetic correlation to the susceptibility to NIDDM. The susceptible genes that predispose to NIDDM have not been identified in most patients. This is due in part to the heterogeneity of the genes responsible for the susceptibility to NIDDM. Obesity is a major predisposing risk factor to NIDDM.

Pathophysiology of NIDDM

Unlike patients with IDDM, individuals with NIDDM have detectable levels of circulating insulin. On the basis of oral glucose tolerance testing the essential elements of NIDDM can be divided into four distinct groups.
  i. Those with normal glucose tolerance
  ii. Chemical diabetes (called impaired glucose tolerance)
  iii. Diabetes with minimal fasting hyperglycemia (fasting plasma glucose <140 mg/dL)

iv. Diabetes mellitus in association with overt fasting hyperglycemia (fasting plasma glucose >140 mg/dL).

The individuals with impaired glucose tolerance have hyperglycemia in spite of having highest levels of plasma insulin, indicating they are resistant to the action of insulin.

In the progression from impaired glucose tolerance to diabetes mellitus, the level of insulin declines indicating that patients with NIDDM have decreased insulin secretion.

Additional studies have subsequently demonstrated that both insulin resistance and insulin deficiency are common in the average NIDDM patient. Many experts conclude that insulin resistance is the primary cause of NIDDM, however, others contend that insulin deficiency is the primary cause because a moderate degree of insulin resistance is not sufficient to cause NIDDM. But, most patients with the common form of NIDDM have both defects.

Recent evidence has demonstrated a role for a member of the nuclear hormone receptor super family of proteins in the etiology of type 2- diabetes. Relatively new classes of drugs used to increase the sensitivity of the body to insulin are the *thiazolidinedione* drugs. These compounds bind to and alter the function of the *peroxisome proliferator-activated receptor g (PPARg)*. PPARg is also a transcription factor and, when activated, binds to another transcription factor known as the *retinoid X receptor (RXR)*. When these two proteins are complexed a specific set of genes becomes activated. PPARg is a key regulator of adipocyte differentiation; it can induce the differentiation of fibroblasts or other undifferentiated cells into mature fat cells. PPARg is also involved in the synthesis of biologically active compounds from vascular endothelial cells and immune cells.

Regulation of Blood Glucose Levels

The blood glucose level is maintained above 90 mg/dL to meet the demands of the brain for oxidizable glucose.

Almost all the carbohydrates ingested in the diet are converted to glucose following transport to the liver. Catabolism of dietary or cellular proteins generates carbon atoms that can be utilized for glucose synthesis via gluconeogenesis. The incompletely oxidize glucose predominantly by skeletal muscle and erythrocytes, provide lactate that is converted to glucose via gluconeogenesis.

Maintenance of blood glucose homeostasis is of paramount importance to the survival of the human organism. The predominant tissue responding to signals that indicate reduced or elevated blood glucose levels is the liver. One of the most important functions of the liver is to produce glucose for the circulation. Both elevated and reduced levels of blood glucose trigger hormonal responses to initiate pathways designed to restore glucose homeostasis. Low blood glucose triggers release of *glucagon* from pancreatic α-cells. High blood glucose triggers release of insulin from pancreatic β-cells. Additional signals: *ACTH and growth hormone*, released from the pituitary act to increase blood glucose by inhibiting uptake by extrahepatic tissues.

Glucocorticoids also act to increase blood glucose levels by inhibiting glucose uptake. *Cortisol*, the major glucocorticoid released from the adrenal cortex, is secreted in response to the increase in circulating ACTH. The adrenal medullary hormone, *epinephrine,* stimulates production of glucose by activating glycogenolysis in response to stressful stimuli.

Glucagon binding to its' receptors on the surface of liver cells triggers an increase in cAMP production leading to an increased rate of glycogenolysis by activating **glycogen phosphorylase** via the PKA-mediated cascade. This is the same response hepatocytes have to epinephrine release. The resultant increased level of G6P in hepatocytes is hydrolyzed to free glucose, by **glucose-6-phosphatase**, which then diffuses to the blood. The glucose enters extrahepatic cells where it is re-phosphorylated by **hexokinase**. Since muscle and brain cells lack glucose-6-phosphatase, the glucose-6-phosphate product of **hexokinase** is retained and oxidized by these tissues.

In opposition to the hepatocyte response to glucagon and epinephrine, insulin stimulates extrahepatic cells to take-up more glucose from the blood for glycogen synthesis and inhibits glycogenolysis. As the glucose enters hepatocytes it binds to **glycogen phosphorylase** and inhibits its activity. The binding of free glucose stimulates the de-phosphorylation of **phosphorylase**, thereby inactivating it. Liver cells contain an isoform of hexokinase called **glucokinase**. Glucokinase has a much lower affinity for glucose than does hexokinase. Therefore, it is not fully active at the physiological ranges of blood glucose. Additionally, glucokinase is not inhibited by its product G6P, whereas, hexokinase is inhibited by G6P.

In non-hepatic tissues, insulin helps recruitment of glucose transporter complexes, to the cell surface. Glucose transporters comprise a family of five members, GLUT-1 is distributed in various tissues, GLUT-2 is found primarily in intestine, kidney and liver, GLUT-3 is found in the intestine and GLUT-5 in the brain and testis. Insulin-sensitive tissues such as skeletal muscle and adipose tissue contain GLUT-4. When the concentration of blood glucose increases in response to food intake, GLUT-2 molecules found in pancreatic cells mediate an increase in glucose uptake that leads to increased insulin secretion.

Unlike most other cells, hepatocytes are freely permeable to glucose and are, therefore, essentially unaffected by the action of insulin. When blood glucose levels are low the liver does not compete with other tissues for glucose since the extrahepatic uptake of glucose is stimulated in response to insulin. Conversely, when blood glucose levels are high, extrahepatic needs are satisfied and the liver takes up glucose for conversion into glycogen for future needs. Since blood glucose level is elevated, hepatic glucokinase is active and the G-6-P produced by glucokinase is rapidly converted to G-1-P by **phosphoglucomutase**, which can be incorporated into glycogen.

Glycogen Metabolism

34

DIGESTION OF CARBOHYDRATES

Dietary carbohydrates from which humans derive energy are in complex forms, such as starch (composed of amylose and amylopectin), glycogen, sucrose and lactose. Cellulose is also consumed but not digested. The first step in the metabolism of digestible carbohydrate is the conversion of higher polymers, to simpler, soluble forms that can be transported across the intestinal wall and delivered to the tissues for immediate use or storage. The hydrolytic breakdown of polymeric sugars begins in the mouth. Saliva has a slightly acidic pH of 6.8 and contains **lingual amylase** that begins the digestion of carbohydrates, but is virtually inactivated by the much stronger acid pH of the stomach. The mixture of saliva, gastric secretions and food; collectively known as **chyme,** moves into the small intestine.

In the small intestine, polymeric-carbohydrates are mainly digested by pancreatic α-amylase, whose activity is similar to salivary amylase. The polymeric-carbohydrates on hydrolysis yield a mixture of disaccharides and trisaccharides, which are further hydrolyzed by *intestinal saccharidases (sucrase, lactase,* and *trehalase)* and *maltases* to yield monosaccharides. The net result is the almost complete conversion of digestible carbohydrate to its constituent monosacc-harides.

The glucose and other simple carbohydrates are transported across the intestinal wall to the hepatic portal vein, and then to liver parenchymal cells and peripheral tissues. There they enter various metabolic pathways depending on the energy charge of the cell, either they are oxidized to yield energy or converted to fatty acids and glycogen for storage.

GLYCOGEN METABOLISM

Glycogen is the storage form of glucose found in liver, muscle, kidney and intestine. Almost 10 percent by weight of liver is glycogen. Muscle has a much lower amount of glycogen per unit mass of tissue, but since the total mass of muscle is so much greater than that of liver, total glycogen stored in muscle is about twice that of liver. The main source of glucose to maintain blood glucose levels comes from liver glycogen. However, muscle glycogen is not available to other tissues, since muscle lacks the enzyme **glucose-6-phosphatase**.

Almost 75 percent of daily glucose is consumed by brain via aerobic pathways. The remainder of it is utilized by erythrocytes, skeletal muscle, and heart muscle. The body obtains glucose either directly from the diet or from amino acids and lactate via gluconeogenesis. Glucose from both exogenous and endogenous source, either remains soluble in the body fluids or is stored in its polymeric form, *glycogen*.

GLYCOGENOLYSIS

Glycogenolysis is the process of cleaving α-1,4 glycosidic linkages in glycogen molecule by phosphorolysis (inorganic Pi is utilized) rather than hydrolysis. This reaction is catalyzed by the enzyme *glycogen phosphorylase*, which sequentially removes single glucose residues from non-reducing end of glycogen, as glucose-1-phosphate.

The Advantages of Phosphorolytic Cleavage of Glycogen

1. The glucose removed from glycogen is in an activated state (glucose-1-phosphate) and this occurs without the hydrolysis of ATP.

2. The concentration of Pi in the cell is high enough to drive the equilibrium of the reaction in the favorable direction. The glucose-1-phosphate released by the action of *glycogen phosphorylase* is isomerized to glucose-6-phosphate by *phosphoglucomutase*; at the active site of phosphoglucomutase a serine residue is in phosphorylated form. During isomerization reaction, the phospho group of phosphoserine is transferred to C-6 of *glucose-1-phosphate* that generates *glucose-1, 6-phosphate* as an intermediate. The phosphate on C-1 of *glucose-1, 6-phosphate* is then transferred to *phosphoglucomutase* to regenerate phosphorylated serine residue, and the final product released is glucose-6-phospahte.

3. The phosphorylase-mediated release of *glucose-1-phosphate* from glycogen is a charged residue, which does not freely diffuse out of the cell. In muscle cells, this is acutely apparent since the purpose of glycogenolysis in muscle cells is to generate glucose for glycolysis. Where as in the liver, kidney and intestine, glucose-6-phospate is dephosphorylated by the action of **glucose-6-phosphatase,** which generate free glucose for maintaining blood glucose level. Free glucose is not formed during glycogenolysis in skeletal muscle, since they lack **glucose-6-phosphatase**.

Glycogen is a highly branched polymer of glucose linked by α-1,4 glycosidic linkages with α-1, 6 branche points (Fig. 34.1). Branches provide multiple free ends for quicker breakdown or for more places to add additional glucose units.

The enzyme *glycogen phosphorylase* sequentially removes glucose residues from non-reducing ends of glycogen, but stops at four glucose

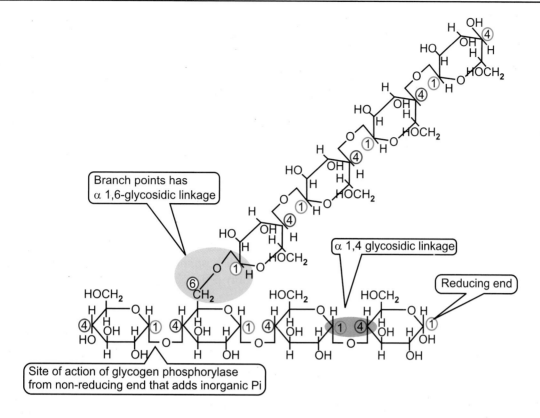

Fig. 34.1: α1,6 glycosidic linkage and α1, 4 glycosidic linkage in glycogen

residues from α-1,6 linkage, which leaves a limit dextran (Fig.34.2). Limit dextran is acted upon by *glycogen-debranching enzyme* that contains two activities: *glucotransferase* and *amylo α-1,6-glucosidase*. The transferase activity removes the terminal three glucose residues of one branch and attaches them to a free C-4 end of a second branch, whereas the amylo α-1,6-glucosidase activity removes the glucose in α-1,6 linkage at the branch. It should be noted that the glucose residue removed by the action of amylo α-1,6-glucosidase is uncharged, since it is not phosphorolytic cleavage reaction. This means, glycogenolysis occurring in skeletal muscle do generate free glucose that could enter the bloodstream. But, **hexokinase** found in muscle has low K_m for glucose, and any free glucose formed is immediately phosphorylated and enters glycolytic pathway.

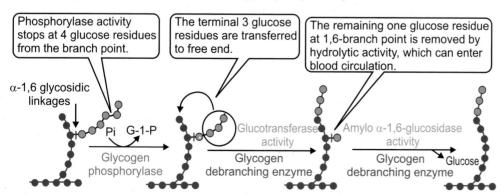

Fig. 34.2: Reactions of glycogenolysis

Regulation of Glycogenolysis

Glycogen phosphorylase is a homodimeric enzyme and its activity is controlled by both allosteric regulation and covalent modification.

Allosteric Regulation

The binding of ATP or glucose to allosteric site of glycogen phosphorylase makes it assume a conformational state T (tense, less active), on the other hand binding of AMP to allosteric site reverts it to R (relaxed, more active) form.

Covalent Modification

Covalent modification by phosphorylation of glycogen phosphorylase is hormonally regulated by epinephrine and glucogon. The phosphorylated form (*Phospharylase-a*) is the active form and the dephosphorylated form (*Phosphorylase-b*) is the inactive form.

Glucagon, released from pancreatic α-cells in response to lowered blood glucose, binds to *glucagon receptors* on the liver cells. Such binding activates the enzyme adenylate cyclase, which is associated with receptors. The activated adenylate cyclase forms large amounts of cAMP, which in turn binds to cAMP-dependent protein kinase (PKA). Now the catalytic subunit of PKA is released that phosphorylates phosphorylase kinase. The phosphorylated form of phosphorylase kinase in turn phosphorylates glycogen phosphorylase-b to switch over to phosphorylase-a form. Enhanced glycogen breakdown by phosphorylase-a restores blood glucose to desired levels.

Epinephrine, released from adrenal glands in response to neural signals, indicating an immediate need for enhanced glucose utilization in muscle, binds to *β-adrenergic receptors* on the surface of *muscle cells* and bring about a cascade of events that culminates in phosphorylation of *glycogen phosphorylase*, which is the active form (Fig. 34.3). The G-1-P released by the action of active form of glycogen phosphorylase immediately enters glycolytic pathway.

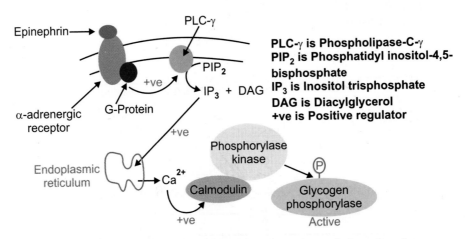

Fig. 34.3: Alpha-receptor mediated response of phosphorylase

Role of Calcium in Regulation of Glycogen Metabolism

Phosphorylase kinase activity is regulated by calcium binding to its *calmodulin subunit*, which induces conformation changes in calmodulin that in turn enhances catalytic activity of phosphorylase kinase.

GLYCOGEN SYNTHESIS

Glycogen synthesis is not the reversal of glycogenolysis since each pathway uses different enzymes. About two-thirds of the dietary glucose we consume is converted to glycogen and stored in our body.

The first step in glycolysis is activation of glucose to glucose 6-phosphate, catalyzed by **hexokinase.**

Synthesis of glycogen also requires activation of glucose to UDP-glucose, catalyzed by *UDPG pyrophosphorylase*. The enzyme UDPG- pyrophosphorylase carries out the activation of glucose to be used for glycogen synthesis. This enzyme exchanges the phosphate on C-1 of glucose-1-phosphate for UDP (Fig. 34.4). The enzyme **glycogen synthase** utilizes UDP-glucose as one substrate and the non-reducing end of glycogen as another. The energy of the phospho-glycosyl bond of UDP-glucose is utilized by glycogen synthase to catalyze the incorporation of glucose into glycogen. UDP is subsequently released from the enzyme. The α-1, 6 branches in glucose are produced by **branching enzymes** also termed the **amylo- (1,4-1,6)-transglycosylase**. This enzyme transfers a terminal fragment of 6 to 7 glucose residues from polymer at least 11 glucose residues long, to an internal glucose residue at the C-6 hydroxyl position (Fig. 34.5).

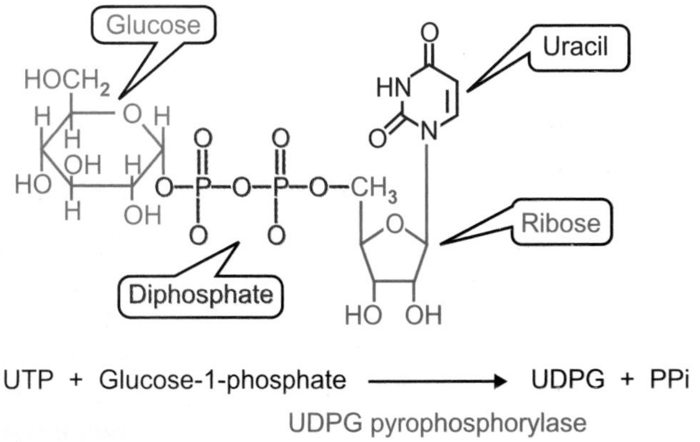

UTP + Glucose-1-phosphate ⟶ UDPG + PPi

UDPG pyrophosphorylase

Fig. 34.4: Uridine diphosphate glucose (UDPG)

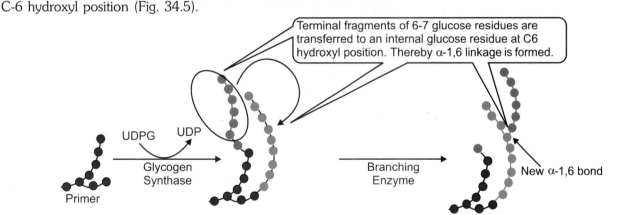

Fig. 34.5: Glycogen synthesis

Until recently, the source of the first glycogen molecule that might act as a primer in glycogen synthesis was unknown. Recently, a protein-enzyme known as **glycogenin** has been discovered at the core of glycogen molecules. Glycogenin has the unusual property of catalyzing its own glycosylation, by attaching C-1 of an UDP-glucose to its tyrosine residue. The attached glucose is believed to serve as the primer required by glycogen synthase.

Glycogenolysis and glycogen synthesis are under the control of three hormones

1. **Insulin:** It is a polypeptide composed of 51 amino acids, secreted by β-cells of pancreas when blood glucose level is high. Insulin increases the rate of glucose transport into muscle and fat cells via glucose transporters (GLUT4) and stimulates glycogen synthesis in liver; thereby blood glucose level is normalized.

2. **Glucagon:** It is a polypeptide composed of 29 amino acids, secreted by α-cells of pancreas when blood glucose level is low. Glucagon restores blood sugar levels by stimulating glycogen degradation in the liver.

3. **Epinephrine:** It stimulates glycogen degradation in liver and releases glucose 1-phosphate and glucose. This results in increased amount of glucose in bloodstream and increased rate of glycolysis in muscle. This kind of response is called **fight-or-flight response**.

Regulation of Glycogen Synthase Activity

Glycogen synthase is a tetrameric enzyme consisting of *four identical subunits*. Phosphorylation of **glycogen synthase** reduces its activity towards UDP-glucose. **Glycogen synthase** in non-phosphorylated state does not require glucose-6-phosphate as an allosteric activator but when phosphorylated it does (Fig. 34.6). The two forms of **glycogen synthase** are identifed by the same nomenclature as used for **glycogen phosphorylase**. The most active and dephosphory-lated form is **synthase-a** and the phosphorylated form that is glucose-6-phosphate-dependent is **synthase-b form**.

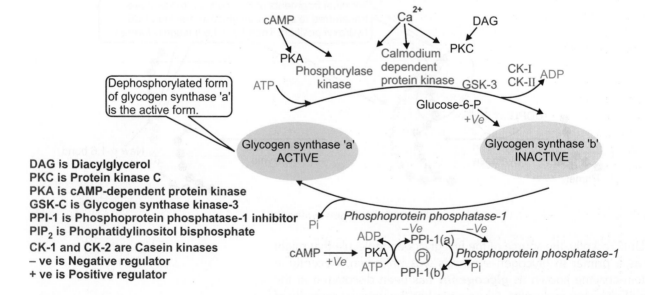

DAG is Diacylglycerol
PKC is Protein kinase C
PKA is cAMP-dependent protein kinase
GSK-C is Glycogen synthase kinase-3
PPI-1 is Phosphoprotein phosphatase-1 inhibitor
PIP₂ is Phophatidylinositol bisphosphate
CK-1 and CK-2 are Casein kinases
– ve is Negative regulator
+ ve is Positive regulator

Fig. 34.6: Regulation of glycogen synthase pathway

Phosphorylation of **synthase-a** occurs primarily in response to hormonal activation of PKA. One of the major kinases active on synthase is **synthase-phosphorylase kinase**, the same enzyme that phosphorylates **glycogen phosphorylase**. However, at least 5 additional enzymes have been identified that phosphorylate **glycogen synthase** directly. One of these enzymes phosphorylating **glycogen synthase** is PKA itself. **Glycogen synthase kinase 3** (**GSK-3**) is an important enzyme that phosphorylates glycogen synthase independent of increases in cAMP levels. Each phosphorylation event occurs at distinct serine residues, which can result in a progressively increased state of synthase phosphorylation.

Glycogen synthase activity can also be affected by epinephrine binding to α-adrenergic receptors through a pathway similar to described earlier that regulate **glycogen phosphorylase**.

When α-adrenergic receptors are stimulated by epinephrine binding, there is an increase in the activity of phospholipase C-γ (PLC-γ) with a resultant increase in PIP_2 (phosphatidylinositol-4,5 bisphosphate) hydrolysis (Fig. 34.7). The products of PIP_2 hydrolysis are DAG (diacylglycerol) and IP_3 (inositoltrisphosphate). DAG and the Ca^{2+} ions released by IP_3 activate PKC, which phosphorylates and inactivates **glycogen synthase**. Additional responses of calcium are the activation of **calmodulin-dependent protein kinase** (calmodulin is a component of many enzymes that are responsive to Ca^{2+}), which phosphorylates **glycogen synthase**.

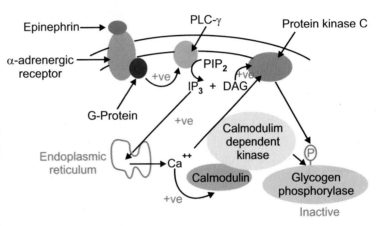

Fig. 34.7: Alpha-receptor mediated response of glycogen synthase

The effects of these phosphorylation reactions lead to:
1. Decreased affinity of synthase for UDP-glucose
2. Decreased affinity of synthase for glucose-6-phosphate and
3. Increased affinity of synthase for ATP and Pi.

Reconversion of **synthase-b** to **synthase-a** requires dephosphorylation. This is carried out predominately by *protein phosphatase-1* (PP-1) the same phosphatase involved in dephosphorylation of glycogen phosphorylase (Fig. 34.7).

The activity of PP-1 is also affected by insulin that exerts an opposing effect to that of glucagon and epinephrine. This should appear obvious since the role of insulin is to increase the uptake of glucose from the blood.

GLYCOGEN STORAGE DISEASES

An inability to degrade glycogen can affect cells in two ways:
a. The cells can become pathologically engorged leading to pressure effects such as cell death and necrosis.
b. Functional loss of glycogen as a source of cell energy and as a blood glucose buffer.

Table of Glycogen Storage Diseases

Type: Name	Enzyme affected	Primary organ	Manifestations
Type 0	Glycogen synthase	Liver	Hypoglycemia, early death, hyperketonemia
Type Ia: von Gierke's	Glucose-6-phosphatase	Liver	Hepatomegaly, renal failure, thrombocyte dysfunction
Type Ib	Microsomal glucose-6-phosphate translocase	Liver bacterial infections	Like Ia, also neutropenia,
Type II: Pompe's	Lysosomal enzymes: α-1,4-glucosidase, Acid α-glucosidase Acid maltase	Skeletal & cardiac muscle	Infantile form = death by 2 years; juvenile form = myopathy; Adult form = muscular dystrophy-like
Type III: Cori's or Forbe's	Debranching enzyme	Liver, skeletal & cardiac muscle	Infant hepatomegaly, myopathy
Type IV: Anderson's	Branching enzyme	Liver, muscle	Hepatosplenomegaly, cirrhosis
Type V: McArdle's	Muscle phosphorylase	Skeletal muscle	Excercise-induced cramps and pain, myoglobinuria
Type VI: Her's	Liver phosphorylase	Liver	Hepatomegaly
Type VII: Tarui's	Muscle PFK-1	Muscle, RBC's	Like V, also hemolytic anemia

Although glycogen storage diseases are quite rare, their effects can be most dramatic. The debilitating effect of many glycogen storage diseases depends on the severity of the mutation causing specific enzyme deficiencies and other events that can cause the same characteristic symptoms. For example, Type I glycogen storage disease (von Gierke's disease) is attributed to lack of **glucose-6-phosphatase**. However, this enzyme is localized on the cisternal surface of the endoplasmic reticulum (ER); in order to gain access to the phosphatase, glucose-6-phosphate must pass through a specific translocase in the ER membrane. Mutation of either the phosphatase or the translocase makes transfer of liver glycogen to the blood a very limited process. Thus, mutation of either gene leads to symptoms associated with von Gierke's disease, which occurs at a rate of about 1 in 200,000 people.

Glucose Metabolism

35

GLYCOLYSIS

Oxidation of glucose to either *pyruvate* or *lactate* is known as glycolysis. Under aerobic conditions, the product of glycolysis in most tissues is *pyruvate* and the pathway is known as *aerobic glycolysis*. When oxygen is depleted, as for instance during prolonged vigorous exercise, the product of glycolysis in muscle tissues is *lactate* and the process is known as *anaerobic glycolysis*.

The reactions of glycolytic pathway take place in the *cytosolic fraction* of cells and have two functions:

a. Oxidation of glucose to provide ATPs and NADH molecules
b. Provide building blocks for anabolic pathways.

The pathway can be visualized as having two separate phases. The first is the *chemical priming phase* that requires ATP as source of energy, and the second is *energy-yielding phase*.

In the chemical priming phase, two equivalents of ATP are required to convert glucose to fructose-1, 6-bisphosphate (F-1, 6-BP).

In the energy-yielding phase F-1, 6-BP is degraded to pyruvates, which yield four equivalents of ATP and two equivalents of NADH.

1. The Hexokinase Reaction

The first reaction of glycolysis is ATP-dependent phosphorylation of glucose to form glucose-6-phosphate (G6P) that is catalyzed by tissue-specific isoenzymes of **hexokinase** (Fig. 35.1). The phosphorylation accomplishes *two goals*:

i. The hexokinase reaction converts uncharged glucose to an anion that is trapped in the cell since cells lack transport systems for phosphorylated sugars.
ii. The biologically inert glucose molecule gets activated to a labile form capable of being further metabolized.

Four mammalian isozymes of hexokinase are known (Types I - IV). The type IV isozyme found in hepatocytes is often referred to as **glucokinase**, which has high K_m for glucose. It means glucokinase is saturated only at very high concentrations of glucose.

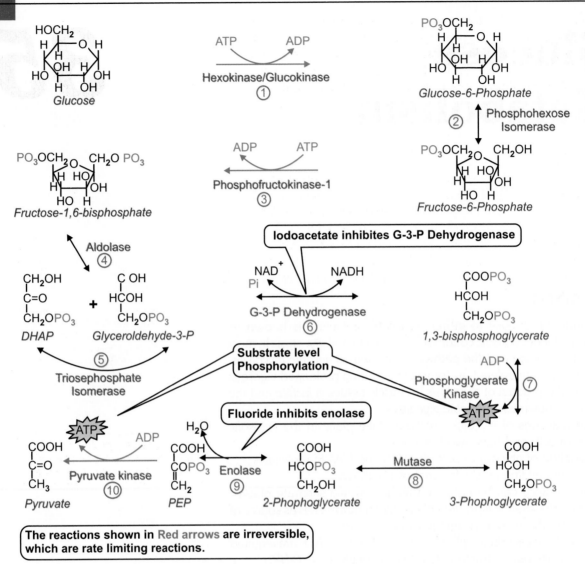

Fig. 35.1: Reactions of glycolytic pathway

This feature of hepatic glucokinase allows the liver to buffer blood glucose. Liver glucokinase is significantly active, only when blood glucose levels are high (after a meal), which causes the liver preferentially to trap and store circulating glucose. When blood glucose levels are very low (fasting), tissues such as liver and kidney (which contain glucokinases) that do not highly dependent on glucose for energy requirements, stops to use the meager glucose supplies that remain available. At the same time, tissues such as the brain, which are critically dependent on glucose, continue to scavenge blood glucose using their *hexokinase* that has low K_m. Under various conditions of glucose deficiency, such as long periods between meals and starvation the liver is stimulated to supply the blood with glucose through the pathway of *gluconeogenesis*. The levels of glucose produced during gluconeogenesis are insufficient to activate glucokinase, thus glucose is allowed to pass out of hepatocytes into the blood.

The regulation of hexokinase and glucokinase activities is different. Hexokinases I, II, and III are allosterically inhibited by product (G6P) accumulation, whereas glucokinases are not. The latter further ensures accumulation of glucose stores in the liver only during times of glucose excess, while favoring glucose utilization by peripheral tissues at other times.

Comparison of the Activities of Hexokinase and Glucokinase (Fig. 35.2)

The K_m for hexokinase is significantly lower (0.1mM) than that of glucokinase (10mM). This difference ensures that nonhepatic tissues (which contain hexokinase) rapidly and efficiently trap blood glucose within their cells by converting it to glucose-6-phosphate. One major function of the liver is to deliver glucose to the blood, this is ensured by having a glucose-phosphorylating enzyme (glucokinase), who's K_m for glucose is sufficiently higher than the normal concentration of blood glucose (5mM).

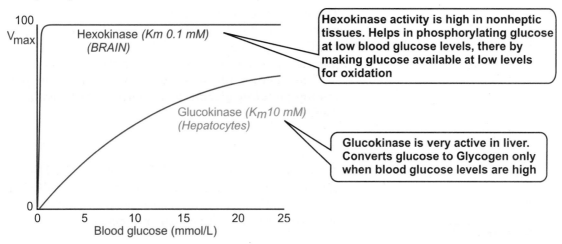

Fig. 35.2: Glucokinase and hexokinase are suited for their functions

2. Phosphohexose Isomerase

The second reaction of glycolytic pthway is isomerization, catalyzed by phosphohexose isomerase (also known as **phosphoglucose isomerase**), in which G6P is isomerized to fructose-6-phosphate (F6P). This reaction is freely reversible at the normal cellular concentrations of these two hexose phosphates.

3. Phosphofructokinase-1 (PFK-1) also called 6 Phosphofructo-1-Kinase

This reaction involves the utilization of a second ATP to convert F6P to fructose-1, 6-bisphosphate (F-1, 6-BP), which is catalyzed by *6-phosphofructo-1-kinase*, better known as phosphofructokinase-1 or PFK-1. This reaction is not readily reversible because of its large positive free energy ($\Delta G^{0'} = +5.4$ kcal/mol) in the reverse direction. Nevertheless, fructose units readily flow in the reverse (gluconeogenic) direction because of the presence of the hydrolytic enzyme, fructose-1, 6-bisphosphatase (F-1, 6-BPase).

The presence of these two enzymes in the same cell compartment provides an example of a metabolic futile cycle, which would rapidly deplete cell energy stores. However, the activity of these two enzymes is so highly regulated that *PFK-1 is considered to be the rate-limiting enzyme of glycolysis and F-1, 6-BPase is considered to be the rate-limiting enzyme in gluconeogenesis.*

4. Aldolase

Aldolase catalyzes the cleavage of F-1, 6-BP to yield two molecules of 3-carbon products: dihydroxyacetone phosphate (DHAP) and glyceraldehyde-3-phosphate (G3P). The aldolase reaction proceeds readily in the reverse direction, since DHAP and G3P are utilized for both glycolysis and gluconeogenesis.

5. Triose Phosphate Isomerase

The two products of the aldolase reaction equilibrate readily in a reaction catalyzed by *triose phosphate isomerase*. Succeeding reactions of glycolysis utilize G3P as a substrate, since mass action principles pull the aldolase reaction in the direction of glycolysis.

The second phase of glucose catabolism features the energy-yielding glycolytic reactions that produce ATP and NADH.

6. Glyceraldehyde -3-Phosphate Dehydrogenase (G3PDH)

In the first of these reactions, *G3PDH* catalyzes the NAD^+-dependent oxidation of G3P to 1, 3-bisphosphoglycerate (1,3-BPG) and NADH. The G3PDH reaction is reversible, since the same enzyme catalyzes the reverse reaction during gluconeogenesis.

7. Phosphoglycerate Kinase (brings about substrate level phosphorylation)

The high-energy phosphate of 1,3-BPG is utilized to form ATP and 3-phosphoglycerate (3PG) by the enzyme phosphoglycerate kinase. *This is the only reaction of glycolysis and gluconeogenesis that involves ATP and yet is reversible under normal cell conditions.*

In erythrocytes, an important reaction catalyzed by *bisphosphoglycerate mutase* leads to formation of 2,3-BPG from 1,3-BPG, which is an important regulator of hemoglobin's affinity for oxygen. Note that *2,3-bisphosphoglycerate phosphatase* degrades 2,3-BPG to 3-phosphoglycerate, without ATP generation. The 2,3-BPG shunt thus operates with the expenditure of 1 equivalent of ATP per triose passed through the shunt. The process is not reversible under physiological conditions. This pathway is called Rapaport-Leubering cycle.

8. Phosphoglycerate Mutase and Enolase

The remaining reactions of glycolysis are aimed at converting the relatively low energy molecule, 3-PG to a high-energy form and harvesting the phosphate as ATP. The 3-PG is first converted to 2-PG by phosphoglycerate mutase.

9. Enolase

Enolase converts 2-PG to phosphoenoylpyruvate (PEP).

10. Pyruvate Kinase (brings about substrate level phosphorylation)

The final reaction of aerobic glycolysis is catalyzed by the highly regulated enzyme pyruvate kinase (PK). In this strongly exergonic reaction, the high-energy phosphate of PEP is conserved as ATP. The loss of phosphate by PEP leads to the production of pyruvate in an unstable enol form, which spontaneously tautomerizes to the more stable keto form of pyruvate. This reaction contributes a large proportion of the free energy of hydrolysis of PEP.

ATP Production Per Molecule of Glucose

Pathway	Reaction catalyzed by	Method of ~P production	No of ~P formed
Glycolysis	Phosphoglycerate kinase	Substrate level phosphorylation	2
	Pyruvate kinase	Substrate level phosphorylation	2
	G-3-P dehydrogenase	Oxidation of 2 NADH by ETC	6*
		TOTAL	**10**
		ATP utilized during initial reactions by HK & PFK	2 (-)
		NET	**8**
TCA cycle		Oxidation of two moles of pyruvate	30
		Total ATP per mole of glucose under aerobic conditions	30 + 8 = 38
		Total ATP per mol of glucose under anaerobic conditions	4 - 2 = 2

*If NADH formed in glycolysis is transported into mitochondria via malate shuttle total ~P formed is 38. Instead if NADH is transported via Glycerophosphate shuttle total ~P formed is 36.

ANAEROBIC GLYCOLYSIS

Under aerobic conditions, in most cells with the exception of erythrocytes, pyruvate is further metabolized via the TCA cycle. Under anaerobic conditions in all cells and under all conditions in erythrocytes, pyruvate is reduced to lactate by the enzyme *lactate dehydrogenase (LDH),* and the lactate is transported out of the cell into the circulation. Conversion of pyruvate to lactate under anaerobic conditions provides the cell with a mechanism for the oxidation of NADH that is formed during the G3PDH reaction. This reaction is necessary since NAD^+ is a required substrate for G3PDH, without which glycolysis will cease to function. During aerobic glycolysis the electrons of cytoplasmic NADH are transferred to mitochondrial ETC, to generate a continuous pool of cytoplasmic NAD^+.

Aerobic glycolysis generates substantially more ATP per mole of glucose oxidized than during anaerobic glycolysis. The significance of anaerobic glycolysis to a muscle cell when it needs large amounts of energy stems from the fact that the rate of ATP production from glycolysis is approximately 100 times faster than that from oxidative phosphorylation. During exercise, muscle cell requires maximum amount of ATP in the shortest time frame. This is why muscle cells derive almost all its ATP requirement during exercise from anaerobic glycolysis.

Regulation of Glycolysis

First line of control is by regulating glucose transport into cells via transporters.
a. Intestinal and renal cells have **Na^+-dependent glucose co-transport system** called **SGLTI** *that* allows movement of glucose by passive transport via facilitated diffusion.
b. Hexose transporters called GLUT (glucose transporters) family:
   GLUT1 and 3 are present in all mammalian cells that continually transport glucose.
   GLUT2 - present in liver cells.
   GLUT4 - present in skeletal muscle cells and adipocytes; insulin increases the number of transporters in the cell membrane that promotes rapid uptake of glucose.
   GLUT 5 - involved in transport of glucose in small intestine.
   GLUT 7 - transports glucose 6-phosphate from cytosol into ER.

Second line of control is by regulation of enzyme activity.

The reactions catalyzed by *hexokinase, PFK-1* and *PK* proceeds with a relatively large free energy decrease. These irreversible reactions are the ideal candidates for regulation of the flux through glycolysis. All three enzymes are allosterically regulated.

Regulation of hexokinase is not the major control point of glycolysis in skeletal muscle. This is due to the fact that large amounts of G6P are derived from glycogenolysis even in the absence of hexokinase activity.

Regulation of pyruvate kinase (PK) is important for reversing glycolysis in order to activate gluconeogenesis, when ATP is high. Activity of PK is regulated by allosteric modulation and covalent modification. Allosterically PK is activated by fructose-1,6-bisphosphate, and inhibited by ATP. Phosphorylation of pyruvate kinase by *protein kinase A* decreases the activity of pyruvate kinase. As such this enzyme-catalyzed reaction is not a major control point in glycolysis.

The rate-limiting step in glycolysis is the reaction catalyzed by PFK-1.

PFK-1 is a tetrameric enzyme that exists in two conformational states termed **R** and **T** that are in equilibrium. ATP is both a substrate and an allosteric inhibitor of PFK-1. Each subunit has two ATP binding sites, a substrate site and an inhibitor site. The substrate site binds ATP equally well when the tetramer is in either conformation. The inhibitor site binds ATP essentially only when the enzyme is in the T state. F6P is the other substrate for PFK-1 and it binds preferentially to the R state enzyme. At high concentrations of ATP, the inhibitor site becomes occupied and shifting the equilibrium of PFK-1 conformation to that of the T state decreasing PFK-1's ability to bind F6P. The inhibition of PFK-1 by ATP is overcome by AMP, which binds to the R state of the enzyme and, thereby, stabilizes the **R** conformation of the enzyme that is capable of binding F6P.

METABOLIC FATES OF PYRUVATE

Pyruvate is the branch point molecule of glycolysis. The ultimate fate of pyruvate depends on the oxidation state of the cell. In the reaction catalyzed by *glyceraldehydes-3-phosphate dehydrogenase* (G3PDH), a molecule of NAD^+ is reduced to NADH. In order to maintain the redox state of the cell, this NADH must be re-oxidized to NAD^+.

During aerobic glycolysis NADH is reoxidized to NAD^+ in the mitochondrial ETC that generate ATP.

During anaerobic glycolysis, the NADH formed by the action of *G3PDH* is reoxidized to NAD^+ in the cytosol catalyzed by LDH, which transferes the electrons of NADH to pyruvate that forms lactate. Thereby NAD^+ is regenerated to keep glycolysis going.

Pyruvate, catalyzed by **pyruvate dehydrogenase** gets converted to acetyl-CoA that is completely oxidized in TCA cycle during which additional NADH molecules are generated.

Pyruvate, catalyzed by *pyruvate carboxylase* gets converted to oxaloacetate that can enter the pathway of gluconeogenesis or it can be utilized for fatty acid and cholesterol synthesis.

LACTATE METABOLISM

Erythrocytes and skeletal muscle under conditions of exertion derive all of their ATP needs through anaerobic glycolysis. Large quantities of NADH formed during this process are re-oxidized by transferring their electrons to pyruvate that generates lactate. This reaction is catalyzed by *lactate dehydrogenase* (LDH). The lactate formed diffuses out of the tissues and is transproted to highly aerobic tissues such as cardiac muscle and liver. In these tissues, LDH catalyzes the oxidation of lactate to pyruvate, which is further oxidized in the TCA cycle. If the energy level in these cells is high the carbons of pyruvate is diverted to gluconeogenic pathway.

Mammalian cells contain two distinct types of LDH subunits, termed M and H. Combinations of these different subunits generates LDH isozymes with different characteristics. The H type subunit predominates in aerobic tissues such as heart muscle (as the H_4 tetramer) while the M subunit predominates in anaerobic tissues such as skeletal muscle and erythrocytes (as the M_4 tetramer). The LDH (H_4) found in heart muscle has a low K_m for pyruvate and is inhibited by high levels of pyruvate. The LDH (M_4) found in skeletal muscle has a high K_m for pyruvate and is not inhibited by pyruvate. This suggests, the M-type LDH is utilized for reducing pyruvate to lactate, whereas the H type for the reverse.

ETHANOL METABOLISM

Animal cells contain **alcohol** *dehydrogenase* (ADH) that oxidizes ethanol to acetaldehyde, which is further oxidized to acetate by *acetaldehyde dehydrogenase* (Fig. 35.3). These reactions also lead to the reduction of NAD^+ to NADH. Acetaldehyde and acetate are toxic, which cause many side effects (hangover) that are associated with alcohol consumption. The metabolic effects of ethanol intoxication are due to generation of large quantities of acetaldehyde, acetate and the resultant cellular imbalance in the $NADH/NAD^+$.

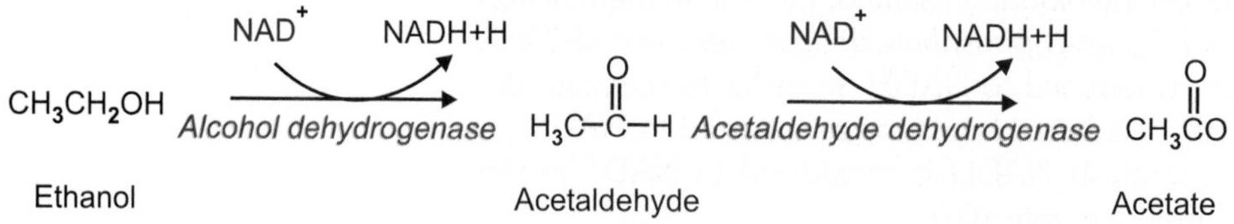

Fig. 35.3: Oxidation of ethanol

The reduction in NAD^+ impairs the flux of glucose through glycolysis at the **glyceraldehyde-3-phosphate dehydrogenase** reaction, thereby energy production gets limited. Additionally, there is an increased rate of lactate production as a consequence to increased NADH formation in the liver. This reversal of the LDH reaction in hepatocytes depletes availability of pyruvate for gluconeogenesis. Thereby glucose production by gluconeogenesis in the liver gets reduced, leading to a reduction in the capacity of the liver to deliver glucose to the blood.

GLUCONEOGENESIS

Synthesis of glucose from non-carbohydrate precursors such as lactate, glycerol, and carbon skeletal of gluconeogenic amino acids (alanine) is termed gluconeogenesis. The major site of gluconeogenesis is the liver, but it also occurs in kidney.

Gluconeogenesis is designed to maintain blood glucose levels that meet the demands of brain, testes, erythrocytes and renal medulla, whose sole energy source is glucose. However, during starvation the brain can utilize ketone bodies for its energy needs.

Synthesis of glucose from three and four carbon precursors is not a simple reversal of glycolysis, because **hexokinase, PFK, and PK** catalyzed reactions are metabolically irreversible. Hence, these steps of glycolysis need to be bypassed to favor gluconeogenesis.

If gluconeogenesis is not a simple reversal of glycolysis, it is very expensive from an energy standpoint, since gluconeogenesis starting from two moles of pyruvate to two moles of 1, 3-bisphosphoglycerate (1,3-BPG) consumes an equivalent of six moles of ATP. Whereas during glycolysis, the conversion of two moles of 1,3-BPG to two moles of pyruvate will only yield four moles of ATP. The stoichiometry for gluconeogenesis:

2 pyruvate + 4 ATP + 2 GTP + 2 NADH + 6 H_2O →glucose + 4 ADP +2 GDP + 6 P_i + 2 NAD^+ + $2H^+$

Several steps are required to convert two moles of 1,3-BPG to one mole of fructose-1,6-bisphosphate (Fig. 35.4).

First there is a reversal of the reaction catalyzed by **glyceraldehyde-3-phosphate dehydrogenase**, which requires NADH to convert 1, 3-BPG to glyceraldehyde-3-phosphate (G-3-P).

Secondly, one mole of G-3-P must be isomerized to DHAP and only then a mole each of DHAP and glyceraldehyde-3-phosphate condenses to form a mole of fructose-1,6-bisphosphate catalyzed by a reversal of the **aldolase** reaction. In most non-hepatic tissues that lack **glucose-6-phosphatase**, the glucose-6-phosphate generated would be a substrate for glycogen synthesis. In hepatocytes, the presence of **glucose-6-phosphatase** allows the dephosphorylation of G-6-P to generate free glucose that is delivered into the blood. Since the liver glucokinase high K_m, most of the glucose is not phosphorylated and flows down its' concentration gradient out of hepatocytes into the blood.

The three metabolically irreversible reactions (*pyruvate kinase, phosphofructokinase-1 (PFK-1)* and *hexokinase /glucokinase*) of glycolysis are bypassed using different enzymes during gluconeogenesis. The glucose-6-phosphate (G6P) produced by gluconeogenesis in the liver, renal cortex and in skeletal muscle (under certain situations) can be incorporated into glycogen. Since skeletal muscle lacks **glucose-6-phosphatase** it cannot deliver free glucose to the blood and the process of gluconeogenesis is exclusively a mechanism to generate glucose for storage as glycogen. In this case, one more bypass occurs at the **glycogen phosphorylase** catalyzed reaction.

Bypass 1: Pyruvate to phosphoenolpyruvate (PEP)

Conversion of pyruvate to PEP requires the action of **two mitochondrial enzymes.**

First is an ATP-requiring reaction catalyzed by *pyruvate carboxylase* (PC). As the name of the enzyme implies, pyruvate is carboxylated to form oxaloacetate (OAA). The CO_2 in this reaction is in the form of bicarbonate (HCO_3^-). This reaction is an anaplerotic reaction since it can be used to *fill-up* the TCA cycle intermediates.

Second enzyme is PEP *carboxykinase* (PEPCK) that catalyze the conversion of oxalate to PEP. The PEPCK requires GTP to decarboxylate oxalloacetate to yield phosphoenolpyruvate. Since CO_2 incorporated into pyruvate, by *pyruvate carboxylase* is subsequently released in the PEPCK catalyzed reaction, there is no net fixation of carbon. *In human cells, PEPCK is equally distributed between mitochondria and cytosol, hence this second reaction can occur in either cellular compartment.*

For gluconeogenesis to proceed, oxaloacetate produced by pyruvate carboxylase needs to be transported to the cytosol.

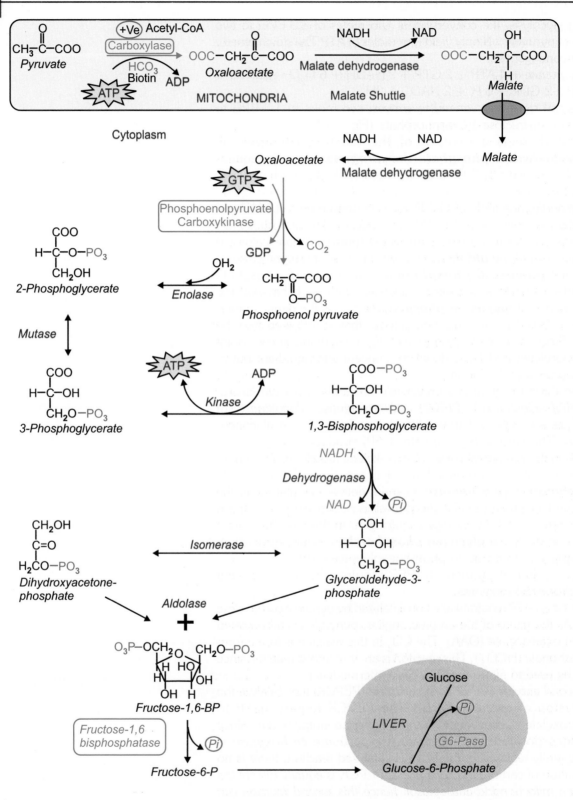

Fig. 35.4: Gluconeogenesis

However, no transport mechanism exist for its' direct transfer and OAA will not freely diffuse. Mitochondrial OAA can become cytosolic via three pathways.

1. Conversion of OAA to PEP (through the action of the mitochondrial PEPCK).
2. Transamination of OAA to aspartate.
3. Reduction of OAA to malate.

All of which are transported to the cytosol, where PEP can directly enter gluconeogenic pathway, aspartate undergoes reverse transamination to form OAA, and malate is oxidized to OAA. The NADH produced during the oxidation of malate to OAA in the cytosol is utilized during the **glyceraldehyde-3-phosphate dehydrogenase** reaction of glycolysis (1,3-BPG to G-3-P). *The coupling of these two oxidation-reduction reactions is required to keep gluconeogenesis functional when pyruvate is the principal source of carbon atoms.*

The utilization of malate to transport OAA to the cytosol is a function of the *malate/aspartate shuttle*, the mechanism used to transport cytosolic reducing equivalents into the mitochondrion for use in *oxidative phosphorylation*. The conversion of OAA to malate predominates when pyruvate is the source of carbon atoms for gluconeogenesis. In the cytoplasm, OAA is converted to PEP by the cytosolic version of PEPCK. Hormonal signals control the level of PEPCK as a means to regulate the flux through gluconeogenesis.

The net result of the pyruvate carboxylase (PC) and PEPCK reactions is:

pyruvate + ATP + GTP + H_2O → PEP + ADP + GDP + P_i + $2H^+$

Bypass 2: Fructose-1,6-bisphosphate to fructose-6-phosphate

Conversion of fructose-1,6-bisphosphate (F-1,6-BP), to fructose-6-phosphate (F-6-P) is the reverse of the rate-limiting step of glycolysis. This simple hydrolytic reaction catalyzed by **fructose-1,6-bisphosphatase** (F-1,6-BPase) is a major control point of gluconeogenesis.

Bypass 3: Glucose-6-phosphate (G6P) to glucose (or glycogen)

G6P is converted to glucose through the action of *glucose-6-phosphatase* (G6Pase). This reaction is also a simple hydrolysis reaction like that of F-1,6-BPase. Since the brain and skeletal muscle, as well as most nonhepatic tissues lack G6Pase activity, any glucose formed by gluconeogenesis in these tissues is not utilized for blood glucose supply. In the kidney, muscle and *especially the liver*, G6P can be shunted toward glycogen if blood glucose levels are adequate.

SUBSTRATES FOR GLUCONEOGENESIS

Lactate

Lactate is the predominant source of carbon atoms for gluconeogenesis. During anaerobic glycolysis in skeletal muscle, pyruvate is reduced to lactate, by *lactate dehydrogenase* (LDH). This reaction serves two important functions during anaerobic glycolysis.

i. It regenerates NAD and makes it available for use by the ***glyceraldehyde-3-phosphate dehydrogenase*** catalyzed reaction of glycolysis.

ii. The lactate produced is released to the bloodstream and transported to the liver where it is converted to glucose.

The glucose is then returned to the blood for use by muscle as an energy source and to replenish glycogen stores. This cycle is termed the Cori cycle (Fig. 35.5).

Gluconeogenic leg of Cori cycle consumes 6ATPs compared to 2ATPs formed during the Glycolytic leg of Cori cycle. The cycle cannot be sustained indefinitely.

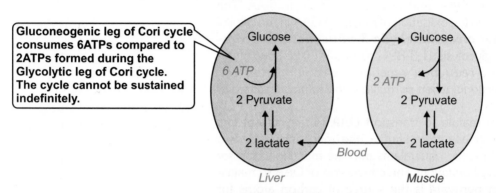

Fig. 35.5: Cori cycle

PYRUVATE

Pyruvate generated in muscle and other peripheral tissues can be transaminated to alanine, which is returned to the liver for gluconeogenesis. The transamination reaction requires an α-amino acid as donor of the amino group to generate an α-keto acid in the process. This pathway is termed the glucose-alanine cycle (Fig. 35.6). Although the majority of amino acids are degraded in the liver some are deaminated in muscle.

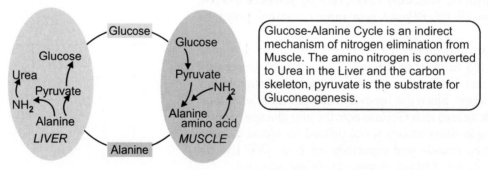

Glucose-Alanine Cycle is an indirect mechanism of nitrogen elimination from Muscle. The amino nitrogen is converted to Urea in the Liver and the carbon skeleton, pyruvate is the substrate for Gluconeogenesis.

Fig. 35.6: Glucose-alanine cycle

The glucose-alanine cycle serves two functions:

i. It is an indirect mechanism for muscle to eliminate nitrogen while replenishing its energy supply.

ii. It allows nonhepatic tissues to deliver the amino portion of catabolized amino acids to the liver for excretion as urea. In the liver, alanine is converted back to pyruvate and used as a gluconeogenic substrate or oxidized in the TCA cycle. The amino nitrogen is converted to urea in the urea cycle and excreted by the kidneys.

AMINO ACIDS

All 20 of the amino acids, with the *exception of leucine and lysine*, can be degraded to TCA cycle intermediates. This allows the carbon skeletons of the amino acids to be converted to oxaloacetate and subsequently into pyruvate, which can be utilized by gluconeogenic pathway. Muscle during exertion and liver during fasting; catabolize muscle proteins to amino acids, which contributes the major source of carbon for gluconeogenesis.

GLYCEROL

Oxidation of fatty acids yields enormous amounts of energy, however, the carbons of the fatty acids cannot be utilized for net synthesis of glucose. The acetyl-CoA derived from β-oxidation of fatty acids can be incorporated into the TCA cycle; however, during the TCA cycle two carbons are lost as CO_2. *This explains why fatty acids do not undergo net conversion to carbohydrate.*

The glycerol backbone of lipids can be used for gluconeogenesis. This requires phosphorylation of glycerol, by *glycerol kinase* to form glycerol-3-phosphate, which is dehydrogenated to dihydroxyacetone phosphate (DHAP) by *glyceraldehyde-3-phosphate dehydrogenase* (G3PDH). The G3PDH reaction is the same as that used in the transport of cytosolic reducing equivalents into the mitochondrion for use in oxidative phosphorylation. This transport pathway is called the **glycerol-phosphate shuttle**. The glycerol backbone of triacylglycerols in adipose tissue is ensured of being used as a gluconeogenic substrate since adipose cells lack *glycerol kinase*. In fact adipocytes require a basal level of glycolysis in order to provide them with DHAP as an intermediate in the synthesis of triacylglycerols.

PROPIONATE

Oxidation of fatty acids having odd number of carbon atoms and the oxidation of certain amino acids generate propionyl-CoA, which is converted to succinyl-CoA (TCA cycle intermediary). This conversion is catalyzed by the concerted action of *propionyl-CoA carboxylase* (an ATP and biotin requiring enzyme), *methylmalonyl-CoA epimerase and methylmalonyl-CoA mutase* (vitamin B_{12} requiring enzyme).

Regulation of Gluconeogenesis

The regulation of gluconeogenesis is in direct contrast to the regulation of glycolysis. In general, negative effectors of glycolysis are positive effectors of gluconeogenesis. Regulation of the *activity F-1,6-BPase is the most significant site* for controlling the flux toward glucose synthesis. This is predominantly controlled by *fructose-2,6-bisphosphate (F-2,6-BP),* which is a powerful negative allosteric effector of F-1,6-BPase activity.

Gluconeogenesis is also controlled at the level of pyruvate to PEP conversion. The hepatic signals elicited by glucagon or epinephrine lead to phosphorylation and inactivation of *pyruvate kinase* (PK), which will allow for an increase in the flux through gluconeogenesis. ATP and alanine also allosterically inhibit PK. The former signals adequate energy and the latter signals that sufficient substrates are available for gluconeogenesis. Conversely a reduction in energy levels as evidenced by increasing concentrations of ADP, leads to inhibition of both PC and PEPCK. Allosteric activation of PC occurs through acetyl-CoA. Each of these regulations occurs on a short time scale, whereas long-term regulation can be effected at the level of PEPCK. The amount of this enzyme increases in response to prolonged glucagon stimulation. This situation would occur in a starving individual or someone with an inadequate diet.

CO-ORDINATED ALLOSTERIC REGULATION OF GLYCOLYSIS AND GLUCONEOGENESIS

The most important allosteric regulator of both glycolysis and gluconeogenesis is *fructose-2, 6-bisphosphate, (F-2, 6-BP)*, which is not an intermediate in glycolysis or in gluconeogenesis.

The bifunctional enzyme PFK-2/F-2,6-BPase catalyzes the synthesis of F-2,6-BP (Fig. 35.7).

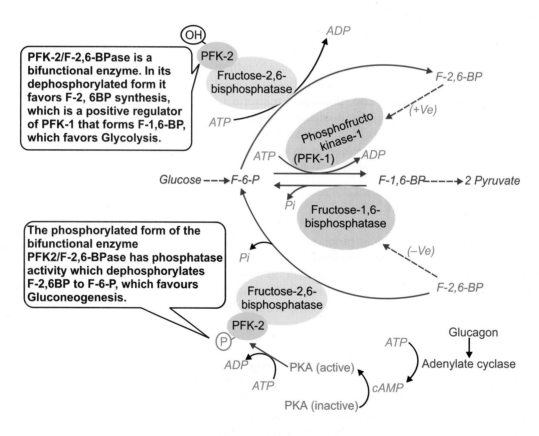

Fig. 35.7: Regulation of glycolysis and gluconeogenesis

In the nonphosphorylated form, the enzyme is known as PFK-2 and serves to catalyze the synthesis of F-2,6-BP. The result is that the activity of PFK-1 is greatly stimulated and the activity of F-1,6-BPase is greatly inhibited.

Under conditions where PFK-2 is active, fructose-6-P is converted to F-1,6-BP by the action of PFK-1. Simultaneously conversion of F-1,6-BP to F-6-P by F-1,6-BPase is inhibited. These two actions together bring about a net production of F-1,6-BP that goes in the direction of glycolysis.

The phosphorylated form of bifunctional enzyme no longer exhibits kinase activity, but a new active site that hydrolyzes F-2,6-BP to F6P and inorganic phosphate. The metabolic effect of the phosphorylation of the bifunctional enzyme is that the allosteric stimulation of PFK-1 ceases, and allosteric inhibition of F-1,6-BPase is eliminated. This results in net formation of F-6-P, which moves in the direction of gluconeogenesis that produces F6P and eventually glucose.

The interconversion of the bifunctional enzyme is catalyzed by *cAMP-dependent protein kinase* (PKA), which in turn is regulated by the circulating peptide hormones. A drop in blood glucose level, leads to a fall in pancreatic insulin secretion and a rise in circulating glucagon. Binding of glucagon to plasma membrane receptors on liver cells, activate membrane-localized *adenylate cyclase* that lead to an increase in the conversion of ATP to cAMP. The cAMP binding to the regulatory subunits of PKA, leads to the release and activation of the catalytic subunits. Numerous enzymes, including the bifunctional PFK-2/F-2,6-BPase are phosphorylated by PKA. Under these conditions, liver becomes metabolically gluconeogenic to produce glucose and reestablish normoglycemia.

Regulation of glycolysis also occurs at the step catalyzed by *pyruvate kinase* (PK), which is inhibited by ATP and acetyl-CoA, but activated by F-1,6-BP. The inhibition of PK by ATP is similar to the effect of ATP on PFK-1. The binding of ATP to the inhibitor site reduces its affinity for PEP. The liver enzyme is also regulated at the level of its synthesis. Increased carbohydrate ingestion induces the PK synthesis that results in elevated cellular levels of the enzyme.

A number of PK isozymes have been described. The liver isozyme (L-type), characteristic of a gluconeogenic tissue, is regulated via phosphorylation by PKA, whereas the M-type isozyme found in brain, muscle, and other glucose requiring tissue is unaffected by PKA. As a consequence of these differences, blood glucose levels and associated hormones can regulate the balance of liver gluconeogenesis and glycolysis while muscle metabolism remains unaffected.

In erythrocytes, the fetal PK isozyme has much greater activity than the adult isozyme; as a result, fetal erythrocytes have comparatively low concentrations of glycolytic intermediates. Because of the low steady-state concentration of fetal 1,3-BPG, the 2,3-BPG shunt is greatly reduced in fetal cells and little 2,3-BPG is formed. Since 2,3-BPG is a negative effector of hemoglobin affinity for oxygen, fetal erythrocytes have a higher oxygen affinity than maternal erythrocytes. Therefore, transfer of oxygen from maternal hemoglobin to fetal hemoglobin is favored, assuring the fetal oxygen supply. In the newborn, an erythrocyte isozyme of the M-type with comparatively low PK activity displaces the fetal type, resulting in an accumulation of glycolytic intermediates. The increased 1,3-BPG levels activate the 2,3-BPG shunt, producing 2,3-BPG needed to regulate oxygen binding to hemoglobin.

Genetic diseases of *adult erythrocyte PK* are known in which the kinase is virtually inactive. The erythrocytes of affected individuals have a greatly reduced capacity to make ATP and thus do not have sufficient ATP to perform activities such as ion pumping and maintaining osmotic balance. These erythrocytes have a short half-life and lyse readily, which is responsible for some cases of *hereditary hemolytic anemia*.

The liver PK isozyme is regulated by phosphorylation, allosteric effectors and modulation of gene expression. The major allosteric effectors are F-1,6-BP, which stimulates PK activity by decreasing its $K_{m (app)}$ for PEP. Expression of the liver PK gene is strongly influenced by the quantity of carbohydrate in the diet. High-carbohydrate diets induce up to 10-fold increases in PK concentration. The PKA inhibits liver PK activity by phosphorylation.

Muscle PK (M-type) is not regulated by the same mechanisms as the liver enzyme. Extracellular conditions that lead to the phosphorylation and inhibition of liver PK, such as low blood glucose and high levels of circulating glucagon, do not inhibit the muscle enzyme. The advantage of such differential regulation is that hormones such as glucagon and epinephrine favor liver gluconeogenesis by inhibiting liver glycolysis, while at the same time muscle glycolysis can proceed in accord with needs directed by intracellular conditions.

PENTOSE PHOSPHATE PATHWAY (PPP) OR HEXOSE MONOPHOSPHATE (HMP) SHUNT

The pentose phosphate pathway is an anabolic pathway that utilizes the six-carbon glucose to generate five-carbon sugars (ribose-5-phosphate) and NADPH (reducing equivalents). This pathway is active in tissues that synthesize fatty acids or sterols (liver, adipose tissue, adrenal cortex, thyroid, erythrocytes, testis and lactating mammary glands), which require large quantities of NADPH. All reactions of the pathway are cytosolic. However, under certain conditions glucose is completely oxidize to CO_2 and water in this pathway.

Primary Functions of HMP

1. To generate reducing equivalents in the form of NADPH for reductive biosynthetic reactions within cells.
2. To provide the cell with ribose-5-phosphate (R5P) for the synthesis of the nucleotides and nucleic acids.
3. Pathway also catalyzes the interconversion of three-, four-, five-, six-, and seven-carbon skeletons of dietary carbohydrates into glycolytic/gluconeogenic intermediates.

Enzymes that function primarily in the reductive direction utilize the $NADP^+$/NADPH cofactor pair, as opposed to oxidative enzymes that utilize the NAD^+/NADH cofactor pair. The reactions of fatty acid biosynthesis and steroid biosynthesis utilize large amounts of NADPH. In liver, 30 percent of glucose is oxidized by HMP. The erythrocytes utilize the reactions of HMP to generate large amounts of NADPH that are required to maintain glutathione in reduced form. The conversion of ribonucleotides to deoxyribonucleotides (through the action of **ribonucleotide reductase**) also requires NADPH as the electron source, therefore all rapidly proliferating cells need large quantities of NADPH.

REACTIONS OF PENTOSE PHOSPHATE PATHWAY

The pentose phosphate pathway has an **oxidative** and a **non-oxidative** phase.

Oxidative Phase

The oxidative steps of the pathway utilize glucose-6-phosphate (G6P) as the substrate. These reactions that occur at the beginning of the pathway generates NADPH (Fig.35.8). Every mole of glucose-6-phosphate (G-6-P) that enters the PPP generates two moles of NADPH by reactions catalyzed by **glucose-6-phosphate dehydrogenase** and **6-phosphogluconate dehydrogenase**.

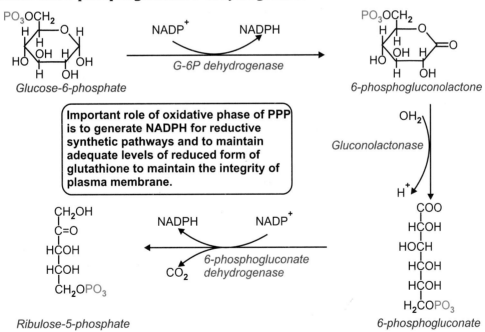

Important role of oxidative phase of PPP is to generate NADPH for reductive synthetic pathways and to maintain adequate levels of reduced form of glutathione to maintain the integrity of plasma membrane.

Fig. 35.8: Reactions of oxidative phase of PPP

Metabolic disorders associated with the oxidative phase of pentose phosphate pathway affect the cellular functions.

Oxidative stress within cells is controlled primarily by the action of the peptide, *glutathione* (GSH). Peroxides that are generated during oxidative stress are reduced by glutathione, to generate water and an alcohol, or two molecules of water if the peroxide is hydrogen peroxide. During this reaction glutathione itself gets oxidized. The reduced form of glutathione is regenerated by the enzyme *glutathione reductase*, which requires NADPH as a cofactor.

Disulfide bonds play a very important role in protein structure and function, but inappropriately introduced disulfides can be detrimental, such disulfide bonds are reduced nonenzymatically by cysteine thiols or glutathione.

Nonoxidative Phase

The nonoxidative steps of the PPP are primarily designed to generate ribose-5-phosphate (R5P). Equally important reactions of the PPP are to convert dietary 5-carbon sugars into both 6-carbon sugars (*fructose-6-phosphate*) and 3-carbon sugars (*glyceraldehyde-3-phosphate*), which can be utilized by the glycolytic pathway. The primary enzymes involved in the nonoxidative steps of the PPP are **transaldolase** and **transketolase (Fig. 35.9)**.

Transketolase 1 and 2 functions to transfer *2-carbon groups* from substrates of the PPP, thus **rearrange** the carbon atoms that enter this pathway. Like other enzymes that transfer 2-carbon groups, transketolase requires **thiamine pyrophosphate** (TPP) as a cofactor in the transfer reaction.

Transaldolase is also involved in the rearrangement of carbon skeletons of the substrates of the PPP by transferring *3-carbon groups*. The transaldolase reaction involves *Schiff base* formation between the substrate and a lysine residue at the active site of the enzyme.

The net result of the PPP, if not used solely for R5P production is the oxidation of G6P, into a 5-carbon sugar. In turn, three moles of 5-carbon sugar are converted, via the enzymes of the PPP, back into two moles of 6-carbon sugars and one mole of 3-carbon sugar. The 6-carbon sugars can be recycled into the pathway in the form of G6P, generating more NADPH. The 3-carbon sugar generated is glyceraldehyde-3-phsphate that can be shunted to glycolysis and oxidized to pyruvate. Alternatively, it is shunted to gluconeogenic pathway to generate 6-carbon sugar (fructose-6-phosphate or glucose-6-phosphate).

Remember that any disruption in the level of NADPH may have a profound effect on the ability of cells to deal with oxidative stress. Erythrocyte is exposed to greater oxidizing conditions than any other cell. After all it is the oxygen carrier of the body.

ERYTHROCYTES AND THE PENTOSE PHOSPHATE PATHWAY

The predominant pathways of carbohydrate metabolism in the erythrocytes are *glycolysis*, the *PPP* and *2,3-bisphosphoglycerate (2,3-BPG)* metabolism.

a. Glycolysis provides ATP for membrane ion pumps and NADH for reoxidation of methemoglobin.
b. The PPP provides NADPH, for the erythrocytes to maintain glutathione in its reduced state (Fig. 35.10). The inability to maintain reduced glutathione in erythrocytes leads to increased

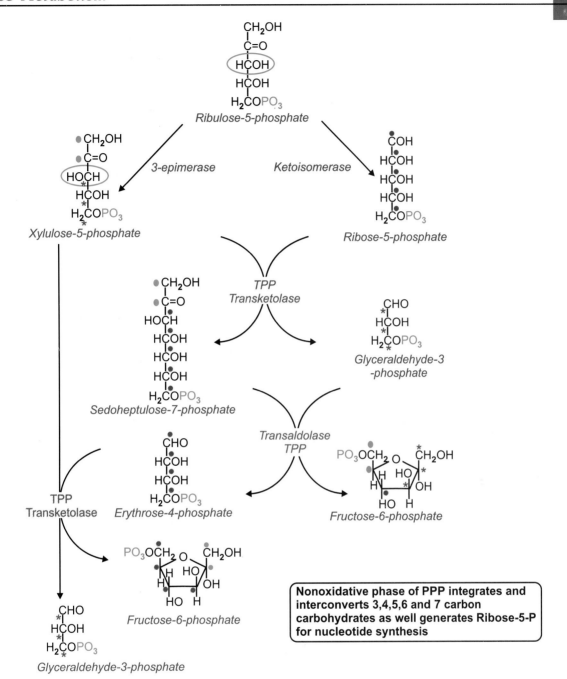

Fig. 35.9: Nonoxidative part of HMP

accumulation of peroxides, predominantly H_2O_2, that in turn results in a weakening of the cell wall and concomitant hemolysis. Accumulation of H_2O_2 also leads to increased rates of oxidation of hemoglobin to methemoglobin that also weakens the cell wall. Glutathione removes peroxides via the action of **glutathione peroxidase**. The PPP in erythrocytes is essentially the only pathway for these cells to produce NADPH. Any defect in the production of NADPH could, therefore, have profound effects on the survival of erythrocytes.

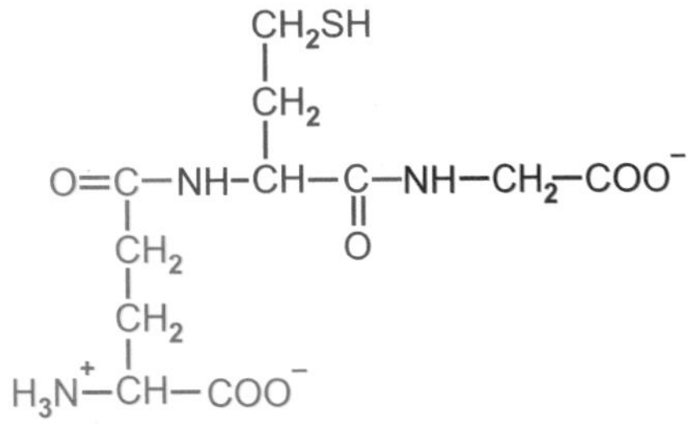

Glutathione (GSH)

Glutathione (GSH) is a tripeptide composed of γ-glutamate, cysteine and glycine. The sulfhydryl side chains of the cysteine residues of two glutathione molecules form a disulfide bond (GSSG) during the course of being oxidized in reactions with various oxides and peroxides in cells.
Reduction of GSSG to two moles of GSH is catalysed by glutathione reductase; an enzyme that requires coupled oxidation of NADPH.

Fig. 35.10: Structure of glutathoine

Several deficiencies in the level of activity (not function) of **glucose-6- phosphatedehydrogenase** have been observed to be associated with resistance to the malarial parasite *Plasmodium falciparum*, among individuals of Mediterranean and African descent. The basis for this resistance is the weakening of the erythrocyte membrane (the erythrocyte is the host cell for the parasite) such that it cannot sustain the parasitic life-cycle long enough for productive growth

c. *2,3-bisphosphoglycerate (2,3-BPG)* helps stabilize the T or deoxygenated form of hemoglobin by cross-linking the β-chains of hemoglobin molecule, thereby decreasing the affinity of hemoglobin for oxygen.

Fructose Metabolism

36

Fructose is the preferred energy source for sperm cells. Metabolism of fructose differs in muscle and liver.

In muscle, the enzyme *hexokinase* phosphorylates fructose to yield fructose-6-phosphate that directly enters glycolytic pathway (Fig. 36.1).

In liver cells, the enzyme *fructokinase* phosphorylates fructose to yield fructose-1-phosphate (F-1-P), which is the specific substrate for *aldolase B*, the predominant form found in liver. Aldolase B cleaves F-1-P to yield dihydroxyacetone phosphate (DHAP) and glyceraldehyde. *Triose phosphate isomerase* catalyzes the isomerization of dihydroxyacetone phosphate to gleceraldehyde-3-phosphate ((G3P), which enters glycolytic pathway. Where as most of the glyceraldehyde is phosphorylated to yield G3P, but to lesser extent glyceraldehyde is also converted to DHAP by the concerted action of 3 enzymes, *alcohol dehydrogenase, glycerol kinase* and *glycerol phosphate dehydrogenase* (Fig. 36.1). Both DHAP and G3P may be degraded in glycolytic pathway or converted to glucose by gluconeogenesis.

CLINICAL SIGNIFICANCE OF FRUCTOSE METABOLISM

Three inherited abnormalities associated with fructose metabolism have been identified.

Essential Fructosuria

It is a benign metabolic disorder caused by the ***lack of fructokinase***, which is normally present in the liver, pancreatic islets and renal cortex. The extent of fructosuria in this disease depends on the time and amount of dietary intake of fructose or sucrose. Since the disorder is asymptomatic and harmless it may go undiagnosed.

Hereditary Fructose Intolerance

It is a potentially lethal disorder resulting from ***lack of aldolase-B***, which is normally present in the liver, small intestine and renal cortex.

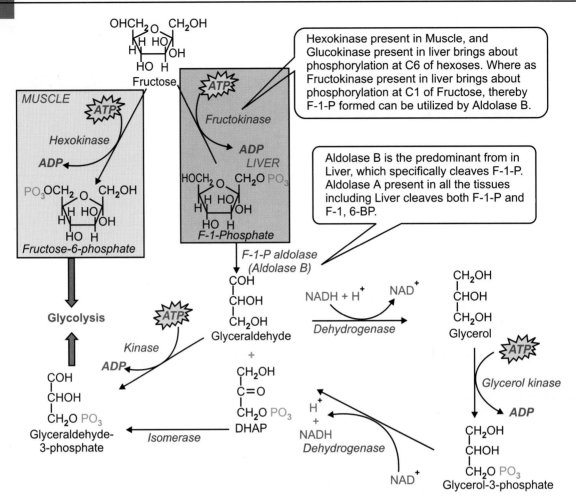

Fig. 36.1: Fructose metabolism

The disorder is characterized by severe hypoglycemia and vomiting following fructose intake. Prolonged intake of fructose by infants with this defect leads to vomiting, poor feeding, jaundice, hepatomegaly, hemorrhage and eventually hepatic failure and death. The hypoglycemia that results following fructose uptake is due *inhibition of glycogenolysis* caused by F-1-P, which interfere with the glycogen phosphorylase reaction, and also *inhibition of gluconeogenesis* at the deficient aldolase step. Such individuals can be managed best by withdrawing foods containing sucrose and fructose.

Hereditary Fructose-1, 6-Bisphosphatase Deficiency

Deficiency of *fructose-1,6-bisphosphatase* severely impairs hepatic gluconeogenesis, hence fructose intake in this condition leads to episodes of hypoglycemia, apnea, hyperventilation, ketosis and lactic acidosis. Hypoglycemia is due to *inhibition of liver glycogen phosphorylase* by elevated F-1-P and F1,6-BP. These symptoms could be lethal in neonates, but in later life episodes are triggered by fasting and febrile infections.

GALACTOSE METABOLISM

Dietary source of galactose is lactose. In the small intestine, the intestinal lactase hydrolyzes lactose to yield galactose and glucose. In the liver, galactose is readily converted to glucose through a series of reactions (Fig. 36.2). The first reaction is phosphorylation of galactose to galactose-1-phosphate catalyzed by *Galactokinase*. In the next step catalyzed by *galactose-1-phosphate uridyltransferase*, galactose-1-phosphate displaces glucose-1-phosphate of UDP-glucose; thereby UDP-glucose becomes UDP-galactose. Then UDP-galactose is epimerized to UDP-glucose by the enzyme *UDP-galactose epimerase*. The glucose-1-phosphate is isomerized to glucose-6-phosphate by the enzyme *phosphoglucomutase*.

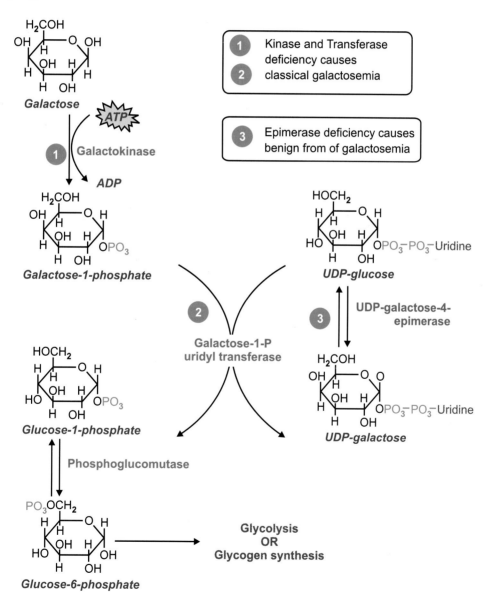

1 Kinase and Transferase
   deficiency causes
2 classical galactosemia

3 Epimerase deficiency causes
   benign from of galactosemia

Fig. 36.2: Galactose metabolism

CLINICAL SIGNIFICANCE OF GALACTOSE METABOLISM

Three inherited disorders of galactose metabolism are known.

Classic galactosemia is a major symptom of two enzyme defects.

One form of galactosemia results from absence of *galactokinase*.

The second form of galactosemia is due to the absence of the enzyme *galactose-1-phosphate uridyl transferase*.

Neonates with these defects fail to thrive and suffer vomiting and diarrhea following milk ingestion. Hence such individuals are termed lactose intolerant. Clinical findings of these disorders include impaired liver function, when left untreated leads to severe cirrhosis, elevated blood galactose (hypergalactosemia), hyperchloremic metabolic acidosis, urinary galactitol excretion and hyperaminoaciduria. All these lead to blindness and liver damage, unless controlled by exclusion of galactose from the diet. Even on a galactose-restricted diet, individuals with transferase deficiency exhibit urinary galactitol excretion and persistently elevated erythrocyte galactose-1-phosphate levels.

The molecular basis of *blindness* in these individuals is due to the conversion of circulating galactose to the sugar-alcohol galactitol, by an NADPH-dependent *galactose reductase* that is present in neural tissue and in the lens of the eye. A high concentration of galactitol in the lens causes osmotic swelling, with the resultant formation of cataracts and other symptoms.

Liver failure and *mental retardation* are due to depletion of inorganic phosphate in liver and brain as a consequence to accumulation of galactose-1-phosphate.

The principal treatment of these disorders is total elimination of lactose from the diet.

The deficiency of *UDP-galactose-4-epimerase* causes benign form of galactosemia. Two different forms of this deficiency have been found. One form, which is benign, affects only erythrocytes and leukocytes. The other form affects multiple tissues and manifests symptoms similar to the transferase deficiency. Treatment involves restriction of dietary galactose.

MANNOSE METABOLISM

The digestion of many dietary polysaccharides and glycoproteins yields mannose, which is phosphorylated by *hexokinase* to generate mannose-6-phosphate (Fig. 36.3). Mannose-6-phosphate is converted to fructose-6-phosphate, by the enzyme *phosphomannose isomerase*, which then enters the glycolytic pathway or is converted to glucose-6-phosphate by the gluconeogenic pathway of hepatocytes. In eukaryotes, mannose is constituent of N- and O-linked glycans. GDP-mannose is the donor form of mannose.

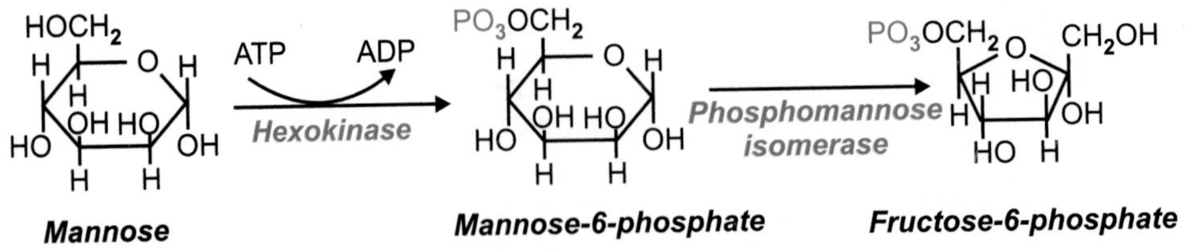

Fig. 36.3: Mannose metabolism

GLUCURONATE METABOLISM (URONIC ACID PATHWAY)

The uronic acid pathway is an alternative pathway for the oxidation of glucose that does not provide any ATP, but is utilized for the generation of the activated form of glucuronate (UDP-glucuronate) that is highly polar (Fig. 36.4).

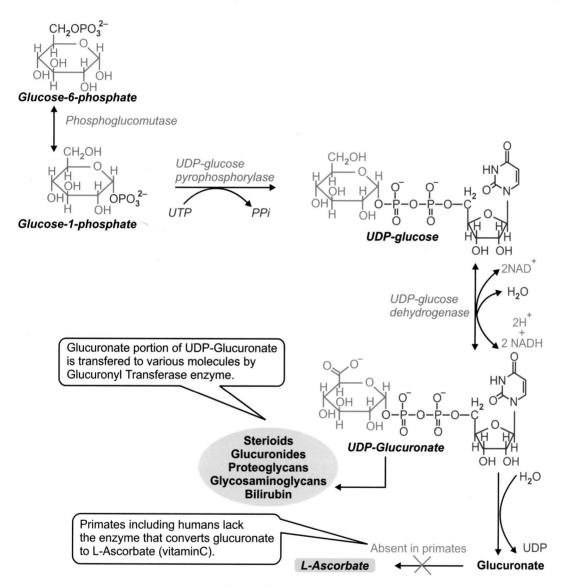

Fig. 36.4: Uronic acid pathway

UDP-glucuronate is used in the synthesis of glycosaminoglycan and proteoglycans as well as to form conjugates with bilirubin, steroids and certain drugs to make them water-soluble that helps their excretion. The synthesis of ascorbate (vitamin C) does not occur in humans and primates since they lack the enzyme **glucunolactone oxidase**.

The uronic acid pathway begins with the conversion of G-6-P to G-1-P catalyzed by *phosphoglucomutase*. The enzyme *UDP-glucose pyrophosphorylase* then activates G-1-P to UDP-glucose, which is oxidized to UDP-glucuronate by a NAD$^+$-requiring enzyme *UDP-glucose dehydrogenase*. UDP-glucuronate serves as a precursor for the synthesis of iduronic acid and UDP-xylose, which are incorporated into proteoglycans and glycoproteins, or forms conjugates with bilirubin, steroids, xenobiotics, drugs and many compounds containing hydroxyl (-OH) groups.

CLINICAL SIGNIFICANCE OF GLUCURONATE METABOLISM

Significant numbers of erythrocytes die each day that releases the iron-free portion of heme, which is subsequently degraded. The primary sites of porphyrin degradation are the reticuloendothelial cells of the liver, spleen and bone marrow. The breakdown of porphyrin yields bilirubin, a product that is nonpolar and therefore, insoluble in aqueous blood. It is transported to the liver via blood, bound to plasma albumin. In the liver, bilirubin is conjugation to glucuronate. The soluble conjugated bilirubin; *diglucuronide* is then secreted into the bile. An inability to conjugate bilirubin, for instance in hepatic disease or when the level of bilirubin production exceeds the capacity of the liver, is a contributory cause of jaundice. The conjugation of glucuronate to certain nonpolar drugs is important for their solubilization in the liver. Drugs conjugated to glucuronate are more easily cleared from the blood into urine by the kidneys. The glucuronate drug-conjugation system can, however, lead to drug resistance; chronic exposure to certain drugs, such as barbiturates and azathioprine (AZT), leads to an increase in the synthesis of the *UDP-glucuronyltransferases* in the liver that are involved in glucuronate drug-conjugation. The increased levels of these hepatic enzymes result in a higher rate of drug clearance leading to a reduction in the effective concentration of drugs in the body.

Chemistry of Nucleotides

37

Nucleotides as a class may be considered one of the most important biomolecules of the cell. Nucleotides are found primarily as the monomeric units of the major nucleic acids, the RNA and DNA. However, they perform numerous other important functions within the cell.

These functions include:

1. Serve as *energy stores* in phosphate transfer reactions. The predominant nucleotide involved in these phosphate transfer reactions is ATP. The ATP is the most commonly used source but other nucleotides are also used as the source of energy that drives most biochemical reactions. For example, GTP is used in protein synthesis as well as a few other reactions, UTP is the source of energy for activating glucose and galactose and CTP is an energy source in lipid metabolism.

2. The adenosine monophosphate (AMP) is part of the structure of some of the coenzymes like NAD^+, $NADP^+$, FAD and coenzyme A.

3. Nucleotides serve as mediators (*second messengers in signal transduction events*) of numerous important cellular processes. The predominant second messenger is cyclic-AMP (cAMP), which is a cyclic derivative of AMP formed from ATP.

Neither the bases nor the nucleotides are required dietary components, since they can be synthesized *de novo*, as well those that are already present can be salvaged and reused.

Nitrogen Bases

There are two kinds of nitrogen-containing bases derived by appropriate substitution on the ring structure of the parent substances, purines and pyrimidines (Fig. 37.1). It is the chemical basicity of purines and pyrimidines that has given them the common term "bases" as they are associated with nucleotides present in DNA and RNA.

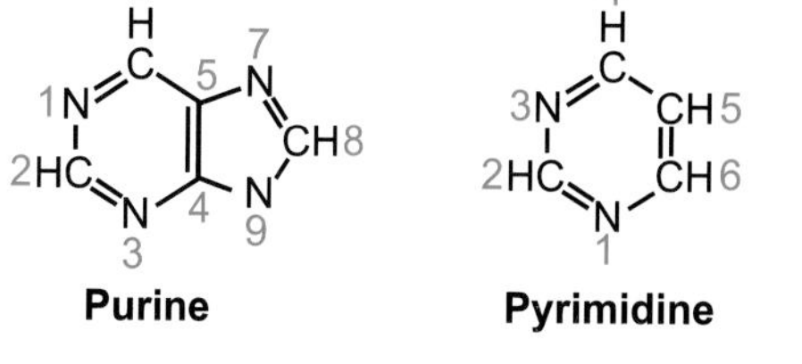

Purine   **Pyrimidine**

Fig. 37.1: Note that the direction of the numbering of the purine ring is different from pyrimidine

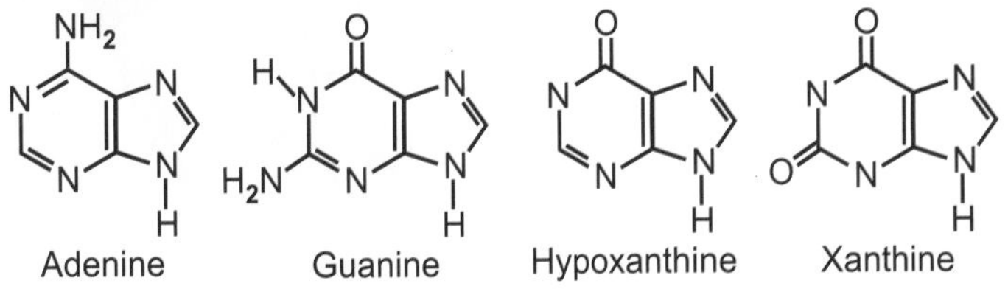

Adenine   Guanine   Hypoxanthine   Xanthine

Fig. 37.2: Purine bases

Purines consist of six-membered and five-membered nitrogen-containing rings, fused together. Pyridmidines have only a six-membered nitrogen-containing ring. There are four purine and four pyrimidine bases that are of concern to us.

Purine bases are adenine (A), guanine (G), hypoxanthine and xanthine (Fig. 37.2).

Adenine and guanine are found in both DNA and RNA. Hypoxanthine and xanthine are not incorporated into the nucleic acids but are important intermediates in the synthesis and degradation of the purine nucleotides.

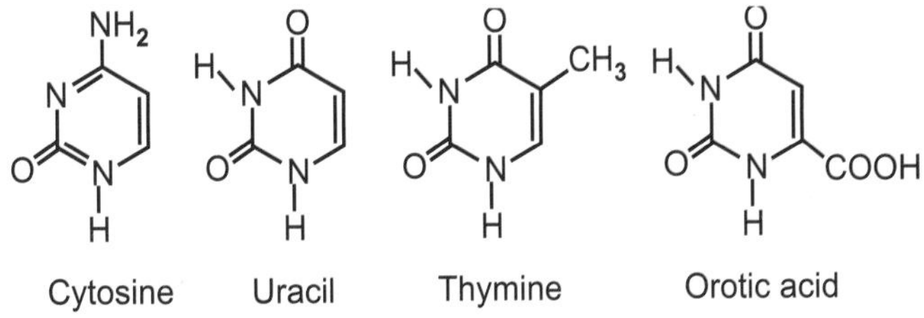

Pyrimidine bases are uracil (U), thymine (T), cytosine (C) and orotic acid (Fig. 37.3).

Cytosine   Uracil   Thymine   Orotic acid

Fig. 37.3: Pyrimidine bases

Cytosine is found in both DNA and RNA. Uracil is found only in RNA. Thymine is normally found in DNA. Sometimes tRNA will contain some thymine as well as uracil (psedouridine). Orotic acid is an intermediate in the biosynthesis of pyrimidine nucleotides.

The purine and pyrimidine bases in cells are linked to carbohydrate (D-ribose or 2'-deoxy-D-ribose) through a β-N-glycosidic bond between the anomeric carbon of the ribose and the N^9 of a purine or N^1 of a pyrimidine and in this form are termed, **nucleosides.** The base can exist in two distinct orientations about the N-glycosidic bond (Fig. 37.4). These configurations are identified as, *syn* and *anti*. It is the anti configuration that predominates in naturally occurring nucleotides

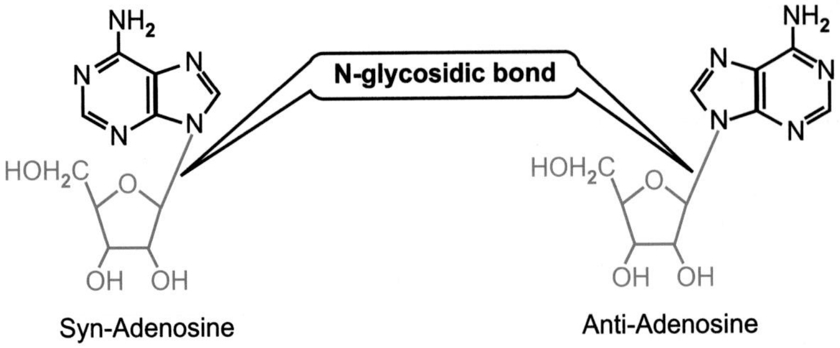

N-glycosidic bond

Syn-Adenosine   Anti-Adenosine

Fig. 37.4: Syn and anti-configuration of adenosine

Nucleosides

When a sugar, either ribose or 2-deoxyribose, is linked to purine or pyrimidine (nitrogen bases) through a β-N-glycosidic bond, the resulting compound is called a *nucleoside*. Carbon 1 of the sugar is attached to nitrogen 9 of a purine base or to nitrogen 1 of a pyrimidine base. The names of *purine nucleosides* end in -osine and the names of *pyrimidine nucleosides* end in -idine.

Purine nucleosides	Pyrimidine nucleosides
Adenosine	Uridine
Guanosine	Thymidine
Inosine -the base in inosine is *hypoxanthine*	Cytidine

The convention is to number the ring atoms of the base normally and to use l', 2', 3' etc. to distinguish the ring atoms of the sugar (Fig. 37.5). Unless otherwise specified, the sugar is assumed to be ribose. To indicate that the sugar is 2'-deoxyribose, a d- is placed before the name.

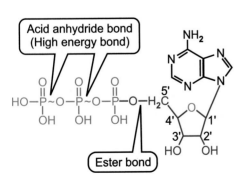

Acid anhydride bond (High energy bond)

Ester bond

Fig. 37.5: ATP structure showing acid anhydride and ester bonds

Nucleotides

Addition of one or more phosphates to the sugar portion of a nucleoside results in a *nucleotide*. Generally, the phosphate is in ester linkage to carbon 5' of the sugar (Fig. 37.5). If more than one phosphate is present, they are generally in acid anhydride linkages to each other. If such is the case, no position designation in the name is required. However, if the phosphate is in any other position, it must be designated. For example, 3'-5' cAMP indicates that a phosphate is in ester linkage to both the 3' and 5' hydroxyl groups of an adenosine molecule and forms a cyclic structure. The 2'-GMP would indicate that a phosphate is in ester linkage to the 2' hydroxyl group of a guanosine. Some representative names are:

AMP = adenosine monophosphate = adenylic acid

CDP = cytidine diphosphate

dGTP = deoxyguanosine triphosphate

dTTP = deoxythymidine triphosphate (more commonly designated TTP)

cAMP = 3'-5' cyclic adenosine monophosphate

Acid anhydride bonds link the di- and triphosphates of nucleotides (Fig. 37.5). Acid anhydride bonds have a high $DG^{0'}$ for hydrolysis imparting upon them a high potential to transfer the phosphates to other molecules. It is this property of the nucleotides that results in their involvement in phospho group-transfer reactions in the cell.

The nucleotides found in DNA are unique from those of RNA in that the ribose exists in *the 2'-deoxy* form and the abbreviations of the nucleotides contain a *-d* designation. The monophosphorylated form of adenosine found in DNA (deoxyadenosine-5'-monophosphate) is written as dAMP.

The nucleotide *uridine is never found in DNA* and *thymine is almost exclusively found in DNA*. Thymine is found in tRNAs but not in rRNAs or mRNAs. There are several less common bases found in DNA and RNA. The primary modified base in DNA is 5-methylcytosine. A variety of modified bases appear in the tRNAs. Many modified nucleotides are encountered outside of the context of DNA and RNA that serve important biological functions.

Adenosine Derivatives

The most common adenosine derivative is its cyclic form, 3'-5'-cyclic adenosine monophosphate (cAMP). This molecule is a very powerful second messenger involved in signal transduction events from the cell surface to internal proteins, e.g. cAMP-dependent protein kinase (PKA) that phosphorylates a number of proteins, thereby their activity is affected either positively or negatively.

Base Formula	Base (X=H)	Nucleoside X=ribose or deoxyribose	Nucleotide X=ribose phosphate
	Cytosine, C	Cytidine, A	Cytidine monophosphate CMP
	Uracil, U	Uridine, U	Uridine monophosphate UMP
	Thymine, T	Thymidine, T	Thymidine monophosphate TMP
	Adenine, A	Adenosine, A	Adenosine monophosphate AMP
	Guanine, G	Guanosine, A	Guanosine monophosphate GMP

Cyclic-AMP is also involved in the regulation of ion channels by direct interaction with channel proteins, e.g., in the activation of odorant receptors by odorant molecules. The cAMP is formed in response to activation of receptor-coupled *adenylate cyclase*. These receptors can be of hormone-receptor or odorant-receptor type.

S-adenosylmethionine (SAM) is a form of "activated" methionine, which serves as a methyl donor in methylation reactions and as a source of propylamine in the synthesis of polyamines.

Guanosine Derivatives

The cyclic form of GMP (cGMP) that is found in cells also functions as a second messenger molecule. In many situations, its' role is to antagonize the effects of cAMP. The cGMP is formed in response to receptor-mediated signals similar to those that activates adenylate cyclase. However, in this case it is *guanylate cyclase* that is coupled to the receptor. The most important cGMP-coupled signal transduction cascade is that of photoreception. However, in photoreception the activation of rhodopsin (in the rods) or conopsins (in the cones) is by the absorption of a photon of light (through 11-*cis*-retinal covalently associated with rhodopsin and opsins) that activates transducin, which in turn activates a cGMP-specific *phosphodiesterase* that hydrolyzes cGMP to GMP. This lowers the effective concentration of cGMP, bound to gated ion channels, resulting in their closure and a concomitant hyperpolarization of the cell.

Synthetic Nucleotide Analogs

Many nucleotide analogues are chemically synthesized and are used for their therapeutic potential. The nucleotide analogues are used to inhibit specific enzymatic activities. Large families of analogues are used as antitumor agents. For example, those that interfere with the synthesis of DNA, preferentially kill rapidly dividing tumor cells. Some of the commonly used nucleotide analogues as chemotherapeutic drugs are 6-mercaptopurine, 5-fluorouracil, 5-iodo-2'-deoxyuridine and 6-thioguanine (Fig. 37.6). Each of these compounds disrupts the normal replication process by interfering with the correct formation of Watson-Crick base-pairing.

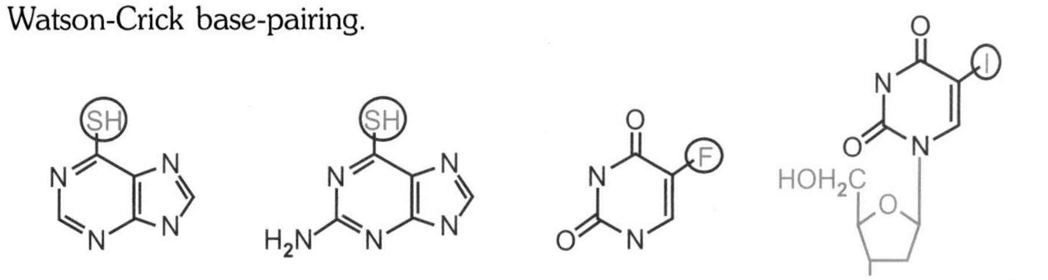

6-Mercaptopurine   6-Thioguanine   5-Flurouracil   5-Iodo-deoxyuridine

Fig. 37.6: Synthetic nucleotide analogs

Nucleotide analogs are used also as antiviral agents. Several analogs are used to interfere with the replication of HIV, such as azothioprine (Fig. 37.7)). Several purine analogs are also used to treat gout. The most common is allopurinol, which resembles hypoxanthine (Fig. 37.7). Allopurinol inhibits the activity of *xanthine oxidase*, an enzyme involved in *de novo* purine biosynthesis.

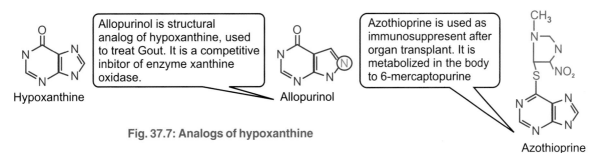

Hypoxanthine

Allopurinol is structural analog of hypoxanthine, used to treat Gout. It is a competitive inbitor of enzyme xanthine oxidase.

Allopurinol

Azothioprine is used as immunosuppresent after organ transplant. It is metabolized in the body to 6-mercaptopurine

Azothioprine

Fig. 37.7: Analogs of hypoxanthine

Administration of allopurinol, which is a structural analog of hypoxanthine, competitively inhibits xanthine oxidase and leads to accumulation of xanthine and hypoxanthine; these compounds being more water-soluble are excreted in urine.

Both cytarabine and vidarabine, the structural analogs of cytosine and adenosine respectively, have arabinose rather than ribose as their sugar moiety (Fig. 37.8). Hence they are used in chemotherapy of cancer and viral infections. 5-deoxyuridine, a structural analog of uracil is used to treat herpetic keratitis.

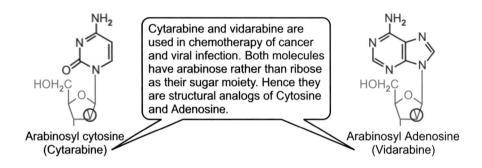

Fig. 37.8: Structural analogs of cytidine and adenosine

Additionally, several nucleotide analogues such as azathioprine (metabolized in the body to 6-mercaptopurine) are used after organ transplantation in order to suppress the immune system and reduce the likelihood of transplant rejection by the host.

Unusual Bases

Unusual bases present in nucleic acids are the result of chemical modification they undergo following their synthesis (Fig. 37.9). Such chemically modified bases.offer protection against the enzymes that hydrolyze nucleic acids; as well they have certain regulatory role in regulation of DNA functions.

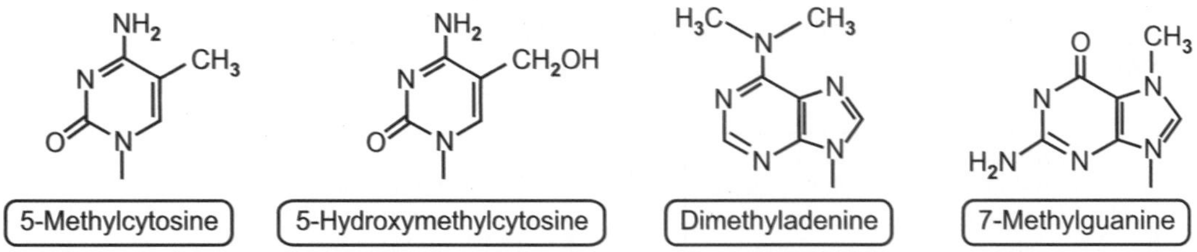

Fig. 37.9: Unusual naturally occurring bases

Nucleotide Metabolism

38

The metabolic requirements for the synthesis of nucleotides and their bases (purines and pyrimidines) are met by both *dietary intake* and *de novo synthesis* from low molecular weight precursors. The ability to salvage nucleotides from sources within the body spares any nutritional requirement for nucleotides, thus the purine and pyrimidine bases are not essentially required in the diet. In fact the salvage pathways are the major source of nucleotides for synthesis of DNA, RNA and enzyme cofactors.

Dietary nucleic acids are degraded in the small intestine by pancreatic enzymes. The combined actions of **endonucleases**, **phosphodiesterases** and **nucleoside phosphorylases** effectively hydrolyze the dietary nucleic acids. Endonucleases degrade DNA and RNA at internal sites leading to the production of oligonucleotides, which are further degraded by phosphodiesterases that act from the ends inward yielding free nucleosides. The bases are removed from nucleosides by the action of phosphorylases that yield ribose-1-P and free bases. Little dietary purine is absorbed and that which is absorbed is largely catabolized to form uric acid in man, which may serve as a scavenger of reactive oxygen species. Pyrimidine catabolism, however, produces β-aminoiosobutyrate, NH_3 and CO_2.

Both, the salvage pathway and *de novo* synthesis of purines and pyrimidines, require *5-phospho-D-ribosyl-1-pyrophosphate (PRPP)* to synthesize nucleoside-5'-phosphates, which is catalyzed by *phosphribosyltransferases*. The PRPP is formed by the action of **PRPP synthetase** that requires ribose-5-phosphate and energy in the form of ATP:

ribose-5-phosphate + ATP → PRPP + AMP

Note that this reaction releases AMP, because two high-energy phosphate equivalents are consumed during the reaction.

DE NOVO BIOSYNTHESIS OF PURINE NUCLEOTIDE

De novo synthesis of purine nucleotides utilizes the entire glycine molecule, the amino nitrogen of aspartate, amide nitrogens of

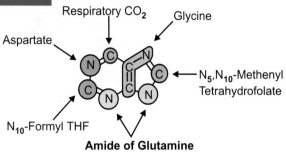

Fig. 38.1: Sources of nitrogen and carbon atoms of purine

glutamine, components of the folate one-carbon pool, carbon dioxide, ribose-5-P and a great deal of energy in the form of ATP (Fig. 38.1). Inosine monophosphate (IMP) is the first nucleotide formed during biosynthesis of purine nucleotides (Fig.38.2), which is then converted to either AMP or GMP (Fig. 38.3).

Since purines are synthesized as ribonucleotides (not as free bases), a necessary prerequisite is the synthesis of *5-phosphoribosyl-1-pyrophosphate (PRPP)*, which occurs in many tissues since PRPP has a number of roles such as nucleotide synthesis, salvage pathway, and NAD and NADP formation. The enzyme is heavily controlled by a variety of compounds such as di- and triphosphonucleotides and 2,3-DPG.

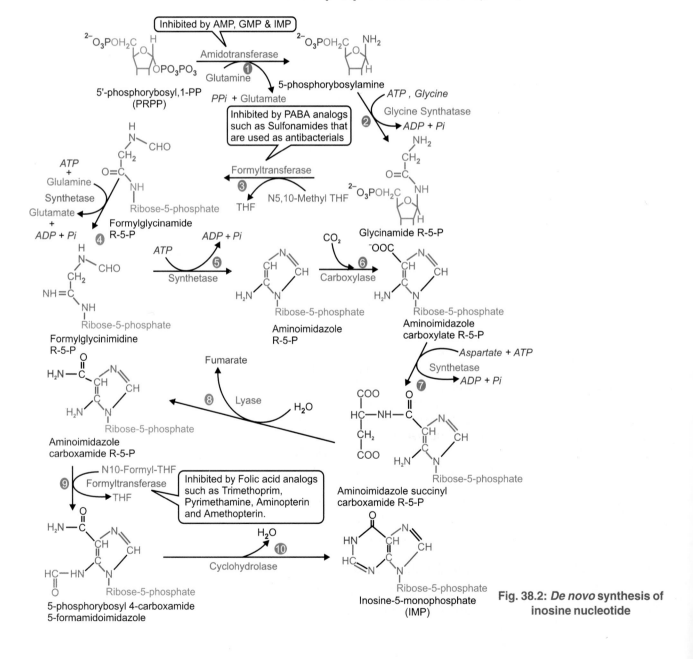

Fig. 38.2: *De novo* synthesis of inosine nucleotide

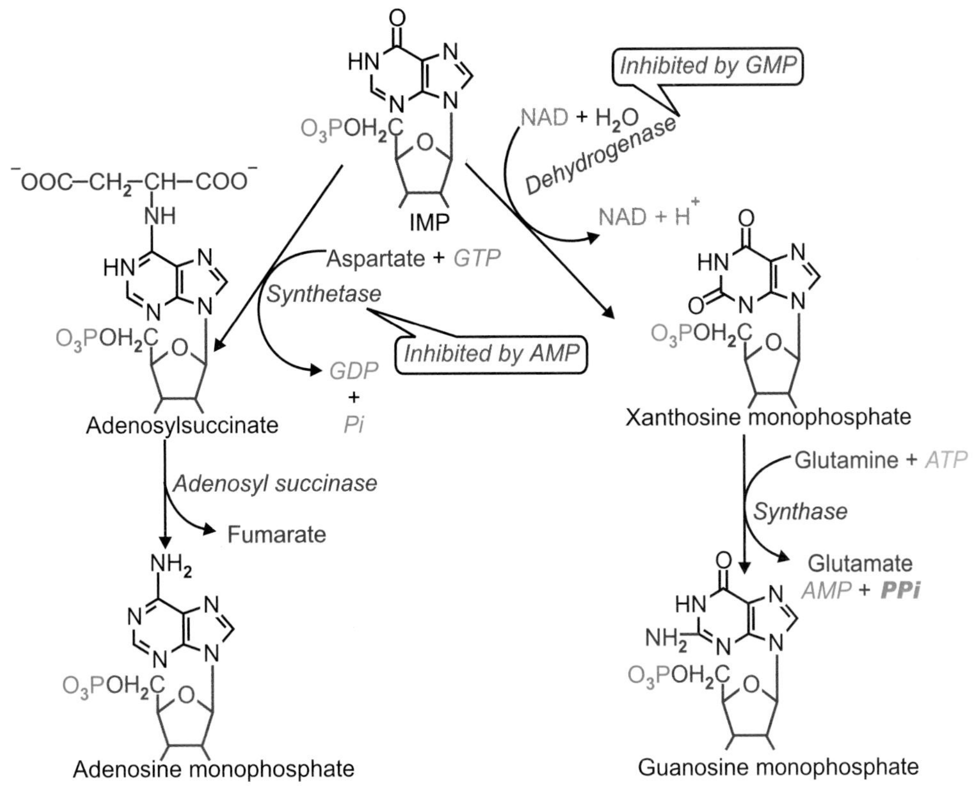

Fig. 38.3: AMP and GMP synthesis from IMP

Commitment Step

De novo synthesis of purine nucleotides occurs actively in the cytosol of the liver where all necessary enzymes are present as a macromolecular aggregate. The first step is replacement of the pyrophosphate of PRPP by the amide group of glutamine, catalyzed by *amidotransferase*. The product of this reaction is 5-phosphoribosylamine. The amine group that has been placed on carbon 1 of the sugar becomes nitrogen 9 of the ultimate purine ring. This is the commitment and rate-limiting step of the pathway.

Amidotransferase activity is under tight allosteric control by feedback inhibition. AMP, GMP, or IMP molecules alone will inhibit the amidotransferase activity, while AMP and GMP together or AMP and IMP together act synergistically to inhibit amidotransferase activity. This is a fine control and probably the major factor in minute-by-minute regulation of the enzyme. The binding of nucleotides to allosteric sites on the enzyme causes the small active enzyme molecules to form inactive macromolecular aggregates.

Intracellular concentrations of PRPP also play a role in regulating the rate. Normal intracellular concentrations of PRPP are below the K_m of the enzyme amidotransferase, hence there is great potential for increasing the rate of the reaction by increasing the PRPP concentration. The enzyme is not particularly sensitive to changes in glutamine concentrations. Very high PRPP concentrations overcome the nucleotide feedback inhibition by dissociating the large inactive aggregates of enzymes, back to the small active molecules.

Synthesis of IMP

Purine *de novo* synthesis is an energy-expensive pathway. Hence, it should be carefully controlled.

Once the 5-phosphoribosylamine is formed by the committing enzyme amidotransferase, the rest of the molecule is formed by a series of additions to make the 5- and then the 6-membered ring (Fig. 38.2). At the expense of an ATP, the whole glycine molecule adds to the amino group to provide what will eventually be atoms 4, 5, and 7 of the purine ring (The amino group of 5-phosphoribosylamine becomes nitrogen N of the purine ring.) One more atom is needed to complete the five-membered ring portion and that is provided by 5,10-methenyl tetrahydrofolate.

Before ring closure occurs, the amide of glutamine adds to carbon 4 to start the six-membered ring portion (that becomes nitrogen 3). This addition requires ATP. Another ATP is required to join carbon 8 and nitrogen 9 to form the five-membered ring.

The next step is the addition of carbon dioxide (as a carboxyl group) to form carbon 6 of the ring. The amine group of aspartate adds to the carboxyl group with a subsequent removal of fumarate. This amino group is the nitrogen 1 of the final ring. This process, which is typical for the use of the amino group of aspartate, requires ATP. The final atom of the purine ring, carbon 2 is provided by N^{10}-formyl tetrahydrofolate. Ring closure produces the purine nucleotide, IMP.

During this entire process, 4 ATPs (4 high energy phospho groups) are consumed and at no time do we have either a free base or a nucleotide.

Formation of AMP and GMP

Both AMP and GMP are formed from IMP (Fig. 38.3). Formation of GMP requires that IMP be first oxidized to xanthosine monophosphate (XMP) by an NAD dependent dehydrogenase. Then the oxygen at position 2 of IMP is substituted by amide nitrogen of glutamine at the expense of ATP. Similarly, GTP provides the energy to convert IMP to AMP, and the oxygen at position 6 of IMP is substituted by α-amino nitrogen of aspartate in a mechanism similar to that used in forming nitrogen 1 of the ring. The carbon skeleton of aspartate is removed as fumarate leaving the nitrogen behind as the 6-amino group of the adenine ring. The monophosphate forms of nucleotides are readily converted to their di- and triphosphates forms by the action of kinases.

Regulation of *De Novo* Synthesis

Regulation of purine nucleotide synthesis has two phases.
a. The first phase of control is at the amidotransferase step by nucleotide inhibition and/or PRPP concentrations regulate the synthesis as a whole.
b. The second phase of control involves the maintenance of an appropriate balance (not equality) between ATP and GTP. Each one stimulates the synthesis of the other by providing energy.

Feedback inhibition controls the branched portion, since GMP inhibits the conversion of IMP to XMP and AMP inhibits the conversion of IMP to adenylosuccinate.

One could imagine the controls operating in such a way that if only one of the two nucleotides are required, there would be a partial inhibition of *de novo* synthesis because of high levels of the other and the IMP synthesized would be directed toward the synthesis of the required nucleotide. If both nucleotides are present in adequate amounts, their synergistic effect on the amidotransferase will result in almost complete inhibition of *de novo* synthesis.

SALVAGE OF PURINE NUCLEOTIDES

Salvage pathway is the process of phosphorybosylation in which free purine bases (adenine, guanine, and hypoxanthine) and purine nucleosides are reconverted to their corresponding purine nucleotides (Fig. 38.4). Two key transferase enzymes are involved in the salvage of purines.

  i. *Adenosine phosphoribosyltransferase* (APRT) catalyzes the reaction:
    Adenine + PRPP $\leftrightarrow$ AMP + PP$_i$
  ii. *Hypoxanthine-guanine phosphoribosyltransferase* (HGPRT) catalyzes the reactions:
    Hypoxanthine + PRPP $\leftrightarrow$ IMP + PP$_i$

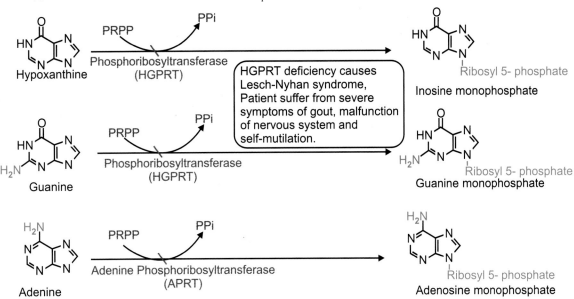

Fig. 38.4: Purine salvage pathway

    Guanine + PRPP $\leftrightarrow$ GMP + PP$_i$

Phosphorylation of purine nucleosides by kinases also contributes to the salvage of purines (Fig. 38.5), but this pathway is less significant than those catalyzed by the phosphoribosyltransferases.

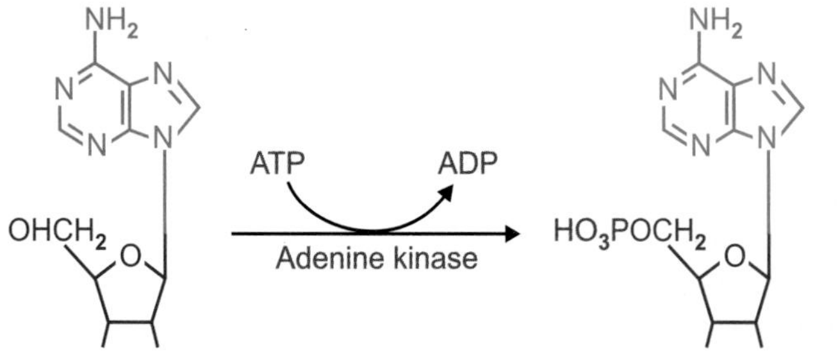

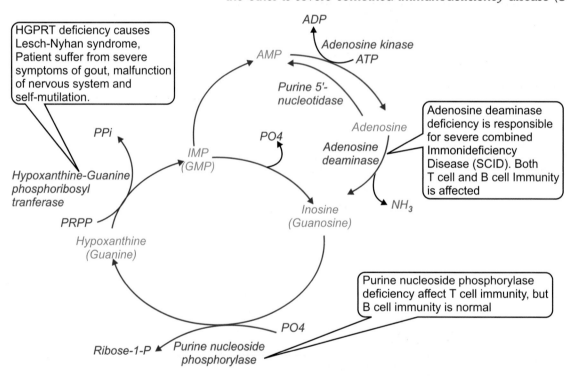

Fig. 38.5: Phosphorylation of
adenosine to AMP

Clinical Significances of Purine Metabolism

Clinical problems associated with nucleotide metabolism in humans are predominantly the result of abnormal purine catabolism. The clinical consequences of which, ranges from mild to severe or even fatal disorders. Clinical manifestations of abnormal purine catabolism arise primarily from the insolubility of the degradation byproduct (uric acid). Excess accumulation of uric acid leads to *hyperuricemia*, which is more commonly known as gout. The precipitation of sodium urate crystals in the synovial fluid of the joints, leads to severe inflammation and arthritis. Most forms of gout are the result of excess purine catabolism or of a partial deficiency in the salvage enzyme, HGPRT. Most forms of gout can be treated by allopurinol administration, which is a structural analog of hypoxanthine that strongly inhibits **xanthine oxidase**.

Two well-described severe disorders are associated with defects in purine metabolism (Fig.38.6). One is Lesch-Nyhan syndrome and the other is severe combined immunodeficiency disease (SCID).

Fig. 38.6: Purine salvage cycle involving interconversion of IMP, AMP and GMP

Lesch-Nyhan syndrome is the result of a loss of functional HGPRT gene on the X chromosome. The disorder is inherited as a sex-linked trait. Patients with this defect exhibit not only severe symptoms of gout but also a severe malfunction of the nervous system. In the most severe form, patients may resort to self-mutilation and die before the age of 20 years.

Severe combined immunodeficiency disease is caused by a deficiency in the enzyme *adenosine deaminase* (ADA) that is responsible for converting adenosine to inosine in the catabolism of the purines (Fig. 38.6). This deficiency selectively leads to destruction of B and T lymphocytes that mount immune responses. In the absence of ADA, deoxyadenosine is phosphorylated to yield levels of dATP that are 50-fold higher than normal. The levels are especially high in lymphocytes, which have abundant amounts of the salvage enzymes, including **nucleoside kinases**. High concentrations of dATP inhibit *ribonucleotide reductase;* thereby the production of other dNTPs is prevented. The net effect is inhibition of DNA synthesis. The normal response of lymphocytes to antigenic challenge is its dramatic proliferation, but the inability to synthesize DNA seriously impairs the immune responses, and the disease is usually fatal in infancy unless special protective measures are taken. A less severe immunodeficiency results when there is a lack of *purine nucleoside phosphorylase* (PNP).

One of the many glycogen storage diseases von Gierke's disease can also lead to excessive uric acid production. This disorder results from a deficiency in **glucose 6-phosphatase** activity. The increased availability of glucose-6-phosphate enhances the rate of flux through the pentose phosphate pathway that yields large quantities of ribose-5-phosphate and consequently PRPP. The increases in PRPP result in excess purine biosynthesis.

CATABOLISM OF PURINE NUCLEOTIDES

The end product of purine catabolism in humans is insoluble uric acid that is excreted in the urine as sodium urate crystals. Other mammals have the enzyme *urate oxidase*, which converts urate to more soluble allantoin as the end product. Uric acid is formed primarily in the liver and excreted by the kidney into the urine.

The catabolism of purine nucleotides has two phases. In the first phase, purine nucleotides are degraded to bases (hypoxanthine and guanine). In the second phase, the bases are converted to xanthine, which is further oxidized to uric acid (Fig. 38.7).

Nucleotides to Bases

Guanine nucleotides are hydrolyzed by 5'nucleotidase to the nucleoside guanosine, which undergoes phosphorolysis to guanine and ribose-1-P. In humans, intracellular nucleotidases are not very active toward AMP, however, AMP is deaminated by the enzyme **adenylate (AMP) deaminase** to IMP. In the catabolism of purine nucleotides, IMP is further degraded by hydrolysis with nucleotidases to **inosine** and then phosphorolysis to **hypoxanthine**.

Adenosine does occur but usually arises from S-adenosylmethionine during the course of transmethylation reactions. Adenosine is deaminated to inosine by an adenosine deaminase.

Deficiencies in either **adenosine deaminase** or in the **purine nucleoside phosphorylase** lead to two different immunodeficiency diseases by mechanisms that are not clearly understood. With **adenosine deaminase** deficiency, both T and B cell immunity is affected (Fig. 38.7). The **phosphorylase deficiency** affects the T

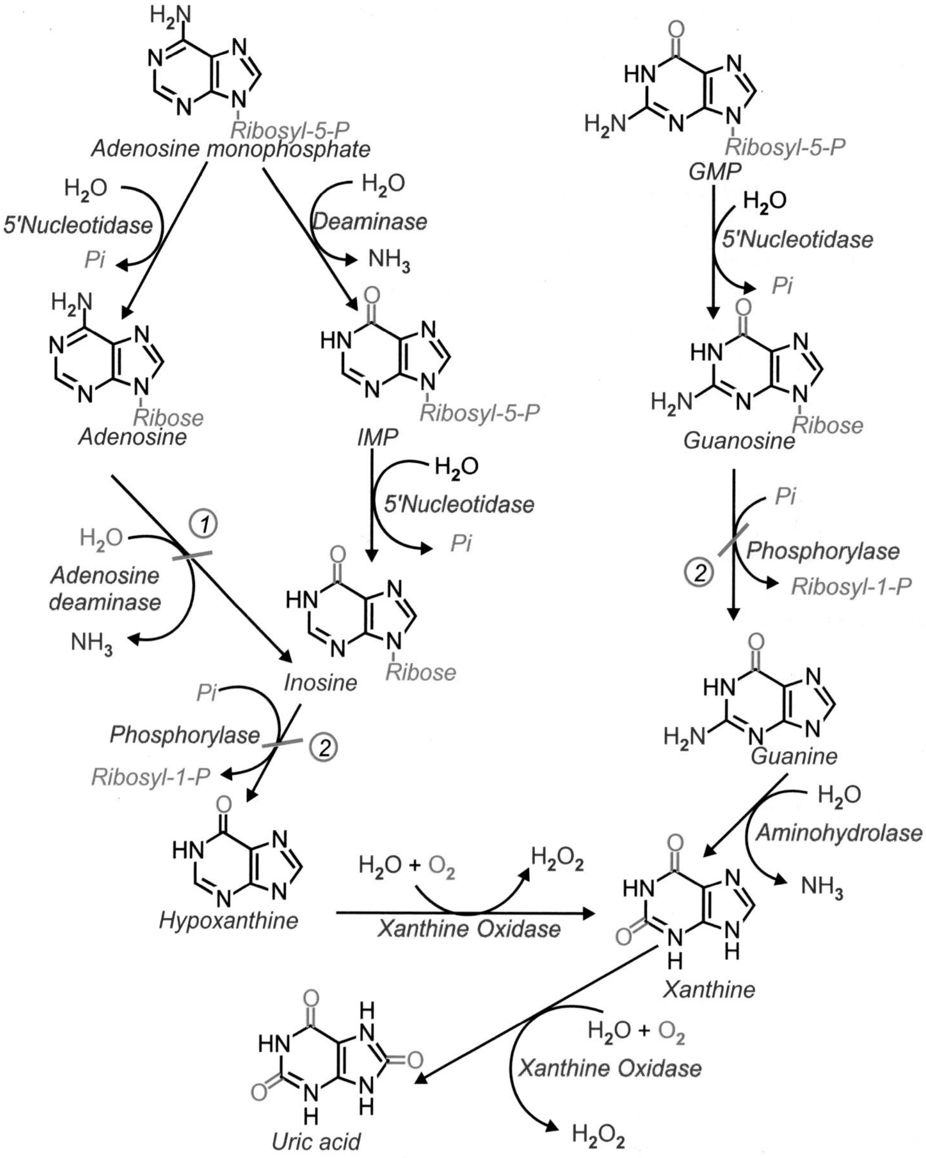

Reaction 1 is Important for T-cell and B-cell function. In severe combined immunodeficiency, build-up of dATP in erythrocytes inhibits ribonnucleotide reductase that affects DNA synthesis.

Reaction 2 is important for only T-cell function. Elevated purine nucleosides and nucleotides. Accumulation of dGTP in erythrocytes that stimulates formation of dATP, which in turn causes hypouricemia.

Hyperuricemia is the result of increased activity of phosphorybosyl synthetase or its' insensitivity to feedback inhibition, and partial deficiency or complete deficiency of HGPRTase.

Fig. 38.7: Catabolism of purine nucleotides

cells but B cells are normal. In September 1990, a 4-year-old girl was treated for *adenosine deaminase deficiency* by genetically engineering her cells to incorporate the gene. The treatment, so far, seems to be successful.

The catabolism of methylated purines depends upon the location of the methyl group. If the methyl is on an -NH₂ group it is removed along with the -NH₂ group and the core is metabolized in the usual fashion. If the methyl is on ring nitrogen, the compound is excreted unchanged in the urine.

Bases to Uric Acid

Both adenine and guanine nucleotides converge at the common intermediate xanthine. Hypoxanthine, representing the original adenine is oxidized to xanthine, by *xanthine oxidase*. Guanine is deaminated to form xanthine, with simultaneous release of the amino group as ammonia. When this process is occurring in tissues other than liver, most of the ammonia is transported to the liver as glutamine for ultimate excretion as urea.

Oxidation of xanthine, by *xanthine oxidase* and oxygen, produces urate and hydrogen peroxide. The urate is excreted in the urine and the hydrogen peroxide is degraded by catalase.

Significant concentration of xanthine oxidase is present only in liver and intestine, whereas the pathway leading to the production of nucleosides and free-bases is present in many tissues.

GOUT AND HYPERURICEMIA

Uric acid and its monosodium salt (primary form in blood) are sparingly water-soluble. Under normal conditions the limited solubility in urine is not a problem, unless the urine is highly acidic or has high calcium concentration, when sodium salts of urate co-precipitate with calcium salts and can form calculi in kidney or bladder. A very high concentration of urate in the blood leads to a fairly common group of diseases referred to as gout.

Gout is a group of pathological conditions associated with markedly elevated levels of urate in the blood (3-7 mg/dl normal). Hyperuricemia is not always symptomatic, but, in certain individuals, something triggers the *deposition of sodium urate crystals* in joints and tissues. In addition to the extreme pain accompanying acute attacks, repeated attacks lead to destruction of tissues and severe arthritic-like malformations. *The term gout should be restricted to hyperuricemia with the presence of tophaceous deposits of urate.*

Urate in the blood could accumulate either through an overproduction and/or an under excretion of uric acid. In gouts caused by an *overproduction* of uric acid, the defects are in the control mechanisms governing the production of the nucleotide precursors. The only major control of urate production that we know so far is the availability of substrates (nucleotides, nucleosides and free bases).

One common approach to the treatment of gout is the use of **allopurinol**, a structural analog of purine that directly inhibits xanthine oxidase.

Allopurinol competes with xanthine for active site on xanthine oxidase, but the product binds so tightly that the enzyme is now unable to oxidize its normal substrate. Uric acid production is diminished and the blood levels of xanthine and hypoxanthine are elevated, which are more soluble than urate and are less likely to deposit as crystals in the joints. Another approach is to stimulate the secretion of urate in the urine.

Summary

In summary, all purines except the ring-methylated purines are deaminated, in which the amino group enters the general ammonia pool and the ring is oxidized to form uric acid. Since the purine ring is excreted intact as uric acid, there is no energy benefit from these carbons.

THE PURINE NUCLEOTIDE CYCLE

During exercise the purine nucleotide cycle serves an important function in the muscle (Fig.38.8). The fumarate formed during the interconversion of IMP to AMP in this cycle provides skeletal muscle the only source of anaplerotic substrate for the TCA cycle. For continued operation of the cycle during exercise, muscle protein is utilized to supply the amino nitrogen for aspartate generation. The regeneration of aspartate occurs by the standard transamination reactions that interconvert amino acids with α-ketoglutarate to form glutamate, which in turn reacts with oxaloacetate to form aspartate.

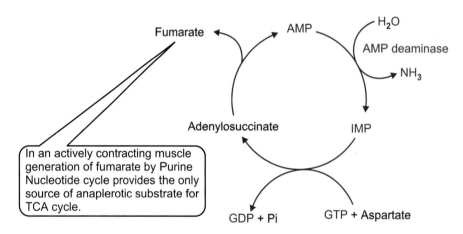

Fig. 38.8: Purine nucleotide cycle

Disorders of Purine Metabolism

Disorder	Defect	Nature of defect	Comments
Gout	PRPP synthetase	Increased enzyme activity due to elevated V_{max}	Hyperuricemia
Gout	PRPP synthetase	Enzyme is resistant to feedback inhibition	Hyperuricemia
Gout	PRPP synthetase	Enzyme has increased affinity for ribose-5-phosphate (lowered K_m)	Hyperuricemia
Gout	PRPP amido-transferase	Loss of feedback inhibition of enzyme	Hyperuricemia
Gout	HGPRT[a]	Partially defective enzyme	Hyperuricemia
Lesch-Nyhan syndrome	HGPRT	Lack of enzyme	See Text
SCID	ADA[b]	Lack of enzyme	See Text

Immuno-deficiency	PNP[c]	Lack of enzyme	See Text
Renal lithiasis	APRT[d]	Lack of enzyme	2,8-dihydroxyadenine renal lithiasis
Xanthinuria	Xanthine oxidase	Lack of enzyme	Hypouricemia and Xanthine renal lithiasis
Von Gierke's disease	Glucose-6-phosphatase	Enzyme deficiency	See above

[a]Hypoxanthine-guanine phosphoribosyltransferase; [b]adenosine deaminase; [c]purine nucleotide phosphorylase; [d]adenosine phosphoribosyltransferase

DE NOVO SYNTHESIS OF PYRIMIDINE NUCLEOTIDES

De novo synthesis of pyrimidine nucleotides is far simpler than purine nucleotides, and is still from readily available components (Fig. 38.9). The carbon dioxide and amide nitrogen of glutamine provide atoms 2 and 3 of the pyrimidine ring. They do so, however, after first being converted to carbamoyl phosphate. The other four atoms of the ring are provided by aspartate. Synthesis of pyrimidine nucleotides differs from purine nucleotides, in that the free-pyrimidine base (orotate) is first synthesized, which is then transferred on to 5'-phosphorybosyl portion of PRPP to form orotate monophosphate (OMP).

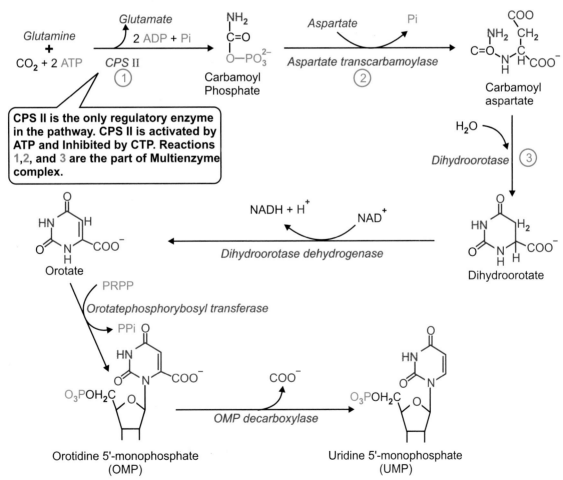

Fig. 38.9: Synthesis of uridine monophosphate (UMP)

For the purpose of understanding the synthesis of pyrimidine, nucleotides can be studied under three headings: synthesis of carbamoyl phosphate, synthesis of orotic acid and the synthesis of pyrimidine nucleotides.

Carbamoyl Phosphate Synthesis

Pyrimidine synthesis begins with the synthesis of *carbamoyl phosphate* in the cytosol of those tissues (highest in spleen, thymus, GI tract and testes) capable of synthesizing pyrimidines. This reaction is catalysed by *carbamoyl phosphate synthetase II* that is different from the mitochondrial *carbamoyl phosphate synthetase I* involved in the synthesis of carbamoyl phosphate for urea synthesis. *Carbamoyl phosphate synthetase II* (CPS II) prefers glutamine rather than free ammonia and has no requirement for N-acetylglutamate as an activator (Fig. 38.9).

Formation of Orotic Acid

Condensation of carbamoyl phosphate with aspartate is catalyzed by **aspartate transcarbamylase** that yields carbamylaspartate, which is then converted to dihydroorotate by dihydroorotase.

In humans **CPSII, asp-transcarbamylase,** and **dihydrooro-tase** activities are part of a **multifunctional enzyme protein**.

The ring of dihydroorotate is oxidized by a complex and poorly understood enzyme *dihydroorotate dehydrogenase* that produces the free orotic acid. This enzyme is located on the outer face of the inner mitochondrial membrane in contrast to the other enzymes, which are cytosolic.

Formation of the Nucleotides

Orotic acid is converted to its nucleotide orotate monophosphate (OMP) with transfer of PRPP catalysed by *orotatephosphoribosyl transferase*. OMP is then converted sequentially to other pyrimidine nucleotides. Decarboxylation of OMP yields UMP (Fig.38.9). Orotatephosphoribosyl transferase and OMP decarboxylases are also part of a multifunctional protein. After conversion of UMP to UTP by the action of kinase, the amide nitrogen of glutamine is added at the expense of ATP that yields CTP (Fig. 38.10).

Synthesis of the Thymine Nucleotides

The *de novo* pathway to dTTP synthesis first requires the use of dUMP from the metabolism of either UDP or CDP. The dUMP is converted to dTMP by the transmethylation reaction of **thymidylate synthase**. The methyl group is donated by tetrahydrofolate in a reaction similar to the donation of methyl groups during the biosynthesis of purines.

The salvage pathway to dTTP synthesis involves the enzyme **thymidine kinase** that can use either thymidine or deoxyuridine as substrate:

thymidine + ATP $\leftrightarrow$ TMP + ADP

deoxyuridine + ATP $\leftrightarrow$ dUMP + ADP

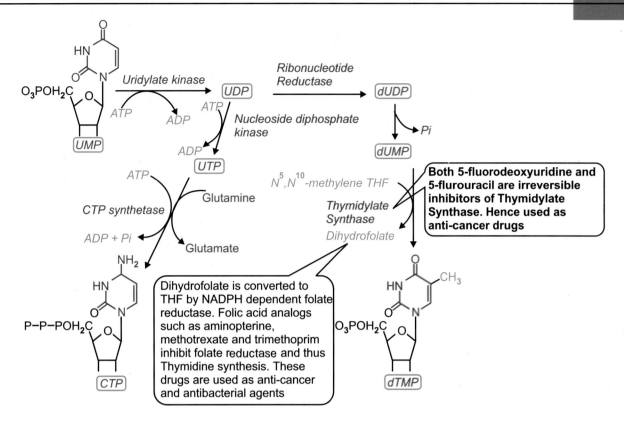

Fig. 38.10: Synthesis of CTP and TMP from UMP

The activity of **thymidine kinase** is unique in that it fluctuates with the cell cycle, the activity rising to peak during the phase of DNA synthesis and is inhibited by dTTP.

Synthesis of Cytidine Nucleotide

UDP is first converted to UTP by *Nucleotide diphosphate Kinase*. In the next step, UTP is aminated to CTP by the amide nitrogen of glutamine that requires ATP.

Clinical Relevance of Tetrahydrofolate

Tetrahydrofolate (THF) is oxidized to dihydrofolate (DHF) during TMP synthesis catalyzed by thymidylate synthase (Fig. 38.10). Tetrahydrofolate is regenerated by an NADPH dependent *dihydrofolate reductase* (DHFR). Cells that are unable to regenerate THF suffer defective DNA synthesis and eventual death. Taking advantage of this, as well as the fact that dTTP is utilized only in DNA, it is possible to therapeutically target rapidly proliferating tumor cells over nonproliferating cells through the inhibition of **thymidylate synthase**. Many anticancer drugs act directly to inhibit *thymidylate synthase*, or indirectly, by inhibiting DHFR.

The class of molecules used, to inhibit **thymidylate synthase** are called the *suicide substrates*, because they irreversibly inhibit the enzyme. Molecules of this class include *5-fluorouracil* and *5-fluorodeoxyuridine*. Both are converted within cells to *5-fluorodeoxyuridylate (FdUMP)* that inhibits **thymidylate synthase**. Many DHFR inhibitors have been synthesized, including *methotrexate*, *aminopterin*, and *trimethoprim*. Each of these is an analog of folic acid.

REGULATION OF PYRIMIDINE BIOSYNTHESIS

Pyrimidine synthesis is regulated mainly at the first step of the pathway catalyzed by *aspartate transcarbamoylase* (ATCase), which is a multifunctional protein capable of catalyzing the formation of *carbamoyl phosphate, carbamoyl aspartate*, and *dihydroorotate*. In mammalian cells ATCase is inhibited by CTP and activated by ATP. The CPS-II domain is activated by ATP and inhibited by UDP, UTP, dUTP, and CTP.

The ATCase activity is also regulated by glycine that acts as a competitive inhibitor of the glutamine-binding site. Similar to purine synthesis, ATP also regulates pyrimidine biosynthesis at the level of PRPP formation. An increase in the level of PRPP results in activation of pyrimidine synthesis.

There is also regulation of OMP *decarboxylase,* which is competitively inhibited by UMP and CMP (to a lesser degree). Finally, *CTP synthase* is feedback-inhibited by CTP and activated by GTP.

CATABOLISM OF PYRIMIDINE NUCLEOTIDES

In contrast to purines, pyrimidines undergo ring cleavage and the usual end products of catabolism are *beta-amino acids* plus *ammonia* and *carbon dioxide*. Pyrimidines are acted upon by *nucleotidases* and *nucleoside phosphorylase* to yield the free bases. The 4-amino group of both cytosine and 5-methyl cytosine is released as ammonia.

In order for the rings to be cleaved, they must first be reduced by NADPH. Atoms 2 and 3 of both rings are released as ammonia and carbon dioxide. The rest of the ring is left as a beta-amino acid (Fig.38.11). Beta-amino isobutyrate from thymine and 5-methyl cytosine is largely excreted. Beta-alanine from cytosine and uracil, may either be excreted or incorporated into the brain and muscle dipeptides, carnosine (his-β-ala) or anserine (methyl his-β-ala).

SALVAGE OF PYRIMIDINE NUCLEOTIDES

The salvage of pyrimidine bases has less clinical significance than that of the purines, since the by-products of pyrimidine catabolism are water-soluble. However, as mentioned earlier, the salvage pathway that leads to thymidine nucleotide synthesis is especially important in the preparation for cell division. Uracil can be salvaged to form UMP by the combined actions of **uridine phosphorylase** and **uridine kinase**:

$$\text{uracil} + \text{ribose-1-phosphate} \leftrightarrow \text{uridine} + P_i$$
$$\text{uridine} + \text{ATP} \rightarrow \text{UMP} + \text{ADP}$$

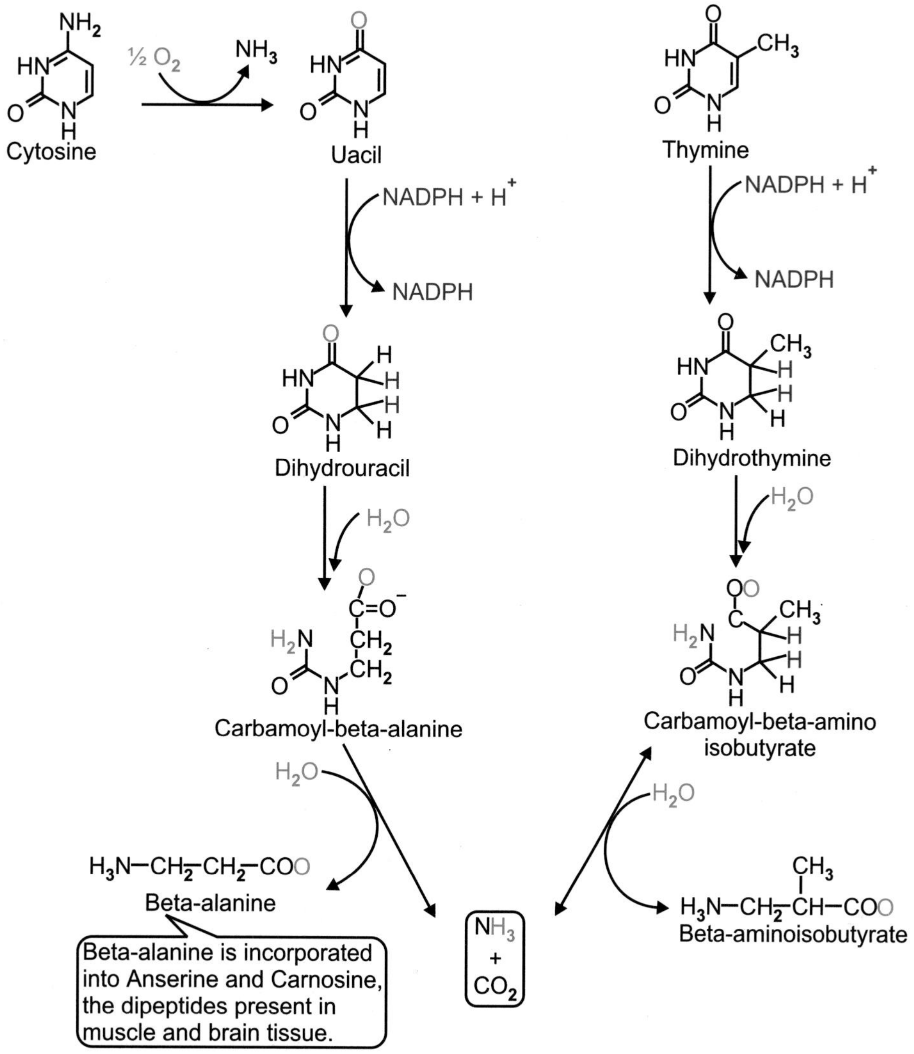

Fig. 38.11: Catabolism of pyrimidine

Deoxyuridine also is a substrate for uridine phosphorylase. Formation of dTMP, by salvage of dTMP requires ***thymine phosphorylase*** and the previously encountered thymidine kinase:

thymine + deoxyribose-1-phosphate ↔ thymidine + P$_i$
thymidine + ATP → dTMP + ADP

The salvage of deoxycytidine is catalyzed by ***deoxycytidine kinase***:

deoxycytidine + ATP ↔ dCMP + ADP

Deoxyadenosine and deoxyguanosine are substrates for deoxycytidine kinase, although the K$_m$ for these substrates is much higher than for deoxycytidine.

The main function of *pyrimidine nucleoside kinases* is to maintain a cellular balance between the concentrations of pyrimidine nucleosides and pyrimidine nucleoside monophosphates, rather than salvage of pyrimidines

Disorders of Pyrimidine Metabolism

Disorder	Defective enzyme	Comments
Orotic aciduria, Type I	Orotate phosphoribosyl transferase and OMP decarboxylase	See Text
Orotic aciduria, Type II	OMP decarboxylase	See Text
Orotic aciduria (mild, no hematologic component)	The urea cycle enzyme, ornithine transcarbamoylase, is deficient	Increased mitochondrial carbamoyl phosphate exits and augments pyrimidine biosynthesis; hepatic encephalopathy
β-aminoisobutyric aciduria	Transaminase, affects urea cycle function during deamination of α-amino acids to of α-keto acids	Benign, frequent in Orientals
Drug induced orotic aciduria	OMP decarboxylase	Allopurinol and 6-azauridine treatments cause orotic acidurias without a hematologic component; their catabolic by-products inhibit OMP decarboxylase

CLINICAL SIGNIFICANCE OF PYRIMIDINE METABOLISM

Very few disorders of pyrimidine catabolism are known, since the catabolites are water-soluble. Two inherited disorders affecting pyrimidine biosynthesis are known, due to the deficiencies in the bifunctional enzyme that catalyze the last two steps of UMP synthesis, ***orotate phosphoribosyl transferase*** and ***OMP decarboxylase***. These enzyme deficiencies result in *orotic aciduria* that causes retarded growth, leukopenia and severe anemia (hypochromic erythrocytes and megaloblastic bone marrow). These disorders can be treated with uridine and/or cytidine administration, which lead to increased UMP production via the action of nucleoside kinases. The UMP then inhibits CPS-II, thus orotic acid production stops.

FORMATION OF DEOXYNUCLEOTIDES

De novo synthesis as well the salvage pathways involve the ribonucleotides with the exception of small amount thymine salvage discussed earlier. Deoxyribonucleotides for DNA synthesis are formed from the ribonucleotide diphosphates

The protein *thioredoxin* and the enzyme *nucleoside diphosphate reductase (NDR),* reduces the 2' position on the ribosyl moiety of nucleotide diphosphate (NDP). During this reaction, the 2 sulfhydryl groups of thioredoxine get oxidized to a disulfide bond. The thioredoxin is restored to its reduced form by *thioredoxin reductase* and NADPH (Fig. 38.12).

This system is very tightly controlled by a variety of allosteric effectors. The dATP is a general inhibitor and ATP is general activator. Apart from this each pair of specific NTP and dNTP act as allosteric effectors of NDR complex. The result is maintenance of an appropriate balance of the deoxynucleotides for DNA synthesis.

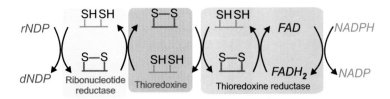

Fig. 38.12: Nucleoside diphosphate reductase complex

Synthesis of dTMP

DNA synthesis also requires dTTP that is not synthesized in the *de novo* pathway and salvage is not adequate to maintain the necessary amount. It is dTMP rather than dTTP that is generated from dUMP by methylation reaction using the folate-dependent one-carbon pool (Fig. 38.10).

Since the nucleoside diphosphate reductase is not very active toward UDP, CDP is reduced to dCDP, which is converted to dCMP. This is then deaminated to form dUMP. In the presence of **5,10-methylene tetrahydrofolate** and **thymidylate synthetase**, the carbon group is transferred to the pyrimidine ring as a reduced methyl group. The **dihydrofolate** formed during this reaction is subsequently reduced to tetrahydrofolate by the action of dihydrofolate reductase.

Regulation of dNTP Formation

All the deoxyribonucleotides are generated by the same ribonucleotide reductase. To ensure balanced production of all four of the dNTPs required for DNA replication, the activity and substrate specificity of *ribonucleotide reductase* must be tightly regulated. Such regulation occurs by nucleoside triphosphate binding to either the activity sites or the specificity sites of the enzyme complex. The ATP or dATP bind to activity site with low affinity, whereas ATP, dATP, dGTP, or dTTP bind to specificity site with high affinity. The ATP binding to activity sites leads to increased enzyme activity, while the dATP binding inhibits the enzyme. The binding of nucleotides at specificity sites effectively allows the enzyme to detect the relative abundance of the four dNTPs and to adjust its affinity for the less abundant dNTPs, in order to achieve a balance of production.

INTERCONVERSION OF NUCLEOTIDES

Nucleoside monophosphate and diphosphates are released during the catabolism of nucleic acids. The nucleosides so formed, do not accumulate to any significant degree, owing to the action of **nucleoside monophosphate (NMP) kinases** and **nucleoside diphosphate (NDP) kinases**. The NMP kinases catalyze ATP-dependent reactions of the type:

(d) NMP + ATP $\leftrightarrow$ (d) NDP + ADP

There are four classes of NMP kinases that catalyze, the phosphorylation of:

i. AMP and dAMP
ii. GMP and dGMP.
iii. CMP, UMP and dCMP.
iv. dTMP.

The enzyme adenylate kinase is important for ensuring adequate levels of energy in cells such as liver and muscle. The predominant reaction catalyzed by adenylate kinase is:

$$\textbf{2ADP} \leftrightarrow \textbf{AMP + ATP}$$

The NDP kinases catalyze reaction of the type:

$$\textbf{N}_1\textbf{TP + N}_2\textbf{DP} \leftrightarrow \textbf{N}_1\textbf{DP + N}_2\textbf{TP}$$

N_1 can represent a purine ribo- or deoxyribonucleotide, N_2 a pyrimidine ribo- or deoxyribonucleotide. The activity of the NDP kinases can range from 10 to 100 times higher than that of the NMP kinases. This difference in activity maintains a relatively high intracellular level of (d) NTPs relative to that of (d)NDPs. Unlike the substrate specificity seen for the NMP kinases, the NDP kinases recognize a wide spectrum of (d)NDPs and (d)NTPs.

Chemotherapeutic Agents

Thymidylate synthetase is particularly sensitive to availability of the folate one-carbon pool. Some of the cancer chemotherapeutic agents interfere with this process as well as with the steps in purine nucleotide synthesis involving the pool.

Cancer chemotherapeutic agents like **methotrexate** (4-amino, 10-methyl folic acid) and **aminopterin** (4-amino, folic acid) are structural analogs of folic acid that inhibit dihydrofolate reductase. Interferes with maintenance of the folate pool affects the *de novo* synthesis of purine nucleotides and of dTMP synthesis. Such agents are highly toxic and need administration under careful control.

Nucleic Acid Structure and Function

39

Nucleic acids are polynucleotides that are formed by the condensation of two or more nucleotides. The condensation occurs between the 5'-phosphate of one nucleotide and the 3'-hydroxyl of a second to form a **phosphodiester bond**. The formation of phosphodiester bonds in DNA and RNA exhibits directionality. The primary structure of DNA and RNA (the linear arrangement of the nucleotides) proceeds in the 5'→ 3' direction. The common representation of the primary structure of DNA or RNA molecules is to write the nucleotide sequences from left to right synonymous with the 5' → 3' direction, e.g.; 5'-pTpCpGpA-3' (Fig. 39.1).

Structure of DNA

Utilizing X-ray diffraction data obtained from crystals of DNA, James Watson and Francis Crick proposed a model for the structure of DNA. This model predicted that DNA would *exist as a helix of two complementary antiparallel strands*, which are wound around each other in a *right-handed direction*. The two strands are held together by *hydrogen bonding between purine and pyrimidine bases* in adjacent strands. In the Watson-Crick model, the *bases are in the interior of the helix* aligned at a nearly 90-degree angle relative to the axis of the helix (Fig. 39.1).

Experimental determination has shown that the concentration of adenine (A) is equal to thymine (T) and the concentration of guanine (G) is equal to cytidine (C) in any given DNA molecule. This means that A will only base pair with T, and G with C. According to this pattern known as *Watson-Crick base pairing*, the base pair G and C form three H-bonds, whereas the base-pair A and T form two H-bonds. This makes G-C base pair more stable than A-T base pair.

From any fixed position in the helix, one strand is oriented in the 5' → 3' direction and the other in the 3' → 5' direction. The *exterior surface* of DNA molecule has two deep grooves formed between the *ribose-phosphate chains*. These two grooves are of unequal size and are termed the *major* and *minor grooves*. The difference in their size

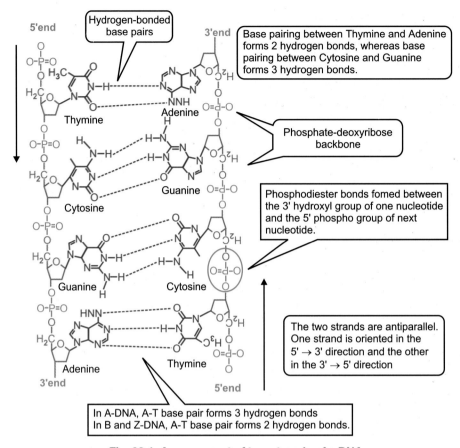

Fig. 39.1: Arrangement of two strands of a DNA

The callout boxes in Fig. 39.1 read:

- Hydrogen-bonded base pairs
- Base pairing between Thymine and Adenine forms 2 hydrogen bonds, whereas base pairing between Cytosine and Guanine forms 3 hydrogen bonds.
- Phosphate-deoxyribose backbone
- Phosphodiester bonds fomed between the 3' hydroxyl group of one nucleotide and the 5' phospho group of next nucleotide.
- The two strands are antiparallel. One strand is oriented in the 5' → 3' direction and the other in the 3' → 5' direction
- In A-DNA, A-T base pair forms 3 hydrogen bonds
  In B and Z-DNA, A-T base pair forms 2 hydrogen bonds.

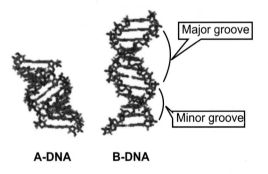

Fig. 39.2: Three different forms of DNA

is due to the asymmetry of the deoxyribose rings and the structurally distinct nature of the upper surface of base pairs relative to their bottom surface.

The double helix of DNA exists in several different forms (Fig. 39.2), depending upon *sequence, content* and *ionic conditions* of crystal preparation.

The *B-form of DNA prevails under physiological conditions* of low ionic strength and a high degree of hydration. Regions of the helix that are rich in pCpG dinucleotides can exist in a novel left-handed helical conformation termed *Z-DNA*. This conformation results from a 180-degree change in the orientation of the bases relative to that of the more common *A-DNA* and *B-DNA*.

PARAMETERS OF MAJOR DNA HELICES

When the cell divides it is necessary that its DNA is replicated (copied), in such a way that each daughter cell acquires the same amount of genetic material. For DNA to replicate, the two strands of the helix must first be separated in a process termed denaturation. The DNA can be denatured *in vitro* by heating, when the H-bonds between bases become unstable and the strands of the helix separate. This process is called thermal denaturation.

The regions of DNA duplex that are rich in G-C base pairs are stable and resistant to thermal denaturation, compared to those regions that are rich in A-T base pairs. During the process of thermal denaturation, the temperature at which 50% of the DNA molecule exists as single strands is termed *melting temperature* (T_M). This is characteristic of the base composition of DNA molecule. Higher the G-C content of DNA, higher is its melting point. The T_M depends upon several factors in addition to the base composition that includes the chemical nature of the solvent and the ionic strength.

Parameters	A Form	B Form	Z-Form
Direction of helical rotation	Right	Right	Left
Residues per turn of helix	11	10	12 base pairs
Rotation of helix per residue (in degrees)	33	36	-30
Base tilt relative to helix axis (in degrees)	20	6	7
Major groove	Narrow and deep	Wide and deep	Flat
Minor groove	Wide and shallow	Narrow and deep	Narrow and deep
Orientation of N-glycosidic Bond	Anti	Anti	Anti for Pyrimidine, Syn for Purine
Comments		Most prevalent within cells	Occurs in stretches of alternating purine-pyrimidine base pairs

When the thermally melted DNA is allowed to cool, the complementary strands will again re-form the duplex with correct base pairs. This process is termed annealing or hybridization.

ANALYSIS OF STRUCTURE OF DNA

Chromatography

Several of the chromatographic techniques available for the characterization of proteins can also be applied to characterize DNA. The most commonly used technique is high performance liquid chromatography (HPLC). Affinity chromatographic techniques can also be employed. The most commonly used affinity matrix is hydroxyapatite (a form of calcium phosphate), which binds double-stranded DNA with greater affinity than single-stranded DNA.

Electrophoresis

The molecular sieve used in electrophoresis of DNA must be different from the one used for proteins, since DNA molecules have much higher molecular weights than proteins. The material of choice is agarose (a carbohydrate polymer purified from salt-water algae), which is a copolymer of mannose and galactose that when melted and re-cooled forms a gel with pores sizes dependent upon the concentration of agarose. The phosphate backbone of DNA is highly negatively charged; therefore DNA will migrate in an electric field. The size of DNA fragments can then be determined by comparing their migration in the gel against known size standards. Extremely large DNA molecules (in excess of 106 base pairs) can also be effectively separated in pulsed-field gel electrophoresis (PFGE) using agarose gels. This technique employs two or more electrodes, placed orthogonally with respect to the gel that receive short alternating pulses of current. PFGE allows whole chromosomes and large portions of chromosomes to be analyzed.

RIBONUCLEIC ACID (RNA)

RNA molecules usually have *secondary structure,* consisting of stem and loop domains.

The *stem* is a double helical structure that arises from base pairing between complementary stretches of bases within the same strand. The presence of modified bases that prevents base pairing and lack of complementary base results in *loop* formation.

The *"cloverleaf"* model of tRNA emphasizes the two major types of secondary structure, *the* **stem** and *the loop* domains.

Transfer RNAs typically include many modified bases, particularly in the loop domains.

Tertiary structure depends on interactions among bases that are at more distant sites. Many of these interactions involve non-standard base pairing and/or interactions involving three or more bases. tRNAs usually fold into an *L-shaped tertiary structure* (Fig. 39.3).

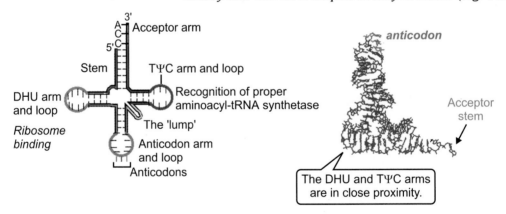

Fig. 39.3: Structure of a typical tRNA and 3D structure of tRNA

Some RNAs, including viral RNAs and segments of ribosomal RNAs fold in *pseudoknots* to form tertiary structures that mimic the 3D structure of tRNA. Pseudoknots are stabilized by tertiary (non-standard) H-bond interactions.

There are four types of ribonucleic acids (RNAs) with different functions. The tertiary structure of these different RNAs appears similar to DNA, but have several important differences:

a. RNA usually forms intramolecular base pairing
b. The information carried by RNA is not altered by these intramolecular base pairs.
c. The major and minor grooves are not pronounced

d. The structural, information adaptor, and information transfer roles of different RNAs are essential in decoding the information encoded in DNA.

The four types of RNAs are: tRNA (transfer RNA), mRNA (messenger RNA), rRNA (ribosomal RNA), and snRNA (small nuclear RNA).

Transfer RNA (tRNA)

Transfer RNA is the information adapter molecule. It is the direct interface between amino acid sequence of a protein and the information in mRNA. Therefore, it decodes the information in mRNA. More than 300 different tRNAs have been sequenced either directly or from their corresponding DNA sequences. The length of tRNAs varies from 60-95 nucleotides. The majority contains 76 nucleotides. The tRNAs from different species of organisms have a similar structure; indeed a human tRNA can function in yeast cells.

The tRNA exhibits a clover leaf-like secondary structure with 4 arms and 3 loops, the acceptor arm, T pseudouridine C (TjC) arm and loop, anticodon arm and loop and DHU arm and loop. Sometimes tRNA molecules have a lump (an extra or variable loop). Synthesis of tRNA is from two genes. The body of tRNA is transcribed from one gene and the acceptor stem of all tRNAs is transcribed by another gene, which is added after the body is transcribed. The acceptor arm is replaced often during the lifetime of a tRNA.

The tRNA molecule in its 3-D structure is folded, such that the DHU and TφC loops are in contact, and the *acceptor stem* and *the anticodon loop* occupy the opposite ends (Fig. 39.3).

The role of tRNAs in translation (protein biosynthesis) is to **carry activated amino** acids to the elongating polypeptide chain.

The features of any tRNA include (Fig. 39.3):

i. A phosphate at the 5' end.

ii. A *stem*, comparising 7 base pairs that includes the 5'-terminal nucleotide. Many base pairs in the stem are non-Watson-Crick base pairs, e.g. GU.

iii. A 3' *hydroxyl end* called the acceptor arm, with the nucleotide sequence 5'-CCA-3'. This end is called acceptor arm, since the amino acid is carried by the tRNA while attached to OH group at the 3'-end.

iv. A *dihydrouracil (DHU) loop*, which helps binding to ribosome during translation.

v. ATψC (thymidine-pseudouridine-cytidine) loop that helps recognition of proper aminoacyl-tRNA .

vi. An *anticodon loop* that has triplet nucleotide sequence, which is complementary to the triplet codon on the mRNA and interacts during translation.

Messenger RNA (mRNA)

Messenger RNA (mRNA) is the copy of the genetic information from a gene in the DNA. The role of mRNA is to carry the information contained in a gene to the translation machinery.

mRNAs are heterogeneous in size and sequence. It always has a 5' cap, composed of 7-methylguanosine and 2' O-methyl purine linked by a 5' to 5' triphosphate. The 5' cap helps the translational machinery to identify this RNA molecule as mRNA. Most mRNA molecules, also has a poly-adenosine tail at the 3' end, composed of 20-200 adenosyl residues. Both the 5' cap and the 3' tail contribute to the stability of the mRNA in the cell.

In eukaryotic cell mRNA is not made directly but is transcribed as heterogeneous nuclear RNA (hnRNA), which contains introns and exons. The introns are removed and exons spliced (joined together) that contain genetic information. Then the 5' cap and 3' tail is added. *In some cases, individual nucleotides can be added in the middle of the mRNA sequence by a process called RNA editing.* In the Figure 39.4, the exons are shown as the region of variable sequence.

The hnRNA and mRNA are always found in cells, bound to cations and proteins. Such complexes are termed ribonucleoproteins or RNPs.

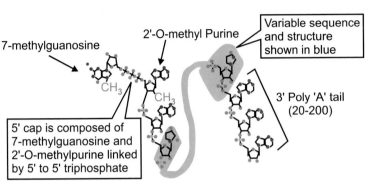

7-methylguanosine

2'-O-methyl Purine

Variable sequence and structure shown in blue

3' Poly 'A' tail (20-200)

5' cap is composed of 7-methylguanosine and 2'-O-methylpurine linked by 5' to 5' triphosphate

Fig. 39.4: Structure of mRNA

Ribosomal RNA (rRNA)

Ribosomal RNA (rRNA) molecules are extremely abundant that make up at least 80 percent of the RNA molecules found in a typical eukaryotic cell. The rRNAs are the components of ribosomes, which are protein synthetic factories (transalational machinery) in the cell. Eukaryotic ribosomes contain four different rRNA molecules designated as 18 S, 5.8 S, 28 S, and 5 S rRNA. Three of the rRNA molecules are synthesized in the nucleolus, and the other is synthesized in the cytoplasm (Fig.39.5).

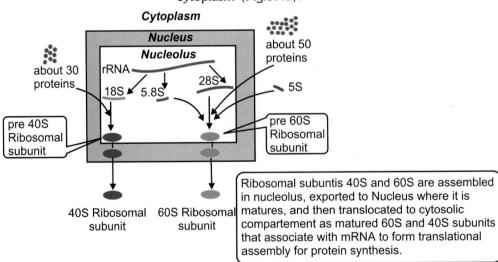

Cytoplasm

Nucleus

Nucleolus

about 30 proteins

about 50 proteins

rRNA

18S 5.8S   28S   5S

pre 40S Ribosomal subunit

pre 60S Ribosomal subunit

40S Ribosomal subunit   60S Ribosomal subunit

Ribosomal subuntis 40S and 60S are assembled in nucleolus, exported to Nucleus where it is matures, and then translocated to cytosolic compartement as matured 60S and 40S subunits that associate with mRNA to form translational assembly for protein synthesis.

Fig. 39.5: Synthesis of ribosomal subunits

Synthesis of the 3 rRNA molecules in the nucleolus is unusual, because they are made from a single primary transcript that is cleaved into three mature rRNA molecules: 18 S, 5.8 S, and 28 S. These three rRNA molecules and the 5 S rRNA synthesized elsewhere combine with ribosomal proteins in the nucleolus to form pre 40 S and pre 60S ribosomal subunits. These pre-subunits are exported to the nucleus where they mature and later transported out into cytoplasm to assume their role in protein synthesis.

The rRNA molecules have several roles in protein synthesis.

i. The 28 S rRNA has a catalytic role, it forms part of the peptidyl transferase activity of the 60 S subunit.

ii. The 18S rRNA has a recognition role, involved in correct positioning of the mRNA and the peptidyl tRNA.

iii. The rRNA molecules have a structural role. They fold into three-dimensional shapes that form the scaffold on which the ribosomal proteins assemble.

Small Nuclear RNS (snRNA)

Small nuclear RNAs (snRNA) are a group of heterogenous small RNA molecules found in the nucleus. These snRNA molecules have several important functions such as RNA splicing (removal of the introns from hnRNA) and maintenance of the telomeres (chromosome ends). They are always found associated with specific proteins and the complexes are referred to as small nuclear ribonucleoproteins (SNRNP/snurps). Many autoimmune diseases are characterized by the presence of antibodies against snurps.

RIBOSOMES

Ribosomes found in eukaryotic cytoplasm are much larger and more complex than prokaryotic ribosomes. Ribosomes found in eukaryotic mitochondria and chloroplast, differ from other ribosomes. The ribosome is the translational machinery, composed of a small subunit and a large subunit.

Ribosome source	Whole ribosome	Small subunit	Large subunit
E.Coli	70 S	30 S 16 S RNA 21 Proteins	50 S
23 S & 5 S RNAs 31 Proteins Rat Cytoplasm	80 S (S values refer to sedimentation coefficients)	40 S 18 S 33 Proteins	60 S 28S, 5.8S, & 5S RNAs 49 Proteins

Structures of the large and small subunits of bacterial and eukaryotic ribosomes have been determined, by X-ray crystallography and by cryo-electron microscopy with image reconstruction.

The schematic cut-section of translational machinery in E.coli is shown in Figure 39.6. The ribosomal assembly (80S) is composed of a large subunit (60S) shown green, and a small subunit (40S) shown blue. The peptidyl-tRNA site ('P' site), and aminoacyl-tRNA site ('A' site) are in a cleft of the smaller 40S subunit.

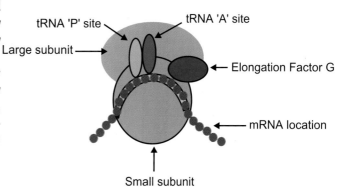

Fig. 39.6: Transalational machinery assembly

Small Ribosomal Subunit

In the translation complex, the **mRNA** threads through a tunnel within the small ribosomal subunit. The binding of mRNA to small ribosomal subunit is the function of 16S rRNA in *E.coli.* The binding sites for **tRNA** are in a cleft in the small subunit. The small ribosomal subunit is relatively flexible and assumes different conformations while interacting with other components of translational machinery. The overall shape of 30S ribosomal subunit is determined by the rRNA, which predominantly consists of double helices connected by single-stranded loops. The ribosomal proteins generally have globular domains as well as long extensions that interact with rRNA and stabilize interactions between helices of RNA.

Large Ribosomal Subunit

The interior of the large subunit is mostly composed of rRNA, while the exterior is composed of proteins. The active site domain for peptide bond formation found in larger subunit is almost devoid of protein. The 23S rRNA is a "ribozyme" that catalyzes the *peptidyl transferase* (peptide bond formation) function. A universally conserved adenosine base functions as a general acid base catalyst during peptide bond formation.

Protein synthesis takes place in a cavity within the ribosome. Nascent polypeptides emerge through a **tunnel** in the large ribosome subunit.

DNA Synthesis (Replication)

40

All living cells undergo a division during their lifespan. Some cells divide continually (e.g. stem cells), others divide a specific number of times before cell death (*apoptosis*), and still others divide a few times and then enter a terminally differentiated or quiescent state. Most cells in the body fall into one of the latter two categories. During the process of cell division, it is necessary that everything within the cell be duplicated for the daughter cells to survive. The process of an accurate, efficient and rapid duplication of the cellular genome termed *DNA replication* is of paramount importance for survival of daughter cells.

Eukaryotic Genome

Due to the complexity of the organization of eukaryotic organisms compared to prokaryotes, eukaryotic genome is also vastly larger than those of prokaryotes. However, the size of a given eukaryotic genome is not directly correlated to the complexity of the organism. This is due to the fact that a large amount of DNA in the genome is noncoding. The biological functions of these noncoding nucleotide sequences are *not fully understood*. However, some sequences are involved in the *control of gene expression* while others may simply act as an *evolutionary buffer* able to *withstand mutations* without disrupting the integrity of the organism.

The coding sequences of the genome are designated as genes. Most genes occur only once in an organism's haploid genome, hence are identified as *nonrepetitive DNA*. However, several genes exist as clusters of 50 to 10,000 copies of the same gene, as is the case for the genes coding rRNAs and histones.

The eukaryotic genes are characterized by the presence of *introns*, which are stretches of noncoding nucleotide sequences that separate the *exons*, which are the coding sequences of a gene. The existence of introns in the genes of prokaryotes is extremely rare. All human genes contain introns, with the notable exception of histone genes that are intronless. The introns separate exons into coding regions with distinct functional domains.

Chromatin Structure

The structural form in which DNA exists within cells is called *chromatin*, which is an ordered association of DNA with DNA-binding proteins. The interaction of DNA-binding proteins with DNA stabilizes the structure and organization of chromatin. There are 2 classes of DNA-binding proteins. The major class is *histones*, which are involved in maintaining the compact structure of chromatin. There are 5 different histone proteins identified as *H1, H2A, H2B, H3* and *H4*.

The other class of DNA-binding proteins is a diverse group of proteins called *nonhistone proteins,* which include various transcription factors, polymerases, hormone receptors and other nuclear enzymes. In any given cell there are more than 1000 different types of nonhistone proteins bound to the DNA.

The double-helical DNA containing approximately 150 bp forms two super helical turns around the histone octomer core, composed of two subunits each of H2A, H2B, H3 and H4 histones that form nucleosome (Fig. 40.2). The DNA stretch of 20 to 200 bp or more in between two nucleosomes is called linker DNA and the H1 histone associated with it is called linker histone. The nucleosomes with intervening linker DNA structure would appear as beads on a string if the DNAs were pulled into a linear structure (Fig. 40.1).

The beads on a string structure of nucleosomes coil into a solenoid shape which itself coils further into compact DNA. These final coils are compacted further into the characteristic chromatin seen in a karyotyping spread. The protein-DNA structure of chromatin is further stabilized by attachment to a nonhistone protein scaffold called the ***nuclear matrix.***

EUKARYOTIC CELL CYCLE

The cell cycle is the sequence of events that occur during the lifetime of a cell. The cell cycle of eukaryote is divided into four phases during which specific sequence of events occurs. The cell cycle ultimately concludes in formation of two identical daughter cells (*cytokinesis*).

The events occurring during each of the four phases of a typical cell cycle are (Fig. 40.3):

1. ***M phase*** stands for mitotic phase or mitosis, during this period cell prepares for and then undergoes cytokinesis. During mitosis, the chromosomes are paired and then divided prior to cell division. The events in this stage of the cell cycle leading to cell division are prophase, metaphase, anaphase and telophase.

2. ***G$_1$ phase*** corresponds to the gap in the cell cycle that occurs following cytokinesis. During this phase, cells make a decision to either exit the cell cycle to become quiescent or terminally differentiated or to continue dividing. Terminal differentiation is identified as a nondividing state for a cell. Quiescent and terminally differentiated cells are identified as being in G$_0$ phase. Cells in G$_0$ can remain in this state for extended periods of time. Specific stimuli may induce the G$_0$ cell to re-enter the cell cycle at the G$_1$ phase or alternatively it may induce permanent terminal differentiation.

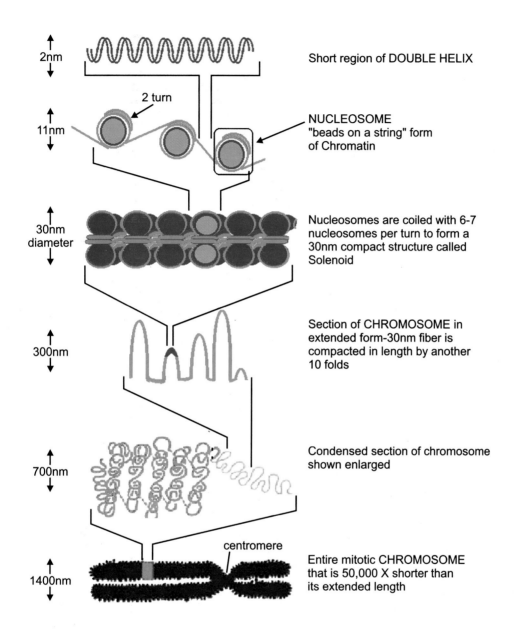

Fig. 40.1: Organization of genetic material (DNA)

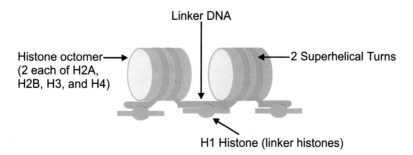

Fig. 40.2: Nucleosome organization

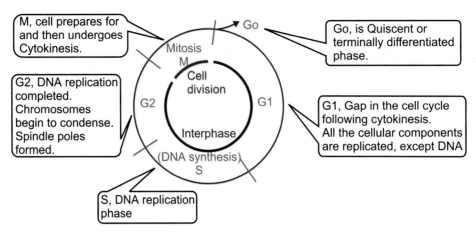

Fig. 40.3: Simple diagram of cell cycle

During G_1 cells begin synthesizing all the cellular components (except DNA replication) that is needed to form two identical daughter cells. As a result the cell size begins to increase during G_1.

3. **S phase** is the DNA synthesis phase of the cell cycle during which the DNA is replicated. Additionally, some specialized proteins particularly histones are synthesized during S phase.

4. **G_2 phase** is reached when DNA replication is completed. During G_2 the chromosomes begin to condens, the nucleoli disappear and two microtubule-organizing centers begin to polymerize tubulins for eventual formation of the spindle poles.

Typical eukaryotic cell cycles occupy approximately 16-24 hours when grown in culture. However, in the context of the multicellular organisms the cell cycles can vary from as short as 6 to 8 hours, to greater than 100 days. The cell cycle times depends on the G_1 phase of the cycle.

DNA REPLICATION

The process of DNA replication is complex that involves the activities of multiple enzymes. The DNA replication must possess a very high degree of fidelity if the daughter cells were to inherit the genetic complement that is the same as the parental cell.

In the bacterium E. coli, three distinct enzymes have been identified capable of catalyzing the DNA replication. These enzymes are designated as DNA polymerase (pol) I, II, and III. Polymerase-I is the most abundant, but its primary function is to ensure the fidelity of replication through repair of damaged and mismatched DNA. Replication of the *E. coli* genome is the job of pol-III, which is much less abundant than pol I, however, its activity is nearly 100 times that of pol I.

In eukaryotes, five distinct DNA polymerases have been identified, designated as α, β, γ, δ and ϵ. The identity of the individual enzymes relates to its subcellular localization as well as its primary replicative activity. The polymerase-α (pol-α) of eukaryotic cells is the equivalent of pol-III in *E. coli*. The pol-β of eukaryotes is equivalent of pol-I in *E.coli*. The Polymerase-γ in eukaryotes is responsible for replication of mitochondrial DNA.

The ability of *DNA polymerases* to replicate DNA requires a number of other accessory proteins. The combination of polymerases with other accessory proteins is identified as *DNA polymerase holoenzyme*. The accessory proteins of DNA replication include:

1. DNA primase
2. Processivity accessory proteins
3. Single strand DNA binding proteins
4. Helicase
5. DNA ligase
6. Topoisomerases
7. Uracil-DNA N-glycosylase

The process of DNA replication begins at specific sites in the chromosomes termed *origins of replication* that requires an RNA primer bearing a free 3'-OH. Replication proceeds specifically in the $5' \rightarrow 3'$ *direction* on both strands of DNA concurrently and results in the copying of the template strands in a *semiconservative* manner. The semiconservative nature of DNA replication means that the newly synthesized daughter strands remain associated with their respective parental template strands.

The large size of eukaryotic chromosomes, make it necessary for *multiple origins of replication* to exist in order to complete replication within a reasonable period of time. At a point of origin of replication the strands of DNA must dissociate and unwind in order to allow access to *DNA polymerase*. Unwinding of the duplex at the origin as well as along the strands as the process of replication proceeds is carried out by **helicases**. The binding of *single-strand binding* proteins to the separated DNA strand stabilizes the resultant regions of single-stranded DNA. The stabilized single-stranded regions are then accessible to the enzyme activities required for DNA replication (Fig. 40.4). The site of the unwound template strands is termed the *replication fork*.

In order for DNA polymerases to synthesize DNA they must encounter a free 3'-OH which is the substrate for attachment of the 5'-phosphate of the incoming nucleotide. During repair of damaged DNA the 3'-OH can arise from the hydrolysis of the backbone of one of the two strands. During replication the 3'-OH is supplied through the use of an *RNA primer*, synthesized by the *primase activity*. The *primase* utilizes the DNA strands as templates and synthesizes a short stretch of RNA generating a primer for DNA polymerase.

Synthesis of DNA proceeds in the $5' \rightarrow 3'$ direction through the attachment of the 5'-phosphate of an incoming dNTP to the existing 3'-OH in the elongating DNA strands with the concomitant release of pyrophosphate. Initiation of synthesis, at origins of replication, occurs simultaneously on both strands of DNA. Synthesis then precedes *bidirectional*, with one strand in each direction being copied

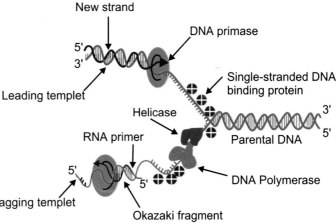

Fig. 40.4: Assembly of replication factors

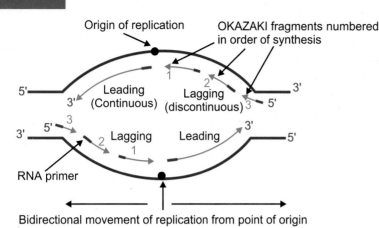

Fig. 40.5: DNA synthesis (Replication) at replication forks

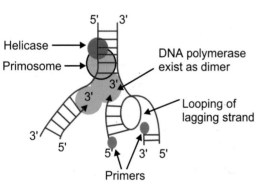

Fig. 40.6: Looping of lagging strand at replisome

continuously and one strand in each direction being copied *discontinuously* (Fig. 40.5). During the process of DNA polymerases incorporating dNTPs into DNA in the 5' →3' direction they are moving in the 3' →5' direction with relation to the template strand.

The strand of DNA synthesized continuously is termed the *leading strand* and the discontinuous strand is termed the *lagging strand*. The lagging strand of DNA is composed of short stretches of RNA primer plus newly synthesized DNA approximately 100-200 bases long (the approximate distance between adjacent nucleosomes). The lagging strands of DNA are called *Okazaki fragments*. The concept of continuous strand synthesis is somewhat of a misnomer since DNA polymerases do not remain associated with a template strand indefinitely. The ability of a particular polymerase to remain associated with the template strand is termed its' *processivity*. The longer it associates the higher the processivity of the enzyme. DNA polymerase processivity is enhanced by additional protein activities of the *replisome* identified as *processivity accessory proteins*.

The DNA polymerase can copy both strands of DNA in the 5' →3' direction simultaneously, because DNA polymerases exist as dimers in association with the other necessary proteins at the replication fork and identified as the *replisome* (Fig. 40.6). The template for the lagging strand is temporarily looped through the replisome such that the DNA polymerases are moving along both strands in the 3' → 5' direction simultaneously for short distances, the distance of an Okazaki fragment. As the replication forks progress along the template strands the newly synthesized daughter strands and parental template strands reform a DNA double helix. The means that only a small stretch of the template duplex is single-stranded at any given time.

The progression of the replication fork requires unwinding of the DNA duplex ahead of it. Since the eukaryotic chromosomal DNA is attached to histones the progressive movement of the replication fork causes severe torsional stress in the duplex ahead of the fork. The **DNA topoisomerases** relieve torsional stresses in DNA duplex by causing either single-stranded (*topoisomerases I*) or double-stranded (*topoisomerases II*) nicks (breaks) in the DNA backbone. These breaks in DNA strands allow unwinding of the duplex and removal of torsions. The nicks are then resealed by the *topoisomerases*.

The RNA primers that are still attached to the leading strands and Okazaki fragments are removed by *repair DNA polymerases*, which simultaneously replace the ribonucleotides with deoxyribonucleotides. The gaps that exist between the 3'-OH and the 5'-phosphate of newly synthesized fragment are sealed by **DNA ligases,** thereby replication process is completed.

Additional Activities of DNA Polymerase

The main function of *DNA polymerase* is synthesis of DNA in $5' \rightarrow 3'$ direction. However, DNA polymerases possess two important additional activities that include a $5' \rightarrow 3'$ and a $3' \rightarrow 5'$ exonuclease (bidirectional) activities (Fig. 40.7).

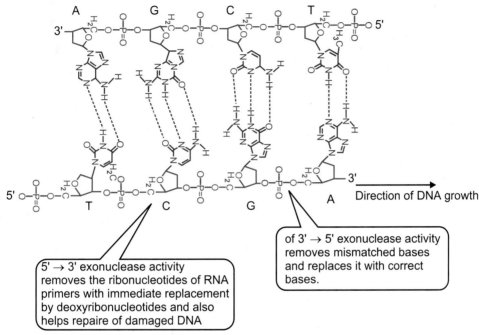

Fig. 40.7: Multifunctional activities of DNA polymerase

The $5' \rightarrow 3'$ *exonuclease activity removes the RNA primer* that initiated DNA synthesis and replaces it with deoxyribonucleotides in the $5' \rightarrow 3'$ direction (polymerase activity). The $5' \rightarrow 3'$ exonuclease activity is also required for the repair of damaged DNA.

The $3' \rightarrow 5'$ *exonuclease activity* is required to remove the mismatched bases that are incorporated during DNA replication. These mismatched bases are recognized by the polymerase immediately, since it fails to form Watson-Crick base-pairing. The mismatched base is then removed by the $3' \rightarrow 5'$ exonuclease activity and the correct base inserted prior to any further progression of replication.

CONTROL OF REPLICATION

Two control mechanisms of DNA replication have been identified, one is *licencing* (positive) and the other geminin (negative). This redundancy probably reflects the crucial importance of precise replication to the integrity of the genome.

Licensing: Positive Control of Replication

In order to be replicated, each origin of replication must be bound by an origin *recognition complex* of proteins (ORC), which remain on the DNA throughout the process (Fig.40.8). Accessory proteins called *licensing factors* accumulate in the nucleus during the G_1 phase of the cell cycle. They licencing factors Cdc6 and Cdt1, which bind

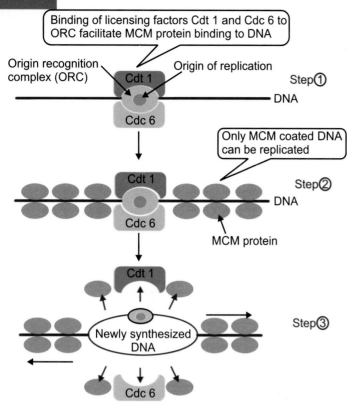

Fig. 40.8: Licensing positive control replication

to the ORC and are essential for coating the DNA with mitosis *control mechanism (MCM) proteins*. Only DNA coated with MCM proteins (there are 6 of them) can be replicated. Once replication begins in S phase, Cdt1 and Cdc6 leave the ORCs. The MCM proteins leave in front of the advancing replication fork.

Geminin: Negative Control of Replication

G_2 nuclei also contain at least one protein— called *geminin*—that prevents assembly of MCM proteins on freshly synthesized DNA (probably by removing Cdt1).

As the cell completes mitosis, geminin is degraded so the DNA of the two daughter cells will be able to respond to licensing factors and be able to replicate their DNA at the next S phase.

Some cells deliberately cut the cell cycle short allowing repeated S phases without completing mitosis and/or cytokinesis. This is called *endoreplication*.

POST REPLICATIVE MODIFICATION OF DNA

One of the major postreplicative chemical modifications the eukaryotic DNA is *methylation* of cytosine residues that are present in CpG dinucleotides. However, it should be noted that not all C residues of CpG dinucleotides are methylated. The cytidine is methylated at the 5 position of the cytosine ring generating 5-methylcytidine (Fig. 40.9).

Postreplicative DNA methylation is also observed in prokaryotic cells. The biological significance of such methylation is to prevent DNA degradation by *restriction endonucleases* that are synthesized by prokaryotes to degrade invading viral DNAs. Since the viral DNAs are not modified by methylation they are degraded by the prokaryotic restriction enzymes. The methylated prokaryotic genome is resistant to the action of these enzymes.

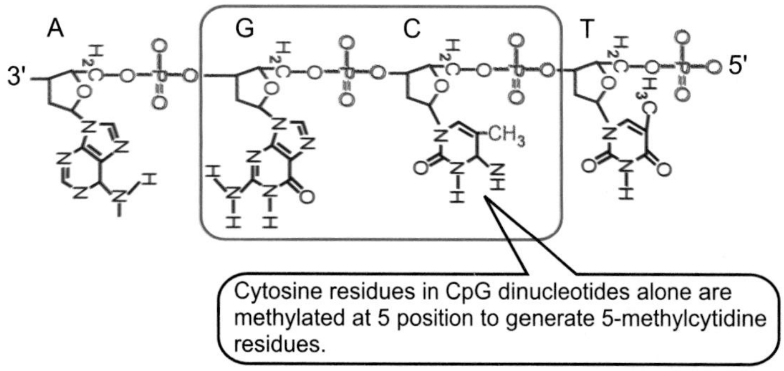

In eukaryotes, methylated DNA would be transcriptionally less active. Under-methylation of the MyoD gene (a master control gene that regulate the differentiation of muscle cells by controlling the expression of muscle-specific genes) is shown to result in the conversion of fibroblasts to myoblasts.

The pattern of methylation is copied postreplicatively by the *maintenance methylase*

Cytosine residues in CpG dinucleotides alone are methylated at 5 position to generate 5-methylcytidine residues.

Fig. 40.9: Postreplicative modification of DNA

system, which recognizes C residue methylation pattern in the maternal DNA strand and methylates the C residue present in the corresponding CpG dinucleotide of the daughter strands.

CHROMOSOMAL RECOMBINATION

The term *chromosomal recombination* refers to a process in which genetic information between two homologous chromosomes are exchanged. The new chromosomes so formed contain a mix of genetic information from each of the original chromosomes. There are three main forms of naturally occurring *genetic recombination*. They are:

i. Homologous recombination,
ii. Site-specific recombination and
iii. DNA transposition.

Homologous recombination is the process of genetic exchange that occurs between two chromosomes, which share region/regions of homologous DNA sequences (Fig.40.10). During meiosis, homologous chromosomes are exactly aligned, so that respective genes appose. Then a process of crossover occurs, so that genetic information is reciprocally exchanged. This form of recombination occurs frequently while sister chromatids are paired *during meiosis*. Indeed, it is this process of homologous *recombination between the maternal and paternal chromosomes* that imparts genetic diversity to an organism. Homologous recombination generally involves exchange of large regions of the chromosomes.

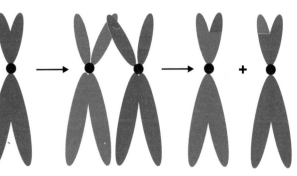

Fig. 40.10: Homologous recombination of DNA by crossing over of chromosomes

Site-specific recombination involves exchange of small regions (20 - 200 base pairs) of DNA sequence, which requires proteins that are capable of recognizing specific nucleotide sequences in the DNA. Site-specific recombination is a mechanism, meant to alter the program of genes expressed at specific stages of development. One such event in humans is the rearrangements of immunoglobulin gene in somatic cell during B cell differentiation in response to antigen presentation. These rearrangements in the immunoglobulin genes result in an extremely diverse antibody production. A typical antibody molecule is composed of both heavy and light chains. The genes coding for chains undergo somatic cell rearrangement yielding the potential for approximately 3000 different light chain combinations and approximately 5000 heavy chain combinations. The possibility of any given heavy chain combining with any given light chain, the potential diversity exceeds 10,000,000 possible different antibody molecules.

DNA Transposition is a unique form of recombination where mobile genetic elements (jumping genes/transposons) can virtually move from one region to another within a chromosome or to another chromosome. Transposition event does not require any sequence homology or specific proteins. Transposition events must be tightly regulated, since there is the possibility of disruption of a vitally important gene during this process. However, the exact nature of how transposition events are controlled is not clear.

The identification of the occurrence of transposition in the human genome resulted when it was found that certain processed genes were present in the genome. These processed genes are nearly identical to the processed mRNA encoded by the normal gene. The processed genes contain the poly (A) tail that would have been present in the RNA and they lack the introns of the normal gene.

These particular forms of genes must have arisen through a reverse transcription event, and then been incorporated into the genome by a transposition event. Since most of the processed genes that have been identified are non-functional they have been termed pseudogenes.

REPAIR OF DAMAGED DNA

The process of DNA repair is essential to correct errors and to fix damages that occur during the course of a cell's lifetime (Fig.40.11). Among all the macromolecules it is only the DNA that is repaired when damaged, instead of being replaced. The errors missed by polymerase proofreading (known to occur in prokaryotes) are removed by postreplicative repair process.

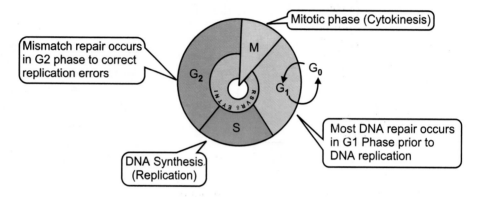

Fig. 40.11: DNA repair

Exposure to the environmental stimuli such as alkylating chemicals, UV radiation, radioactive irradiation and free radicals that are generated spontaneously in the oxidizing environment of the cell can all cause DNA damage. These phenomena lead to mutations in the coding capacity of the DNA. In addition, the spontaneous tautomerization of the bases in DNA can also cause mutations.

Multiple mutations of DNA in somatic cells can lead to the genesis of transformed phenotypes. An inability to repair DNA damage can even cause a severe condition such as nonviral induced cancer. Proper understanding of DNA repair mechanisms is essential in the design of potential therapeutic agents in the treatment of cancer.

Modification of the DNA bases by alkylation (predominately the incorporation of -CH_3 groups) occurs on purine residues. Deamination of cytidine residues generates uracil, which is an unusual base in DNA (Fig. 40.12). Methylation of G residues allows them to base pair with T instead of C. A unique activity called O^6-*alkylguanine transferase* removes the alkyl group from G residues. The protein itself becomes alkylated and is no longer active, thus, a single protein molecule can remove only one alkyl group.

Mutations in DNA are of two types. **Transition mutations** result from the exchange of one purine for another purine or one pyrimidine for another pyrimidine. ***Transversion mutations*** result from the exchange of a purine for a pyrimidine or visa versa.

The prominent by-product from **UV irradiation** of DNA is the formation of thymine dimmers (Fig. 40.13). These form two adjacent T residues in the DNA. Repair of thymine dimers is most understood from consideration of the mechanisms used in *E. coli.* However, several mechanisms are common to both prokaryotes and eukaryotes.

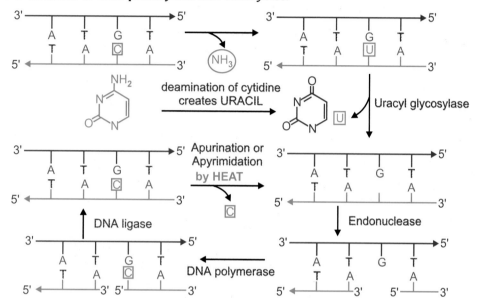

Fig. 40.12: Deamination, apurination/apyrimidation and its repair

Thymine dimers are removed by several mechanisms. Specific ***glycohydrolases*** recognize the dimer as abnormal and cleave the N-glycosidic bond of the bases in the dimer. This results in the base leaving and generates an apyrimidine site in DNA that is repaired by DNA polymerase and ligase. Glycohydrolases are also responsible for the removal of other abnormal bases, not just thymine dimers.

Another, widely distributed activity is **DNA photolyase** or **photo reactivating enzyme**, which binds to thymine dimers in the dark and cleaves pyrimidine rings in response to visible light stimulation. The chromophore associated with this enzyme that allows visible light activation is $FADH_2$.

Xeroderma pigmentosa (XP) is an autosomal recessive genetic disease due to a defect in DNA repair of thymine dimmers induced by UV radiation (Fig. 40.13). There are at least nine distinct genetic defects associated with this disease. One of these is due to a defect in the gene coding for the glycohydrolase that cleaves the N-glycosidic bond of the thymine dimers. There are two major clinical forms of XP, one that leads to progressive degenerative changes in the eyes and skin, and the other that causes progressive neurological degeneration.

Another inherited disorder affecting DNA repair in which patients suffer from sun sensitivity, short stature and progressive neurological degeneration without an increased incidence of skin cancer is *Cockayne syndrome.*

Ataxia telangiectasia (AT) is an autosomal recessive disorder

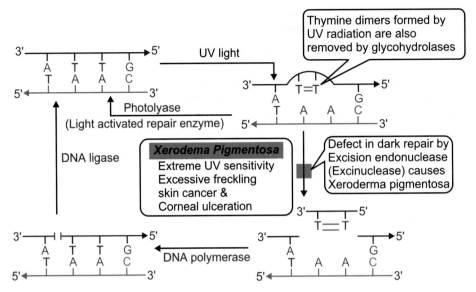

Fig. 40.13: Thymine dimer formation and repair

Ataxia telangiectasia (AT) is an autosomal recessive disorder characterized by neurological disability and suppressed immune function. These patients develop a disabling cerebellar ataxia early in life and have recurrent infections. Patients suffering from AT, also suffer from an increased sensitivity to X-irradiation, suggesting a role for the AT gene in DNA repair.

Damage	Cause	Recognition/ Excision enzyme	Repair enzyme
Thymine dimers	UV radiation	Excision endonuclease (Photolyase) activity is deficient in xeroderma pigmentosa	DNA polymerase DNA ligase
Cytosine deamination	Chemicals	Uracil glycosylase	Endonuclease DNA polymerase DNA ligase
Apurination or Apyrimidation	Spontaneous, Heat	Endonuclease	DNA polymerase DNA ligase
Mismatched bases	DNA replication error	HMSH2, hMLH1 deficient in hereditary nonpolyposis colorectal cancer (HNPCC)	DNA polymerase DNA ligase

MUTATIONS

Mutations are the permanent changes that occur in the sequence of nucleotides in a DNA molecule. Such mutations occurring in germ line are the essence of evolution; where as high rates of mutations occurring in somatic cells are undesirable.

Mutations are the result of errors in replication or recombination, or even the chemical modifications the DNA structure undergoes spontaneously or by chemicals and irradiation.

Errors in replication are mostly corrected by proof reading activity of replication and postreplicative repair system.

Errors in chromosomal recombination events (observed during translocation and rearrangement of genes as in the case of immunoglobulin gene, chromosomal crossover during meiosis, viral DNAs moving in and out of host genome, movement of mobile genes to different locations in the gene, and occasionally DNA formed by reverse transcription getting incorporated into host genome) cause no changes or a minimal change that can be repaired. However, some of the changes in DNA rearrangement cannot be repaired that lead to lethal mutations.

Mutations caused by chemicals, irradiation and spontaneous changes are discussed earlier (Repair of damaged DNA).

Types of Mutations

What ever is the cause of mutations, the types of mutations are limited. They are broadly grouped under three classes (Fig. 40.14).
i.   Substitution of base
ii. Deletion of base
iii. Insertion of base

The base substitution could be *transition* (one purine substituted by another purine or one pyrimidine substituted by another pyrimidine) or *transversion* (purine substituted by pyrimidine or vice versa). Such substitutions can result in missense, nonsense or silent mutations.

Missense mutations lead to changed codon, which results in a changed amino acid in the gene product (protein). Such a change can be of no consequence or of serious consequences as seen in sickle cell anemia.

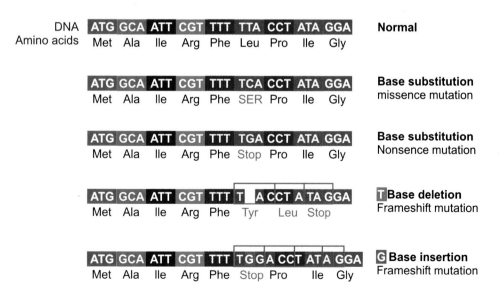

Fig. 40.14: Common types of mutations

Nonsense mutation is the result of changed codon, wherein an amino acid codon is changed to stop codon. Such mutations result in premature termination of protein synthesis that are mostly nonfunctional and can have serious consequences as seen in thalassemias.

Silent mutations are the result of base substitution that forms codon synonym, which will not alter the amino acid sequence and have no effect on the gene products.

Deletion or insertion of one or more base shifts the reading frame of codon. This results in the production of nonfunctional gene product.

RNA Synthesis (Transcription)

41

Synthesis of RNA or transcription is a polymerization reaction in which individual ribonucleotides link sequentially into a linear chain to generate one of the three different classes of RNA.

Transcription requires specific RNA polymerases, DNA template, Mg^{2+} or Mn^{2+} and four types of ribonucleotide triphosphates (rATP, rGTP, rCTP and rUTP).

The three classes of RNA are:

1. *Messenger RNAs (mRNAs)* are the genetic coding templates of the translational machinery, which determine the order of amino acids to be incorporated into an elongating polypeptide during translation.

2. *Transfer RNAs (tRNAs)* form covalent attachment to individual amino acids and recognize the encoded sequences of the mRNAs to allow insertion of correct amino acids into the elongating polypeptide chain.

3. *Ribosomal RNAs (rRNAs)* associate with numerous ribosomal proteins to form the ribosomes. Ribosomes engage the mRNAs and form a catalytic field into which the tRNAs enter with their attached amino acids. The proteins of the ribosomes catalyze all of the functions of translation.

The RNA synthesized by transcription is complimentary to the template strand of the DNA duplex and similar to the *nontemplate strand* with the exception that all the T are substituted by U. Hence the nontemplate strand is designated as coding strand.

Synthesis of RNA requires accurate and efficient initiation, elongation in the 5' → 3' direction (i.e. the polymerase moves along the template strand of DNA in the 3' →5' direction) and distinct and accurate termination.

Transcription exhibits several features that are distinct from replication.

1. Transcription does not require a primer.

2. The number of transcription initiation sites are many more than replication sites.

3. The number of RNA polymerase molecules out numbers the DNA polymerase in a given cell.
4. RNA polymerase proceeds at a rate much slower (about1/10th) than DNA polymerase.
5. The fidelity of RNA polymerization is much lower than DNA.

RNA Polymerases

RNA polymerases are some of the largest and most complex proteins in the living organisms. The overall structure of these enzymes in both prokaryotes and eukaryotes are similar; each polymerase is composed of two large polypeptides and about 6 to 10 small peptides. The two large polypeptides together with few smaller polypeptides form the enzyme core that is capable of transcribing any natural or artificial DNA sequence, into an RNA copy. The remaining smaller polypeptides restrict the enzyme capabilities, to transcribe only those natural DNAs containing a promoter and to certain gene types.

In prokaryotes, a single type of *RNA polymerase* transcribes all classes of RNA. Whereas in eukaryotes three types of RNA polymerases designated as RNA polymerase I, II and III, are involved in transcribing different classes of RNA (Table 41.1).

Table 41.1: Eukaryotic RNA Polymerase

RNA polymerase types	RNAs transcribed	Ionic requirements
I	28S, 18S, and 5.8S rRNAs	Mg^{2+}
II	mRNAs, and most snRNA	Mg^{2+}
III	tRNAs, 5SrRNA, one snRNA and scRNAs	Mn^{2+}

UPSTREAM ACTIVATION OF TRANSCRIPTION

Transcriptional *activators* bind to specific nucleotide sequence of DNA, upstream of transcriptional site to form *activator-DNA complex*. The complex so formed can recruit *chromatin remodeling* and *modifying complexes* that influence chromatin structure locally (Fig. 41.1). The chromatin remodeling increases the stability of the activator-DNA complex and also facilitates access of *promoter sequences* for binding of the *transcription apparatus*. Activators help to bind and recruit the *transcription initiation apparatus* to promoter site. Most of these processes are reversible and are regulated by *transcriptional repressors*. Activators may also influence events subsequent to assembly of the initiation apparatus such as promoter clearance and RNA polymerase processivity. The Figure 41.1 shows a single activator bound at promoter site, but promoters typically contain multiple activator binding sites.

MECHANISM OF TRANSCRIPTION

The process of replication starts when an RNA polymerase binds to the DNA template and recognizes the first base to be copied. In both

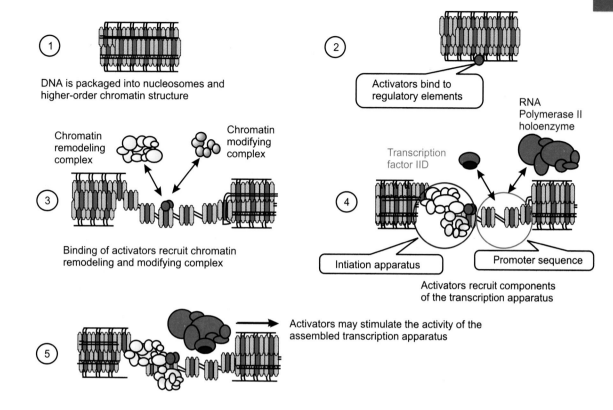

Fig. 41.1: Upstream activation of transcription

prokaryotic and eukaryotic transcription the first ribonucleotide that is incorporated is a *purine triphosphate* (rATP or rGTP). According to base-pairing rules, if guanine is present at this site, the *RNA polymerase* binds rCTP from among a pool of four ribonucleotide triphosphates (rATP, rGTP, rCTP, rUTP). The enzyme undergoes a conformational change causing it to read the next base exposed on the DNA template, which is adenine. The presence of adenine at the second site induces the enzyme to bind rUTP from the nucleotide pool. RNA polymerase then catalyzes the linking reaction, in which the last two phosphates of the second nucleotide (rUTP) are cleaved and the remaining phosphate binds to the 3'-carbon of the first nucleotide (rGTP). The reaction creates a phosphodiester linkage between the 3'-carbon of the first sugar and the 5'-carbon of the second sugar (Fig. 41.2). Removing the terminal phosphates from rUTP releases large amount of free energy that favors formation of phosphodiester linkage that is essentially irreversible. The process is then repeated and polymerization continues, by adding one nucleotide at a time into the growing chain (3' end) until the enzyme reaches the termination signal in the DNA template. Since a 5'-carbon marks the beginning and the 3'-OH marks the end of a newly synthesized RNA chain, transcription is said to proceed in the 5'→ 3' direction.

The process of transcription proceeds in three distinct phases:
Initiation: Binding of RNA polymerase to template DNA.
Elongation: Ribonucleotides are added along the DNA template.

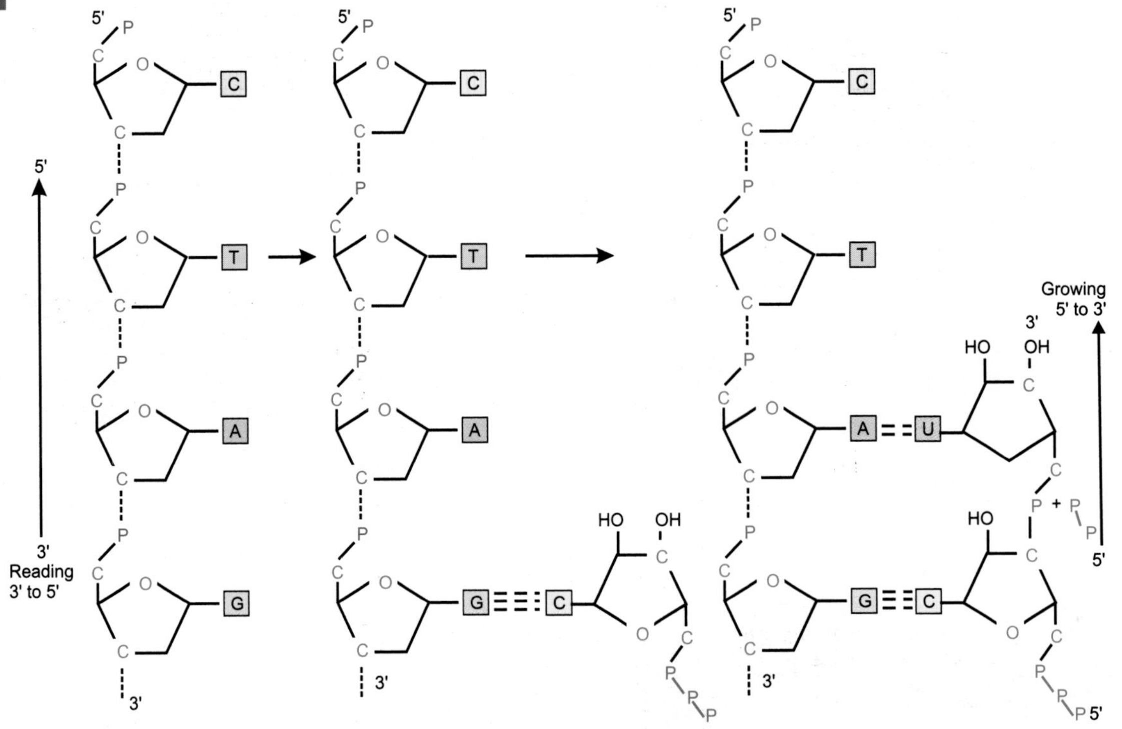

Fig. 41.2: Overall mechanism of transcription

Termination: The enzyme and the newly formed RNA are released from DNA template.

INITIATION

Random collisions between *RNA polymerase* and *DNA* lead to initiation if they occur in a specific region on the DNA designated as *promoter sequence*. This region contains *sequence elements* (TATA) that bind several transcription factors in combination with RNA polymerase and indicates the first base to be copied into an RNA transcript. The promoter sequence also includes sequences involved in regulation of transcription.

Several transcription factors called *initiation factors* are necessary for RNA polymerases to recognize and bind tightly to the promoter. Without these factors an RNA polymerase may bind loosely to DNA sequences of essentially any type without initiating RNA transcription. Evidently the initiation factors bind first to the promoter, forming an active complex that fits one or more sites on the RNA polymerase enzyme. The RNA polymerase then binds tightly to the initiation factors and the promoter that unwinds DNA in their promoter region. The transcription initiation of mRNA genes in particular, involves participation of a number of regulatory proteins that indicate, which of the many protein-encoding genes are to be copied. These proteins recognize sequences located primarily outside, but near the promoter site.

Assembly of the Transcriptional Apparatus

The promoter sequence in the template-strand of DNA contains both the TATA motif and the initiation start (Inr) region (Fig. 41.3). The

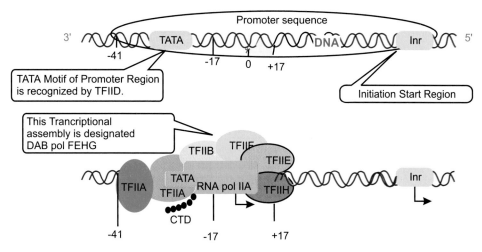

Fig. 41.3: Assembly of transcriptional apparatus

TFIID factor recognizes the TATA motif and binds to DNA that forms TATA/TFIID complex, which is recognized by TFIIA and TFIIB that binds and stabilizes the protein/DNA interaction, thereby creating the *DAB complex*. The TFIIF mediates the association of RNA polymerase II with the DAB complex to form *DABpolF*. Finally DABpolF complex is recognized by factors TFIIE, TFIIH and TFIIJ that together form DABpolFEHJ, which unwinds the DNA duplex and is capable of RNA elongation in presence of ribonucleotide triphosphates.

Of the two DNA strands fully exposed by the unwinding, only one contains the correct promoter sequences and acts as a template (Fig. 41.4). The location of the promoter sequences indicates which chain is the template by allowing attachment of the initiation complex.

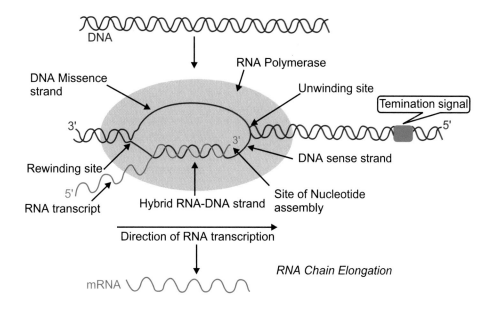

Fig. 41.4: RNA chain elongation

The template is not always the same nucleotide chain of the DNA double helix; different genes may have their template chains on either side of the DNA helix. For a given gene, however, the nucleotide chain being copied remains the same; RNA polymerase does not switch, back and forth between the two chains of the double helix within the boundaries of a gene.

Binding between *RNA polymerase* and the *promoter* is tight enough to protect the DNA in the region of contact from attack by enzymes or strong bases. This characteristic is used to identify and determine the length of the promoter through a technique called DNA footprinting. The footprint made by RNA polymerase indicates that during initiation the enzyme binds tightly to a DNA segment of about 75 base pairs, extending from about 55 nucleotides in advance of and 20 nucleotides past the first nucleotide to be copied.

In *E.coli* bacilli, RNA polymerase is composed of five distinct polypeptide chains. Association of several of these generates the *RNA polymerase holoenzyme*. The **sigma** subunit is only transiently associated with the holoenzyme. This subunit is required for accurate initiation of transcription by providing the proper cues to polymerase that a start site has been encountered. In *E.coli* several additional nucleotides are added before the *sigma subunit* disassociates.

ELONGATION

Once the first base is added, elongation begins and ribonucleotides are sequentially added that involve the addition of the 5'-phosphate of ribonucleotides to the 3'-OH of the elongating RNA with the concomitant release of pyrophosphate until the polymerase reaches the specific termination signal (Fig. 41.4). During addition of each ribonucleotide the enzyme binds a nucleotide triphosphate and matches it to the template, splits pyrophosphate (two phosphate) groups from the nucleotide, and moves to the next template base to be copied.

TERMINATION

Termination signaling sequences appear in some eukaryotic genes, such as those encoding rRNAs. In eukaryotic mRNA genes, termination may be coupled to processing reactions rather than occurring in response to specific signal sequences in the DNA. In prokaryotes, termination of transcription and separation and release of RNA polymerase, elongating factors and the transcript from the template are carried out by termination factors.

In *E.coli,* transcriptional termination occurs by both *factor-dependent* and *factor-independent* means.

Factor-dependent termination requires the termination protein rho (Fig. 41.5). The *rho factor* recognizes and binds to *termination sequences* in the 3' portion of the RNA transcript. This binding destabilizes the interaction between the *RNA*

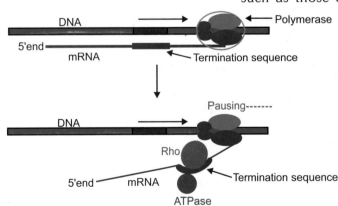

'RHO' attaches to termination sequence and interacts with polymerase. Polymerase stalls, then falls off. This reaction is ATPase dependent

Fig. 41.5: 'Rho' dependent termination of transcription

polymerase and the DNA template, leading to dissociation of the polymerase and termination of transcription. Following termination the core polymerase dissociates from the template. The core and sigma subunit can then reassociate forming the holoenzyme again ready to initiate another round of transcription.

The factor-independent termination of gene transcription in *E. coli* has two structural features (Fig. 41.6). One feature is the presence of *two symmetrical GC-rich segments* that are capable of forming a *stem-loop structure* in the RNA transcript and the second is a downstream *A rich sequence* in the template. The formation of the stem-loop in the RNA destabilizes the association between polymerase and the DNA template. This is further destabilized by the weaker nature of the AU base pairs that are formed, between the template and the RNA, following the stem-loop. This leads to dissociation of polymerase and termination of transcription. Most gene transcriptions in *E. coli* terminate by this method.

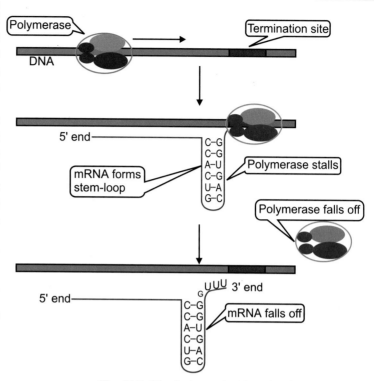

Fig. 41.6: Rho-independent termination

POSTTRANSCRIPTIONAL PROCESSING OF RNA

In bacteria, when transcription of rRNA and tRNA is completed they are ready for use in translation without any processing. Bacterial mRNA is ready for translation even before transcription is completed, because they lack nuclear-cytoplasmic separation that exists in eukaryotes. The ability of prokaryotic mRNAs to initiate translation while transcription is still in progress affords a unique opportunity for regulating the transcription of certain genes. Most of the bacterial mRNAs are *polycistronic*. This means that multiple polypeptides can be synthesized from a single primary transcript that does not occur in eukaryotic mRNAs.

All three classes of eukaryotic RNAs are transcribed from genes that contain *introns* and the initial transcript undergoes significant post-transcriptional processing. The sequences encoded by the introns of DNA must be removed from the primary transcript, before the RNAs become biologically active. The process of intron removal and joining of exons is called *RNA splicing*. The initial mRNA transcript undergoes additional processing. The 5' ends of all eukaryotic mRNAs are *capped* with a unique 5' → 5' linkage to a *7-methylguanosine* residue (Fig. 41.7). The 5' capping has two important functions, one is, it protects the capped end of mRNA from the action of exonucleases and the other is, it is recognized by specific proteins of the translational machinery

The initial mRNA transcript also undergoes polyadenylation at the 3' end. A specific sequence, *AAUAAA* is recognized by the endonuclease activity of ***polyadenylate polymerase*** that cleaves

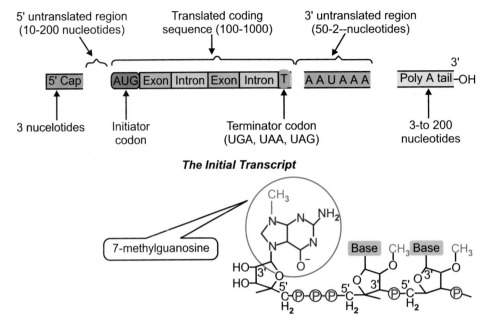

Fig. 41.7: The 5' cap of eukaryotic mRNA

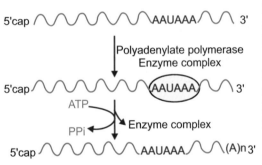

Fig. 41.8: Polyadenylation of 3' end of mRNA

the primary transcript approximately 11 - 30 bases 3' of the sequence element. A stretch of 20 - 250 A residues is then added to the 3' end by the polyadenylate polymerase activity (Fig. 41.8).

The initial tRNA transcripts, undergoes several addition processing apart from intron removal. That include cleaving of extranucleotides at both the 5' and 3' ends, addition of a *5'-CCA-3'* sequence to the 3' end of all tRNAs and chemical modification of several nucleotides. More than 60 different modified bases are identified in tRNAs.

Both prokaryotic and eukaryotic rRNAs are synthesized as long precursors termed *preribosomal RNAs*. In eukaryotes a 45S preribosomal RNA serves as the precursor for the 18S, 28S and 5.8S rRNAs.

SPLICING OF RNA

Many genes that code for proteins in eukaryotes are interrupted by regions called *introns* that do not appear in the mature mRNA. The process of intron removal from initial transcript and joining of *exons* (coding regions) is called *splicing*. The splicing mechanism must be able to recognise exon/intron boundaries so that cuts and joins can be made at the correct place.

The only feature, which is 100% conserved at intron/exon junctions is that introns begin with GU and end in AG (Fig. 41.9). The other nucleotides that are found more frequently at particular positions is shown as percentages in the Figure 41.9. Vertebrates also usually have a pyrimidine rich sequence (12Py) close to the 3' end of the intron. The intron size varies widely; only 30-40 nucleotides at each end of an intron are required for its efficient removal.

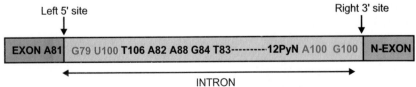

Fig. 41.9: The ends of nuclear introns are defined by GU and AG

There are four different classes of introns. The two most common are the *group I* and *group II* introns. Group I introns are found in nuclear, mitochondrial and chloroplast rRNA genes, where as group II introns are found in mitochondria and chloroplast mRNA genes. Many of the group I and group II introns are *self-splicing*, which do not require any additional protein factors for an efficient and accurate removal of introns.

Group-I Self-Splicing Introns

Group-I introns require an external guanosine nucleotide as a cofactor. The 3'-OH of the guanosine nucleotide acts as a *nucleophile* to attack the 5'-phosphate of the 5' nucleotide of the intron (Fig. 41.10). The resultant 3'-OH at the 3' end of the 5' exon then attacks the 5' nucleotide of the 3' exon releasing the intron and covalently attaching the two exons together. The 3' end of the 5' exon is termed the *splice donor site* and the 5' end of the 3' exon is termed the *splice acceptor site*.

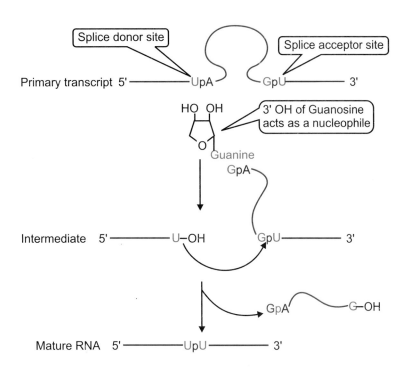

Fig. 41.10: Group I self-splicing intron

Group-II Self-Splicing Introns

Group II introns are spliced similarly except that instead of an external nucleophile the 2'-OH of an adenine residue within the intron is the nucleophile. This residue attacks the 3' nucleotide of the 5' exon forming an internal loop called a *lariat structure* (Fig. 41.11). The 3' end of the 5' exon then attacks the 5' end of the 3' exon releasing the intron and covalently attaching the two exons together.

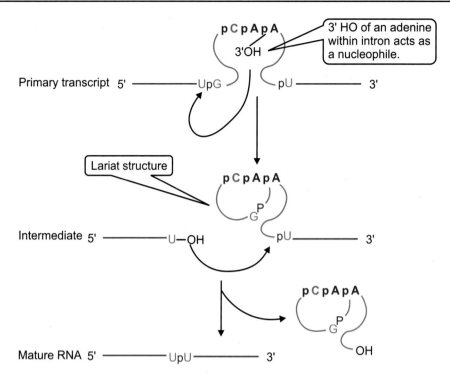

Fig. 41.11: Group-II self-splicing intron

Third Class of Introns

This class of introns found in nuclear mRNAs undergo a splicing reaction similar to group II introns, in that an internal lariat structure is formed catalyzed by specialized RNA-protein complexes called *small nuclear ribonucleoprotein particles* (snRNPs, pronounced **snurps**). The RNAs found in snRNPs are identified as U1, U2, U4, U5 and U6. The genes encoding these snRNAs are highly conserved in vertebrate and insects and are also found in yeasts and slime molds indicating their importance.

Analysis of a large number of mRNA genes has led to the identification of highly conserved consensus sequences at the 5' and 3' ends of essentially all mRNA introns.

The RNA found in U1 has sequences that are complimentary to sequences near the 5' end of the intron. The binding of U1 RNA distinguishes the GU at the 5' end of the intron from other randomly placed GU sequences in mRNAs (Fig. 41.12). The RNA found in U2 also recognizes sequences near the 3' end of intron. The addition of U4, U5 and U6 RNAs forms a complex identified as the *spliceosome* that then removes the intron and joins the two exons together.

Fourth Class of Introns

These introns found in certain tRNAs are spliced by a specific splicing endonuclease that utilizes the energy of ATP hydrolysis to catalyze intron removal and ligation of the two exons together.

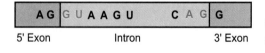

Fig. 41.12: Splicing consesus sequence

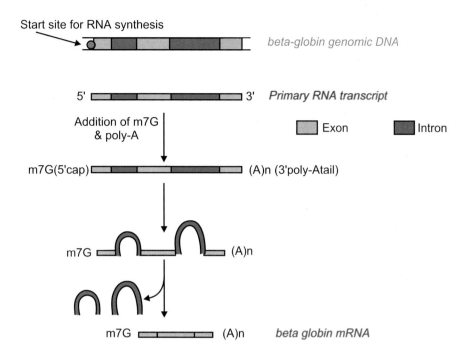

Start site for RNA synthesis

beta-globin genomic DNA

5' ⬛ 3' *Primary RNA transcript*

Addition of m7G & poly-A

☐ Exon   ⬛ Intron

m7G(5'cap) ⬛ (A)n (3'poly-Atail)

m7G ⬛ (A)n

m7G ⬛ (A)n   *beta globin mRNA*

Summary of RNA processing in eukaryotes using beta-globin gene as an example. The beta-globin gene contains three protein coding segments called exons and two intervening noncoding segments called introns. After addition of 5' methyl cap and poly-A tail, the introns are removed during splicing of exons. The sequence of the resulting mRNA corresponds to that of the protein beta-globin.

Fig. 41.13: Summary of RNA processing

CLINICAL SIGNIFICANCE OF ALTERNATE AND ABERRANT SPLICING

The presence of introns in eukaryotic genes can protect the genetic makeup of an organism from genetic damage by outside influences such as chemical or radiation. An equally important function of introns is to allow *alternative splicing*, which increases the genetic diversity of the genome without increasing the overall number of genes.

Different processed mRNAs can be obtained from a single primary transcript by altering the pattern of exons that are spliced together. Thereby different proteins can arise from a single gene. Alternative splicing can occur either at specific developmental stages or in different cell types.

Alternative splicing is known to occur in the primary transcripts from at least 40 different genes. Depending on the site of transcription, a given gene can yield different mRNA (Fig. 41.14). For example, the *calcitonin gene* in thyroid gland yields an mRNA that synthesizes *calcitonin*, whereas the same gene in brain yields *calcitonin-gene related peptide (CGRP)*. The alternative splicing that occurs in the *α-tropomyosin transcript* is more complex. At least 8 different alternatively spliced α-tropomyosin mRNAs have been identified.

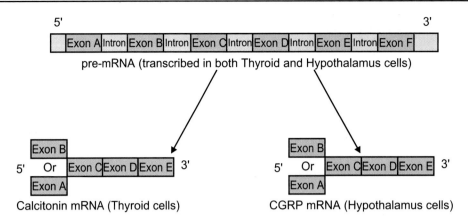

Fig. 41.14: Alternative splicing

Abnormalities in the splicing process can lead to various disease states. Many defects in the β-globin genes are known to cause β-thalassemias. Some of these defects are the result of mutations in the sequences of the gene required for intron recognition and therefore result in abnormal processing of *β-globin primary transcript*.

Patients suffering from a number of different connective tissue diseases exhibit humoral autoantibodies that recognize RNA-protein complexes. Patients suffering from systemic lupus erythematosus have autoantibodies that recognize the U1 RNA of the spliceosome that is required for splicing third class of introns discussed earlier.

Protein Biosynthesis (Translation)

42

Although the chemistry of peptide bond formation looks very simple, the biosynthetic processes leading to peptide bond formation are exceedingly complex. The RNA directed synthesis of polypeptide chain that requires all three classes of RNA is called translation. The mRNA is the *template* that decides the content and sequence of amino acid in the polypeptide chain. Yet both tRNAs and rRNAs are required for the process of translation. The tRNAs carry activated amino acids into the ribosome that associates with the mRNA to ensure access of correct activated tRNAs and possess the necessary enzymatic activities to catalyze peptide bond formation.

Genetic Code

Genetic code is the information contained in the mRNA that is needed to direct protein biosynthesis.

The genetic code is in the form of *triplet of nucleotides (codons).*

The triplets of nucleotides are groups of three adjacent bases in mRNA that specify the amino acids of protein.

Genetic code is read in a sequential manner starting near the 5' end of the mRNA. This means that translation proceeds along the mRNA in the *5'→ 3' direction that corresponds to the N-terminal to C-terminal* direction of the amino acid sequences within proteins.

Because mRNAs are composed of four different bases and each codon is a triplet of nucleotides, there are 4^3 or 64 possible codon sequences (Fig. 42.1).

Of the 64 triplets of nucleotides, 61 specify for 20 amino acids. The remaining three codons UAA, UAG and UGA are stop codons, which facilitate or code for termination of translation.

Codons are unambiguous but are degenerate. A given code either designates an amino acid or a stop signal. However, there are 61 codons for 20 amino acids, that means more than one codon can specify the same amino acid, hence code is said to be degerate.

	U		C		A		G	
U	UUU	Phe	UCU	Ser	UAU	Try	UGU	Cys
	UUC	Phe	UCC	Ser	UAC	Try	UGC	Cys
	UUA	Leu	UCA	Ser	UAA	End	UGA	End
	UUG	Leu	UCG	Ser	UAG	End	UGG	Trp
C	CUU	Leu	CCU	Pro	CAU	His	CGU	Arg
	CUC	Leu	CCC	Pro	CAC	His	CGC	Arg
	CUA	Leu	CCA	Pro	CAA	Gln	CGA	Arg
	CUG	Leu	CCG	Pro	CAG	Gln	CGG	Arg
A	AUU	Ile	ACU	Thr	AAU	Asn	AGU	Ser
	AUC	Ile	ACC	Thr	AAC	Asn	AGC	Ser
	AUA	Ile	ACA	Thr	AAA	Lys	AGA	Arg
	AUG Start	Met	ACG	Thr	AAG	Lys	AGG	Arg
G	GUU	Val	GCU	Ala	GAU	Asp	GGU	Gly
	GUC	Val	GCC	Ala	GAC	Asp	GGC	Gly
	GUA	Val	GCA	Ala	GAA	Glu	GGA	Gly
	GUG	Val	GCG	Ala	GAG	Glu	GGG	Gly

Fig. 42.1: The genetic code

The codes do not overlap. During translation the codes are read sequentially, one codon after another without spacer bases, from a fixed starting point.

Genetic code is universal. With only a very few exceptions the codons (triplet of nucleotides) are universal, that means a given code represent the same amino acid across all the living forms.

Overlapping genes. In some viruses, the expressed portions of viral genome overlap and code for multiple proteins in different reading frames.

Wobble hypothesis. As discussed earlier, 3 of the possible 64 triplet codons are translational termination codons. The remaining 61 codons are considered as being recognized by individual tRNAs. Most cells contain different tRNAs that are specific for the same amino acid. Such tRNAs are designated as **isoaccepting tRNAs**. It means, many tRNAs bind to two or three codons specifying their cognate amino acids. For example, yeast tRNAphe has the anticodon 5'-GmAA-3', which can recognize the codons 5'-UUC-3' and 5'-UUU-3'. It is therefore possible for non-Watson-Crick base pairing to occur at the third codon position, i.e. the 3' nucleotide of the *mRNA codon* and the 5' nucleotide of the *tRNA anticodon*. This phenomenon has been termed the **wobble hypothesis.**

The precise dictionary of the genetic code was determined *in vitro* with the use of translation systems and polyribonucleotides. The results of these experiments confirmed that some amino acids are encoded by more than one triplet codon, hence the degeneracy of the genetic code. These experiments also established the identity of translational termination codons.

Activation of Amino Acids

The role of tRNAs in translation is to **carry activated amino** acids to the elongating polypeptide chain. Activation of amino acids is a two-step process catalyzed by **aminoacyl-tRNA synthetases** that carries out activation of amino acids. Each tRNA, and the amino acid it carries, is recognized by individual aminoacyl-tRNA synthetases (Fig. 42.2). This means there exists at least 20 different aminoacyl-tRNA synthetases; there are actually 21 of them, since the *initiator met-tRNA of both prokaryotes and eukaryotes is distinct from noninitiator met-tRNAs.*

Activation of amino acid is the process of linking an amino acid to an appropriate tRNA. This is a two-step reaction catalyzed by *aminoacyl-tRNA synthetases* as summarized below (Fig. 42.3).

amino acid + ATP → aminoacyl-AMP + PP$_i$

aminoacyl-AMP + tRNA → aminoacyl-tRNA + AMP

In step one; the oxygen of the α-carboxyl group on the amino acid attacks the α-phosphorus of ATP that yields aminoacyl-AMP and pyophosphate.

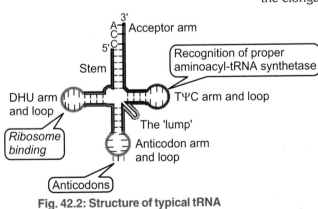

Fig. 42.2: Structure of typical tRNA

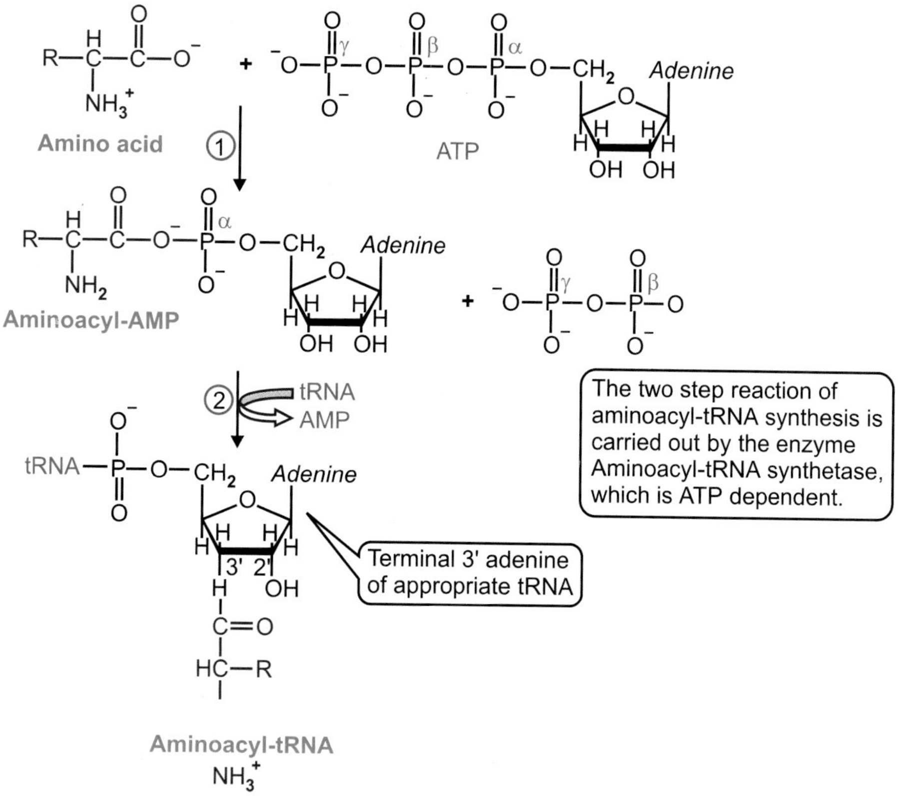

Fig. 42.3: Aminoacyl tRNA synthesis

In step two; the 2' or 3' hydroxyl of the terminal adenosine of tRNA attacks the carbonyl carbon of aminoacyl-AMP to yield aminoacyl-tRNA.

Accurate recognition of the correct amino acid and tRNA by *aminoacyl-tRNA synthetase* is an absolute prerequisite for translation process. Since R groups of amino acids differ from each other, the amino acid binding pocket on different aminoacyl-tRNA synthetases is different from one another. The exact mechanism is not known for all synthetases. However, it is likely to be a combination of the presence of specific modified bases and the secondary structure of the tRNA that is correctly recognized by the synthetases. It is absolutely necessary that the discrimination of correct amino acid and correct tRNA be made by a given synthetase prior to release of the aminoacyl-tRNA from the enzyme. Once the aminoacyl-tRNA is released there is no further way to **proofread** whether a given tRNA is coupled to its corresponding amino acid. Erroneous coupling would lead to the wrong amino acid getting incorporated into the polypeptide chain during translation. The discrimination of amino acid during protein synthesis comes from the recognition of the anticodon of a tRNA by the codon of the mRNA and not by recognition of the amino acid.

Ribosomes perform the all important functions of bringing together the charged aminoacyl-tRNAs and the mRNAs, to translate the nucleotide sequences of mRNA to amino acid sequences of polypeptide chain. Ribosomes are composed of proteins and rRNAs. The cells of all living organisms need to synthesis proteins, therefore, ribosomes are a major constituent of all cells. The make up of the ribosomes (rRNA and associated proteins) are slightly different between prokaryotes and eukaryotes.

ORDER OF TRANSLATIONAL EVENTS

Protein synthesis can take place, following assembly of small and large subunits of ribosome onto the mRNA, and an adequate supply of charged tRNAs. To review the process of protein synthesis:

1. Protein biosynthesis proceeds from the N-terminus to the C-terminus of the protein.
2. The ribosomes "read" the mRNA in the 5' → 3' direction.
3. Active translation occurs on polyribosomes (also termed polysomes). This means, at any given time more than one ribosome can be bound to and translate a given mRNA.
4. Chain elongation occurs by sequential addition of amino acids to the C-terminal end of the ribosome bound polypeptide.

Translation proceeds in an ordered process. First, an accurate and efficient *initiation* occurs, and then chain *elongation* proceeds and finally it terminates accurately and efficiently. All three of these processes require specific proteins, some of which are ribosome-associated and the others are separate from the ribosome, but may be temporarily associated with it during translation.

INITIATION

In both prokaryotes and eukaryotes, initiation of translation requires a *specific initiator tRNA*, $tRNA^{met}_i$ that incorporates the initial methionine residue into all polypeptides. In prokaryotes, a specific version of $tRNA^{met}_i$ is required to initiate translation, [$tRNA^{f\,met}_i$]. The methionine attached to this initiator tRNA is formylated. Formylation of methionine takes place after the $tRNA^{met}_i$ is formed, which requires N^{10}-formyl-THF. The $tRNA^{f\,met}_i$ is still able to recognize the AUG codon. Although $tRNA^{met}_i$ is specific for initiation it is not formylated in eukaryotes.

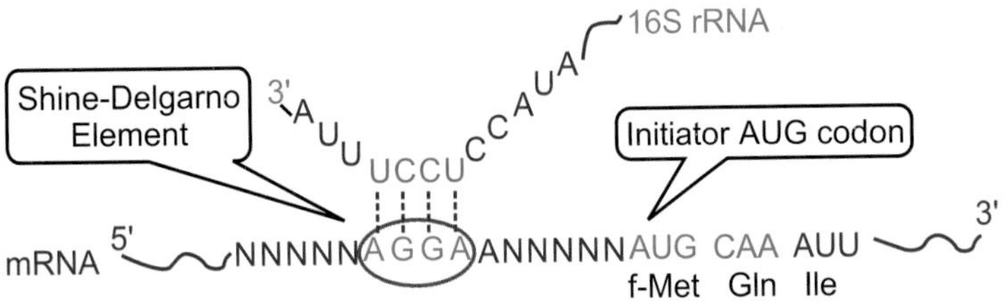

The initiation of translation requires recognition of an *initiator AUG codon*. In prokaryotic mRNAs, this initiator AUG is located on the 3' side of a *Shine-Delgarno element* (Fig. 42.4). The Shine-Delgarno element is recognized by complimentary sequences in the 16S rRNA of small subunit. In eukaryotes, a specific sequence context surrounding the initiator AUG aids ribosomal discrimination. This context is $^A/_G$**CC$^A/_G$CCAUG$^A/_G$** in most mRNAs.

An accurate initiation of translation also requires specific non-ribosomal associated proteins termed *initiation factors*. In prokaryotes, they are designated as *IFs* and in eukaryotes, they are designated as **eIFs**. Numerous eIFs have been identified.

Fig. 42.4: The Shine-Delgarno element is found on the 5' side of initiator AUG codon in prokaryotic mRNA. This element is comlementary to sequences present near the 3' end of the 16S rRNA of small ribosomal subunit of prokaryotes

Initiation Factor	Activity
eIF-1	Repositioning of met-tRNA to facilitate mRNA binding
eIF-2	Tertiary complex formation
eIF-2A	AUG dependent met-tRNA$_{met}$ binding to 40S ribosome
eIF2B (also called GEF)	GTP/GDP exchange during elf-2 recycling
eIF-3	Ribose subunit antiassociation, binding to 40S subunit
eIF-4F	mRNA binding to 40S subunit, ATPase dependent RNA helicase
eIF-A	ATPase dependent RNA helicase activity
eIF-E	5' cap recognition
eIF-G	Acts as a scaffold for the assembly of eIF-4e, 4a, and 4f complex
eIF-B	Stimulates helicase, binds simultaneously with eIF-4F
eIF-5	Release of eIF-2 and eIF-3, ribosome dependent ATPase
eIF-6	Ribosome subunit antiassociation

Initiation of translation proceeds in four specific steps:

i. Ribosome dissociate into its' 40S and 60S subunits.
ii. The preinitiation complex is formed consisting of initiator tRNA, GTP, eIF-2 and the 40S subunit.
iii. The mRNA binds to the preinitiation complex.
iv. The 60S subunit associates with the preinitiation complex to form the 80S initiation complex.

The binding of initiation factors eIF-1 and eIF-3 to the 40S subunit of the ribosome causes dissociation of 40S and 60S subunit, which allows the preinitiation complex to form.

The first step in the formation of the preinitiation complex is the binding of GTP to eIF-2 to form a binary complex, which then binds to the activated initiator tRNA^{met} to form a ternary complex. The binding of ternary complex to the 40S subunit forms the 43S pre-initiation complex. The eIF-3 and eIF-1 that are already bound to the 40S subunit stabilizes the preinitiation complex.

Specific eIFs bind to cap structure of eukaryotic mRNAs prior to its association with the preinitiation complex. Cap binding is accomplished by the initiation factor *eIF-4F*. This factor is actually a complex of 3 proteins, eIF-4E, eIF-4A and eIF-4G. The protein eIF-4E physically recognizes and binds to the cap structure, eIF-4A binds and hydrolyzes ATP and exhibits RNA helicase activity. Unwinding of the secondary structure of mRNA is necessary to allow access of the ribosomal subunits. The binding of the mRNA to the 43S preinitiation complex is facilitated by *eIF-4G*.

Once the mRNA is properly aligned to the preinitiation complex, the eIF-1 facilitates the binding of initiator met-tRNA$_{met}$ to the initiator AUG codon and the 60S subunit associates with the complex (Fig. 42.5). The association of the 60S subunit requires the activity of eIF-5, which has first bound to the pre-initiation complex. The energy needed to stimulate the formation of the 80S initiation complex comes

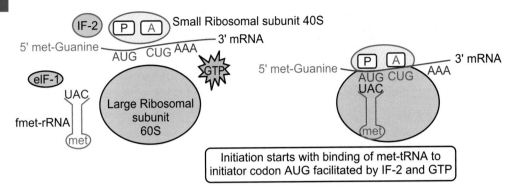

Initiation starts with binding of met-tRNA to initiator codon AUG facilitated by IF-2 and GTP

Fig. 42.5: Initiation

from the hydrolysis of the GTP bound to eIF-2. The GDP bound form of eIF-2 then binds to eIF-2B that stimulates the exchange of GTP for GDP on eIF-2. When GTP is exchanged eIF-2B dissociates from eIF-2. This is termed the *eIF-2 cycle*. This cycle is absolutely required in order for eukaryotic translational initiation to occur. The GTP exchange reaction can be affected by phosphorylation of the α-subunit of eIF-2.

At this stage the initiator met-tRNA^{met} is bound to the mRNA within a site of the ribosome termed the *P-site* (peptide site). The other site within the ribosome to which incoming charged tRNAs bind is termed the **A-site** (amino acid site).

ELONGATION

The process of elongation requires specific nonribosomal proteins called *elongation factors*. In prokaryotes, they are designated as *EFs* and in eukaryotes, they are designated as **eEFs**. Elongation of polypeptide chain occurs in a cyclic manner, such that at the end of one complete round of amino acid addition, the *A site* will be empty and ready to accept the incoming *aminoacyl-tRNA* as dictated by the next codon of the mRNA. This means that not only does the incoming amino acid need to be attached to the peptide chain but also the ribosome must move down the mRNA to the next codon. Each incoming aminoacyl-tRNA is brought to the ribosome by an *eEF-1α-GTP complex*. When the correct tRNA is deposited into the A site the GTP is hydrolyzed and the *eEF-1α-GDP complex* dissociates. In order for additional translocation events, the GDP must be exchanged for GTP. This is carried out by *eEF-1βγ* similarly to the GTP exchange that occurs with eIF-2 catalyzed by eIF-2B.

The peptide attached to the tRNA in the P site is transferred to the amino group at the aminoacyl-tRNA in the A site (Fig.42.6). This reaction is catalyzed by *peptidyltransferase*. This process is termed *transpeptidation*. The elongated peptide now resides on a tRNA in the A site. The A site needs to be freed in order to accept the next aminoacyl-tRNA.

The process of moving the peptidyl-tRNA from the A site to the P site is termed, *translocation*. Translocation is catalyzed by *eEF-2* coupled to GTP hydrolysis. In the process of translocation, the

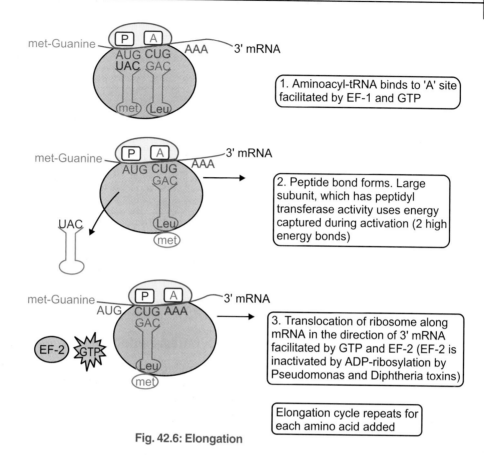

Fig. 42.6: Elongation

1. Aminoacyl-tRNA binds to 'A' site facilitated by EF-1 and GTP

2. Peptide bond forms. Large subunit, which has peptidyl transferase activity uses energy captured during activation (2 high energy bonds)

3. Translocation of ribosome along mRNA in the direction of 3' mRNA facilitated by GTP and EF-2 (EF-2 is inactivated by ADP-ribosylation by Pseudomonas and Diphtheria toxins)

Elongation cycle repeats for each amino acid added

ribosome is moved along the mRNA such that the next codon of the mRNA resides under the A site. Following translocation eEF-2 is released from the ribosome. The cycle can now begin all-again.

TERMINATION

The specific protein factors required for termination of translational are identified as *releasing factors*. There are two RFs in prokaryotes and one eRFs in eukaryotes. The termination signals are present in the mRNA as termination codons, which are same in both prokaryotes and eukaryotes (Fig. 42.7). There are three termination codons, UAG, UAA and UGA.

In prokaryotes, RF-1 recognizes the termination codons UAA and UAG, whereas RF-2 recognizes the termination codons UAA and UGA. The eRF along with GTP binds to the A site of the ribosome. The binding of eRF to the ribosome stimulates the peptidyltransferase activity to release the peptidyl group into surrounding water. The resulting uncharged tRNA left in the P site is expelled with simultaneous GTP hydrolysis. The inactive ribosome then releases its mRNA and the 80S complex dissociates to 40S and 60S subunits, which are ready for another round of translation.

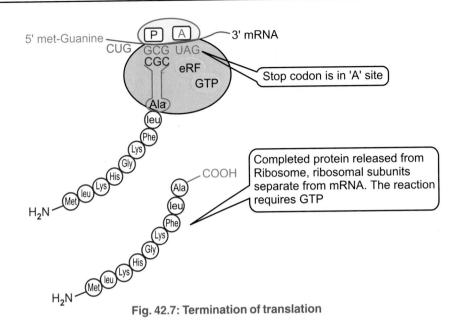

Fig. 42.7: Termination of translation

Protein Synthesis Inhibitors

Many of the antibiotics utilized for the treatment of bacterial infections as well as certain toxins function through the inhibition of translation. Inhibition can be effected at all stages of translation from initiation to elongation to termination.

Several Antibiotic and Toxins inhibit Translation

Inhibitor	Comments
Chloramphenicol	Inhibits prokaryotic peptidyltransferase
Streptomycin	Inhibits prokaryotic peptide chain initiation, also induces mRNA misreading
Tetracycline	Inhibits prokaryotic aminoacyl-tRNA binding to the ribosome small unit
Neomycin	Similar in activity to streptomycin
Erythromycin	Inhibits prokaryotic translocation through the ribosome large subunit
Fusidic acid	Similar to erythromycin only by preventing EF-G from disassociating from the large subunit
Puromycin	Resembles an aminoacyl-tRNA, interferes with peptide transfer resulting in premature termination in both prokaryotes and eukaryotes
Diphtheria toxin	Catalyzes ATP ribosylation and inactivation of eEF-2
Ricin	Found in castor beans, catalyzes cleavage of the eukaryotic large subunit rRNA
Cycloheximide	Inhibits eukaryotic peptidyltransferase

Synthesis of Selenoprotein

Selenium is a trace element and is found as a component of several prokaryotic and eukaryotic enzymes that are involved in redox reactions. The selenium in these selenoproteins is incorporated as a unique amino acid, selenocysteine during translation. A particularly important eukaryotic selenoenzyme is *glutathione peroxidase*. This enzyme is required during the oxidation of glutathione by hydrogen peroxide (H_2O_2) and organic hydroperoxides.

Incorporation of selenocysteine by the translational machinery occurs via an interesting and unique mechanism. The tRNA for selenocysteine is charged with serine and then enzymatically selenylated to produce the selenocysteinyl-tRNA.

The anticodon of selenocysteinyl-tRNA interacts with a stop codon in the mRNA (UGA) instead of a serine codon. The selenocysteinyl-tRNA has a unique structure that is not recognized by the termination machinery and is brought into the ribosome by a dedicated specific elongation factor. An element in the 3' non-translated region (UTR) of *selenoprotein mRNAs* determines whether UGA is read as a stop codon or as a *selenocysteine codon*.

Regulation of Translation

Regulation of initiation in eukaryotes is effected by phosphorylation of a ser (S) residue in the α subunit of *eIF-2*. Phosphorylated eIF-2 in the absence of eIF-2B is just as active an initiator as nonphosphorylated eIF-2. However, when eIF-2 is phosphorylated the GDP-bound complex is stabilized and exchange for GTP is inhibited. The exchange of GDP for GTP is mediated by *eIF-2B* (also called guanine nucleotide exchange factor-*GEF*). When eIF-2 is phosphorylated it binds eIF-2B more tightly thus slowing the rate of exchange. It is this inhibited exchange that affects the rate of initiation.

The phosphorylation of eIF-2 is the result of an activity called **heme-controlled inhibitor (HCI)**, which is a mitochondrial product that is generated in the absence of heme. Removal of phosphate is catalyzed by a specific *eIF-2 phosphatase* that is unaffected by heme (Fig. 42.8).

In virally infected cells, translation is regulated by induced proteins interferons, which would benefit the virally infected cell to turn off protein synthesis to prevent propagation of the viruses. In response to viral infection, the cells are induced to synthesize three classes of **interferons (IFs)**. The *leukocyte* or *α-IFs*, the *fibroblast* or *β-IFs* and the *lymphocyte* or *γ-IFs*, which are induced by dsRNAs and themselves induce a specific kinase termed **RNA-dependent protein kinase (PKR)** that phosphorylates eIF-2 thereby shutting off translation in manner similar to that of heme control of translation. Additionally, IFs induce the synthesis of **2'-5'-oligoadenylate, pppA (2'p5'A) n**, that activates a pre-existing ribonuclease, RNase L. RNase L degrades all classes of mRNAs thereby shutting off translation.

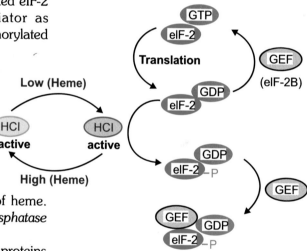

Fig. 42.8:
Regulation of translation by heme controlled inhibitor (HCI)

Protein Modifications and Targeting

43

Following translation proteins undergo proteolytic cleavage and various types of chemical modifications that make them biologically functional. The simplest form of proteolytic cleavage is the removal of methionine that is introduced to initiate translation. Many proteins of the enzyme class are synthesized as inactive precursors called **zymogens** or *proproteins*. Such proteins are activated under proper physiological conditions by limited proteolysis. Pancreatic enzymes and enzymes involved in clotting are the best examples of limited hydrolysis of proteins.

Proteolytic Cleavage

Most of the cellular proteins are synthesized in the cytosol, but those proteins destined for secretion and incorporation into membranes are synthesized by ribosomes associated with the membranes of the endoplasmic reticulum (ER). The ER associated with ribosomes is termed rough endoplasmic reticulum (RER). All proteins of this class contain an N-terminus sequence termed **signal sequence** or **signal peptide**. The signal peptide is a short stretch of 13-36 aminoacyl residues that are predominantly hydrophobic. Following the passage of this signal peptide through the ER membrane, it is recognized by a multiprotein complex termed the **signal recognition particle (SRP)** and is removed by **signal peptidase**. Proteins that contain a signal peptide are called **preproteins** to distinguish them from **proproteins**. Some secreted proteins having pro-sequences are further proteolyzed and are termed **preproproteins**.

A complex example of post-translational processing of a preproprotein is the cleavage of **prepro-opiomelanocortin (POMC)** synthesized in the pituitary. This preproprotein undergoes complex cleavages, the pathway of which differs depending upon the cellular location of POMC synthesis.

Another example of a preproprotein is **insulin**. When insulin is secreted from the pancreas it has a prepeptide. Following cleavage of the 24 amino acid signal peptide the protein folds into proinsulin, which is further cleaved to yield active insulin that is composed of two peptide chains linked together through disulfide bonds.

Glycosylation

Membrane associated carbohydrates are exclusively in the form of oliogsaccharides that are covalently attached to membrane proteins to form **glycoproteins.** To a lesser extent carbohydrates are covalently attached to membrane lipids to form **glycolipids**. The predominant sugars found in glycoproteins are glucose, galactose, mannose, fucose, GalNAc, GlcNAc and NANA. The distinction between *proteoglycans* and *glycoproteins* resides in the level and types of carbohydrate modification.

The carbohydrates are linked to protein component through either *O-glycosidic* or *N-glycosidic* bonds (Fig. 43.1). The latter is the predominant form found in mammalian cells. The N-glycosidic linkage is through the amide group of asparagine. The O-glycosidic linkage is to the hydroxyl of serine, threonine or hydroxylysine. The linkage of carbohydrate to hydroxylysine is generally found only in the collagens. The linkage of carbohydrate to 5-hydroxylysine is either the single sugar galactose or the disaccharide glucosylgalactose. In ser-and thr-type of O-linked glycoproteins, the carbohydrate that is directly attached to the protein is GalNAc. Where as in N-linked glycoproteins, it is GlcNAc.

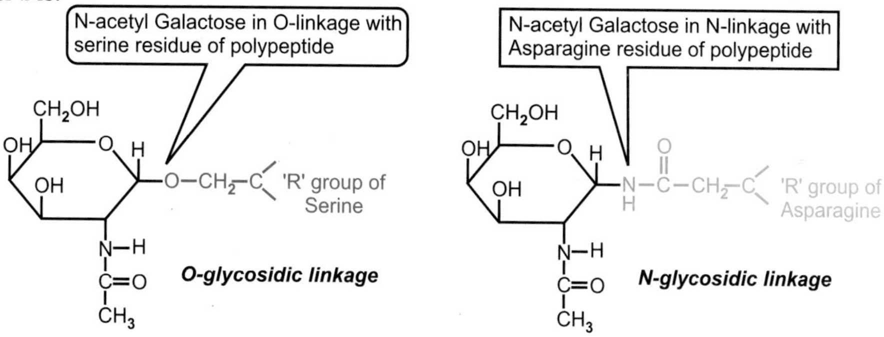

Fig. 43.1: O-glycosidic and N-glycosidic linkages

Target asparagine (Asn) residues are in the tripeptide sequence Asn-X-Ser or Asn-X-Thr where X is any amino acid other than proline. All N-linked glycoproteins contain a common core of carbohydrate attached to the polypeptide. This core consists of three mannose residues and two GlcNAc (N-acetyl galactose). A variety of other sugars are attached to this core and comprise three major N-linked families:

I. High-mannose type contains all mannose outside the core in varying amounts.

II. Hybrid type contains various sugars and amino sugars.

III. Complex type is similar to the hybrid type, but in addition, contains sialic acids to varying degrees.

Most of the secreted and membrane bound proteins are modified by carbohydrate attachment. It is always the extracellular portion of the membrane bound proteins that is modified. Intracellular proteins are less frequently modified by glycosylation.

Mechanism of Carbohydrate Linkage to Protein

The O-linked glycosylation occurs post-translationally in the Golgi apparatus, where as the N-linked glycosylation occurs *co-translationally* in the lumen of the ER and the Golgi apparatus.

O-linked sugars: Attachment of oligosaccharide chains to proteins via O-link is usually through the hydroxyl groups of the side chains of serine or threonine. Attachment of the chains is via carbon-1 of an N-acetylgalactosamine residue derived from activated N-acetylgalactosamine (UDP- acetylgalactosamine) and attached to the protein chain through the action of specific transferases. The sites of attachment are on the exterior of the protein and a proline residue is always close to the serine or threonine residues that act as sites of attachment. The carbohydrate chain is assembled by the stepwise action of membrane bound glycotransferases that use nucleotide sugars as substrate. These sugars are synthesized in the cytoplasm whereas O-linked glycosylation usually occurs in the Golgi apparatus. Nucleotide sugars are transported into the Golgi apparatus via transport proteins that act bi-directionally. The final residue of the carbohydrate chain is often sialic acid, which prevents degradation of proteins. The *asialoglycoprotein receptors* found on the cell surface of hepatocytes bind and degrade glycoproteins that have lost their sialic acid residue.

N-linked sugars: In contrast to the step-wise addition of sugar groups to the O-linked class of glycoproteins, N-linked glycoprotein synthesis requires dolichol phosphate. Dolichols are polyprenols (C80-C100) containing 17 to 21 isoprene units, in which the terminal unit is saturated and hydroxylated (Fig.43.2).

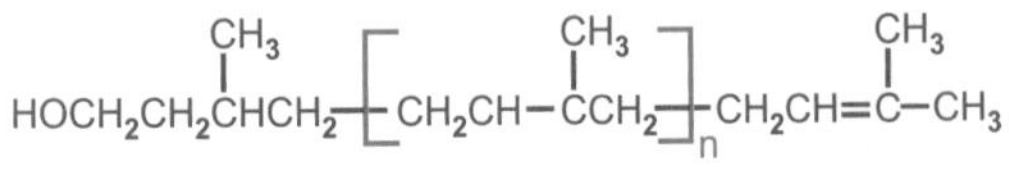

Fig. 43.2: Dolichol (the red bracket denotes the isoprene unit)

Synthesis of the carbohydrate chain commences on the cytoplasmic side of the ER. To begin with the terminal hydroxyl group of dolichol is phosphorylated by a specific kinase. Then N-acetylglucosamine phosphate is transferred from UDP-n-acetyl-glucosamine to yield *dolichol pyrophosphate-n-acetylglucosamine*. A second molecule of n-acetylglucosamine is added from UDP-n-acetylglucosamine. This is followed by the sequential addition of 5 mannose residues using GDP-mannose as the donor molecule for these additions. The complex then translocates across the membrane to the luminal side of the ER. Here four more mannose residues and three glucose residues are added before the complex is transferred to selected asparagine residues. After this the protein passes into the Golgi apparatus where sugar residues may be added or removed. This whole sequence of events is termed *oligosaccharide processing*.

Clinical Significances of Glycoproteins

Glycoproteins on cell surfaces are important for communication between cells, to maintain cell structure and for self-recognition by the immune system. The alteration of cell-surface glycoproteins can therefore, produce profound physiological effects, of which several are listed below.

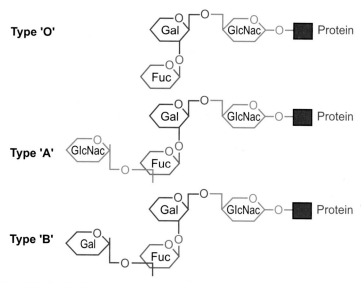

Fig. 43.3: Carbohydrate portion of ABO blood group glycoproteins

1. The ABO blood group antigens are the carbohydrate moieties of glycolipids on the surface of cells as well as the carbohydrate portion of serum glycoproteins. When present on the surface of cells the ABO carbohydrates are linked to sphingolipid and are therefore of the glycosphingolipid class. When the ABO carbohydrates are associated with protein in the form of glycoproteins they are found in the serum and are referred to as the secreted forms. Some individuals produce the glycoprotein forms of the ABO antigens while others do not. This property distinguishes **secretors** from **non-secretors**, a property that has forensic importance such as in cases of rape.

2. The truncation of surface glycoproteins on erythrocyte leads to cell clumping, as in congenital dyserythropoietic anemia type II.

3. Several viruses, bacteria and parasites have exploited the cell-surface carbohydrates associated with protein (glycoproteins), as portals of entry into the cell

    i. **Human immunodeficiency virus (HIV)**, the causative agent of **AIDS**, gains entry into cells of the immune system by attaching to a class of cellular receptors known as the chemokine receptors, most notably CXCR4 and CCR5.

    ii. **Poxvirus family of viruses** gain entry into cells, most frequently migratory leukocytes, by attaching to chemokine receptors including CCR1, CCR5 and CXCR4.

    iii. **Dystroglycan (DG)** is a component of the dystrophin-glycoprotein complex. It is composed of two proteins, one is *peripheral membrane* called α-DG and the other is *trans-membrane* called β-DG. The α-DG interacts with laminin-2 in the basal lamina and β-DG binds to dystrophin containing cytoskeletal proteins in muscle and peripheral nerves. DG is involved in agrin- and laminin-induced acetylcholine receptor clustering at neuromuscular junctions, morphogenesis, early development, and the pathogenesis of muscular dystrophies.

Recent evidence demonstrates that α-DG present on Schwann cell membranes is the receptor for **Mycobacterium leprae** and also serves as the receptor for the arenavirus class of pathogens.

iv. **Human parvovirus, B19**, attaches to the erythrocyte-specific cell-surface globoside identified as erythrocyte P antigen to infect erythrocytes.

v. **Malarial parasite Plasmodium vivax**, binds to the erythrocyte *chemokine receptor* known as the *Duffy blood group antigen* (also known as the erythrocyte receptor for interleukin-8) to infect erythrocytes.

vi. **The MN blood group system** is a well-characterized set of erythrocyte surface antigens that represent the variable carbohydrate modifications of the transmembrane glycoprotein designated as glycophorin. Glycophorin is the cellular receptor for influenza virus as well as the receptor for erythrocyte invasion by the malarial parasite **Plasmodium falciparum**.

vii. **Helicobacter pylori** is the bacterium responsible for chronic active gastritis and gastric and duodenal ulcers; it is also the causative agent for one of the most common forms of cancer in humans, adenocarcinoma. This bacterium attaches to the *Lewis blood group antigen* on the surfaces of gastric mucous cells.

viii. **Rabies virus binds** to cells through interactions with neural cell adhesion molecule (N-CAM).

ix. **Fibroblast growth factor (FGF) receptor** has been reported to be the portal of entry for human herpes virus Type I. Recent new evidence indicates that the portal of entry for human herpes simplex Type I viruses is *3-O-sulfated heparan sulfate*.

x. *Human herpes virus 6 (HHV-6)* infection occurs in virtually all persons within the first 2 years of life and persists the entire lifetime. In immunocompromised patients HHV-6 causes opportunistic infections and is the causative agent of *exanthema subitum*. HHV-6 has been linked to multiple sclerosis and to the progression of AIDS. The cellular receptor for HHV-6 is the cell-surface type-I glycoprotein, CD46.

4. Some glycoproteins are bound to membrane by a lipid linkage: the protein is attached to the carbohydrate through phosphatidylethanolamine (PE) linkage, and the carbohydrate is in turn attached to the membrane via phosphatidylinositol (PI) linkage, which anchors the structure within the membrane. This type of linkage is called a *glycosylphosphatidylinositol (GPI) anchor*, and proteins that are anchored in this way are termed *glypiated proteins*. Paroxysmal nocturnal hemoglobinuria, results from the loss of an erythrocyte surface glycoprotein called *decay-accelerating factor* (DAF), which prevents erythrocyte lysis by complement.

Other important GPI linked proteins are the enzymes *acetylcholinesterase*, intestinal and placental *alkaline phosphatase* and *5'-nucleotidase*, the cell adhesion molecule N-CAM (neural cell adhesion molecule) and the T-cell markers Thy-1 and LFA-3 (lymphocyte function associated antigen-3).

5. The proper degradation of glycoproteins has medical relevance. Glycoproteins are degraded within lysosomes that require specific lysosomal hydrolases, termed *glycosidases*. *Exoglycosidases* remove sugars sequentially from the nonreducing end and exhibit restricted substrate specificities. In contrast, *endoglycosidases* cleave carbohydrate linkages from within and exhibit broader substrate specificities. Several inherited storage disorders involving the glycoprotein degradation products have been identified in humans. These disorders result from defects in the genes encoding specific glycosidases, which lead to incomplete degradation and over-accumulation of partially degraded glycoproteins. Such disorders are generally known as *lysosomal storage diseases* that include *mucolipidoses* that result from incomplete degradation of the carbohydrate portions of glycolipids.

Enzyme Defects in Degradation of Asn-GlcNAc Type Glycoproteins

Disease	Enzyme seficiency	Symptoms/Comments
Aspartylglycosaminuria	Aspartylglycosaminidase	Progressive mental retardation, delayed speech and motor development, coarse facial features
β-mannosidosis	β-mannosidase	Primarily neurological defects, speech impairment
α-mannosidosis	α-mannosidase	Mental retardation, dystosis multiplex, hepatosplenomegaly, hearing loss, delayed speech
GM$_1$ gangliosidosis	β-galactosidase	Also identified as a glycosphingolipid storage disease
GM$_2$ gangliosidosis (Sandhoff-Jatzkewitz disease)	β-N-acetylhexosaminidases A and B	Also identified as a glycosphingolipid storage disease
Sialidosis (Mucolipidosis-I)	Neuraminidase (sialidase)	Myoclonus, congenital ascites, hepatosplenomegaly, coarse facial features, delayed mental and motor development
Fucosidosis	α-fucosidase	Progressive motor and mental deterioration, growth retardation, coarse facial features, recurrent sinus and pulmonary infections

6. Defects in the export of glycoproteins to lysosomes can also lead to clinical complications. Deficiency of *GlcNAc phosphotransferase* in lysosomes leads to the formation of dense inclusion bodies in the fibroblasts. Two disorders related to defects in the export of lysosomal enzymes have been identified, one is *I-cell disease* (mucolipidosis II) that is characterized by severe psychomotor retardation, skeletal abnormalities, coarse facial features, painful restricted joint movement, and early mortality and the other is *pseudo-Hurler polydystrophy* (mucolipidosis III, also called mucolipidosis-HI) that is less severe; it progresses more slowly, and afflicted individuals live to adulthood

Acylation

Following synthesis many proteins undergo chemical modification at their N-termini. In most cases an acetyl group, donated by acetyl-CoA replaces the initiator methionine. In some proteins, the myristoyl group is added to the N-termini, which allows the modified protein to associate with membranes. For example, the catalytic subunit of *cAMP-dependent protein kinase (PKA)* is myristoylated.

Methylation

Methylation of lysine residues in some proteins such as calmodulin and cytochrome c occurs post-translationally. The activated methyl donor is ***S-adenosylmethionine***.

Phosphorylation

In animal cells, one of the most common types of protein modification that occurs, is phosphorylation. A vast majority of such phosphorylations occurs as a transient mechanism of physiologically relevant examples are: the phosphorylation of *glycogen synthase* and *glycogen phosphorylase* in hepatocytes in response to *glucagon* release from the pancreas.

The phosphorylated form of *glycogen synthase* is inactive, whereas, the phosphorylated form of *glycogen phosphorylase* is active. The phosphorylated form of these two enzymes leads to an increased hepatic glucose delivery to the blood.

The amino acylresidues, subject to phosphorylation in animal cells are serine, threonine and tyrosine in the ratio of approximately 1000/100/1 for serine/threonine/tyrosine.

Although the level of tyrosine phosphorylation is minor, the importance of its phosphorylation is profound. The activity of numerous growth factor receptors is controlled by tyrosine phosphorylation.

Sulfation

Fibrinogen and some secreted proteins (*e.g, gastrin*) undergo sulfation at their tyrosine residues. The universal sulfate donor in such a reaction is *3'-phosphoadenosyl-5'-phosphosulfate* (Fig. 43.4). Sulfation of tyrosine residues is not a regulatory modification as that of phosphorylation. Sulfation of proteins is permanent, since it is necessary for their biological activity.

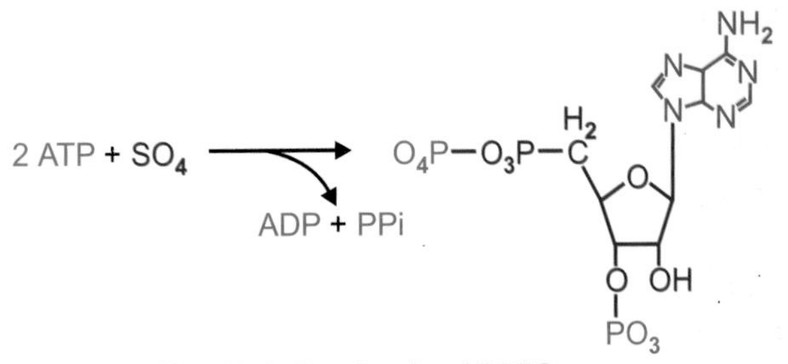

Prenylation

The addition of isoprenoid compounds, a 15-carbon *farnesyl group* or a 20-carbon *geranylgeranyl group* to an acceptor protein is referred to as prenylation. The isoprenoid groups are attached to cysteine residues at the carboxy terminus of proteins in a thioether linkage (C-S-C). Important examples of prenylated proteins include the oncogenic GTP-binding

$$2\,ATP + SO_4 \longrightarrow O_4P{-}O_3P{-}C \quad (ADP + PPi)$$

Fig. 43.4: Synthesis of PAPS

and hydrolyzing protein **Ras** and the γ-subunit of the visual protein *transducin*, both of which are farnesylated. The γ-subunit of numerous G-proteins of signal transduction cascades is modified by geranylgeranylation.

Ascorbic acid-Dependent Modifications

Protein modifications that require ascorbate as a cofactor include *hydroxylation* and *carboxy terminal amidation of proline* and *lysine residues*. The hydroxylating enzymes are identified as **prolyl hydroxylase** and **lysyl hydroxylase**. The donor of the amide for C-terminal amidation is glycine.

The most important proteins, which are extensively hydroxylated, are the collagens. Several peptide hormones such as *oxytocin* and *vasopressin* have C-terminal amidation.

Vitamin K-Dependent Modifications

Vitamin K is a cofactor for protein carboxylase that carboxylates glutamyl residues in proteins. The result of this reaction is glutamyl residues are converted to γ-carboxyglutamate residues (Fig. 43.5).

The formation of gla residues within several proteins of the blood-clotting cascade is critical for their normal function. The presence of γ-carboxyglutamate residues allows the protein to chelate calcium ions and thereby render an altered conformation and biological activity to the protein. The coumarin-based anticoagulants, *warfarin* and *dicumarol* function by inhibiting the carboxylation reaction.

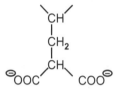

Fig. 43.5: Gamma-carboxyglutamyl residue

PROTEIN TARGETING

Within the cells, proteins are synthesized on free ribosomes are those anchored to endoplasmic reticulum (ER). Consequent to synthesis the proteins need to be directed to their correct location such as ER, cell membrane, mitochondria, lysosome or the nucleus. In many instances, the newly synthesized protein is required to cross a membrane barrier.

The proteins that are to cross into the ER en route to their final destination have an N-terminal sequence of about 20 amino acids that are predominantly hydrophobic. These residues are designated as *signal peptide*, which is removed during protein processing. Once the signal peptide has been synthesized and extruded from the ribosome, it binds to a complex termed the *signal recognition particle* (Fig. 43.6). When the signal recognition particle (SRP) binds to the signal peptide of the protein, the synthesis stops and the SRP-ribosome complex moves to the cytoplasmic surface of the ER, where the complex binds to a receptor called the *docking protein* or *translocon*. The ribosome is anchored to the ER surface by translocon and the signal peptide locates into a pore that is part of the translocon. When the ribosome-SRP complex binds to the membrane the SRP dissociates and protein synthesis resumes. As the signal peptide is now through the ER membrane it allows the protein to pass into the

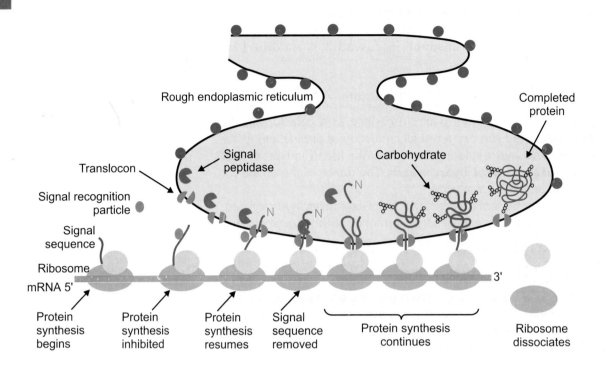

Fig. 43.6: Synthesis of secreted proteins

ER lumen. The signal peptide is then cleaved off by *signal peptidase* that is part of the pore complex.

Proteins that are part of the membrane have a stop *transfer sequence*. When their N terminus is in the ER and the C terminus in the cytoplasm, the arrival of *stop transfer sequence* at the membrane stops the protein transfer. Some proteins span the membrane several times but the mechanisms through which this is achieved are yet to be elucidated.

Import of Proteins into the Mitochondria Matrix

The proteins destined for mitochondrion have to cross both the outer and inner mitochondrial membranes. Passage across the inner membrane is complicated, because this membrane has to maintain an electrochemical potential for ATP synthesis. Proteins destined for mitochondrial import combine with specialized protein complex termed *mitochondrial stimulation factor* (MSF). This complex specifically recognizes *mitochondrial import sequences* (basic amino acids on the pre-sequence of the newly synthesized proteins) and targets these proteins to receptors on the mitochondrial surface. Both *mitochondrial stimulation factor* and the *signal recognition particle,* act as adaptors to translocate proteins across membrane. In addition MSF helps to disperse aggregated proteins using ATP, since aggregation prevents importation.

Targeting to the Mitochondrial Outer Membrane

The proteins destined for mitochondrial outer membrane, bind to the *import mechanisms proteins*, and then pass into vesicles. These vesicles have two regions, the cis and trans sites, to which the proteins bind sequentially. The cis-site is on the cytoplasmic side of the mitochondria and have many negatively charged residues that may interact with the basic residues in the pre-sequence of proteins for mitochondrial import. The trans-site is on the inner surface of the membrane and translocation from the cis- to the trans-site depends on the pre- sequence and does not require ATP.

Transport to the Mitochondrial Inner Membrane

Proteins for these regions transllocate across the outer membrane and interact with specific recognition sites on the inner membrane. Proteins involved with this are Mim (mitochondrial inner membrane) 17, 23 and 44 and heat shock protein (hsp) 70. Mim 17 and 23 may form a channel through which proteins bound to hsp 70 pass into the inner membrane and mitochondrial matrix. The hsp is thought to be the driving force for getting the proteins through the channel by the hydrolysis of ATP.

Lysosomal Targeting

In the Golgi apparatus, mannose-6-phosphate is covalently attached to enzymes, destined for the lysosomes. These proteins then bind to transmembrane receptors via the mannose-6-phosphate, which promotes the vesicles formation that detach from the membrane and fuse with a specialized vesicle termed the **C**ompartment of **U**ncoupling of **R**eceptor and **L**igand (CURL). The acidic pH of vesicles promotes dissociation of the receptor-ligand complex allowing the protein to fuse with the lysosomal membrane and enter into the lysosome.

Nuclear Transport

A variety of RNAs (mRNA, tRNA, rRNA) move from nucleus to cytoplasm and proteins move from cytoplasm to nucleus. In addition, many proteins shuttle between cytoplasm and nucleus.

Aqueous channels in the nuclear membrane called *nuclear pore complexes* or *nucleophorins* allow diffusion of ions, metabolites, small proteins (<60K) and the transport of larger molecules that are energy dependent. Many nucleophorins have the sequence F-X-F-G (where X is any amino acid) and/or G-L-F-G repeated many times. These sequences interact with transport factors but their precise function is unclear. Proteins that are to be imported into the nucleus have clusters of basic amino acids (e.g. K-K-K-R-K) and proteins that are to be both imported and exported have sequences L-X-X-X-L-X-X-X-L-X-I.

Transport into the nucleus involves the proteins *importin* α and β that form a heterodimeric carrier in which importin-α binds to the protein and importin β strengthens this binding and interacts with the nuclear pore complex. Transportin, which is structurally related to importin-β is also involved in protein import into the nucleus.

Translocation through the nuclear pore complex requires energy that is provided by a small GTPase termed *Ran*, which is a highly abundant protein that cycles between *Ran-GTP* and *Ran- GDP*.

Control of Gene Expression

44

Gene expression is the ability of a gene to produce a biologically active protein. The regulatory mechanisms that control gene expression in eukaryotes is much more complex than in prokaryotes. The major difference between the two is the presence of nuclear membrane in eukaryotes, which prevents the simultaneous transcription and translation that occurs in prokaryotes. The major point of regulatory control in prokaryotes is transcriptional initiation. Where as in eukaryotes, the gene expression is regulated at many different points.

GENE CONTROL IN PROKARYOTES

In prokaryotes, the genes that encode different proteins necessary to perform coordinated functions, such as biosynthesis of a given amino acid are clustered together as operons. The mRNA that is transcribed from such operon is polycistronic, which means the genetic information for multiple proteins are encoded in a single transcript.

In prokaryotes, **the predominant site** for control of gene expression is **transcriptional initiation**. The transcriptional initiation is controlled by two DNA sequence elements, which are approximately 35 and 10 bases, upstream of the transcriptional initiation site. These two sequence elements are required for recognition of transcriptional start sites by **RNA polymerase**, hence are termed *promoter sequences*. The consensus sequence for the *-35 position is TTGACA*, and for the *-10 position is TATAAT*. The -10 position is also known as the **Pribnow-box**.

The **RNA polymerases** recognize and bind to these promoter sequences. The activity of **RNA polymerase** at a given promoter site is in turn regulated by its interaction with other accessory proteins (regulatory proteins), which are of two types, one is positive regulator (**activator**) and the other is negative regulator (**repressor**). The accessibility of promoter sequences is regulated by the interaction of proteins with sequences termed *operators*. In most operons, the *operator sequences* are adjacent to the *promoter sequences*. Operator sequences are the binding site for repressor protein. However, there are several operons in *E. coli* that contain overlapping sequence elements, one that binds a repressor and one that binds an activator.

In prokaryotes (*E.coli*), the expression of operons is controlled by two major modes of transcriptional regulation. Both the mechanisms involve repressor proteins. One mode of control regulates the operons that produce enzymes necessary for the utilization of energy; the expression of these operons is regulated by catabolites, hence called *catabolite-regulated operons*. The other mode regulates operons that produce enzymes necessary for the synthesis of small biomolecules such as amino acids; the expression of these operons is *attenuated* by sequences within the transcribed RNA.

A classic example of a catabolite-regulated operon is the ***lac operon***, which is responsible for obtaining energy from β-galactosides such as lactose. A classic example of an attenuated operon is the ***trp operon***, responsible for the biosynthesis of tryptophan.

The lac Operon

The *lac* operon consists of one regulatory gene (the *i gene*) and three structural genes (z, y, and a). The *i gene* codes for the repressor protein of the *lac* operon (Fig. 44.1). The z gene codes for the enzyme **β-galactosidase** that is responsible for the hydrolysis of lactose to galactose and glucose. The y gene codes for *permease* that increases cell permeability for β-galactosides. The a gene encodes a ***transacetylase***.

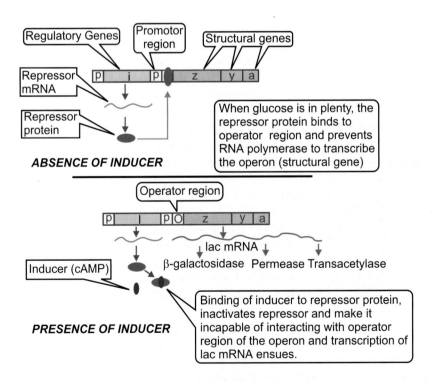

Fig. 44.1: lac operon

During normal growth of *E.coli* in a glucose-based medium, the *lac* repressor is bound to the operator region of the *lac* operon, preventing transcription. However, in the presence of an inducer (e.g. cAMP) of the *lac* operon, the inducer binds to repressor protein and makes it incapable of interacting with the operator region of the operon. RNA polymerase is thus able to bind at the promoter region, and transcription of the operon ensues.

The *lac* operon is repressed, even in the presence of lactose, if glucose is also present. This repression is maintained until the glucose supply is exhausted. The repression of the *lac* operon under these conditions is termed *catabolite repression* and is the result of the low levels of cAMP that result from an adequate glucose supply. The repression of the *lac* operon is relieved even in the presence of glucose if excess cAMP is added. As the level of glucose in the medium falls, the level of cAMP increases. Simultaneously there is an increased binding of cAMP to the *lac* repressor. The complex formed by cAMP binding to repressor protein is incapable of interacting with operator site. The net result is an increase in transcription from the operon.

The ability of cAMP to activate expression from the *lac* operon results from an interaction of cAMP with a protein termed CRP (*cAMP receptor protein*), which is also called *CAP* (*catabolite activator protein*). The cAMP-CRP complex binds to a region of the *lac* operon just upstream of the region bound by RNA polymerase and that somewhat overlaps that of the repressor-binding site of the operator region. The binding of the cAMP-CRP complex to the *lac* operon stimulates RNA polymerase activity 20-to-50-fold.

GENE CONTROL IN EUKARYOTES

In eukaryotic cells, gene expression is regulated at several points:

i. *Chromatin structure:* The compact physical structure of chromatin and the presence of histones and CpG methylation affect the accessibility of the chromatin to RNA polymerases and transcription factors.

ii. *Transcriptional initiation:* This is the most important mode of regulating eukaryotic gene expression. Specific factors that exert control include the strength of *promoter elements* within the DNA sequences of a given gene, the presence or absence of enhancer sequences and the interaction between multiple activator proteins and inhibitor proteins.

iii. *Processing and modification of transcript:* Eukaryotic mRNAs are subjected to post-transcriptional processing such as capping, polyadenylation and accurate splicing. Several genes have been identified that undergo tissue-specific patterns of alternative splicing, which generate biologically different proteins from the same gene.

iv. *Transcript stability:* Unlike prokaryotic mRNAs, whose half-lives are all in the range of 1 to 5 minutes, eukaryotic mRNAs can vary greatly in their stability. Certain unstable transcripts have sequences that are signals for rapid degradation.

v. *Translational initiation:* Since many mRNAs have multiple methionine codons, the ability of ribosomes to recognize and initiate synthesis from the correct AUG codon can affect the expression of a gene product. Only recently several examples have emerged demonstrating that some eukaryotic proteins initiate at non-AUG codons.

vi. *Post-translational modification of proteins:* Common modifications include glycosylation, acetylation, fatty acylation and disulfide bond formations.

vii. *Protein transport:* In order for proteins to express their biologically activity following translation and processing, they must be transported to their site of action.

viii. *Control of protein stability:* Many proteins are rapidly degraded, whereas others are highly stable. Specific amino acid sequences in some proteins have been shown to bring about rapid degradation

Control of Transcription Initiation in Eukaryotes

Transcription of the different classes of RNAs in eukaryotes is carried out by three different polymerases.

i. RNA pol I synthesizes the rRNAs, except for the 5S species.

ii. RNA pol II synthesizes the mRNAs and some small nuclear RNAs (snRNAs) involved in RNA splicing.

iii. RNA pol III synthesizes the 5S rRNA and the tRNAs. The vast majority of eukaryotic RNAs are subjected to post-transcriptional processing.

The most complex controls observed in eukaryotic genes are those that regulate the expression of RNA pol II-transcribed mRNA genes. Almost all eukaryotic mRNA genes contain basal promoters of two types and any number of different transcriptional regulatory domains (Fig. 44.2). The basal promoter elements are termed *CCAAT-boxes* (pronounced "cat") and *TATA-boxes* because of their sequences. The TATA-box is similar in sequence to the prokaryotic Pribnow-box. Numerous proteins identified as *TFIIA, B, C,* etc. (transcription factors regulating RNA pol II), have been observed to interact with the TATA-box. The protein identified as C/EBP (CCAAT-box/Enhancer Binding Protein) binds to the CCAAT-box element.

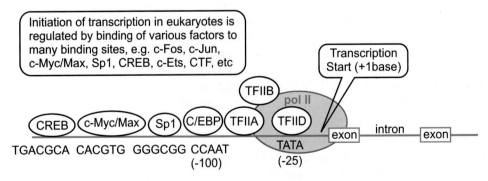

Fig. 44.2: Control of transcription initiation

There are many other regulatory sequences in mRNA genes that bind various transcription factors. Theses regulatory sequences are predominantly located upstream (5') of the transcription initiation site, although some elements occur downstream (3') or even within the genes themselves. Different combinations of transcription factors also can exert differential regulatory effects upon transcriptional initiation. Each of the different cell types express characteristic combinations of transcription factors, which is the major mechanism for cell-type specificity in the regulation of mRNA gene expression.

Structural Motifs of Transcription Factors in Eukaryotes

The transcriptional factors (proteins) of eukaryotes have certain conserved structural motifs, which are important for the regulation of gene expression. Few such examples are:

Homeodomain The homeodomain is a highly conserved domain (sequence) of 60 amino acids found in a large family of transcription factors. This group of genes, when altered, would cause transformations of one body part for another, hence called homeotic transformations. This class of genes has been identified in both invertebrate and vertebrate organisms. The principal function of all homeodomain-containing proteins is to establish pattern in an organism such as that of the spinal column in vertebrates.

POU domain The POU domain is a domain that is a hybrid between a domain related to the homeodomain and a POU-specific domain. The term POU was derived from the names of the first three factors shown to have a region of similarity, **P**it-1 (a pituitary-specific transcription factor), **O**ct-1 (an octamer binding protein first shown to regulate immunoglobulin gene transcription) and **U**nc-86 (a nematode gene).

Helix-loop-helix (HLH) The HLH domain is required for protein dimerization. The HLH motif is composed of two regions of α-helix separated by a region of variable length, which forms a loop between the two alpha-helices. The α-helical domains are structurally similar and are necessary for protein interaction with sequence elements that exhibit a twofold axis of symmetry. This class of transcription factor most often contains a region of basic amino acids located on the N-terminal side of the HLH domain (termed bHLH proteins) that is necessary in order for the protein to bind DNA at specific sequences. The HLH domain is necessary for homo- and heterodimerization. Examples of bHLH proteins include MyoD (a myogenesis inducing transcription factor) and c-Myc (originally identified as a retroviral oncogene). Several HLH proteins that do not contain the basic region act as repressors. These HLH proteins repress the activity of other bHLH proteins by forming heterodimers with them and preventing DNA binding.

Zinc fingers The zinc finger domain is a DNA-binding motif consisting of specific spacings of cysteine and histidine residues that allow the protein to bind zinc atoms. The metal atom coordinates the sequences around the cysteine and histidine residues into a finger-like domain. The finger domains can "interdigitate" into the major groove of the DNA helix. The spacing of the zinc finger domain in this class of transcription factor coincides with a half-turn of the double helix. The classic example is the RNA pol III transcription factor (TFIIIA). Proteins of the steroid/thyroid hormone family of transcription factors also contain zinc fingers.

Leucine zipper The leucine zipper domain is necessary for protein dimerization. It is a motif generated by a repeating distribution of leucine residues spaced 7 amino acids apart within α-helical regions of the protein. These leucine residues end up with their R-groups protruding from the α-helical domain in which the leucine residues reside. The protruding R-groups are thought to "interdigitate" with leucine R-groups of another leucine zipper domain, thus stabilizing homo- or heterodimerization. The leucine zipper domain is present in many DNA-binding proteins, such as c-Myc, and C/EBP.

Winged helix The winged helix is a DNA-binding motif composed of an α/β structure. This structure contains 3 N-terminal α-helices and a 3-stranded antiparallel β-sheet. The folding of the β-sheet region about the α-helices gives the appearance of wings on the helices, hence the term "winged-helix". This motif was first identified in the transcription factor HNF-3γ. HNF-3γ is a member of a large family of transcription factors that are related to the *Drosophila* gene *fork head*; hence the gene family is termed the fork head (FKH) family.

Table of Representative Transcription Factors

Factor	Sequence Motif	Comments
c-Myc and Max	CACGTG	c-Myc first identified as retroviral oncogene; Max specifically associates with c-Myc in cells
c-Fos and c-Jun	TGA$^C/_G$T$^C/_A$A	Both first identified as retroviral oncogenes; associate in cells, also known as the factor AP-1
CREB	TGACG$^C/_T$$^C/_A$$^G/_A$	Binds to the cAMP response element; family of at least 10 factors resulting from different genes or alternative splicing; can form dimers with c-Jun
c-ErbA; also TR (thyroid hormone receptor)	GTGTCAAAGGTCA	First identified as retroviral oncogene; member of the steroid/thyroid hormone receptor superfamily; binds thyroid hormone
c-Ets	$^G/_C$$^A/_CGGA^A/_T$$^G/_C$	First identified as retroviral oncogene; predominates in B- and T-cells
GATA	$^T/_A$GATA	Family of erythroid cell-specific factors, GATA-1 to -6
c-Myb	$^T/_C$AAC$^G/_T$G	First identified as retroviral oncogene; hematopoietic cell-specific factor
MyoD	CAACTGAC	Controls muscle differentiation
NF-(kappa)B and c-Rel	GGGA$^A/_C$TN$^T/_C$CC[1]	Both factors identified independently; c-Rel first identified as retroviral oncogene; predominate in B- and T-cells
RAR (retinoic acid receptor)	ACGTCATGACCT	Binds to elements termed RAREs (retinoic acid response elements) also binds to c-Jun/c-Fos site
SRF (serum response factor)	GGATGTCCATATTAG-GACATCT	Exists in many genes that are inducible by the growth factors present in serum

Proto-oncogenes and Cancer

45

The normal cells can be transformed to malignant cells by activation of oncogenes, or deletion of onco-suppressor genes. The etiological factors are spontaneous mutations, XX chromosomal translocation, chemical carcinogens, physical agents that damage the chromatin, and oncogenic viruses.

ONCOGENES

Genetic damage appears to be the single most common event that causes tumor genesis. Any genetic damage that may be present in a parental tumorogenic cell cannot be corrected and all cells of subsequent generations inherit it. The genes that are found to suffer genetic damage in cancer cells are of two types, one is the proto-oncogene (dominant gene) and the other is onco-suppressor gene (recessive gene).

Proto-oncogenes are the genes present in normal cells, which when sustain damage produce a protein that is capable of inducing cellular transformation. An oncogene is a gene that has already sustained some genetic damage and, is producing a protein capable of inducing cellular transformation.

The various processes that transforms a proto-oncogene to an oncogene, includes retroviral transduction, retroviral integration, point mutations, insertion mutations, gene amplification, chromosomal translocation and/or protein-protein interactions.

Proto-oncogenes that were originally identified as cellular genes that got transformed by retroviral transduction are designated as c- indicative of the cellular origin. Whereas those that were originally identified as retroviral genes that got integrated into cellular gene are designated as v- to signify viral origin.

Once-suppressor genes are variously termed as *tumor suppressors*, *growth suppressors, recessive oncogenes or anti-oncogenes*. These are the genes that normally protect the cells from getting infected with cancer. When these genes are mutated are deleted, cancer results. Damage to genes that encode growth factors, growth factor receptors and proteins of the various signal transduction cascades would lead to cellular transformation. Anti-oncogenes are written with capital letters, whereas small letters abbreviates oncogens.

TUMOR VIRUSES

Tumor viruses are of two distinct types. One type of viruses has DNA genomes (e.g. papilloma and adenoviruses) and the other type of viruses has RNA genomes (termed *retroviruses*). RNA tumor viruses are common in chickens, mice and cats but rare in humans. The only retroviruses currently known to affect humans are the ***human T-cell leukemia viruses (HTLVs)*** and the related retrovirus, ***human immunodeficiency virus (HIV)***.

Cellular transformations by RNA viruses (retroviruses) are by mechanisms that are related to the life cycle of these viruses.

i. When a cell is infected by a retrovirus, the viral RNA genome is converted into DNA by the viral encoded RNA-dependent DNA polymerase (***reverse transcriptase***). The DNA so formed, integrates into the host genome (Fig. 45.1). When the host genome is duplicated during the process of cellular division the newly integrated viral DNA also gets copied. The ends of retroviral genome, within the host genome contain powerful transcriptional promoter sequences termed *long terminal repeats (LTRs)*, ***which*** promote the transcription of the integrated viral DNA leading to the production of new virus particles.

The integration process leads to rearrangement of the viral genome and the consequent incorporation of a portion of the host genome into the viral genome. This process is termed *transduction*. At some frequency, transduction process can make the virus acquire a gene from the host that is normally involved in cellular growth control. Because of the alteration of the host gene during the transduction process as well as the gene being transcribed at a higher rate due to its association with the retroviral LTRs, the transduced gene confers a growth advantage to the infected cell. The end result of this process is unrestricted cellular proliferation leading to tumorigenesis. The transduced genes are termed oncogenes. The normal cellular gene in its unmodified, non-transduced form is termed a proto-oncogene since it has the capacity to transform cells if altered in some way or expressed in an uncontrolled manner. Numerous oncogenes have been discovered in the genomes of transforming retroviruses.

ii. In the second mechanism, the powerful transcription promoting effect of the retroviral LTRs can transform the host cells. When a retrovirus genome with LTRs, integrates into a host genome close to a gene that encodes a *growth regulating protein* can result in abnormally elevated level of this protein and cellular transformation. This is termed ***retroviral***

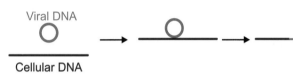

Viral DNA

Cellular DNA

Fig. 45.1: Process of viral DNA integration into cellular DNA

integration induced transformation. It has been shown recently that HIV induces certain forms of cancers by this process.

Cellular transformation by *DNA tumor viruses* has been shown to be the result of *protein-protein interaction*. Proteins called **tumor antigens** (T antigens), encoded by the DNA tumor viruses can interact with cellular proteins. Such interaction removes the cellular proteins away from their normal functional locations within the cell. The cells normally have proteins called tumor suppressor protein, which suppresses cellular transformation. When viral T antigens predominantly interact with this protein, it can results, in cellular transformation.

Classification of Proto-oncogenes

Proto-oncogenes are classified into many different groups based on their normal function within cells or based on sequence homology to other known proteins. Proto-oncogenes have been identified at all levels of signal transduction cascades that control *cell growth, proliferation* and *differentiation*. The list of proto-oncogenes identified to date and the new genes that are being isolated continuously are too large, and only those genes that have been highly characterized are described.

Growth Factors

The c-Sis gene encodes the PDGF β chain. The v-sis gene was the first oncogene to be identified as having homology to a known cellular gene. The int-2 gene encodes an FGF-related growth factor. The KGF (also called Hst) gene also encodes an FGF-related growth factor and was identified in gastric carcinoma and Kaposi's sarcoma cells.

Receptor Tyrosine Kinases

The c-Fms (*fims*) gene encodes the *colony stimulating factor-1 receptor* and was first identified as a retroviral oncogene. The Flg (*flag*) gene encodes a form of the FGF receptor. The Neu (*new*) gene was identified as an EGF receptor-related gene in an ethylnitrosourea-induced **neu**roblastoma. The conversion of proto-oncogenic to oncogenic Neu requires only a single amino acid change in the transmembrane domain. The Trk (*track*) genes encode the NGF receptor-like proteins. The first Trk gene was found in a pancreatic cancer. Subsequently, two additional Trk-related genes were identified. These three are now identified as TrkA, TrkB and TrkC. The Met gene encodes the *hepatocyte growth factor receptor*. The c-Kit gene encodes the *mast cell growth factor receptor*.

Membrane Associated Non-Receptor Tyrosine Kinases

The v-src gene was the first identified oncogene. The c-Src gene is the archetypal protein tyrosine kinase. The Lck gene was isolated from a T cell tumor line (**L**ymphocyte **c**ell **k**inase) and has been shown to be associated with the CD4 and CD8 antigens of T cells.

G-Protein Coupled Receptors

The Mas gene was identified in a mammary carcinoma and has been shown to be the angiotensin receptor.

Membrane Associated G-Proteins

There are three different homologous of the c-Ras gene, each of which was identified in a different type of tumor cell. The Ras gene is one of the most frequently disrupted genes in colorectal carcinomas.

Serine/Threonine Kinases

The Raf gene is involved in the signaling pathway of most RTKs. It is likely responsible for threonine phosphorylation of MAP kinase following receptor activation.

Nuclear DNA-Binding/Transcription Factors

A disrupted human c-Myc gene has been found to be involved in numerous hematopoietic neoplasias. Disruption of c-Myc has been shown to be the result of retroviral integration and transduction as well as chromosomal rearrangements. The Fos gene was identified in the **fe**line **os**teosarcoma virus. The protein interacts with a second proto-oncogenic protein, Jun to form a transcriptional regulatory complex.

Cancer Syndromes of Hereditary Origin

Syndrome	Cloned gene	Function	Chromosomal location	Tumor types
Familial retinoblastoma	RB1	Cell cycle regulation	13q14	Retinoblastoma, osteogenic sarcoma
Wilms tumor	WT1	Transcriptional regulation	11p13	Pediatric kidney cancer
Neurofibromatosis type 1	NF1 protein = neurofibromin 1	Catalysis of RAS inactivation	17q11.2	Neurofibromas, sarcomas, gliomas
Familial adenomatous Polyposis	APC	Signaling through adhesion molecules to nucleus	5q21	Colon cancer
Deleted in pancreatic carcinoma 4	DPC4 also known as Smad4	Regulation of TGF-b/BMP signal transduction	18q21.1	Pancreatic carcinoma, colon cancer
Familial breast cancer	BRCA1	Repair of double strand breaks by association with Rad51 protein	17q21	Breast and ovarian cancer
Hereditary nonpolyposis colorectal cancer	MSH2	DNA mismatch repair	2p16	Colorectal cancer
Familial melanoma	CDKN2A protein = cyclin-dependent kinase inhibitor 2A	Cell-cycle regulation	9p21	Melanoma, pancreatic cancer, others
Hereditary papillary renal cancer (HPRC)	MET	Transmembrane receptor for hepatocyte growth factor (HGF)	7q31	Renal papillary cancer
Ataxia telangiectasia (AT)	ATM	DNA repair	11q22.3	Lymphoma, cerebellar ataxia, immunodeficiency
Xeroderma pigmentosum (XP)	Several complementation groups: XPA, XPC, XPD, XPE, XPF	DNA repair helicases, nucleotide excision repair	XPA = 9q22.3 XPC = 3p25 XPD = 19q13.2-q13.3 XPE = 11p12-p11 XPF = 16p13.3-p13.13	Skin cancer

TUMOR SUPPRESSORS AND CANCER

Tumor suppressor genes were identified, by making cell hybrids between normal and tumor cells. On some occasions a chromosome from the normal cell was able to revert the transformed phenotype.

Several tumor suppressor genes have been isolated. They include genes identified through the study of familial cancers such as the retinoblastoma (RB), Wilms' tumors (WT1), neurofibromatosis type-1 (NF1), familial adenomatosis polyposis coli (FAP or APC), and those identified through loss of heterozygosity such as in colorectal carcinomas (called DCC for detected in colon carcinoma) and p53, which was originally thought to be a proto-oncogene. However, the wild-type p53 protein suppresses the activity of mutant alleles of p53, which are the oncogenic forms of p53.

p53

The p53 gene was originally discovered because the protein product complexed with the SV40 large T antigen. It was first thought that p53 was a proto-oncogene.

Subsequent analysis of several murine leukemia cell lines showed that the p53 locus was lost by either insertions or deletions on both alleles. This suggested that wild-type p53 might be a tumor suppressor not a dominant proto-oncogene. Direct confirmation came when it was shown that wild-type p53 could suppress transformation in oncogene cooperation assays with mutant p53 and ras.

It has now been demonstrated that mutation at the p53 locus occurs in cancers of the colon, breast, liver and lung. Involvement of p53 in neoplasia is more frequent than any other known tumor suppressor or dominant proto-oncogene.

The p53-encoded protein is a nuclear localized phosphoprotein. This suggests that p53 may be involved in transcriptional regulation.

p53 protein forms a complex with SV40 large T antigen, as well as the E1B transforming protein of adenovirus and E6 protein of human papilloma viruses. Complexing with tumor antigens increases the stability of the p53 protein. This increased stability of p53 protein is characteristic of mutant forms found in tumor lines. The complexes of T antigens and p53 render p53 incapable of binding to DNA and inducing transcription.

The activity of p53 appears to be regulated also by phosphorylation. The level of p53 is low after mitosis but increases during G1 phase. During S phase the protein becomes phosphorylated by cdc2 kinase and CKII. Sequences at the N-terminus of the p53 protein function as a transcription activator suggesting p53 may activate the transcription of genes involved in suppression of cell growth. Additionally, p53 protein has been shown to block the binding of DNA polymerase-a to SV40 large T, blocking replication of SV40 DNA. It is suggested that p53 may also regulate the initiation of DNA synthesis.

Familial cancer syndrome	Tumor suppressor gene	Function	Chromosomal location	Tumor types observed
Familial retinoblastoma	RB1	Cell cycle regulation	13q14.1-q14.2	Retinoblastoma, osteogenic sarcoma
Wilms tumor	WT1	Transcriptional regulation	11p13	Pediatric kidney cancer
Neurofibromatosis type 1	NF1 protein = neurofibromin 1	Catalysis of RAS inactivation	17q11.2	Neurofibromas, sarcomas, gliomas
Familial adenomatous polyposis	APC	Signaling through adhesion molecules to nucleus	5q21-q22	Colon cancer
Deleted in pancreatic carcinoma 4	DPC4 also known as Smad4	Regulation of TGF-b/BMP signal transduction	18q21.1	Pancreatic carcinoma, colon cancer
Familial breast cancer	BRCA1	Repair of double strand breaks by interaction with Rad51 protein	17q21	Breast and ovarian cancer
Familial breast cancer	BRCA2	Similar to BRCA1 activity?	13q12.3	Breast and ovarian cancer
Hereditary nonpolyposis colon cancer	MSH2	DNA mismatch repair	2p22-p21	Colon cancer
Familial melanoma	CDKN2A protein = cyclin-dependent kinase inhibitor 2A	Cell-cycle regulation	9p21	Melanoma, pancreatic cancer, others

Retinoblastoma (RB)

In the familial form of retinoblastoma, individuals inherit a mutant allele with loss of function from an affected parent. A subsequent somatic mutation inactivates the normal allele also resulting in the development of retinoblastoma. This leads to an apparently dominant mode of inheritance.

In sporadic forms of tumors involving the RB locus, two somatic mutational events must occur, the second of which must occur in the descendants of the cell receiving the first mutation. This combination of mutational events is extremely rare.

The RB RNA encodes a nuclear localized phosphoprotein. pRB is not detectable in any retinoblastoma cells. Surprisingly, detectable levels of pRB can be found in most proliferating cells even though there is a restricted number of tissues affected by mutations in the RB gene (i.e. retina, bone and connective tissue).

Many different types of mutations result in loss of RB function. Splicing errors, point mutations and small deletions in the promoter region have also been observed in some retinoblastomas.

The germ line mutations at RB occur predominantly during spermatogenesis as opposed to oogenesis. However, the somatic mutations occur with equal frequency at the paternal or maternal locus.

pRB functions at some capacity in the regulation of cell cycle progression. Its ability to regulate the cell cycle correlates to the state of phosphorylation of pRb. Phosphorylation is maximal at the start of S phase and lowest after mitosis and entry into G_1.

Stimulation of quiescent cells with mitogen induces phosphorylation of pRB, in contrast, differentiation induces hypophosphorylation of pRB. It is, therefore, the hypophosphorylated form of pRB that suppresses cell proliferation.

Wilms' Tumor (WT1)

Genetic evidence indicates that chromosomal deletions at three distinct loci may be involved in the development of Wilms' tumors, a kidney cancer found in children, which involve either one or both kidneys. Only a single candidate locus has thus far been characterized. The potential Wilms' tumor gene at 11p13 is found in a deleted region. This region contains a single transcription unit identified as WT1 that spans 50-60 kb. The WT1 gene codes for a protein containing four zinc finger domains suggesting it may be a transcription factor. Expression of WT1 is very restrictive, unlike the RB gene that is expressed everywhere. Wilms' tumors that are homozygous for 11p13 deletions do not contain WT1 mRNA. Most other Wilms' tumors show high expression of WT1 mRNA but these are likely to be produced from mutated WT1 genes.

Molecular Tools in Medicine

46

RECOMBINANT DNA

In the practice of modern molecular medicine, many techniques of molecular biology are utilized for the analysis of disease, disease causing genes and gene functions. Particularly the developments in the field of *cloning* and **recombinant DNA** techniques have made it possible the study of disease genes and their function in unaffected individuals.

The term **recombinant DNA** refers to manipulations by which different segments of DNA are covalently recombined. **Cloning** refers to the process of preparing identical multiple copies of an individual type of recombinant DNA molecule. Clone refers to cells with identical genotype.

The classical mechanisms of producing recombinant DNA, involves the insertion of an exogenous fragments of DNA into a **vector** (The term **vector** refers to the DNA molecule used, to **carry** or **transport** DNA of interest into cells), which is either bacterially derived **plasmid** (the self-replicating, circular double stranded DNAs found in bacteria) or viral based **bacteriophage** (viruses that infect bacteria).

Many enzymes are used in the process of recombinant DNA technology and cloning. A list of such commonly used enzymes is given in the Table 46.1.

Table 46.1: Commonly used enzymes in recombinant DNA technology

Enzyme(s)	Activity	Comments
Restriction endonucleases	Recognize specific nucleotide sequences and cleaves the DNA within or near to the recognition sequences	See below
Reverse transcriptase (RT)	Retrovirally encoded RNA-dependent DNA polymerase	Used to convert mRNA into a complimentary DNA (**cDNA**) copy for the purpose of cloning cDNAs
RNase H	Recognizes RNA-DNA duplexes and randomly cleaves the phosphodiester backbone of the RNA	Used primarily to cleave the mRNA strand that is annealed to the first strand of cDNA generated by reverse transcription

Contd...

Contd...

DNA polymerase	Synthesis of DNA	Used during most procedures where DNA synthesis is required, also used *in vitro* mutagenesis
Klenow DNA into polymerase	Proteolytic fragment of DNA polymerase that lacks the 5' → 3' exonuclease activity	Used to incorporate radioactive nucleotides restriction enzyme generated ends of DNA, also can be used in place of DNA polymerase
DNA ligase	Covalently attaches a free 5' phosphate to a 3' hydroxyl	Used in all procedures where to molecules of DNA need to be covalently attached
Alkaline phosphatase	Removes phosphates from 5' ends of DNA molecules	Used to allow 5' ends to be subsequently radio-labeled with the γ-phosphate of ATP in the presence of polynucleotide kinase, also used to prevent self-ligation of restriction enzyme digested plasmids and lambda vectors
Polynucleotide kinase	Introduces γ-phos-phate of ATP to 5 ends of DNA	Used for labeling the 5' ends of DNA with radio-labeled γ-phosphate of ATP in the presence of polynucleotide kinase.
DNase I	Randomly hydrolyzes the phosphodiester bonds of double-stranded DNA	Is used in the identification of regions of DNA that are bound by protein and thereby protected from DNase I digestion, also used to identify transcriptionally active regions of chromatin since they are more susceptible to DNase I digestion
S₁ nuclease	Exonuclease that recognizes single-stranded regions of DNA	Used to remove regions of single strandedness in DNA or RNA-DNA duplexes
Exonuclease III	Exonuclease that removes nucleotides from the 3' end of DNAs	Used to generate deletions in DNA for sequencing, or to map functional domains of DNA duplexes
Terminal transferase	DNA polymerase that requires only a 3'-OH, lengthens 3' ends with any dNTP	Used to introduce homopolymeric (same dNTP) & quottails onto the 3' ends of DNA duplexes, also used to introduce radio-labeled nucleotides on the 3' ends of DNA
T3, T7, and SP6 RNA polymerases	Bacterial virus encoded RNA polymerase, recognize specific nucleotide sequences for initiation of transcription	Used to synthesize RNA *in vitro*
Taq and Vent DNA polymerase	Thermostable DNA polymerases	Used in PCR
Taq and Vent DNA ligases	Thermostable DNA ligases	Used in LCR

Restriction Endonucleases

Restriction endonucleases are bacterial enzymes that hydrolyze specific nucleic acid sequences within the double-stranded DNA. These bacterial enzymes are called restriction endonucleases, since they restrict the growth of certain viruses that infect bacteria.

Restriction endonucleases are unique in their ability to recognize specific sequences that are **palindromes**, i.e. they are the same sequences in the 5' → 3' direction (**5'-GAATTC-3'**) of both strands.

Some restriction endonucleases cause **staggered symmetrical cuts** away from the center of their recognition site within the DNA duplex; some make **blunt symmetrical cuts** in the middle of their recognition site while still others cleave the DNA at a distance from the recognition sequence. Enzymes that make staggered cuts leave the resultant DNA with cohesive or **sticky ends** (Fig. 46.1). Enzymes that cleave the DNA at the center of the recognition sequence leave **blunt-ended** fragments of DNA (Fig. 46.2).

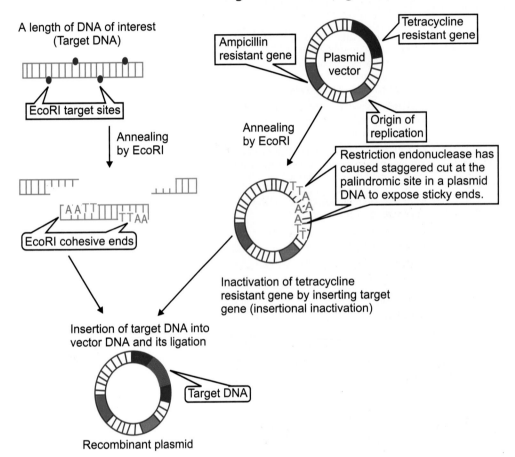

Fig. 46.1: Use of restriction endonuclease to make recombinant DNA

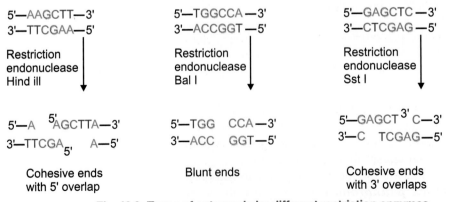

Fig. 46.2: Types of cuts made by different restriction enzymes

Any two pieces of DNA containing the complementary sequences within their sticky ends can come together and covalently ligated according to base pairing rule. In the presence of **DNA ligase,** any two blunt-ended fragments of DNA can be ligated together irrespective of the sequences at the ends of the duplexes.

CLONING

Any fragment of DNA can be cloned once it is introduced into a suitable vector and transferred into a bacterial host. Cloning refers to the production of large quantities of identical DNA molecules that involves the use of a bacterial cell as a host for replication of vector DNA.

cDNA cloning refers to the production of a library of cloned double-stranded DNAs, which represent all mRNAs present in a particular cell or tissue.

Genomic cloning refers to the production of a library of cloned double-stranded DNAs representing the entire genome of a particular organism. From either of these types of libraries one can isolate a single cDNA or gene clone by using a variety of screening protocols.

In order to clone either cDNAs or copies of genes a vector is required to carry the DNA to be cloned. Vectors used are of two types.

One type of vectors is derived from bacterial *plasmids*. Plasmids are circular DNAs found in bacteria that replicate autonomously from the host genome. These DNAs were first identified because they harbored genes that conferred antibiotic resistance to the bacteria. The antibiotic resistance genes found on the original plasmids are presently used to allow selection of bacteria that have taken up the plasmids containing the DNAs of interest. Plasmids are of limited use, because only those DNA fragments having less than 10,000 base pairs (bp) can be cloned. But in practice fragments of around 5,000 bp are the limit.

The second class of vectors is derived from the bacterial virus (**bacteriophage lambda**), which is capable of both integration into the host genome (*lysogeny*) and lysis of the infected host (*lysis*). The genes required for lysogeny are removed from the lambda-based vectors in order to allow only the lytic life cycle to take place. The advantage of using lambda-based vectors is that they can carry fragments of DNA up to 25,000 bp.

In the analysis of the human genome even lambda-based vectors are limiting and a *yeast artificial chromosome (YAC)* vector system has been developed for the cloning of DNA fragments up to 500,000 bp.

cDNA CLONING

The cDNA cloning technique consists of; first reverse transcription of the mRNA, followed by synthesis of the second strand of DNA, and insertion of the double-stranded cDNA into either a plasmid or lambda vector for cloning (Fig. 46.3).

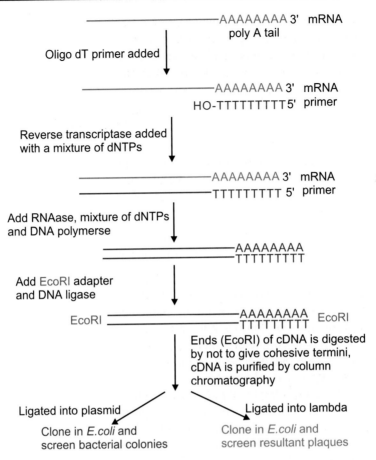

—AAAAAAAA 3' mRNA
poly A tail

Oligo dT primer added

—AAAAAAAA 3' mRNA
HO-TTTTTTTTT 5' primer

*Reverse transcriptase added
with a mixture of dNTPs*

—AAAAAAAA 3' mRNA
—TTTTTTTTT 5' primer

*Add RNAase, mixture of dNTPs
and DNA polymerse*

——AAAAAAAA
——TTTTTTTT

*Add EcoRI adapter
and DNA ligase*

EcoRI ——AAAAAAAA EcoRI
——TTTTTTTT

Ends (EcoRI) of cDNA is digested
by not to give cohesive termini,
cDNA is purified by column
chromatography

Ligated into plasmid   Ligated into lambda
Clone in *E.coli* and   Clone in *E.coli* and
screen bacterial colonies   screen resultant plaques

Fig. 46.3: cDNA cloning

The *first step* of cDNA cloning is to synthesize a complementary DNA copy of the mRNA using a polyT primer and reverse transcriptase.

The *second step* is to make a DNA strand that is complementary to the DNA strand made in the first step using DNA polymerase. The mRNA should be removed before initiating the synthesis of second strand of DNA, which can be achieved by addition of RNase, heat denaturation or alkaline hydrolysis.

The *third step* is the blunt-end ligation of small pieces (10bp) of double-stranded DNA containing restriction enzyme sites (EcoRI) called linkers or adopters to the double stranded DNA synthesized in step two, by use of DNA ligase.

The *fourth step* is the digestion of the ends (EcoRI) of double stranded cDNA by appropriate restriction enzyme (Not I) to give cohesive termini, which are complementary to the cloning site in the vector (plasmid or bacteriophage lambda).

The *fifth step* is cloning of cDNA like any other DNA into vector.

This process creates a *library* of cloned cDNA representing all the mRNA species. Screening of the library for a particular cDNA clone is accomplished using nucleic acid or protein-based (proteins or antibodies) probes. The cDNA libraries can also be screened by biological assay of the products produced by the cloned cDNAs. Screening with proteins, antibodies or by biological assay are mechanisms for analysis of the expression of proteins from cloned cDNAs and is given the term *expression cloning*. Nucleic acid probes can be generated from DNA or RNA. Nucleic acid probes can be radioactively labeled or labeled with modified nucleotides that are recognizable by specific antibodies and detected by colorimetric or chemiluminescent assays.

GENOMIC CLONING

Genomic library refers to a library of clones that contain every sequence of the genome from a specific organism. These libraries are used as a source for clones of genes of the specific organism. The preferred vector for establishment of such libraries is bacteriophage lambda, since these vector systems are capable of carrying 15-25,000 bp of DNA. Cloning slightly larger fragments of genomic DNA can be accomplished using a chimeric plasmid-lambda vector system termed a **cosmid**. Cosmid vectors contain only the **cos** (cohesive) ends of the lambda genome (required for packaging the DNA into infectious virus particles) along with a plasmid antibiotic resistance gene and origin of DNA replication. Since approximately 30,000 bp of lambda DNA have been removed from cosmid vectors, larger genomic DNA fragments can be cloned. Still larger genomic DNA fragments can be cloned into **YAC** vectors (see below).

The basic steps of generating recombinant DNA with lambda DNA are the same as with plasmid DNA.

Genomic DNA can be isolated from any cell or tissue for cloning. The genomic DNA is first digested with restriction enzymes to generate fragments in the size range that are optimal for the vector being utilized for cloning. Given that some genes encompass many more base pairs than can be inserted into conventional lambda or cosmid vectors, the clones that are present in a genomic library must be overlapping. In order to generate overlapping clones, the DNA is only partially digested with restriction enzymes. This means that not every restriction site, present in all the copies of a given gene in the preparation of DNA, is cleaved. The partially digested DNA is then size-selected by a variety of techniques (e.g. gel electrophoresis or gradient centrifugation) prior to cloning. Screening of genomic libraries is accomplished primarily with nucleic acid-based probes. However, they can be screened with proteins that are known to bind specific sequences of DNA (e.g. transcription factors).

CLONING GENOMIC DNA IN YAC VECTORS

Yeast artificial chromosome vectors (YAC vctors) allow, within yeast cells, the cloning of genomic DNA fragments that approach 500,000 bp. These vectors contain several elements of typical yeast chromosomes, hence the term YAC (Fig. 46.4). The YAC vectors contain a **yeast centromere (CEN), yeast telomeres (TEL)** and an **autonomously replicating sequence (ARS)**. Yeast ARSs are essentially origins of replication that function in yeast cells autonomously from the replication of yeast chromosomal replication

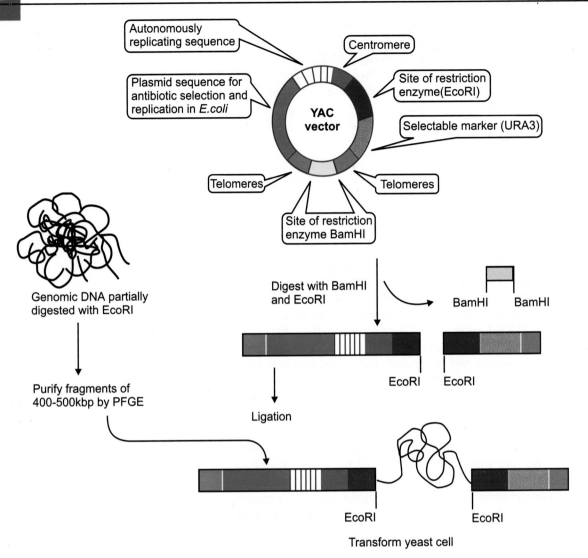

Fig. 46.4: Use of YAC vector to clone genomic DNA

origins. YAC vectors also contain genes (e.g. URA3 gene, a gene involved in uracil synthesis) that allow selection of yeast cells that have taken up the vector.

In the cloning of genomic DNA in a typical YAC vector, the genomic DNA is partially digested with EcoRI and fragments in the range of 400 - 500 kilobase pairs (kbp) are purified by pulsed field gel electrophoresis *(PFGE)*. The YAC vector is digested with EcoRI and BamHI that places the telomere sequences at the ends of the linearized vector. The small BamHI fragment is separated from the rest of the YAC vector by standard gel electrophoresis. The genomic DNA is then ligated into the vector and then used to transform yeast cells.

ANALYSIS OF CLONED PRODUCTS

Cloned cDNAs and genes can be analyzed by numerous techniques. The initial characterization usually involves mapping of the number and location of different restriction enzyme sites. This information is useful for DNA sequencing since it provides a means to digest the clone into specific fragments for sub-cloning, a process that involve the cloning of fragments of a particular cloned DNA. Once the DNA is fully characterized, the cDNA clones can be used to produce mRNA *in vitro*. In turn mRNA is translated *in vitro* to protein. Clones of cDNAs can also be used as probes to analyze the structure of a gene by *Southern blotting* or to analyze the size of the RNA and pattern of its expression by Northern blotting. *Northern blotting* is also a useful tool in the analysis of the exon-intron organization of gene clones since only fragments of a gene that contain exons will hybridize to the RNA on the blot.

Southern Blotting

Southern blotting is the *analysis of DNA structure*, following its attachment to a solid support (Fig. 46.5). The DNA to be analyzed is first digested with a given restriction enzyme then the resultant DNA

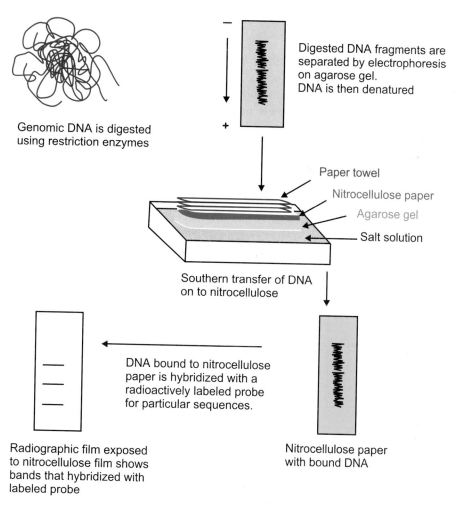

Genomic DNA is digested using restriction enzymes

Digested DNA fragments are separated by electrophoresis on agarose gel. DNA is then denatured

Paper towel
Nitrocellulose paper
Agarose gel
Salt solution

Southern transfer of DNA on to nitrocellulose

DNA bound to nitrocellulose paper is hybridized with a radioactively labeled probe for particular sequences.

Nitrocellulose paper with bound DNA

Radiographic film exposed to nitrocellulose film shows bands that hybridized with labeled probe

Fig. 46.5: Southern blotting

fragments are separated by electrophoresis on agarose gel. The gel is then treated with sodium hydroxide to denature the DNA. The DNA is transferred from the gel to nitrocellulose or nylon filter paper by either capillary diffusion or under electric current. The DNA is fixed to the filter by baking or ultraviolet light treatment. The filter can then be probed for the presence of a given fragment of DNA by various radioactive or nonradioactive means.

Southern blot analysis is usually done to identify the number of genes in the genome and it forms the basis of restriction fragment length polymorphism and DNA fingerprint analysis.

Northern Blotting

Northern blotting involves the *analysis of RNA* following its attachment to a solid support. The RNA is sized by gel electrophoresis then transferred to nitrocellulose or nylon filter paper as for Southern blotting. Probing the filter for a particular RNA is done similar to probing of Southern blots. Northern blot analysis is primarily used to detect and quantitate specific mRNAs from different tissues.

Western Blotting

Western blotting involves the *analysis of proteins* following attachment to a solid support. The proteins are separated by size SDS-PAGE and electrophoretically transferred to nitrocellulose or nylon filters. The filter is then probed with antibodies raised against a particular protein.

RESTRICTION FRAGMENT LENGTH POLYMORPHISM (RFLP) ANALYSIS

The genetic variability at a particular locus (gene) due to even minor base changes can alter the pattern of fragments obtained from DNA digestion by restriction enzyme. Alterations to the genotype can be due to deletions, insertions or even single nucleotide substitutions within the gene being analyzed, which can create a new **restriction enzyme recognition site** or delete an existing **restriction enzyme recognition site**. Taking advantage of this and making use of southern blotting, the pattern of DNA fragments obtained by restriction enzyme digestion is analyzed to detect familial patterns of the fragments of a given gene, by screening the Southern blot with a probe corresponding to the gene of interest. A classic example of a disease that can be detected by RFLP is **sickle cell anemia** (Fig. 46.6).

Sickle cell anemia results from a single nucleotide change (**A to T**) at codon 6 within the β-globin gene. This alteration leads to substitution of amino acid **glutamate to valine**; this substitution abolishes an *MstII* restriction site. As a result, a β-globin gene probe can be used to detect the different *MstII* restriction fragments. It should be recalled that there are two copies of each gene in all human cells, therefore, RFLP analysis detects both copies: the affected allele and the unaffected allele.

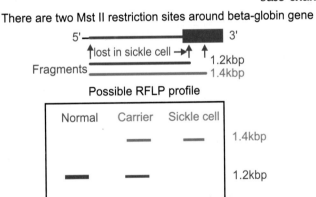

Fig. 46.6: Restriction fragment length polymorphism analysis

An RFLP analysis of genomic DNA for the presence of the sickle-cell locus involves isolation of genomic DNA and it's digestion with the restriction enzyme MstII. In sickle cell carriers or disease, one of the two MstII site is lost at the sickle-cell locus. The DNA is then Southern blotted and analyzed with a beta-globin-specific probe corresponding to sequences at the 5'-end of the gene. Individuals homozygous for the normal globin genes will exhibit a single hybridization band since both maternal and paternal genes are unaffected. Heterozygotes will exhibit the normal band and the larger sickle-cell gene band. Homozygous sickle-cell individuals will exhibit a single larger hybridization band (Fig. 46.6).

Size variability in detectable fragments within a family pedigree indicates differences in the pattern of restriction sites within and around the gene being analyzed. The patterns of RFLP are inherited and segregate according to Mendelian law, which allow their use in genotyping of paternity dispute cases, in criminal investigations and in determining the probability of occurrence of genetic diseases in the offspring of two individuals.

Another form of DNA polymorphism detectable by classical RFLP mapping results from the inherited variations in the number of tandemly repeated DNA sequence elements that are from 2 to 60 bp in length. The number of repeats is also variable from 2 to 40 copies. These elements are termed *variable number tandem repeats (VNTRs)*. When restriction enzyme digestion cuts DNA flanking the VNTRs, the lengths of the resultant fragments will be variable depending upon the number of repeats at a given locus. Many different VNTR loci have been identified and are extremely useful for **DNA fingerprint analysis** in forensic and paternity identity cases.

DNA SEQUENCING

Sequencing of DNA can be accomplished by either chemical or enzymatic methods. The original technique for sequencing by **Maxam and Gilbert** relies on the nucleotide-specific chemical cleavage of DNA and is not routinely used any more. The enzymatic technique of **Sanger's sequencing,** involves the use of 3'-dideoxynucleotidtriphosphates (ddNTP) that terminate DNA synthesis and is, therefore, also called *dideoxy chain termination sequencing.* This method is actually the replication of a DNA strand from a precise start point and its termination at specific base point by use of specific ddNTP (Fig. 46.7).

The Sanger DNA sequencing protocol requires four separate sequencing reactions run simultaneously with cloned DNA templates. Each reaction contains different ddNTP, a mix of all four dNTPs that are radioactive, DNA polymerase and specific oligonucleotide primer that ensures all

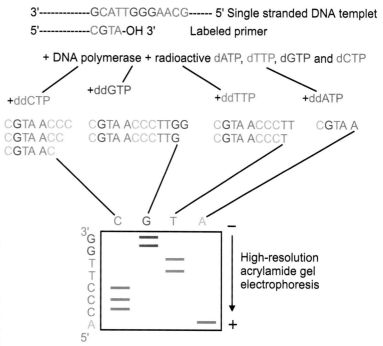

Fig. 46.7: Sanger's DNA sequencing by ddNTP chain termination

sequence reactions start from the same point. The higher the concentration of ddNTP the more frequently chain elongation will terminate. The ddNTP act as terminators of DNA synthesis because they have no 3'hydroxyl group that is required to continue chain elongation. Thereby, one can regulate the extent of sequence elongation by varying the dNTP/ddNTP ratio. Following the chain elongation reactions the products are separated by high-resolution acrylamide gel electrophoresis in adjacent lanes under denaturing conditions. The gel is exposed to radiographic film, and bands appear for each oligonucleotide synthesized. The sequences are read from bottom to top. Bands near the bottom of the gel represent short reaction products (i.e. closest to the 3'-end of the primer) and those near the top the longest products (Fig.46.7).

THE POLYMERASE CHAIN REACTION (PCR)

The PCR is a powerful technique by which both double and single stranded DNAs can be replicated millions of fold in a short time (Fig. 46.8). The process requires a set of specific opposing primes. The design of the primers depends upon the sequences of the DNA that is required to be analyzed. The technique involves mixing the DNA to be amplified, with specific primers, dNTPs, buffer including $MgCl_2$ and thermostable DNA polymerase. The reaction mixture is subjected to many cycles (usually 20 - 50) of melting the template DNA at

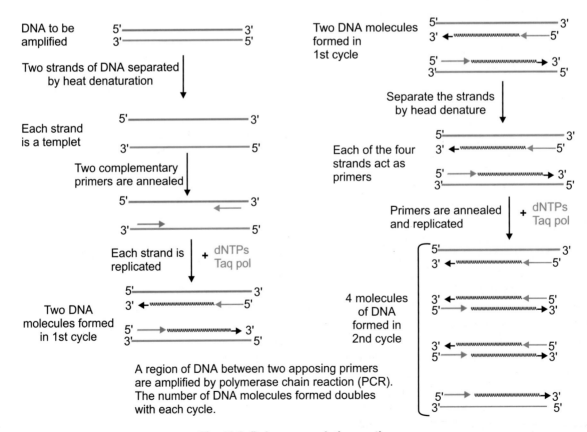

A region of DNA between two apposing primers are amplified by polymerase chain reaction (PCR). The number of DNA molecules formed doubles with each cycle.

Fig. 46.8: Polymerase chain reaction

95°C and then cooled to a temperature that will allow optimal primer binding. The reaction temperature is then raised to 72^0C that is optimal for DNA polymerase whereby primers are extended along the template. The process has been automated with the use of **thermostable DNA polymerases** (Taq pol) isolated from bacteria that grow in thermal vents in hot springs. During the first round of replication a single copy of DNA is converted to two copies and so on resulting in an exponential increase in the number of copies of the sequences targeted by the primers. After just 20 cycles, a single copy of DNA is amplified over 2 million folds.

The products of PCR reactions are analyzed by separation in agarose gels followed by ethidium bromide staining and visualization with UV transillumination. Alternatively, radioactive dNTPs can be added to the PCR in order to incorporate label into the products. In this case, the products of the PCR are visualized by exposure of the gel to X-ray film. The added advantage of radio-labeling PCR products is that the levels of individual amplification products can be quantitated.

The diagnostic uses of PCR include quick amplification and sequencing of genes in which particular mutations are known to cause a disease and detection of bacterial and viral infection.

In forensic practice, PCR is used for quick amplification and sequencing of known hypervariable regions in the nuclear and mitochondrial DNA obtained from extremely small samples of blood, semen and hair.

Examples of Inherited Disorders Detectable by PCR

Disease	Affected Gene
Adenosine deaminase deficiency	Adenosine deaminase (ADA)
Lesch-Nyhan syndrome	Hypoxanthine-guanine phosphoribosyltransferase (HGPRT)
α-1-antitrypsin deficiency	α-1-antitrypsin
Cystic fibrosis	Cystic fibrosis transmembrane conductance (CFTR) protein
Fabry disease	α-galactosidase
Gaucher's disease	Glucocerebrosidase
Sandhoff-Jatzkewitz disease	Hexosaminidase A and B
Tay-Sachs disease	Hexosaminidase A
Familial hypercholesterolemia (FH)	LDL receptor
Glucose-6-phosphate dehydrogenase deficiency	Glucose-6-phosphate dehydrogenase
Maple syrup urine disease	α-keto acid decarboxylase
Phenylketonuria (PKU)	Phenylalanine
Ornithine transcarbamylase deficiency	Ornithine transcarbamylase
Retinoblastoma (Rb)	Rb gene product
Sickle-cell anemia	Point mutation in β-globin gene resulting in improper folding of protein
β-thalassemia	Mutations in β-globin gene that result in loss of synthesis of protein
Hemophilia A	Factor VIII
Hemophilia B	Factor IX
von Willebrand disease	von Willebrand factor (vWF)

TRANSGENESIS

Transgenesis or transfection is the process by which exogenous genes (recombinant DNA) are introduced into the germ line of an organism, which then becomes heritable DNA.

To create a transgenic animal the gene of interest must be passed from generation to generation, i.e. it must be inherited in the germ line. To accomplish this, for example in livestock animals, vectors containing the gene of interest with appropriate regulatory elements (e.g. the β-lactoglobulin promoter if expression of the transgene in the milk is desired) are injected into the nucleus of fertilized eggs. The eggs are then transplanted into the uterus of receptive females for development of the potential transgenic offspring. In order to test the resultant animal for germ line transmission of the transgene the chromosomal DNA of their offspring is tested for the presence of the transgene. If the transgene exhibits Mendelian inheritance then it is being transmitted in the germ line.

Currently the process of transgenesis is being utilized in both the plant and livestock industries. The aim of the majority of these experiments is to generate plants and animals that are more resistant to diseases and infections. However, some transgenic farm animal such as sheep and cows are being developed in order to obtain high levels of expression of therapeutically important proteins in their milk. This allows the animals to secrete large amounts of the protein of interest in the milk, which can be harvested and purified easily.

GENE THERAPY

Disease genes in a population of human off springs can be eliminated by transgenesis, however, technical as well as ethical issues are likely to prevent any transgenic experiments to be carried out with human eggs. Therefore, somatic cell gene therapy is likely to become a common therapeutic approach for the treatment of a number of metabolic disorders. The principle of gene therapy protocols aims to introduce correcting copies of disease genes into somatic cells of the affected individual. Expression of a correct copy of an affected gene in somatic cells prevents transmission through the germ line, thereby, avoiding many of the ethical issues of transgenesis. This is analogous to treatment of individuals by organ or tissue transplantation.

The most common techniques utilized in gene therapy studies are the introduction of the corrected gene into bone marrow cells, skin fibroblasts or hepatocytes. The most commonly used vectors are derived from retroviruses that contain only, the transcriptional promoter regions of these viruses, which drive expression of the gene of interest. The advantage of retroviral-based vector systems is that, it can express in most types of cells.

Human Disorders Treated in Cultured Cells by Gene Therapy

Disorder	Affected gene
SCID	Adenosine deaminase (ADA)
SCID	Purine nucleoside phosphorylase (PNP)
Lesch-Nyhan syndrome	Hypoxanthine-guanine phosphoribosyltransferase (HGPRT)
Gaucher's disease	Glucocerebrosidase
Familial hypercholesterolemia (FH)	LDL receptor
Phenylketonuria (PKU)	Phenylalanine hydroxylase
β-thalassemia	β-globin
Hemophilia B	Factor IX

A number of human inherited disorders have been corrected in cultured cells and several diseases such as malignant melanoma and severe combined immunodeficiency disease are currently being treated by gene therapy techniques. The results are encouraging and that gene therapy is likely to be a powerful therapeutic technique against a host of diseases in the future.

Appendix

Recommended Daily Allowance (RDA) of Essential Nutrients

Nutrient	Male	Female	Pregnancy	Children	Infants
Proteins	1 g/kg	1 g/kg	2 g/kg	1.8 g/kg	2.4 g/kg
Phenylalanine	14 mg/kg				
Leucine	11 mg/kg				
Lysine	9 mg/kg				
Valine	14 mg/kg				
Isoleucine	10 mg/kg				
Threonine	6 mg/kg				
Tryptophan	3 mg/kg				
Vitamin-A	750 ug		1000 ug	400-600 ug	
Vitamin D	5 ug		1200 ug	10 ug	
Vitamin E	10 mg	8 mg	11 mg		
Vitamin K	50-100 ug			1 ug/kg	
Thiamine	1-1.5 mg				
Riboflavin	1.5 mg		2 mg		
Niacin	20 mg		22 mg		
Pyridoxine	2 mg		2.25 mg		
Pantothenate	10 mg				
Biotin	200-300 ug				
Folic acid	100 ug		300 ug		
Vitamin B_{12}	1 ug		1.5 ug		
Ascorbate	70 mg		100 mg		
Calcium	0.5 g		1.5 g	1 g	
Phosphorus	500 mg				
Magnesium	400 mg				
Manganese	5-6 mg				
Sodium	5-0 g				
Potassium	3-4 g				
Iron	15-20 mg	20-25 mg	40-50 mg		
Copper	1.5-3 mg				

Contd...

Contd...

Iodine	150-200 ug
Zinc	10-15 mg
Selenium	50-100 ug

Tumor Markers in Serum

Analyte	Old units	SI units
Alpha-fetoprotein (AFP)	5-15 ng/ml	5-15 ug/L
Carcinoembryonic antigen (CEA)	3-5 ng/ml	3-5 ug/L
Cancer antigen 25 (CA125)	0.35 IU/ml	
Prostate specific antigen (PSA)	100-500 ng/dl	1-5 ug/L

Serum Enzymes

Analyte	Old units	SI units	Enzyme units
Acid phosphatase (Total)	0.5-4KAU/dl	2.5-12 IUL/L	40-200 nkat/L
Acid phosphatase (tartarate labile)	< 0.9KAU/dl	< 1 IU/L	<13 nkat/L
Alanine aminotransferase (ALT/S GPT)		10-40 IU/L	220-680 nkt/L
Aldolase		1.5-7 IU/L	20-117 nkat/L
Alkaline phosphatase (ALP)	3-13 KAU/dl	40-125 IU/L	500-1400 nkat/L
Amylase	80-180 somo gyi U/dl	50-20 IU/L	2.5-5.5 ukat/L
An giotensin converting enzyme		10-50 IU/L	200-800 nkat/L
Aspartate aminotransferase (AST/S GOT)		8-20 IU/L	140-340 nkat/L
Complement-1-esterase	5-10 mg/dl		
Creatine kinase	10-100 U/L		
γ-glutamyl transpeptidase (GGT)		10-30 IU/L	0.2-0.5 ukat/L
Glucose 6-P-dehydrogenase	125-250 U/10^{12} cells	4-10 U/g Hb	
Gluca gon	2-10 ng/dl		
Lactate dehydrogenase		100-200 IU/L	1.7-3.2 ukat/L
Lipase		50-175 IU/L	0.6-3 ukat/L
Nucleotide phosphatase		2-10 IU/L	0.02-0.18 ukat/L
Psedocholinesterase	8-18 IU/ml		
Transketolase in blood		150-200 umol/L	

Hormones

Analyte	Sample	Old units	SI units
ACTH (Corticotrophin)	Plasma	2.5-10 n g/dl	2-10 pmol/L
Aldosterone (standing)	Serum	6-20 n g/dl	0.17-0.6 nmol/L
Antidiuretic hormone (ADH)	Plasma	1-13 p g/ml	
Calcitonin	Serum	0-20 p g/ml	0-20 n g/L

Contd...

Contd...

Analyte	Sample	Old units	SI units
Calcitriol	Serum	1.5-6 ug/dl	50-160 pmol/L
Chorionic gonadotropin beta-HC G (non-pregnant)	Serum	<10 mU/ml	< 10 U/L
Cortisol 9 AM Midnight	Plasma	5-15 ug/dl 2-5 ug/dl	130-600 nmol/L 30-130 nmpl/L
Epinephrine	Plasma Urine	10-00 pg/ml 2-22 ug/day	0-500 pmol/L 10-100 nmol/day
FSH : Male Female (midcycle)	Serum		4-10 IU/L 0-20 IU/L
Growth hormone	Serum		2-6 ug/L
17-hydroxy corticosteroids : Female Male	Urine Urine	2-8 mg/day 3-0 mg/day	5.5-2 pmol/day 8-28 pmol/day
5-hydroxy indole acetic acid (HIAA)	Urine	2-9 mg/day	10-47 umol/day
Insulin	Serum	5-15 uU/ml	30-100 umol/L
17-ketogenic steroids: Females Males	Urine	3-5 mg/day 5-23 mg/day	10-5 umol/day 7-80 umol/day
17-ketosteroids: upto 1 year 1-4 year 5-8 years 8-2 years 13-6 years Male adult Female adult	Urine	< 1 mg/day <2 mg/day <3 mg/day 3-0 mg/day 5-2 mg/day 8-20 mg/day 6-5 mg/day	
LH Male Female (midcycle)	Serum		5-7 IU/L 20-50 IU/L
Norepinephrine	Plasma Urine	70-700 pg/ml 15-80 ug/day	1-4 nmol/L 100-500 nmol/day
Parathyroid hormone (PTH)	Serum		0-25 ng/L
Placental lactogen(HPL) pregnant	Serum	0.5-10 mg/L	20-500 nmol/L
Progesterone: Male Female (after midcycle)	Serum	12- 30 ng/dl 0.6-3 ug/dl	0.3-0.9 nmol/L 19-95 nmol/L
Prolactine : Male Female normal Female (after midcycle)	Serum		0-5 ug/L 10-20 ug/L 90-400 ug/L
Prostaglandin E	Plasma	2.5-20 ng/dl	70-550 pmol/L
Tri-iodothyronine (T3)	Plasma	120-190 ng/dl	1-8-3 nmol/L
Renin	Plasma		0.5-1 ng/L/sec
Reverse T3 (rT3)	Plasma	10-25 ng/dl	0.15-0.4 nmol/L
Thyroxine (T4)	Plasma	5-12 ug/dl	65-150 nmol/L
Testosterone: Male –morning Female- morning	Plasma	300-1000 ng/dl 25-45 ng/dl	10-38 nmol/L 1-1.5 nmol/L
TSH-releasing hormone (TRH)	Plasma		5-60 ng/L
Thyroid stimulating hormone (TSH)	Plasma	0.5-5 uU/ml	0.5-5 mU/L
Thyroxine binding globulin (TB G)	Plasma	1-2 mg/dl	
Transcortin	Plasma	3-3.5 mg/dl	
Vanillyl mandelic acid (VMA)	Urine	2-6 mg/day	7-32 umol/day

Electrolytes and Blood Gases

Analyte	Sample	Old unit	SI units
pH	Blood	7.4	[H+] = 40 nmol/L
Osmaolality	Serum	280-296 mosmol/kg	280-296 mmol/kg
Anion gap	Blood	± 5 mmol/L	
PCO_2 arterial	Blood	35-45 mmH g 4.76 kPa	
PO_2 arterial	Blood	90-100 mmH g 11-3 kPa	150-220 ml/L
Bicarbonate (HCO_3^-)	Serum	22-26 mEq/L	22-26 mmol/L
Sodium (Na^+)	Serum	136-145 mEq/L	136-145 mmol/L
Potassium (K^+)	Serum	3.5-5 mEq/L	3.5-5 mmol/L
Chloride (Cl^-)	Serum CSF Urine	96-106 mEq/L 120-130 mmol/L	96-06 mmol/L 120-130 mmol/L 10-200 mmol/L
Calcium (Ca^{2+})	Serum	9-11 mg/dl	2.-2.5 mmol/L
Magnesium (mg^{2+})	Serum	1.8-2.2 mg/dl	0.7-0.9 mmol/L
Phosphate	Serum Blood Urine	3-4 mg/dl 40 mg/dl 1 g/day	1-.5 mmol/L 32 mmol/day
Sulfate	Serum	0.5-1.5 mEq/L	

Normal Reference Range of Important Biochemical Parameters

Analyte	Sample	Old unit	SI units
Ammonia	Plasma	< 50 ug/dl	
Albumin	Serum CSF	3.5-5 gm/dl 10-30 mg/dl	35-50 gm/L 100-300 mg/L
α-1-acid glycoprotein	Serum	55-40 mg/dl	13.4-34 umol/L
α-1-antitrypsin	Serum	75-200 mg/dl	0.75-2 g/L
Amino acids, total	Serum	30-50 mg/dl	
Angiotensine -I	Plasma	1.8-8 ng/dl	
Angiotensin-II	Plasma	1-6 ng/dl	
Ascorbic acid	Serum	0.4-1.5 mg/dl	23-85 umol/L
Bilirubin, total	Serum	0.2-1 mg/dl	4-17 umol/L
Ceruloplasmin	Serum	25-50 mg/dl	
Cholesterol	Serum	150-200 mg/dl	4-6 mmol/L
Cholesterol (HDL fraction): Male Female	Serum	30-60 mg/dl 35-75 mg/dl	0.75-1.58 mmol/L 0.98-1.95 mmol/L
Cholesterol (LDL fraction)	Serum	60-200 mg/dl	
Complement C1	Plasma	80-120 mg/dl	
Complement C4	Plasma	25-40 mg/dl	
Copper	Plasma	70-150 ug/dl	16-30 umol/L

Contd...

Contd...

Analyte	Sample	Old unit	SI units
C-reactive protein (CRP)	Serum	0.5-1 mg/dl	
Creatine	Serum	0.2-0.4 mg.dl	15-30 umol/L
Creatinine	Serum	0.7-1.4 mg/dl	60-125 umol/L
Cyanocobalamine (Vit B$_{12}$)	Serum	20-80 ng/dl	150-600 pmol/L
Serum electrophoresis fractions	Serum		
Albumin		3.5-4.7 g/dl	
Alpha 1		0.2-0.3 g/dl	
Alpha 2		0.4-0.9 g/dl	
Beta		0.5-1.0 g/dl	
Gamma		0.7-1.5 g/dl	
Fibrinogen	Plasma	200-400 mg/dl	5.8-8.5 umol/L
Ferritin : Male	Serum	3-30 ug/dl	30-300 ug/L
Female		2-12 ug/dl	20-120 ug/L
Folic acid	Serum	5-20 ng/ml	10-40 nmol/L
Galactose	Serum	1-5 mg/dl	0.05-0.25 mmol/L
Globulins	Serum	2.5-3.5 g/dl	25-35 g/L
Glucose (Fastin g)	Plasma	75-0 mg/dl	4.-6.1 mmol/L
	Blood	65-100 mg/dl	3.5-5.6 mmol/L
	CSF	50-70 mg/dl	2.8-4.2 mmol/L
Glutamic acid	Serum	8-10 mg/dl	
Glutathione	RBCs	20-40 mg/dl	2 mmol/L
Hapto globulin	Serum	40-175 mg/dl	400-1750 mg/L
HbA$_{1c}$ (Glycohemo globin)	RBCs	4-8 % of total	
Immuno globulins Total	CSF	4-5 mg/dl	
Immuno globulins I g G	Serum	800-1200 mg/dl	
Immuno globulins I g G1	Serum	800 mg/dl	
Immuno globulins I g G2	Serum	200 mg/dl	
Immuno globulins I g G3	Serum	100 mg/dl	
Immuno globulins I g G4	Serum	50 mg/dl	
Immuno globulins I gM	Serum	50-200 mg/dl	
Immuno globulins I gA	Serum	150-300 mg/dl	
Immuno globulins I gD	Serum	1-10 mg/dl	
Immuno globulins I gE	Serum	1.5-4.5 ug/dl	
Iodine	Serum	5-10 ug/dl	
Iron, whole blood	Blood	5 mg/dl	
Iron serum	Serum	100-150 ug/dl	20-30 umol/L
Iron binding capacity (TIBC)	Serum	250-400 ug/dl	44-70 umol/L
Lactic acid	Plasma	4-20 mg/dl	0.4-2.0 mmol/L
Lipids- total	Serum	400-600 mg/dl	4-6 g/L
Lipoprotein-alpha	Serum	40 mg/dl	

Contd...

Contd...

Analyte	Sample	Old unit	SI units
Lipoprotein- beta	Serum	180 mg/dl	
Nonesterified fatty acids (Free fatty acids)	Plasma	10-20 mg/dl	0.3-0.7 mEq/L
Phenylalanine	Serum	0.75-1.15 mg/dl	0.05-0.1 mmol/L
Phospholipids	Plasma	150-200 mg/dl	2-2.5 mmol/L
Plasmino gen	Serum	10-30 mg/dl	
Pre-albumin	Serum	25-30 mg/dl	
Proteins -total	Serum	6-8 g/dl	60-80 g/L
Prothrombin	Plasma	10-15 mg/dl	
Retinol bindin g protein	Serum	3-6 mg/dl	
Selenium	Serum	50-100 ug/dl	0.5-1 umol/L
Serotonin	Blood	4-36 mg/dl	0.2-2 umol/L
Thyro globulin	Serum	3-5 ug/dl	3-50 ug/L
Transferrin	Serum	200-300 mg/dl	23-35 umol/L
Tri glycerides (fastin g): Male Female	Serum	50-200 mg/dl 40-150 mg/dl	0.5-2.3 mmol/L 0.4-1.6 mmol/L
Troponin I	Serum		1-10 ug/L
Urea	Serum	20-40 mg/dl	2.4-4.8 mmol/L
Urea nitro gen	Serum	8-20 mg/dl	3-9 mmol/L

Uric acid: Male
                       Female
                       Children
	Serum	3.5-7 mg/dl
		3 – 6 mg/dl
		2.0-5.5 mg/dl
			0.21-0.4 mmol/L
			0.18-0.35 mmol/L
			0.2-0.32 mmol/L

Vanil mandelic acid (VMA)	Urine	2-6 mg/dl	7-32 umol/L